THE SKELETON

The Skeleton

Biochemical, Genetic, and Molecular Interactions in Development and Homeostasis

Edited by

Edward J. Massaro

and

John M. Rogers

Developmental Biology Branch,
Reproductive Toxicology Division,
The National Health and Environmental Effects
Research Laboratory, Office of Research Development,
United States Environmental Protection Agency,
Research Triangle Park, NC

Springer Science+Business Media, LLC

Originally published by Humana Press Inc. in 2004
Softcover reprint of the hardcover 1st edition 2004

www.humanapress.com

Production Editor: Jessica Jannicelli.
Cover design by Patricia F. Cleary.

Cover Illustration: Artwork supplied by József Zakany.

For additional copies, pricing for bulk purchases, and/or information about other Humana titles, contact Humana at the above address or at any of the following numbers: Tel.: 973-256-1699; Fax: 973-256-8341; E-mail: humana@humanapr.com or visit our website: http://humanapress.com

This publication is printed on acid-free paper. ∞
ANSI Z39.48-1984 (American National Standards Institute) Permanence of Paper for Printed Library Materials.

Library of Congress Cataloging-in-Publication Data

ISBN 978-1-61737-427-2　　ISBN 978-1-59259-736-9 (eBook)
DOI 10.1007/978-1-59259-736-9

The skeleton : biochemical, genetic, and molecular interactions in development and homeostasis / edited by Edward J. Massaro and John M. Rogers.
p. ; cm.
Includes bibliographical references and index.

1. Bone. 2. Bones--Physiology. 3. Bones--Growth.
[DNLM: 1. Bone and Bones--embryology. 2. Bone Development. 3. Molecular Biology. WE 200 S6276 2004] I. Massaro, Edward J. II. Rogers, John M.
QP88.2.S54 2004
612.7'5--dc22

2003027149

Preface

The skeleton is a complex multifunctional system. In addition to its mechanical/structural support function, it contains the marrow in which blood cells are made and, therefore, is a critical part of the circulatory and immune systems. Also, in that it is the major reservoir for the essential element calcium, a critical component of intracellular signaling pathways, the skeleton is an integral component of the endocrine system. Furthermore, the skeleton is a dynamic system that is subject to modification (remodeling) throughout life under the influence of both intrinsic (chemical) signals and extrinsic (mechanical) signals. Therefore, it is axiomatic that properly regulated crosstalk between the biochemistry and physiology of the skeleton and the chemical biology of the organism is of critical importance both in the complex processes of development and the maintenance of physiologic homeostasis. Thus, gaining insight in the nature and regulation of these interactions is of considerable interest to researchers and clinicians in a broad spectrum of biomedical disciplines.

Bone is formed during embryonic life and grows (formation exceeds resorption) rapidly through childhood. In humans, growth peaks around 20 yr of age. Thereafter, the skeleton enters a prolonged period (lasting approx 40 yr) when bone mass remains relatively stable. During this period, resorption and reformation (remodeling) of both cortical and trabecular bone occur continuously and contemporaneously, resulting in an annual turnover of approx 10% of the adult skeleton with essentially no net effect on bone mass. The maintenance of skeletal mass is regulated through a balance between the activity of cells that resorb bone (osteoclasts) and those that form bone (osteoblasts). Unfortunately, the balance between resorption and formation degenerates with age and, if uncompensated, can have debilitating consequences. For women, the balance terminates at menopause. Bone loss also occurs in men, but usually later in life. Clinical disorders in which bone resorption exceeds formation are common and include osteoporosis, Paget's disease of bone, and bone wasting secondary to such cancers as myeloma and metastatic breast cancer. Osteoporosis is the most common bone resorption disorder. It affects one in three women after the fifth decade of life. The pathophysiology of this condition includes genetic predisposition and alteration of systemic and local hormone levels coupled with environmental influences. Treatment is based on drugs that inhibit bone resorption either directly or indirectly: bisphosphonates, calcitonin, estrogens, and synthetic estrogen-related compounds (SERMs—selective estrogen receptor modulators). The search for more effective anti-osteoporosis drugs with fewer side effects continues. In this regard, it is of both great interest and potentially enormous import to note that recent evidence indicates that low bone mineral density (BMD) appears to protect women over the age of 65 from primary breast cancer. It was reported that women in the highest BMD quartile have approximately three times the risk of developing bone cancer than those in the lowest quartile. Also, those with the highest BMD, obtained from measurements of the wrist, forearm and heel, have almost six times the risk of advanced disease.

Less prevalent than disorders of bone loss are clinical disorders of reduced bone resorption, such as osteopetrosis, and pycnodysostosis (owing to cathepsin K deficiency), that are the consequence of genetic defects. Unfortunately, progress in the search for effective treatments for these orphan diseases often is stymied by lack of support.

Significant insight into many aspects of vertebrate skeletal development has been obtained through molecular and genetic studies of animal models and humans with inherited disorders of skeletal morphogenesis, organogenesis, and growth. Morphogenesis, the developmental process of pattern formation and the establishment of the body plan that is the template for the architecture of the adult form, is an exquisitely complicated program. Our understanding of it contains many gaps. The information for the pattern and form of the vertebrate skeleton emanates from mesenchymal cells during embryonic development. Morphogenesis requires three key ingredients: inductive signals, responding stem cells and a supportive extracellular matrix. Within the vertebrate morphogenetic program, skeletal development is controlled by sequence-dependent activation/inactivation of specific genes that results in the distribution of cells from cranial neural crest, sclerotomes, and lateral plate mesoderm into a pattern of mesenchymal condensations at sites in which skeletal elements will develop. Condensation is the earliest stage of organ formation at which tissue-specific genes are upregulated. It is generated through interactions between molecules in the extracellular matrix such as the cell adhesion molecules fibronectin, N-CAM and N-cadherin. Cell adhesion also is mediated, albeit indirectly, via activation of particular CAM genes by the products of the Hox genes, Hoxa-2 and Hoxd-13. Cells proliferate and differentiate, under the control of transcription factors, into chondrocytes or osteoblasts forming, respectively, cartilage or bone. Proliferation within the condensations is mediated through the activation of cell surface receptors such as syndecan-3, a receptor for fibroblast growth factor 2 (FGF-2), the antiadhesive matrix component, tenascin-C, a ligand for the epidermal growth factor (EGF) receptor (EGFR), the Hox genes, Hoxd-11-13 and transcription factors such as CFKH-1, MFH-1, and osf-2. Growth of condensations is regulated by BMPs, which activate a number of genes including Pax-2, Hoxa-2, and Hoxd-11. Conversely, growth is blocked via inhibition of BMP signaling by the BMP antagonist, Noggin. Defects in the formation of specific bones and joints can occur through mutation of genes involved in the control of bone and joint development. Information derived from ongoing and future research focused on the identification of the genes/gene targets involved in skeletal development and maintenance should open new avenues for the development of therapeutic measures for treating defects resulting either from mutation or trauma.

For most of the skeleton, bones develop from cartilage models comprised of assemblies of chondrocytes in an extracellular collagen-containing matrix that they secrete. The replacement of cartilage by bone is the result of a genetic master program that controls and coordinates chondrocyte differentiation, matrix alteration and mineralization. During the conversion of the cartilage model into bone, the composition of the matrix, including collagen types, is modified, ultimately becoming mineralized through a process termed endochondral ossification and populated by osteocytes. Disruption of the rate, timing, or duration of chondrocyte proliferation and differentiation results in shortened, misshapen skeletal elements. In the majority of such disruptions, vascularization also is perturbed. It has been proposed that vascularization plays a key role in the synchronization of the processes involved in endochondral ossification. Bone formation also occurs via intramembranous ossification, in which bone cells arise directly from mesenchyme without an intermediate cartilage anlage. Data indicate that this process is the result both of a positive selection for osteogenic differentiation and a negative selection against the progressive growth of chondrogenic cells in the absence of a permissive or inductive environment. In any case, through the processes of bone growth and remodeling, an adult skeleton is shaped and molded and continually remolded in response to environmental alterations. In effect, the adult skeleton is not a static entity. Bone is metabolically active throughout life and, under the influence of mechanical stress, nutrition, and hormones, bone remodeling occurs continually. However, bone remodeling is compromised as a function of both post menopausal hormonal changes and aging, resulting in health problems of increasing magnitude as the proportion of the aged in the global population increases.

Mutations in genes encoding structural proteins of the extracellular matrix can perturb the coordination of events necessary for normal skeletal development. The magnitude of the disruption of the process of ordered skeletal development is dependent on both the role of the mutated gene product in the developmental process and the degree of its functional perturbation. The range of mutational consequences is broad, including disruption of ossification/mineralization and linear growth and the structural integrity and stability of articular cartilage. Evidence indicates that osteochondrodysplasias resulting from defects in structural proteins are inherited in an autosomal dominant manner and that a spectrum of related clinical phenotypes can be produced by different mutations in the same gene. In addition, as might be expected, haploinsufficiency of a gene product usually produces a milder clinical phenotype than do mutations resulting in the synthesis of highly structurally abnormal proteins. The synthesis of structurally abnormal protein can produce a dominant-negative effect that is the primary determinant of phenotype. Thus, inherited defects that interfere with post-translational modification of matrix proteins such as hydroxylation, sulfation and/or proteolytic cleavage, can result in distinct osteochondrodysplasias. In the future, it may be possible to identify genes and pathways that can maintain, repair, or stimulate the regeneration of bone and joint structures at post patterning stages of development.

In this regard, it is to be noted that metabolites of vitamin A, including retinoic acid (RA), comprise a class of molecules that are of critical importance in development and homeostasis. Retinoic acid functions through a class of nuclear hormone receptors, the RA receptors (RARs), to regulate gene transcription. Retinoic acid receptor-mediated signaling plays a fundamental role in skeletogenesis. In the developing mammalian limb, RA induces the differentiation of a number of cell lineages including chondrocytes. However, excess RA is a potent teratogen that induces characteristic skeletal defects in a stage- and dose-dependent manner. Genetic analyses have shown that RAR deficiency results both in severe deficiency of cartilage formation in certain anatomical sites and the promotion of ectopic cartilage formation in other sites. In the developing limbs of transgenic mice expressing either dominant-negative or weakly constitutively active RARs, chondrogenesis is perturbed, resulting in a spectrum of skeletal malformations. Recently, RA was reported to bind two circadian clock proteins, Clock and Mop4, and may play a role in regulating circadian rhythms. Thus, it may be possible to utilize these interactions to manipulate the body's response to therapeutic drugs, which is entrained in the circadian flow.

A number of growth factors interact with osteoblasts or their precursors during bone development, remodeling or repair. Traditionally, morphogenetic signals have been studied in embryos. However, it was observed that implantation of demineralized adult bone matrix into subcutaneous sites in a variety of species resulted in local bone induction. Not only did this model system mimic the process of limb morphogenesis, it also permitted the isolation of bone morphogenetic proteins (BMPs). The BMPs constitute a large family of morphogenetic proteins within the transforming growth factor-β (TGF-β) superfamily. It is to be emphasized that these morphogens and related cartilage-derived morphogenetic proteins (CDMPs) that initiate, promote, and maintain chondrogenesis, have actions on systems other than bone. Indeed, bone morphogenetic proteins are multifunctional growth factors involved in many aspects of tissue development and morphogenesis, including, for example, regulation of FSH action in the ovary. The mechanism underlying the phenomenon of bone matrix-induced bone induction is under intense investigation by biomedical engineers and orthopedic researchers.

Growth/differentiation factor-5 (GDF-5), a BMP family member, has been shown to be essential for normal appendicular skeletal and joint development in humans and mice. It has been reported that GDF-5 promotes the initial stages of chondrogenesis by promoting cell adhesion and increased cell proliferation. In the mouse GDF-5 gene mutant brachypod, the defect is manifested early in chondrogenesis (embryonic day [E]12.5) as a reduction in the size of the cartilage blastema. The defect is associated with a decrease in the expression of cell surface molecules resulting in a decrease in cell adhesiveness and, consequently, perturbation of cartilage model competence. Another member of the family, BMP-6, has been shown to be overexpressed in prostate cancer and appears to be associated with bone-forming skeletal metastases. In the United States, prostate cancer became the number one cancer among white males in the mid-1980s and has increased dramatically since then. A study of benign and malignant prostate lesions by *in situ* hybridization showed that BMP-6 expression was high at both primary and secondary sites in cases of advanced cancer with metastases. Does upregulation of BMP-6 promote metastasis or is it involved in the body's defense armamentarium? Is it a target for therapeutics? Such questions are under active investigation by cancer researchers.

Two families of growth factors, the TGF-β superfamily and the insulin-like growth factors (IGF) superfamily, appear to be the principal proximal regulators of osteogenesis. However, these growth factors are not specific for cells of the osteoblast lineage. The mechanism by which skeletal tissue is specifically induced and maintained involves both complex interactions among circulating hormones, growth factors, and regulators of the activity of specific genes. For example, nuclear transcription factors such as core binding factor a1 (Cbfa1), a transcription factor essential for osteoblast differentiation and bone formation, and CCAAT/enhancer binding protein δ (C/EBPδ), that function as regulators of the expression/activity of specific bone growth factors and receptors, are activated in response to glucocorticoids, sex steroids, parathyroid hormone (PTH), and prostaglandin E2 (PGE2). Many environmentally available chemicals, both natural and man-made, have either sex steroid or anti-sex steroid activity. Evidence suggests that such chemicals have negatively impacted fish populations and other animals by interfering with the mechanism of action of reproductive hormones. However, their impact on other mechanisms such as growth have not been thoroughly investigated.

Members of the tumor necrosis factor (TNF) family of ligands and receptors have been identified as critical regulators of osteoclastogenesis. Osteoprotegerin (OPG), a member of the TNF receptor family, plays a key role in the physiological regulation of osteoclastic bone resorption. OPG, a secreted decoy receptor produced by osteoblasts and marrow stromal cells, acts by binding to its natural ligand, OPGL (also known as RANKL [receptor activator of NF-κB ligand]), thereby preventing OPGL from activating its cognate receptor RANK, the osteoclast receptor vital for osteoclast differentiation, activation and survival. In vitro studies have suggested that estrogen stimulates OPG expression whereas parathyroid hormone (PTH) inhibits its expression and stimulates the expression of RANKL. This construct provides a molecular mechanism for the regulation of the osteoclastic bone resorption and osteoblastic bone formation couple and basis for the bone loss of postmenopausal osteoporosis, aging and pathologic skeletal changes (e.g., osteopetrosis, glucocorticoid-induced osteoporosis, periodontal disease, bone metastases, Paget's disease, hyperparathyroidism, and rheumatoid arthritis). Environmental toxicants and endocrine disruptors also may perturb the normal balance between osteoclastic and osteoblastic activity by interfering with homeostasis and/or accelerating aging processes. With regard to endocrine disruption, OPG has been linked to vascular disease, particularly arterial calcification in estrogen-deficient individuals, the aged, and those afflicted with immunological deficits.

During skeletogenesis, cartilage matures either into permanent cartilage that persists as such throughout the organism's life or transient cartilage that ultimately is replaced by bone. How cartilage phenotype is specified is not clear. In vitro studies have shown that Cbfa1 is involved in induction of chondrocyte maturation. In this regard, it is of interest to note that transgenic mice overexpressing either Cbfa1 or a dominant-negative (DN)-Cbfa1 in chondrocytes exhibit dwarfism and skeletal malformations. These phenotypes are mediated through opposing mechanisms. In the former case, Cbfa1 overexpression accelerates endochondral ossification resulting from precocious chondrocyte maturation whereas in the latter, DN-Cbfa1 overexpression suppresses maturation and delays endochondral ossification. In addition, mice overexpressing Cbfa1 fail to form most of their joints and what would be permanent cartilage in normal mice enters the endochondral pathway of ossification. In contrast, in DN-Cbfa1 transgenic mice, most chondrocytes exhibit a marker for permanent cartilage. It may be concluded from these observations that proper temporal and spatial expression of chondrocyte Cbfa1 is required for normal skeletogenesis, including formation of joints, permanent cartilage, and endochondral bone.

Both gain-of-function and loss-of-function mutations in fibroblast growth factor receptor 3 (FGFR3) have revealed unique roles for this receptor during skeletal development. Loss-of-function alleles of FGFR3 lead to an increase in the size of the hypertrophic zone, delayed closure of the growth plate and the subsequent overgrowth of long bones. Gain-of-function mutations in FGFR3 have been linked genetically to autosomal dominant dwarfing chondrodysplasia syndromes in which both the size and architecture of the epiphyseal growth plate are altered. Analysis of these phenotypes and the biochemical consequences of the mutations in FGFR3 demonstrate that FGFR3-mediated signaling is an essential negative regulator of endochondral ossification.

Thorough understanding of bone physiology and how it is modified throughout all stages of life, from *in utero* development to advanced age, is of great current interest for its potential application to the establishment of criteria for the achievement and maintenance of bone health and the reestablishment of bone health following trauma and disease. Other clinical applications include:

• Establishment of criteria for the achievement of optimal bone strength throughout life, its maintenance in such long-term microgravity situations as space travel, and the facilitation of readjustment to normogravity upon return to earth. This will require establishment of rapid and precise methods for distinguishing mechanically competent bone from incompetent bone.

- Establishment of optimal conditions for the healing of fractures, osteotomies, and arthrodeses.
- Understanding the mechanics of induction by falling of metaphyseal and diaphyseal fractures of the radius in children, but primarily metaphyseal fractures in the aged.
- Improvement of the endurance of load-bearing implants.
- Understanding the mechanism(s) of osteopenia and osteoporosis and how and why, during menopause, healthy women lose only bone adjacent to marrow.

Furthermore, because of the multifunctionality and interactions of the skeletal system, biomedical researchers and practitioners of almost every clinical discipline have great interest in bone biology. Even a cursory review of the bone biology literature will reveal the depth of interest in the field. Publications emanate from a broad spectrum of biomedical areas that include: adolescent medicine, anatomy, anthropology, biochemistry, biomechanics, biomedical engineering, biophysics, cardiology, cell and molecular biology, clinical nutrition research, dentistry, developmental biology, endocrinology, enzymology, epidemiology, food science, genetics, genetic counseling, gerontology, hematology, histology, human nutrition, internal medicine, medicinal chemistry, metabolism, microbiology, neurology, oncology, orthopedics, pediatric medicine, pharmacology and therapeutics, physical and rehabilitation medicine, physiology, plastic surgery, public health, radiology and imaging research, space and sports medicine, trace/essential element research, vascular biology, vitaminology and cofactor research, women's health, teratology, and toxicology.

Bone biology is a diverse field, and our goal in developing *The Skeleton: Biochemical, Genetic, and Molecular Interactions in Development and Homeostasis* was to provide researchers and students with an overview of selected topics of current interest in bone biology and to stimulate their interest in this fascinating and diverse field.

Edward J. Massaro
John M. Rogers

Contents

VI. Skeletal Dysmorphology

Contributors

Rosalie Anderson • *Department of Biological Sciences, Loyola University, New Orleans, LA*

Siegfried Arnold • *Large Area Electronics, PerkinElmer Optoelectronics, Wiesbaden, Germany*

Deborah S. Best • *Reproductive Toxicology Division, National Health and Environmental Effects Research Laboratory, Office of Research and Development, US Environmental Protection Agency, Research Triangle Park, NC*

Jean-Pierre Bonnamy • *Department of Molecular and Human Genetics, Baylor College of Medicine, Houston, TX*

Qian Chen • *Department of Orthopaedics, Brown Medical School, Rhode Island Hospital, Providence, RI*

Neil Chernoff • *Developmental Biology Branch, Reproductive Toxicology Division, National Health and Environmental Effects Research Laboratory, Office of Research Development, US Environmental Protection Agency, Research Triangle Park, NC*

Simon J. Conway • *Department of Cell Biology and Anatomy, Institute of Molecular Medicine and Genetics, Medical College of Georgia, Augusta, GA*

Jan Christian • *Department of Cell and Developmental Biology, Oregon Health and Science University, Portland, OR*

Catherine Degnin • *Department of Cell and Developmental Biology, Oregon Health and Science University, Portland, OR*

Dana L. Di Nino • *Department of Anatomy and Cellular Biology, Tufts University Medical School, Boston, MA*

M. Hicham Drissi • *Center for Musculoskeletal Research, University of Rochester, Rochester, NY*

Denis Duboule • *Department of Zoology and Animal Biology and NCCR 'Frontiers in Genetics,' University of Geneva, Geneva, Switzerland*

Patricia Ducy • *Department of Molecular and Human Genetics, Baylor College of Medicine, Houston, TX*

Jennifer Farrington • *Division of Developmental Biology, Department of Cell and Molecular Biology, Tulane University, New Orleans, LA*

Chiara Gentili • *Centro di Medicina Rigenerativa, Istituto Nazionale Ricerca sul Cancro, Genova, Italy*

Françoise Gofflot • *Unit of Developmental Genetics, Université Catholique de Louvain, Bruxelles, Belgium*

Eleanor Golden • *Department of Anatomy and Cell Biology, School of Dental Medicine, University of Pennsylvania, Philadelphia, PA*

Giedre Grigelioniene • *Paediatric Endocrinology Unit, Karolinska Hospital, Stockholm, Sweden*

Renee Hackenmiller • *Department of Cell and Developmental Biology, Oregon Health and Science University, Portland, OR*

Bonnie T. Hamby • *RTI International, Center for Life Sciences and Technology, Research Triangle Park, NC*

MANJONG HAN • *Division of Developmental Biology, Department of Cell and Molecular Biology, Tulane University, New Orleans, LA*
YUJI HATAKEYAMA • *Cartilage Biology and Orthopaedics Branch, National Institute of Arthritis, and Musculoskeletal and Skin Disease, National Institutes of Health, Bethesda, MD*
HANS J. HÖHLING • *Institut für Medizinische Physik und Biophysik, Westfälische Wilhelms-Universität Münster, Germany*
ANDREIA M. IONESCU • *Center for Musculoskeletal Research, University of Rochester, Rochester, NY*
GERARD KARSENTY • *Department of Molecular and Human Genetics, Baylor College of Medicine, Houston, TX*
ROBERT J. KAVLOCK • *Reproductive Toxicology Division, National Health and Environmental Effects Research Laboratory, Office of Research and Development, US Environmental Protection Agency, Research Triangle Park, NC*
MARIE KMITA • *Department of Zoology and Animal Biology and NCCR "Frontiers in Genetics," University of Geneva, Geneva, Switzerland*
CHRISTOPHER S. KOVACS • *Faculty of Medicine—Endocrinology, Memorial University of Newfoundland Health Sciences Centre, St. John's, Newfoundland, Canada*
EIKI KOYAMA • *Department of Orthopaedic Surgery, Thomas Jefferson University Medical School, Philadelphia, PA*
JOHN C. LEE • *Department of Biochemistry, University of Texas Health Science Center, San Antonio, TX*
JULIUS LEYTON • *Cartilage Biology and Orthopaedics Branch, National Institute of Arthritis, and Musculoskeletal and Skin Disease, National Institutes of Health, Bethesda, MD*
SHAOGUANG LI • *The Jackson Laboratory, Bar Harbor, Maine*
THOMAS F. LINSENMAYER • *Department of Anatomy and Cellular Biology, Tufts University Medical School, Boston, MA*
PIERRE J. MARIE • *INSERM U349 Lariboisière Hospital, Paris, France*
MELISSA C. MARR • *RTI International, Center for Life Sciences and Toxicology, Research Triangle Park, NC*
EDWARD J. MASSARO • *Developmental Biology Branch, Reproductive Toxicology Division, National Health and Environmental Effects Research Laboratory, Office of Research Development, US Environmental Protection Agency, Research Triangle Park, NC*
THATO MATSABA • *Bone Research Unit, Medical Research Council/University of the Witwatersrand, Johannesburg, South Africa*
CHRISTINA B. MYERS • *RTI International, Center for Life Sciences and Toxicology, Research Triangle Park, NC*
KEN MUNEOKA • *Division of Developmental Biology, Department of Cell and Molecular Biology, Tulane University, New Orleans, LA*
JOHANNA MYLLYHARJU • *Collagen Research Unit, Biocenter Oulu and Department of Medical Biochemistry and Molecular Biology, University of Oulu, Oulu, Finland*
MICHAEL G. NAROTSKY • *Reproductive Toxicology Division, National Health and Environmental Effects Research Laboratory, Office of Research and Development, US Environmental Protection Agency, Research Triangle Park, NC*
VALERIE NGO-MULLER • *ICGM Cochin Port-Royal, Paris France*

Kazuaki Nonaka • *Section of Pediatric Dentistry, Division of Oral Health, Growth, and Development, Faculty of Dental Science, Kyushu University, Fukuoka, Japan*
Regis J. O'Keefe • *Center for Musculoskeletal Research, University of Rochester, Rochester, NY*
Minoru Omi • *Division of Developmental Biology, Department of Cell and Molecular Biology, Tulane University, New Orleans, LA*
Michael J. Owen • *Imperial Cancer Research Fund, London, UK*
Nathalie Pacico • *Unit of Developmental Genetics, Université Catholique de Louvain, Bruxelles, Belgium*
Maurizio Pacifici • *Department of Orthopaedic Surgery, Thomas Jefferson University Medical School, Philadelphia, PA*
Janet Patton • *Bone Research Unit, Medical Research Council/University of the Witwatersrand, Johannesburg, South Africa*
Jacques J. Picard • *Unit of Developmental Genetics, Université Catholique de Louvain, Bruxelles, Belgium*
Ulrich Plate • *Klinik und Poliklinik für Mund- und Kiefer-Gesichtschirurgie, Westfälische Wilhelms-Universität Münster, Germany*
Hulbert A. P. Pols • *Department of Internal Medicine, Erasmus Medical Center Rotterdam, Rotterdam, The Netherlands*
Nathaniel L. Ramoshebi • *Bone Research Unit, Medical Research Council/University of the Witwatersrand, Johannesburg, South Africa*
Sakamuri V. Reddy • *Center for Bone Biology, Division of Hematology-Oncology, Department of Medicine, University of Pittsburgh, Pittsburgh, PA*
Louise Renton • *Bone Research Unit, Medical Research Council/University of the Witwatersrand, Johannesburg, South Africa*
Ugo Ripamonti • *Bone Research Unit, Medical Research Council/University of the Witwatersrand, Johannesburg, South Africa*
John M. Rogers • *Developmental Biology Branch, Reproductive Toxicology Division, National Health and Environmental Effects Research Laboratory, Office of Research Development, US Environmental Protection Agency, Research Triangle Park, NC*
G. David Roodman • *Center for Bone Biology, Division of Hematology-Oncology, Department of Medicine, University of Pittsburgh, Pittsburgh, PA*
Scott A. Schaller • *Department of Cell and Molecular Biology, Division of Developmental Biology, Tulane University, New Orleans, LA*
R. Woodrow Setzer • *Pharmacokinetics Branch, Experimental Toxicology Division, National Health and Environmental Effects Research Laboratory, Office of Research and Development, US Environmental Protection Agency, Research Triangle Park, NC*
Lillian Shum • *Cartilage Biology and Orthopaedics Branch, National Institute of Arthritis and Musculoskeletal and Skin Diseases, National Institutes of Health, Bethesda, MD*
Shu Takeda • *Department of Molecular and Human Genetics, Baylor College of Medicine, Houston, TX*
June Teare • *Bone Research Unit, Medical Research Council/University of the Witwatersrand, Johannesburg, South Africa*

Rocky S. Tuan • *Cartilage Biology and Orthopaedics Branch, National Institute of Arthritis and Musculoskeletal and Skin Diseases, National Institutes of Health, Bethesda, MD*

Rochelle W. Tyl • *RTI International, Center for Life Sciences and Toxicology, Research Triangle Park, NC*

T. Michael Underhill • *Department of Physiology, and Division of Oral Biology, Faculty of Medicine and Dentistry, University of Western Ontario, London, Ontario, Canada*

Jacqueline C. van der Linden • *Orthopedic Research Laboratory, Erasmus University Rotterdam, Rotterdam, The Netherlands*

Marjolein van Driel • *Department of Internal Medicine, Erasmus Medical Center Rotterdam, Rotterdam, The Netherlands*

Johannes P. T. M. van Leeuwen • *Department of Internal Medicine, Erasmus Medical Center Rotterdam, Rotterdam, The Netherlands*

Jan A. N. Verhaar • *Orthopedic Research Laboratory, Erasmus University Rotterdam, Rotterdam, The Netherlands*

Cun-Yu Wang • *Department of Biologic and Materials Sciences, University of Michigan School of Dentistry, Ann Arbor, MI*

Harrie Weinans • *Orthopedic Research Laboratory, Erasmus University Rotterdam, Rotterdam, The Netherlands*

Nathalie Wéry • *Unit of Developmental Genetics, Université Catholique de Louvain, Bruxelles, Belgium*

Andrea D. Weston • *Department of Physiology, Faculty of Medicine and Dentistry, University of Western Ontario, London, Ontario, Canada*

Lee-Chuan C. Yeh • *Department of Biochemistry, University of Texas Health Science Center, San Antonio, TX*

József Zákány • *Department of Zoology and Animal Biology and NCCR 'Frontiers in Genetics,' University of Geneva, Geneva, Switzerland*

I

Chondrogenesis, Chondrocytes, and Cartilage

1

Molecular Basis of Cell–Cell Interaction and Signaling in Mesenchymal Chondrogenesis

Rocky S. Tuan

INTRODUCTION

Chondrogenesis, the first step in embryonic skeletal development, involves a series of highly regulated events, encompassing recruitment and condensation of mesenchymal chondroprogenitor cells and subsequent differentiation into chondrocytes. This chapter deals with the molecular events contributing to the above processes, specifically cell–cell interactions, cellular signaling pathways, and regulation of gene expression.

PRECARTILAGE CONDENSATION OF MESENCHYMAL CHONDROPROGENITOR CELLS

The cells that contribute to the skeletal elements of the embryonic limb are derived from the lateral plate mesoderm. These cells migrate into the limb field and undergo a phenomenon termed "precartilage condensation," first described by Fell *(1)*. These condensations are easily visualized using standard light or transmission electron microscopy and appear as closely packed mesenchymal cells in the chondrogenic regions when compared with the surrounding nonchondrogenic mesenchyme. Another method of visualizing cellular condensations is by taking advantage of a characteristic specific to condensing, precartilage mesenchymal cells. These cells bind the lectin peanut (*Arachis hypogaea*) agglutinin (PNA) that recognizes the glycosyl terminal of the disaccharide Gal(β1,3)GalNAc, thereby demarcating cellular condensations during the development of skeletal tissues *(2)*. Evidence suggests that PNA binds to some cell-surface component(s) of the condensing mesenchymal cells *(3,4)*. After chondrogenic differentiation, these cells are no longer able to bind PNA, further illustrating the utility of PNA binding as a method for identifying precartilage cells.

The appearance of precartilage condensations is one of the earliest morphological events in skeletogenesis. This is a transient stage of skeletogenesis that provides the scaffold for the formation of the endochondral skeletal elements. It is at this time that the shape, size, position, and number of skeletal elements are established. Cellular condensations form as a result of altered mitotic activity, failure of cells to move away from a center or, as in the limb, aggregation of cells toward a center. This active cell movement causes an increase in mesenchymal cell-packing density, that is, an increase in cells/unit area or volume without an increase in cell proliferation *(2,5–9)*. Evidence supporting the

From: *The Skeleton: Biochemical, Genetic, and Molecular Interactions in Development and Homeostasis*
Edited by: E. J. Massaro and J. M. Rogers © Humana Press Inc., Totowa, NJ

importance of cellular condensation in chondrogenesis has come from both in vivo and in vitro observations. Many classical studies have demonstrated a high cell density requirement for chondrogenesis to occur *(10)*, correlated the extent of cell condensation with the level of chondrogenesis *(11,12)*, demonstrated the initiation of gap-junction-mediated cell–cell communication in condensing mesenchyme *(13,14)*, and described characteristic limb skeletal abnormalities in genetic mutants defective in mesenchymal cell condensation (reviewed in refs. *2* and *15*).

The process of mesenchymal cell condensation is directed by cell–cell and cell–matrix interactions as well as secreted factors interacting with their cognate receptors. Before condensation, mesenchymal cells present in the limb secrete an extracellular matrix (ECM) rich in hyaluronan and collagen type I that prevents intimate cell–cell interaction. As condensation begins, an increase in hyaluronidase activity is observed with a decrease in hyaluronan in the ECM. Hyaluronan is thought to facilitate cell movement, and the increase in hyaluronidase and subsequent decrease in hyaluronan allows for close cell–cell interactions *(16–18)*. The establishment of cell–cell interactions is presumably involved in triggering one or more signal transduction pathways that initiates chondrogenic differentiation. Two cell adhesion molecules implicated in this process are N-cadherin and neural cell adhesion molecule (N-CAM). Both of these molecules are expressed in condensing mesenchyme and then disappear in differentiating cartilage *(19,20)* and later are detectable only in the perichondrium. Perturbing the function(s) of N-cadherin *(21)* or N-CAM *(22)* causes reduction or alterations in chondrogenesis both in vitro and in vivo, further supporting a role for these cell adhesion molecules in mediating the mesenchymal condensation step.

In addition to cell–cell interactions, cell–matrix interactions also appear to play an important role in mesenchymal cell condensation. One ECM component implicated in this process is fibronectin. Fibronectin expression is increased in areas of cellular condensation *(23,24)* and decreases as cytodifferentiation proceeds. Fibronectin may facilitate a matrix-driven translocation of mesenchymal cells into cellular condensations, and this process may be mediated by the amino terminal heparin binding domain *(25,26)*. Recent studies in our laboratory have demonstrated that fibronectin mRNA undergoes alternative splicing during chondrogenesis *(27–29)*. The isoform containing exon EIIIA is present during condensation but disappears once differentiation begins, suggesting that this isoform switching is important for cytodifferentiation to occur. Antibodies specific for the region encoded by exon EIIIA of the fibronectin gene inhibited chondrogenesis of limb micromass cultures in vitro, and when injected into chick limb buds in vivo, caused moderate to severe skeletal malformations *(27,28)*.

CELL ADHESION IN MESENCHYMAL CELL CONDENSATION

Cell adhesion is mediated by two major groups of cell–cell adhesion molecules, the Ca^{2+}-independent and the Ca^{2+}-dependent adhesion molecules *(30–38)*. The Ca^{2+}-independent group is composed of the large immunoglobulin supergene family of membrane glycoproteins known as CAMs, and the Ca^{2+}-dependent group consists largely of a class of transmembrane glycoproteins called the cadherins. Two adhesion molecules, N-cadherin and N-CAM, have been shown to have an important role during the precartilaginous condensation phase during endochondral ossification *(21,22)*.

N-Cadherin

The cadherin superfamily has many members and can be divided into six gene subfamilies based on structural homology: classical cadherins type I (e.g., E-, N-, P-, R-cadherin), classical cadherins type II (cadherin-6 to -12), cadherins found in desmosomes (desmocollins, desmogleins), cadherins with a very short cytoplasmic domain or none (LI-, T-cadherin), protocadherins, and the more distantly related gene products, including the *Drosophila* fat tumor-suppressor gene, the *dachsous* gene, and the *ret*-proto-oncogene *(39)*.

The classical cadherins are a group of Ca^{2+}-dependent, single transmembrane glycoproteins that mediate cell–cell adhesion by homotypic protein–protein interactions through their extracellular domain.

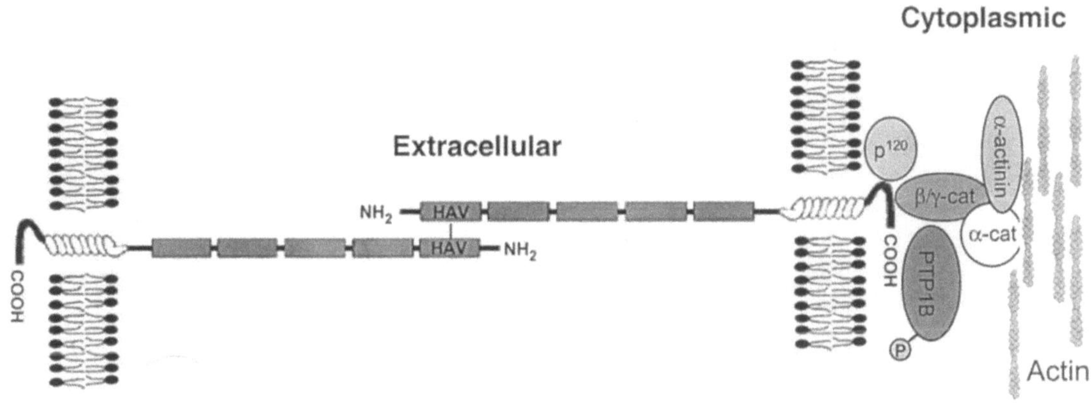

Fig. 1. Schematic of N-cadherin–catenin complex. N-cadherin is a Ca^{2+}-dependent, single-pass transmembrane protein that mediates cell–cell adhesion by homotypic protein–protein interactions through its extracellular domain. The extracellular domain is composed of five tandem repeats, termed cadherin repeats, that form four Ca^{2+} binding sites. The fifth cadherin repeat confers its homotypic specificity by the HAV (histidine–alanine–valine) amino acid sequence. The cytoplasmic domain binds the actin cytoskeleton via interactions with the catenin family of proteins. The cytoplasmic domain binds β/γ-catenin (β/α-cat) directly, which in turn binds α-catenin (α-cat). Subsequently, α-cat binds the actin cytoskeleton directly or in conjunction with α-actinin. Other proteins also bind the cytoplasmic domain of N-cadherin, such as $p120^{ctn}$ and the nonreceptor protein tyrosine phosphatase 1B (PTP1B). Both of these proteins bind the cytoplasmic domain and regulate cell adhesion.

Classic cadherins are synthesized as precursor polypeptides and are then processed into their mature form. The extracellular domain of the mature protein consists of five tandem repeat domains termed cadherin repeats, each of which consists of approx 110 amino acids. The cadherin repeats form four Ca^{2+}-binding domains, and the N-terminal repeat confers the cadherin-specific adhesive property of the molecule. Classic cadherins have a single transmembrane domain followed by a highly conserved cytoplasmic domain responsible for binding to the actin cytoskeleton via the catenin molecules (Fig. 1; ref. *40*).

The cadherin family of molecules exhibit spatiotemporally unique patterns of gene expression *(37)* and demonstrate homotypic binding through their extracellular domain, suggesting that cadherins may function as morphoregulatory molecules during development. N-Cadherin, named for its initial identification in neural tissues, was one of the first identified cadherins, and its functional involvement in cell–cell adhesion and development has been extensively studied *(41–48)*. N-Cadherin plays a major role in neural development but has also been shown to be expressed in other mesodermal tissues, including developing limb mesenchyme. N-Cadherin is expressed in the developing embryonic limb bud in a manner suggestive of a role in cellular condensation (Fig. 2; ref. *21*). Immunohistochemical localization of N-cadherin in the embryonic chick limb reveals a sparsely scattered expression pattern in the central core mesenchyme during the precartilage stage (Hamburger–Hamilton stages 17/18 through 22/23; ref. *49*). Expression dramatically increases in the condensing central core at stage 24/25, and by stage 25/26, the condensed central core region begins to lose N-cadherin expression, whereas cells along the periphery of the limb bud begin to express N-cadherin. By stage 29/30, the mature cartilage is completely devoid of N-cadherin whereas the condensing, perichondral cells surrounding the forming cartilage still exhibit high levels of N-cadherin. As the limb bud continues to develop, the cartilaginous core region continues to grow appositionally, and it is likely that the N-cadherin–positive cells along the periphery contribute to this growth *(21)*.

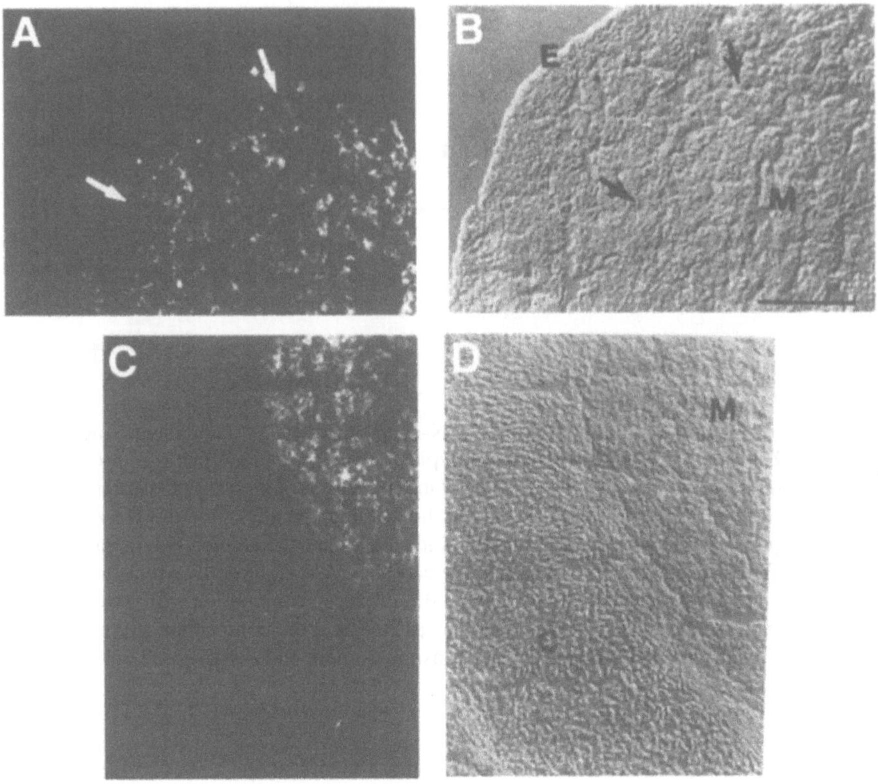

Fig. 2. Spatiotemporal specificity of N-cadherin expression in the developing chick embryonic limb bud. **A** and **B**, Hamburger–Hamilton Stage 24/25. NCD-2 immunofluorescent staining reveals N-cadherin expression to be localized exclusively with the condensing mesenchyme (M; arrows). E, ectoderm. **A**, epifluorescent optics; **B**, Nomarski optics. **C** and **D**, Stage 29/30. Mature cartilage (C) is formed and is negative for N-cadherin, whereas the surrounding mesenchyme (M) remains positive. **C**, epifluorescent optics; **D**, Nomarski optics. Magnification: bar = 100 μm. (Taken from ref. *21*.)

In high-density micromass cultures in vitro, dissociated limb mesenchymal cells aggregate to form cellular condensations that ultimately differentiate into cartilaginous nodules, separated by fibroblasts and myocytes *(10)*. N-Cadherin protein is synthesized by the aggregating (condensing) mesenchyme by 12 h after initiation of the culture, whereas the cells outside of the condensation centers display no evident N-cadherin expression. Expression of N-cadherin becomes more intense as a function of time with maximal expression at 18 h. As the cells in the center of the condensations differentiate, they lose their N-cadherin protein, and the cells along the immediate periphery of the forming nodules maintain N-cadherin expression. Thus, the expression pattern of N-cadherin in vitro recapitulates that in the developing limb *in situ (21)*.

N-Cadherin expression is localized to the prechondroblastic cells of the limb bud, and maximal expression is seen during mesenchymal cell condensation, after which it is downregulated, suggesting that cellular condensation is dependent on N-cadherin–mediated cell–cell interactions *(19,21)*. Evidence to support this theory comes from studies designed to perturb N-cadherin function. We *(19)* were able to demonstrate a significant inhibition of cellular condensation and chondrogenesis in vitro and in vivo using a function-blocking monoclonal antibody, NCD-2, directed against N-cadherin *(42)*. These findings correlate well with previous findings that exogenous Ca^{2+} significantly stimulates chondrogenesis in vitro when added before condensation but has little effect when added after condensation *(11,12)*. In similar studies, the addition of transforming growth factor-β family member, BMP-2, to chick limb bud or the C3H10T1/2 murine multipotential cell line plated at high-density micromass cultures stimulated chondrogenesis on the basis of Alcian blue staining, collagen type II, and link protein expression and led to an increase in [^{35}S]sulfate incorporation *(50–53)*. Further investigation revealed that BMP-2 treatment of C3H10T1/2 cells stimulated N-cadherin mRNA levels fourfold within 24 h and protein levels eightfold by day 5 in culture, whereas an N-cadherin peptidomimic containing the His-Ala-Val sequence was able to inhibit chondrogenesis in a dose-dependent manner *(54)*. To specifically examine the influence of altered N-cadherin expression or activity on chondrogenesis, C3H10T1/2 cells were stably transfected with N-cadherin wild-type or dominant-negative N-terminal deletion constructs. Cells expressing the wild-type N-cadherin at a moderate level (twofold) increased chondrogenesis, whereas cells expressing a fourfold increase in N-cadherin or the dominant-negative construct had an initial, inhibitory effect on BMP-2 stimulation of chondrogenesis *(54)*. In recent studies *(55,56)* we have further examined the functional role of N-cadherin by analyzing the effect of transfecting chick embryonic limb mesenchymal cells with expression constructs that encode for wild-type or amino-deleted/carboxy-deleted mutant forms of N-cadherin. Plasmid and retroviral (RCAS) vectors were used for transient and stable misexpression, respectively. Our results showed that N-cadherin is crucial in mediating the initial cell–cell interaction in mesenchymal condensation and requires both the extracellular homotypic binding site and the intracellular site involved in adhesion complex formation. However, proper chondrogenic progression requires a subsequent downregulation of N-cadherin and cell adhesion, such that prolonged overexpression of wild-type N-cadherin in the stable transfectants actually results in a significantly reduced level of chondrogenesis. Taken together, these data strongly support a functional and activity-dependent role for N-cadherin in cellular condensation and chondrogenesis.

N-CAM

The glycoprotein N-CAM is a member of the immunoglobulin superfamily *(57)*. N-CAM is composed of five immunoglobulin-like domains, each consisting of aprrox 100 amino acids folded into β sheets usually linked by a disulfide bond *(58)*. There is only one N-CAM gene; however, different forms of N-CAM can be generated through alternative splicing of its mRNA as well as varying degrees of glycosylation (sialic acid; refs. *59–61*). The major mRNA splicing differences occur near the carboxy-terminal with some forms displaying altered cytoplasmic domains or missing the transmembrane domain. Homotypic binding of N-CAM occurs near the amino terminal *(62)* and does not appear to be affected by alternative splicing.

N-CAM expression in the developing chick limb follows that of the previously described N-cadherin; however, the expression of N-cadherin mRNA occurs earlier than that of N-CAM mRNA *(20)*. N-CAM expression in vivo is observed in all limb bud cells by stage 22 *(63)*. N-CAM expression increases and is enriched in the condensing mesenchyme at stage 27. By stage 30, the cells in the center of the condensations differentiate and N-CAM expression is lost in mature cartilage, but strong N-CAM expression is maintained in the surrounding perichondrium *(22,63,64)*. The in vitro N-CAM expression pattern parallels that of the in vivo expression. In micromass cultures in vitro, N-CAM is expressed after 1.5 d in the aggregating, precartilage condensations, with a zone of moderately N-CAM–expressing cells surrounding the condensations. By 4 d in culture, the condensations have differentiated into cartilaginous nodules and lose the expression of N-CAM in their center but retain N-CAM expression at their periphery *(22)*.

The functional role of N-CAM in cellular condensation and chondrogenesis was determined by perturbation studies in vitro by using aggregation assays and micromass cultures. Aggregation of dissociated stage 23 chick limb bud cells was reduced when incubated with anti-N-CAM antibodies in suspension culture compared with cells incubated with nonimmune Fab fragments *(22)*. In the presence of anti-N-CAM antibodies, both the number and size of aggregates is reduced 50–60%. Micromass cultures of chick limb bud mesenchyme demonstrated a reduction in both the area occupied by condensations and the degree of cartilage differentiation when incubated with anti-N-CAM antibodies compared with the control cultures incubated with nonimmune Fab or antifibroblast Fab. The effect observed was dose dependent *(22,63)*. Overexpression of N-CAM in micromass cultures results in enhanced aggregation of mesenchymal cells, forming large cell aggregates that differentiate into cartilaginous nodules and are collagen type II positive *(22)*.

A naturally occurring genetic mutation, *Talpid*, is an autosomal-recessive disorder that manifests multiple skeletal disorders, including poly- and syndactyly *(65)*. The limb buds exhibit abnormally large precartilage condensations and the mesenchymal cells are shown to have greater adhesiveness than control cells *(66)*. Micromass cultures of *Talpid* limb bud cells revealed fused precartilage condensations and a much greater amount of chondrogenesis compared with cultures from normal embryos. In addition, anti-N-CAM antibodies reduced the size of cellular condensations and the degree of chondrogenesis in the *Talpid* cultures, suggesting that the increased condensations and chondrogenesis observed in the *Talpid* chicks appear to be at least partially mediated by an increase in N-CAM expression *(64)*.

SIGNALING PROCESSES IN MESENCHYMAL CONDENSATION AND CHONDROGENESIS: ROLE OF WNTS

Although cell–cell adhesion plays an integral part in the condensation stage of chondrogenesis, it has been shown that a number of signaling molecules, such as growth factors (transforming growth factor-βs, growth differentiation factors [GDFs], fibroblast growth factors), and their downstream effectors (homologs of *Drosophilia* Mothers Aganist Decapentaplegic [SMADs], mitogen-activated protein kinases) are responsible for initiation and maintenance of the chondrogenic activity within the developing limb. Similarly, transcription factors, such as Hox, En, and LEF-1, also are important for limb patterning, whereas members of the Wnt family may be involved in limb initiation and maintenance, as well as chondrogenic differentiation and chondrocyte maturation. The current understanding of the action of these signaling molecules is summarized below.

As stated previously, cadherin-dependent adhesion and function appear to be regulated in part via the cytoplasmic associated proteins, α-, β-, γ-catenin, and the newly identified p120ctn *(39,67–79)*. Interestingly, β-catenin is known to exist in three subcellular pools: membrane that is bound in association with adhesion molecules *(39)*, a cytoplasmic pool where β-catenin binds the adenomatous polyposis coli (APC) tumor suppressor protein through an internal repeat with amino acid homology to the catenin binding region of E-cadherin *(80,81)*, and a nuclear pool in association with lymphoid-enhancing factor and T-cell factors (LEF-1/TCF; refs. *82–84*). Because of the apparent "promiscuity" of the β-catenin molecule and the plausible titration between various pools in either a signaling or adhesive capacity, it is possible that mesenchymal condensation may also be dependent on the temporal and spatial availability of β-catenin, possibly through regulation via Wnt signaling.

Recently, it was determined that the interaction of APC with β-catenin is regulated by glycogen synthase kinase 3β (GSK-3b, a key mediator of the Wnt (*Drosophila* wingless: Wg) signaling pathway *(85,86)*. The Wnt family consists of at least 15 cysteine-rich-secreted glycoprotein members that are involved in cell fate determination, induction of neural tissue, kidney tissue, and muscle and mammary glands and have been shown to effect axis determination in early embryos *(87,88)*. Wnt signaling is mediated by interaction with its membrane receptor (*Drosophila* frizzled: DFz2; refs. *89* and *90*), and after regulation of various intermediate effectors, functions to inactivate GSK-3β serine/threonine kinase activity *(91–93)*. In the absence of Wnt signal, GSK-3β phosphorylates APC, causing increased β-catenin binding to the GSK-3β-APC complex *(87)*, and this binding is quickly followed by N-terminal phosphorylation of β-catenin *(94)* via GSK-3β *(86)*. The subsequent phosphorylation of β-catenin serves as a tag that targets the molecule for degradation by the ubiquitin/proteosome pathway (Fig. 3; refs. *95–97*).

Both GSK-3β and the ubiquitin pathway involved in degradation of β-catenin are regulated by protein kinase C (PKC) activity *(92,95,98)*, and serine/threonine phosphorylation of β-catenin may be

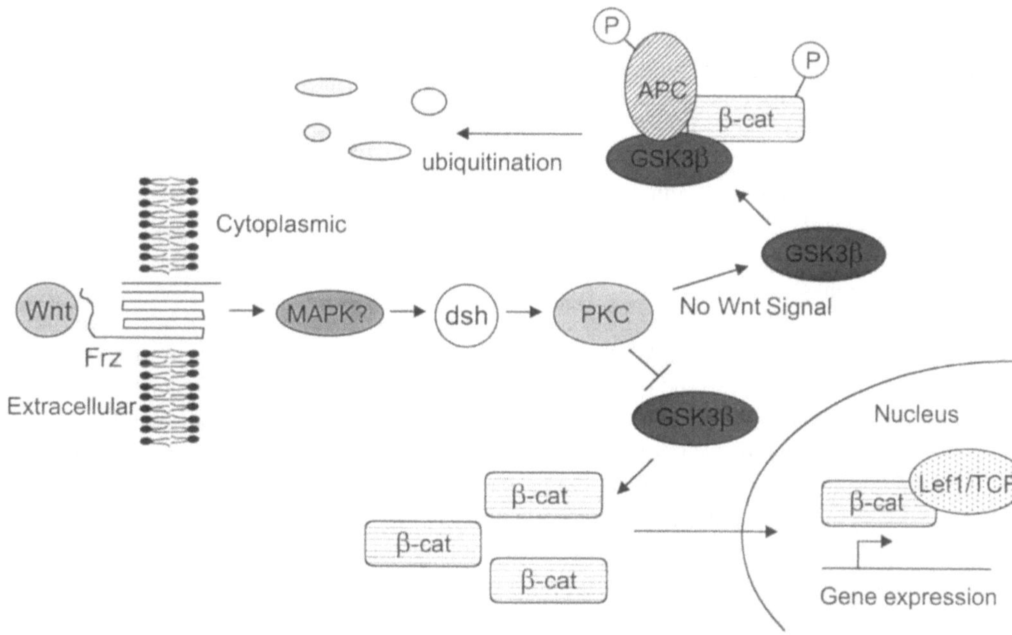

Fig. 3. Wnt-signaling pathway. Wnt signaling is mediated by its interaction with its membrane receptor frizzled (Frz). Upon Wnt ligand binding, glycogen synthase kinase 3β (GSK-3β) is inactivated by a series of kinases and β-catenin (β-cat) accumulates in the cytoplasm and translocates into the nucleus, where it interacts with Lef1/TCF transcription factors, and initiates gene transcription. In the absence of Wnt binding, GSK-3β phosphorylates adenomatous polyposis coli tumor suppressor gene (APC), causing an increased binding of β-cat to the APC-GSK-3β complex followed by phosphorylation of β-cat. This complex is quickly degraded by the ubiquitin/proteosome pathway.

reversed by the protein phosphatase type 1 and 2 family of phosphatases *(86)*. In the presence of Wnt and an inactive GSK-3β, β-catenin accumulates in the cytoplasm, presumably in a signaling capacity, and eventually translocates to the nucleus via binding to nucleoporins *(99)*, where it interacts with LEF-1/TCFs in an active transcription complex (Fig. 3; refs. *82–84,100*). The pool of β-catenin available for Wnt signaling is considered to be of a very low level, and β-catenin nuclear signaling also may be regulated by adhesion molecules that sequester catenins *(101)*.

Interestingly, Wnts may not be the only regulators of β-catenin and LEF-1 activity. As mentioned earlier, overexpression of ILK-1 is able to increase expression levels of LEF-1 and concomitantly to downregulate E-cadherin in epithelial cells *(102)*. The increased levels of LEF-1 caused translocation of β-catenin to the nucleus and activation of LEF-1 responsive promoters. Although Wnts have been identified as the primary candidates in regulation of β-catenin, this recent evidence indicates that at least one, and possibly more pathways, intersects with the β-catenin-LEF-1 complex regulation. While LEF-1/TCF-β-catenin has been shown to have a positive regulatory effect on certain promoters when present together, it has not been disproven that β-catenin and LEF-1 in complex may also have inhibitory qualities. Recently, it was determined that at times when there are low levels of β-catenin in the nucleus, the cAMP response element binding protein binding protein, a factor known exclusively for its coactivation properties, binds and acetylates TCF, causing decreased affinity for β-catenin and inhibition of transcription from TCF-responsive promoters *(103)*. LEF-1 and TCF-1 have been identified in developing mouse limb bud mesenchymal cells and in tail prevertebrae *(104)* and are induced by BMP-4 during murine tooth and hair development *(105)*. Furthermore, the LEF-1-β-catenin complex has recently been shown to bind the E-cadherin promoter *(83)*.

Wnt-1 in PC12 cells has been shown to increase cell adhesion through β-catenin–cadherin interaction *(106,107)* and has been found to cause skeletal abnormalities in developing mouse limb when ectopically expressed in transgenic mice *(108)*. Interestingly, some Wnts have been postulated to exert antagonistic effects towards each other in regulation of embryonic responses, possibly through influencing adhesion. Specifically, Wnt-5A appears to block *Xenopus* dorsalizing response to Wnt-1, causing decreased Ca^{2+}-dependent cell adhesion, an effect mimicked by overexpression of a dominant-negative N-cadherin *(109)*. However, in this report, Wnt-5A was unable to block dorsalization induced by injection of dominant-negative GSK-3β or β-catenin, indicating that antagonism may occur before the Wnt pathway reaches GSK-3β.

Various Wnts are found throughout the developing limb. Wnt-3, -4, -6, and -7B are expressed uniformly throughout the limb ectoderm, Wnt-5A is expressed throughout the distal mesenchyme *(110, 111)*, and Wnt-7A, which is expressed in the dorsal ectoderm *(110)*, appears to act as dorsalizing signal *(110,112, 113)* on the basis of the fact that mice lacking Wnt-7A develop ventralized paws *(110)*. Both Wnt-7A and Wnt-1 have been shown to inhibit chondrogenesis in chick limb bud micromass cultures, and the inhibition by these Wnts occurs after induction of adhesion molecules and aggregation at the late-blastema/early-chondroblast stage apparently by inhibition of chondroblast differentiation *(114)*. Wnt-4 has been implicated in mesenchymal condensation in kidney development *(115)* and Wnt-3A, which has been isolated in the apical ectodermal ridge (AER) *(116,117)*, leads to induction of BMP-2 *(116)*. Although the conserved nature of Wnt proteins implies that they act through similar pathways, Wnt-7A was recently found to exert its dorsoventral influence through a pathway other than the β-catenin/LEF-1 complex, whereas Wnt-3A in the AER appears to use β-catenin and LEF-1 in signaling *(116)*. Our recent findings provide further support for the functional involvement of Wnt signaling in chondrogenesis. In high-density micromass cultures of chick embryonic limb mesenchyme cells, expression of Wnt-3, -5A, and -7A is observed, with Wnt-7A expression showing downregulation over the course of chondrogenesis (Woodward and Tuan, unpublished data). In addition, in cultures of the murine multipotent C3H10T1/2 mesenchymal cells, maintained as high-density micromass to enhance cell–cell interaction and cellular condensation, Wnt-3 expression is upregulated in response to the chondro-enhancer BMP-2 whereas the Wnt-7A message is downregulated upon addition of BMP-2 to cultures *(118,119)*. Furthermore, lithium, a Wnt mimetic by virtue of its inhibition of GSK-3β, inhibits chondrogenesis in both embryonic chick limb mesenchyme (Woodward and Tuan, unpublished data) and in BMP-2–treated C3H10T1/2 micromass cultures *(120)*. In our most recent study, retrovirally mediated misexpression of Wnt-7a in these cultures strongly suppresses chondrogenesis, accompanied by prolonged expression of N-cadherin and stabilization of the N-cadherin/B-catenin adhesion complex *(121)*. However, similar misexpression of Wnt-5a did not affect chondrogenesis. It is noteworthy that a recent study suggests that Wnt-5a acts to regulate chondrocyte maturation and hypertrophy in the developing limbs in vivo *(122)*.

Taken together, these observations strongly implicate the integral involvement of members of the Wnt family of signaling factors in the regulation of cartilage development and limb formation. The emerging information suggests that there are at least two groups of Wnt members that act at the early stage of chondrogenic differentiation (e.g., Wnt-7a) and at the late stage of chondrocyte maturation (e.g., Wnt-5a), respectively. The basis of this difference most likely lies in the cellular mechanism of signaling, for example, involvement of β-catenin/LEF vs intracellular $[Ca^{2+}]$ flux, perhaps mediated via differential interaction between specific Wnt members and cognate, frizzled receptors. This area is certainly worthy of further investigation.

CONCLUSION

The transformation of loosely packed mesenchymal cells into highly organized and patterned skeletal structures requires the careful orchestration of cell–cell interaction and signaling events that ultimately result in the regulation of gene transcription and function. This review highlights the key molecular and cellular components involved in these events, specifically their functional crosstalk. The interconnected nature of these pathways underscores the effects of genetic and teratogenic perturbations that result in skeletal birth defects. Analysis of the cellular and molecular basis of the mechanistic steps initiated by cell–cell interactions and carried out via specific signal transduction pathways should provide a rational basis for understanding normal skeletogenesis as well as determining the cause of developmental defects of the skeleton.

ACKNOWLEDGMENTS

The author wishes to thank all past and current members of the laboratory for their contributions to the advancement of the understanding of limb mesenchymal chondrogenesis, and the National Institutes of Health for continuing support.

REFERENCES

1. Fell, H. B. (1925) The histogenesis of cartilage and bone in the long bones of the embryonic fowl. *J. Morphol.* **40,** 417–451.
2. Hall, B. and Miyake, T. (1992) The membranous skeleton: the role of cell condensations in vertebrate skeletogenesis. *Anat. Embryol.* **186,** 107–124.
3. Aulthouse, A. L. and Solursh, M. (1987) The detection of a precartilage, blastema-specific marker. *Dev. Biol.* **120,** 377–384.
4. Gotz, W., Fischer, G., and Herken, R. (1991) Lectin binding pattern in the embryonal and early fetal human vertebral column. *Anat. Embryol.* **184,** 345–353.
5. Ede, D. (1983) *Cellular Condensations and Chondrogenesis.* Academic Press, New York.
6. Ede, D. A., Flint, O. P., Wilby, O. K., and Colquhoun, P. (1977) The development of precartilage condensations in limb-bud mesenchyme of normal and mutant embryos *in vivo* and *in vitro*, in *Vertebrate Limb and Somite Morphogenesis* (Balls, M., ed). Cambridge University Press, London and New York, pp. 161–179.
7. Newman, S., Frenz, D., Tomasek, J., and Rabuzzi, D. (1985) Matrix-driven translocation of cells and nonliving particles. *Science* **228,** 885–889.
8. Oster, G. (1984) On the crawling of cells. *J. Embryol. Exp. Morphol.* **83,** 329–364.
9. Oster, G. F., Murray, J. D., and Maini, P. K. (1985) A model for chondrogenic condensations in the developing limb: the role of extracellular matrix and cell tractions. *J. Embryol. Exp. Morphol.* **89,** 93–112.
10. Ahrens, P. B., Solursh, M., and Reiter, R. S. (1977) Stage-related capacity for limb chondrogenesis in cell culture. *Dev. Biol.* **60,** 69–82.
11. San Antonio, J. and Tuan, R. (1986) Chondrogenesis of limb bud mesenchymal in vitro: stimulation by cations. *Dev. Biol.* **115,** 313–324.
12. Evans, M. S. and Tuan, R. S. (1988) Cellular condensation and collagen Type II expression during chondrogenesis in vitro. *J. Cell Biol.* **107,** 163a.
13. Coelho, C. N. and Kosher, R. A. (1991) Gap junctional communication during limb cartilage differentiation. *Dev. Biol.* **144,** 47–53.
14. Coelho, C. N. and Kosher, R. A. (1991) A gradient of gap junctional communication along the anterior-posterior axis of the developing chick limb bud. *Dev. Biol.* **148,** 529–535.
15. Mundlos, S. and Olsen, B. R. (1997) Heritable diseases of the skeleton. Part I: Molecular insights into skeletal development-transcription factors and signaling pathways. *FASEB J.* **11,** 125–132.
16. Toole, B. P., Jackson, G., and Gross, J. (1972) Hyaluronate in morphogenesis: inhibition of chondrogenesis in vitro. *Proc. Natl. Acad. Sci. USA* **69,** 1384–1386.
17. Toole, B. and Linsenmayer, T. (1977) Newer knowledge of skeletogenesis: macromolecular transitions in the extracellular matrix. *Clin. Orthop.* **Nov-Dec.,** 258–278.
18. Knudson, C. B. and Toole, B. P. (1987) Hyaluronate-cell interactions during differentiation of chick embryo limb mesoderm. *Dev. Biol.* **124,** 82–90.
19. Oberlander, S. and Tuan, R. (1994) Spatiotemporal profile of N-cadherin expression in the developing limb mesenchyme. *Cell Adhes. Commun.* **2,** 521–537.
20. Travella, S., Raffo, P., Tacchetti, C., Cancedda, R., and Castagnola, P. (1994) N-CAM and N-cadherin expression during in vitro chondrogenesis. *Exp. Cell Res.* **215,** 354–362.
21. Oberlander, S. and Tuan, R. (1994) Expression and functional involvement of N-cadherin in embryonic limb chondrogenesis. *Development* **120,** 177–187.
22. Widelitz, R. B., Jiang, T. X., Murray, B. A., and Chuong, C. M. (1993) Adhesion molecules in skeletogenesis: II. Neural cell adhesion molecules mediate precartilaginous mesenchymal condensations and enhance chondrogenesis. *J. Cell. Physiol.* **156,** 399–411.
23. Dessau, W., von der Mark, H., von der Mark, K., and Fischer, S. (1980) Changes in the patterns of collagens and fibronectin during limb-bud chondrogenesis. *J. Embryol Exp. Morphol.* **57,** 51–60.

24. Kulyk, W. M., Upholt, W. B., and Kosher, R. A. (1989) Fibronectin gene expression during limb cartilage differentiation. *Development* **106,** 449–455.
25. Frenz, D., Akiyama, S., Paulsen, D., and Newman, S. (1989) Latex beads as probes of cell surface-extracellular matrix interactions during chondrogenesis: evidence for a role for amino-terminal heparin-binding domain of fibronectin. *Dev. Biol.* **136,** 87–96.
26. Frenz, D., Jaikaria, N., and Newman, S. (1989) The mechanism of precartilage mesenchymal condensation: a major role for interaction of the cell surface with the amino-terminal heparin-binding domain of fibronectin. *Dev. Biol.* **136,** 97–103.
27. Gehris, A. L., Oberlender, S. A., Shepley, K. J., Tuan, R. S., and Bennett, V. D. (1996) Fibronectin mRNA alternative splicing is temporally and spatially regulated during chondrogenesis in vivo and in vitro. *Devel. Dynamics* **206,** 219–230.
28. Gehris, A. L., Stringa, E., Spina, J., Desmond, M. E., Tuan, R. S., and Bennett, V. D. (1997) The region encoded by the alternatively spliced exon IIIA in mesenchymal fibronectin appears essential for chondrogenesis at the level of cellular condensation. *Dev. Biol.* **190,** 191–205.
29. Bennett, V. D., Pallante, K. M., and Adams, S. L. (1991) The splicing pattern of fibronectin mRNA changes during chondrogenesis resulting in an unusual form of the mRNA in cartilage. *J. Biol. Chem.* **266,** 5918–5924.
30. Edelman, G. M. (1986) Cell adhesion molecules in the regulation of animal form and tissue pattern. *Annu. Rev. Cell Biol.* **2,** 81–116.
31. Edelman, G. M. and Crossin, K. L. (1991) Cell adhesion molecules: implications for a molecular histology [Review]. *Annu. Rev. Biochem.* **60,** 155–190.
32. Grunwald, G. (1996) *Discovery and Analysis of the Classical Cadherins.* JAI Press, Greenwich.
33. Marrs, J. A. and Nelson, W. J. (1996) Cadherin cell adhesion molecules in differentiation and embryogenesis. *Int. Rev. Cytol.* **165,** 159–205.
34. Takeichi, M. (1988) The cadherins: cell–cell adhesion molecules controlling animal morphogenesis. *Development* **102,** 639–655.
35. Takeichi, M. (1990) Cadherins: a molecular family important in selective cell-cell adhesion. *Ann. Rev. Biochem.* **59,** 237–252.
36. Takeichi, M. (1991) Cadherin cell adhesion receptors as a morphogenetic regulator [Review]. *Science* **251,** 1451–1455.
37. Takeichi, M. (1995) Morphogenetic roles of classic cadherins. *Curr. Opin. Cell Biol.* **7,** 619–627.
38. Rutishauser, U. (1990) Neural cell adhesion molecule as a regulator of cell-cell interactions. *Adv. Exp. Med. Biol.* **265,** 179–183.
39. Aberle, H., Schwartz, H., and Kemler, R. (1996) Cadherin-catenin complex: protein interactions and their implications for cadherin function. *J. Cell. Biochem.* **61,** 514–523.
40. Suzuki, S. T. (1996) Structural and functional diversity of cadherin superfamily: are new members of cadherin superfamily involved in signal transduction pathway? *J. Cell. Biochem.* **61,** 531–542.
41. Grunwald, G. B., Pratt, R. S., and Lilien, J. (1982) Enzymic dissection of embryonic cell adhesive mechanisms. III. Immunological identification of a component of the calcium-dependent adhesive system of embryonic chick neural retina cells. *J. Cell Sci.* **55,** 69–83.
42. Hatta, K. and Takeichi, M. (1986) Expression of N-cadherin adhesion molecules associated with early morphogenetic events in chick development. *Nature* **320,** 447–449.
43. Hatta, K., Takagi, S., Fujisawa, H., and Takeichi, M. (1987) Spatial and temporal expression pattern of N-cadherin cell adhesion molecules correlated with morphogenetic processes of chicken embryos. *Dev. Biol.* **120,** 215–227.
44. Hatta, K., Nose, A., Nagafuchi, A., and Takeichi, M. (1988) Cloning and expression of cDNA encoding a neural calcium-dependent cell adhesion molecule: its identity in the cadherin gene family. *J. Cell. Biochem.* **106,** 873–881.
45. Inuzuka, H., Redies, C., and Takeichi, M. (1991) Differential expression of R- and N-cadherin in neural and mesodermal tissues during early chicken development. *Development* **113,** 959–967.
46. Fujimori, T., Miyatani, S., and Takeichi, M. (1990) Ectopic expression of N-cadherin perturbs histogenesis in Xenopus embryos. *Development* **110,** 97–104.
47. Fujimori, T. and T akeichi, M. (1993) Disruption of epithelial cell-cell adhesion by exogenous expression of a mutated nonfunctional N-cadherin. *Mol. Biol. Cell* **4,** 37–47.
48. Radice, G. L., Rayburn, H., Matsunami, H., Knudsen, K. A., Takeichi, M., and Hynes, R. O. (1997) Developmental defects in mouse embryos lacking N-cadherin. *Dev. Biol.* **181,** 64–78.
49. Hamburger, V. and Hamilton, H. L. (1951) A series of normal stages in development of the chick embryo. *J. Morphol.* **88,** 49–92.
50. Duprez, D. M., Coltey, M., Amthor, H., Brickell, P. M., and Tickle, C. (1996) Bone morphogenetic protein-2 (BMP-2) inhibits muscle development and promotes cartilage formation in chick limb bud cultures. *Dev. Biol.* **174,** 448–452.
51. Tyndall, W. A. and Tuan, R. S. (1994) Involvement of N-cadherin mediated cell adhesion in TGF-B1 stimulation of limb mesenchymal chondrogenesis. *Mol. Biol. Cell* **5,** 103A.
52. Tyndall, W. and Tuan, R. (1994) Effect of TGF-β1/BMP-2 on limb mesenchyme chondrogenesis in vitro: modulation of N-cadherin and certain association. *Trans. Ortho. Res. Soc.* **21,** 179.
53. Denker, A. E., Haas, A. R., Nicoll, S. B., and Tuan, R. S. (1999) Chondrogenic differentiation of murine C3H10T1/2 multipotential mesenchymal cells: I. Stimulation by bone morphogenetic protein-2 in high-density micromass cultures. *Differentiation* **64,** 67–76.

54. Haas, A. R. and Tuan, R. S. (1999) Chondrogenic differentiation of murine C3H10T1/2 multipotential mesenchymal cells: II. Stimulation by bone morphogenetic protein-2 requires modulation of N-cadherin expression and function. *Differentiation* **64,** 77–89.
55. DeLise, A. M. and Tuan, R. S. (2002) Perturbing N-cadherin function inhibits cellular condensation and chondrogenesis of limb mesenchymal cells in vitro. *Devel. Dyn.* **225,** 195–204.
56. DeLise, A. M. and Tuan, R. S. (2002) Alterations in the spatiotemporal expression pattern and function of N-cadherin inhibit cellular condensation and chondrogenesis of limb mesenchymal cells in vitro. *J. Cell. Biochem.* **87,** 342–359.
57. Chothia, C. and Jones, E. (1997) The molecular structure of cell adhesion molecules. *Annu. Rev. Biochem.* **66,** 823–862.
58. Cunningham, B., Hemperly, J., and Murray, B. (1987) Neural cell adhesion molecule: structure, immunoglobulin-like domains, cell surface modulation, and alternative RNA splicing. *Science* **236,** 799–806.
59. Murray, B., Hemperly, J., Prediger, E., Edelman, G., and Cunningham, B. (1986) Alternatively spliced mRNAs code for different polypeptide chains of the chicken neural cell adhesion molecule (N-CAM). *J. Cell. Biol.* **102,** 189–193.
60. Nelson, R., Bates, P., and Rutishauser, U. (1995) Protein determinants for specific polysialylation of the neural cell adhesion molecule. *J. Biol. Chem.* **270,** 17171–17179.
61. Rutishauser, U. (1996) Polysialic acid and the regulation of cell interactions. *Curr. Opin. Cell. Biol.* **8,** 679–684.
62. Rao, Y., Wu, X., Gariepy, J., Rutishauser, U., and Siu, C. (1992) Identification of a peptide sequence involved in homophilic binding in the neural cell adhesion molecule NCAM. *J. Cell. Biol.* **118,** 937–949.
63. Chuong, C. (1990) Adhesion molecules (N-CAM and tenascin) in embryonic development and tissue regeneration. *J. Craniofac. Genet. Dev. Biol.* **10,** 147–161.
64. Chuong, C. M., Widelitz, R. B., Jiang, T. X., Abbott, U. K., Lee, Y. S., and Chen, H. M. (1993) Roles of adhesion molecules NCAM and tenascin in limb skeletogenesis: analysis with antibody perturbation, exogenous gene expression, talpid mutants and activin stimulation. *Prog. Clin. Biol. Res.* **383B,** 465–474.
65. Abbott, U., Taylor, L., and Abplanalp, H. (1959) Studies with talpid2, an embryonic lethal of the fowl. *J. Heredity* **383B,** 465–474.
66. Niederman, R. and Armstrong, P. (1972) Is abnormal limb bud morphology in the mutant talpid 2 chick embryo a result of altered intercellular adhesion? Studies employing cell sorting and fragment fusion. *J. Exp. Zool.* **181,** 17–32.
67. Matsuyoshi, N., Hamaguchi, M., Taniguchi, S., Nagafuchi, A., Tsukita, S., and Takeichi, M. (1992) Cadherin-mediated cell-cell adhesion is perturbed by v-src tyrosine phosphorylation in metastatic fibroblasts. *J. Cell. Biol.* **118,** 703–714.
68. Balsamo, J., Leung, T., and Ernst, H. (1996) Regulated binding of PTP1B-like phosphatase to N-cadherin: control of cadherin-mediated adhesion by dephosphorylation of beta-catenin. *J. Cell. Biol.* **134,** 801–813.
69. Lilien, J., Balsamo, J., Hoffman, S., and Eisenberg, C. (1997) β-catenin is a target for extracellular signals controlling cadherin function: the neurocan-GalNAcPTase connection. *Curr. Top Dev. Biol.* **35,** 161–189.
70. Balsamo, J., Ernst, H., Zanin, M. K., Hoffman, S., and Lilien, J. (1995) The interaction of the retina cell surface N-acetylgalactosaminylphosphotransferase with an endogenous proteoglycan ligand results in inhibition of cadherin-mediated adhesion. *J. Cell. Biol.* **129,** 1391–401.
71. Hoschuetzky, H., Aberle, H., and Kemler, R. (1994) β-catenin mediates the interaction of the cadherin-catenin complex with epidermal growth factor receptor. *J. Cell. Biol.* **127,** 1375–1380.
72. Shibamoto, S., Hayakawa, M., Takeuchi, K., Hori, T., Miyazawa, K., Kitamura, N., et al. (1995) Association of p120, a tyrosine kinase substrate, with E-cadherin/catenin complexes. *J. Cell. Biol.* **128,** 949–957.
73. Daniel, J. M. and Reynolds, A. B. (1997) Tyrosine phosphorylation and cadherin/catenin function. *Bioessays* **19,** 883–891.
74. Hazan, R. and Norton, L. (1998) The epidermal growth factor receptor modulates the interaction of E-cadherin with the actin cytoskeleton. *J. Biol. Chem.* **273,** 9078–9084.
75. Papkoff, J. (1997) Regulation of complexed and free catenin pools by distinct mechanisms. *J. Biol. Chem.* **272,** 4536–4543.
76. Kinch, M., Clark, G., Der, C., and Burrridge, K. (1995) Tyrosine phosphorylation regulates the adhesion of ras-transformed breast epithelia. *J. Cell. Biol.* **130,** 461–471.
77. Mo, Y. and Reynolds, A. (1996) Identification of murine p120^{cas} isoforms in human tumor cell lines. *Cancer Res.* **56,** 2633–2640.
78. Ohkubo, T. and Ozawa, M. (1999) p120(ctn) binds to the membrane-proximal region of the E-cadherin cytoplasmic domain and is involved in modulation of adhesion activity. *J. Biol. Chem.* **274,** 21409–21415.
79. Aono, S., Nakagawa, S., Reynolds, A. B., and Takeichi, M. (1999) p120(ctn) acts as an inhibitory regulator of cadherin function in colon carcinoma cells. *J. Cell. Biol.* **145,** 551–562.
80. Rubinfeld, B., Souza, B., and Albert, I. (1993) Association of AP gene product with β-catenin. *Science* **262,** 1731–1734.
81. Su, L., Vogelstein, B., and Kinzler, K. (1993) Association of the APC tumor supressor protein with catenins. *Science* **262,** 1734–1737.
82. Behrens, J., von Kries, J. P., Kuhl, M., Bruhn, L., Wedlich, D., Grosschedl, R., and Birchmeier, W. (1996) Functional interaction of beta-catenin with the transcription factor LEF-1. *Nature* **382,** 638–642.
83. Huber, O., Korn, R., and McLaughlin, J. (1996) Nuclear localization of β-catenin by interaction with transcription factor LEF-1. *Mech. Dev.* **59,** 3–10.
84. Moolenar, M., van de Wetering, M., and Oosterwegel, M. (1996) XTcf-3 transcription factor mediates β-catenin-induced axis formation in *Xenopus* embryos. *Cell* **86,** 391–399.

85. Peifer, M., Pai, L.-M., and Casey, M. (1994) Phosphorylation of the Drosophila adherens junction protein armadillo: roles for wingless signal and zeste-white 3 kinase. *Dev. Biol.* **166,** 543–556.
86. Rubinfeld, B., Albert, I., and Porfiri, E. (1996) Binding of GSK-3β to the APC-β-catenin complex and regulation of complex assembly. *Science* **272,** 1023–1026.
87. Cadigan, K. and Nusse, R. (1997) Wnt signaling: a common theme in animal development. *Genes Dev.* **11,** 3286–3305.
88. Nusse, R. and Varmus, H. (1992) *Wnt* genes. *Cell* **60,** 1073–1087.
89. Bahnot, P., Brink, M., and Samos, C. (1996) A new member of the frizzled family from *Drosophila* functions as a wingless receptor. *Nature* **382,** 225–230.
90. Klingensmith, J., Yand, Y., and Axelrod, D. (1996) Conservation of dishevelled structure and function between flies and mice: isolation and characterization of dvl-2. *Mech. Dev.* **58,** 15–26.
91. Siegfried, E., Chou, T., and Perrimon, N. (1992) Wingless signaling acts through zeste-white 3, the *Drosophila* homologue of glycogen synthase kinase 3 to regulate engrailed and establish cell fate. *Cell* **71,** 1167–1179.
92. Tomlinson, A., Strapps, W., and Heemskerk, J. (1997) Linking frizzled and Wnt signaling in Drospohila. *Development* **124,** 4515–4521.
93. Cook, D., Fry, M., and Hughes, L. (1996) Wingless inactivities glycogen synthase kinase-3 via an intracellular signaling pathway which involves a protein kinase C. *EMBO J.* **15,** 4526–4536.
94. Munemitsu, S., Albert, I., Rubinfeld, B., and Polakis, P. (1996) Deletion of an amino-terminal sequence stabilizes β-catenin in vivo and promotes hyperphosphorylation of the adenomatous polyposis coli tumor suppressor protein. *Mol. Cell. Biol.* **16,** 4088–4094.
95. Salomon, D., Sacco, P., and Roy, S. (1997) Regulation of β-catenin levels and localization by overexpression of plakoglobin and inhibition of the ubiquitin-proteasome system. *J. Cell. Biol.* **139,** 1325–1335.
96. Orford, K., Crockett, C., Jensen, J., Weissmann, M., and Byers, S. (1997) Serine phosphorylation-regulated ubiquitination and degradation of β-catenin. *J. Biol. Chem.* **272,** 2473–2478.
97. Aberle, H., Bauer, A., Stappert, J., Kispert, A., and Kemler, R. (1997) β-catenin is a target for the ubiquitin-proteasome pathway. *EMBO J.* **16,** 3797–3804.
98. Goode, N., Hughes, K., Woodgett, J., and Parker, P. (1992) Differential regulation of glycogen synthase kinase-3 beta by protein kinase C isotypes. *J. Biol. Chem.* **267,** 16878–16882.
99. Fagatto, F., Gluck, U., and Gumbiner, B. (1998) Nuclear localization signal—independent and importin/karyopherin—independent nuclear import of beta-catenin. *Curr. Biol.* **8,** 181–190.
100. Korinek, V., Barker, N., and Willert, K. (1998) Two members of the TCF family implicated in Wnt/beta-catenin signaling during embryogenesis in the mouse. *Mol. Cell. Biol.* **18,** 1248–1256.
101. Fagatto, F. and Gumbiner, B. (1994) Beta-catenin localization during Xenopus embryogenesis: accumulation at tissue and somite boundaries. *Development* **120,** 3667–3679.
102. Novak, A., Shu, C., and Chungyee, L. (1998) Cell adhesion and the integrin-linked kinase regulate the LEF-1 and β-catenin signaling pathways. *Proc. Natl. Acad. Sci. USA* **95,** 4374–4379.
103. Waltzer, L. and Bienz, M. (1998) CBP represses the transcription factor TCF to antagonize wingless signaling. *Nature* **395,** 521–525.
104. Oosterwegel, M., van de Wetering, M., and Timmerman, J. (1993) Differential expression of the HMG box factors TCF-1 and LEF-1 during murine embryogenesis. *Development* **118,** 439–448.
105. Kratochwil, K., Dull, M., Farinas, I., Galceran, J., and Grosschedl, R. (1996) Lef1 expression is activated by BMP-4 and regulates inductive tissue interactions in tooth and hair development. *Genes Dev.* **10,** 1382–1394.
106. Bradley, R. S., Cowin, P., and Brown, A. M. (1993) Expression of Wnt-1 in PC12 cells results in modulation of plakoglobin and E-cadherin and increased cellular adhesion. *J. Cell. Biol.* **123,** 1857–1865.
107. Hinck, L., Nelson, W. J., and Papkoff, J. (1994) Wnt-1 modulates cell-cell adhesion in mammalian cells by stabilizing beta-catenin binding to the cell adhesion protein cadherin. *J. Cell. Biol.* **124,** 729–741.
108. Zakany, J. and Duboule, D. (1993) Correlation of expression of Wnt-1 in developing limbs with abnormalities in growth and skeletal patterning. *Nature* **362,** 546–549.
109. Torres, M., Yang-Snyder, J., Purcell, S., DeMarais, A., and McGrew, L. (1996) Activities of the Wnt-1 class of secreted signaling factors are antagonized by the Wnt-5A class and by a dominant negative cadherin in early Xenopus development. *J. Cell. Biol.* **133,** 1123–1137.
110. Parr, B. A. and McMahon, A. P. (1995) Dorsalizing signal Wnt-7a required for normal polarity of D-V and A-P axes of mouse limb. *Nature* **374,** 350–353.
111. Gavin, B., McMahon, J., and McMahon, A. (1990) Expression of multiple novel Wnt-1/int-1-related genes during fetal and adult mouse development. *Genes Dev.* **4,** 2319–2332.
112. Yang, Y. and Niswander, L. (1995) Interaction between the signaling molecules WNT7a and SHH during vertebrate limb development: dorsal signals regulate anteroposterior patterning. *Cell* **80,** 939–947.
113. Riddle, R. D., Ensini, M., Nelson, C., Tsuchida, T., Jessell, T. M., and Tabin, C. (1995) Induction of the LIM homeobox gene Lmx1 by WNT7a establishes dorsoventral pattern in the vertebrate limb. *Cell* **83,** 631–640.
114. Rudnicki, J. A. and Brown, A. M. (1997) Inhibition of chondrogenesis by Wnt gene expression in vivo and in vitro. *Dev. Biol.* **185,** 104–118.
115. Stark, K., Vainio, S., Vassileva, G., and McMahon, A. (1994) Epithelial transformation of mesonephric mesenchyme in the developing kidney regulated by wnt-4. *Nature* **372,** 679–683.
116. Kengaku, M., Capdevila, J., and Rodriguez-Esteban, C. (1998) Distinct Wnt pathways regulating AER and dorsoventral polarity in the chick limb bud. *Science* **280,** 1274–1277.

117. Roelink, H. and Nusse, R. (1990) Expression of two members of the Wnt family during mouse development-restricted temporal and spatial patterns in the developing neural tube. *Genes Dev.* **5,** 381–388.
118. Fischer, L., Boland, G., and Tuan, R. S. (2002) Functional involvement of Wnt signaling in BMP-2 stimulation of mesenchymal chondrogenesis. *J. Cell. Biochem.* **84,** 816–831.
119. Fischer, L., Boland, G., and Tuan, R. S. (2002) Wnt-3a enhances BMP-2 mediated chondrogenesis of murine C3H10T1/2 mesenchymal cells. *J. Biol. Chem.* **277,** 30870–30878.
120. Fischer, L., Haas, A., and Tuan, R. (2001) Cell adhesion and signaling mechanisms in BMP-2 induction of mesenchymal chondrogenesis. *Signal Transduction* **2,** 66–78.
121. Tufan, A. and Tuan, R. (2001) Wnt regulation of limb mesenchymal chondrogenesis is accompanied by altered N-cadherin-related functions. *FASEB J.* **15,** 1436–1438.
122. Hartmann, C. and Tabin, C. (2000) Dual roles of Wnt signaling during chondrogenesis in the chicken limb. *Development* **127,** 3141–3159.

2

Chondrocyte Cell Fate Determination in Response to Bone Morphogenetic Protein Signaling

Lillian Shum, Yuji Hatakeyama, Julius Leyton, and Kazuaki Nonaka

INTRODUCTION

Advances in the understanding of the molecular determinants of skeletal morphogenesis are facilitated by investigating growth and transcription factor regulation of cartilage patterning, chondrocyte cell fate determination, differentiation, and maturation *(1)*. The development of the skeleton is regulated by interacting signaling pathways composed of extrinsic and intrinsic factors. These factors function in synergistic or antagonistic combinations, and some act as rate-limiting elements to regulate cellular development. An understanding of the mechanisms by which these multiple and diverse pathways interact as networks contributes to early gene- or biomarker-based detection and diagnosis of diseases and disorders that affect cartilage, such as osteoarthritis. Furthermore, the knowledge base provides the necessary foundation for prevention and treatment strategies, such as gene therapy, tissue engineering, and other orthopedic applications.

During skeletal morphogenesis, patterning of the skeletal elements is often mediated by differential segments of chondrogenesis and apoptosis. It is through chondrogenesis that skeletal elements arise and differentiate, and it is through apoptosis that these elements are delineated and shaped into templates that would allow them to undergo endochondral ossification into the bony skeleton. Certain pieces of cartilage are maintained as cartilage in adulthood. In essence, chondrocyte cell fate determination impacts on the initial formation of the skeleton, as well as the maintenance of the cartilage phenotype. In this review, we compare and contrast how the craniofacial and limb skeleton is patterned and developed through a combination of chondrogenic and apoptotic events and how mesenchymal cells are fated toward these two divergent pathways.

PATTERNING FORMATION AND CELL FATE DETERMINATION

Patterning and cell fate determination are two independent yet interdependent processes that produce the intricate design of an organ in which multiple highly specific cell types are organized. Patterning is the delineation of number, size, and shape of the tissue, whereas cell fate determination is the commitment of multipotential cells into lineage specific differentiated cells. These processes culminate in the formation and establishment of tissue boundaries. A feed-forward mechanism of interactions across tissue limits, for example, epithelial–mesenchymal interactions, reinforces the commitment of tissue differentiation. Consequently, the establishment of structural integrity ensures functional fidelity and performance.

From: *The Skeleton: Biochemical, Genetic, and Molecular Interactions in Development and Homeostasis*
Edited by: E. J. Massaro and J. M. Rogers © Humana Press Inc., Totowa, NJ

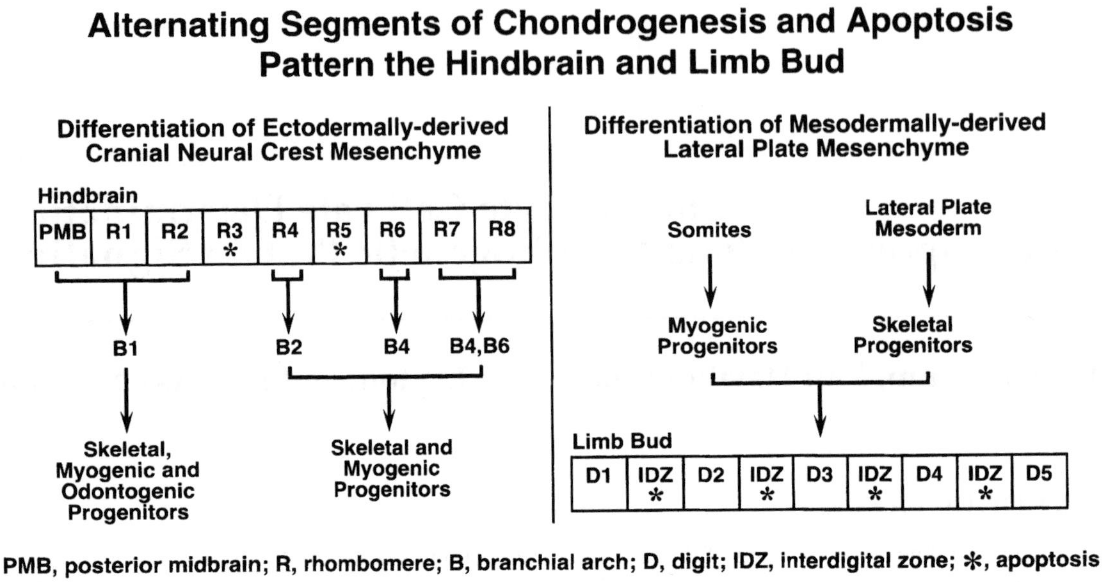

Fig. 1. Alternating segments of chondrogenesis and apoptosis pattern the hindbrain and limb bud.

Development is loaded with exquisite models that exemplify patterning and cell fate determination. Asymmetric divisions of the blastomeres and the formation of the primary embryonic germ layers are some of the earliest developmental events. The setting up of the body plan and segmentation that are associated with the manifestation of *Hox* gene expression reflective of a colinear code in the chromosomes also reveal the beauty of fate determination. The arborization of the hematopoietic cell lineages and the differentiation of highly specific cell types display the road map of the formation and maintenance of the hematopoietic system. Recently, cell fate determination of mesenchymal stem cells into multiple lineages (e.g., bone, cartilage, muscle, fat, tendon, nerves) has been a focus of research efforts in an attempt to define the precise morphoregulatory formulae that channel these cells into lineage-specific progenitors. Among these models, skeletogenesis is particularly interesting because the shaping of the skeleton is a sequence of events that on one hand lead to the birth of osteo- and chondroprogenitor cells and, on the other hand, the death of mesenchymal cells, to define the boundaries for skeletogenesis. Therefore, cell death, or apoptosis, becomes a significant differentiation pathway of mesenchymal cells in addition to osteogenic and chondrogenic differentiation in the system.

APOPTOSIS AND CHONDROGENESIS

Apoptosis, or programmed cell death, is a physiological process during which signal transduction elicits cellular responses that result in cell death *(2)*. It is a regulated event that is observed in many developmental systems, most notably during the formation of the nervous system, craniofacial complex, and limb in vertebrates *(3,4)*. Apoptosis is applied in these embryonic systems for patterning purposes (Fig. 1). Recurrent themes appear as we compare craniofacial and limb patterning. First, the cellular origins for these structures are compartmentalized. Cranial neural crest cells populating the craniofacial region arise from the posterior midbrain and the hindbrain that is segmented into eight pairs of rhombomeres. The limb paddle contains intercalating segments of digital and interdigital zones. Second, the delimitation of the structures is in part caused by alternating segments of apoptosis and survival. Extensive apoptosis in rhombomeres 3 and 5 allows for the distinction of three major migrating streams of neural crest cells, and apoptosis of the interdigital mesenchyme defines the digits. Third, cells destined for apoptosis can be diverted away from their doom fate when isolated and allowed to develop in vitro, suggesting that neighboring surviving segments play a significant role in the determination of apoptosis. For example, when rhombomere 3 is isolated and cranial neural crest cells are allowed to develop from the explants, most of the cells survive *(5)*. Similarly, the interdigital mesenchyme is not predetermined to undergo apoptosis because the isolation of this tissue and its development in vitro freed from adjacent digits allows it to produce cartilage *(6,7)*. This also suggests that cells at this patterning stage have tremendous plasticity and that their fates are regulated by cell–cell interactions.

Bone morphogenetic proteins (BMPs) are key regulators of both apoptosis and chondrogenesis, which are intimately related to each other during morphogenesis. Therefore, disruption to BMP signaling often leads to developmental defects. The disruption can be at the level of the ligand, such as mutations to the molecules that result in changes in binding specificity or affinity, or perturbations of BMP-binding proteins that lead to changes in ligand presentation. Defects can also occur in any of the downstream signaling components; receptors, cytoplasmic transducers, transcription factors, and target genes that are regulated by or interact with BMPs. Because most of the adult skeleton arises from endochondral ossification of a cartilaginous template, defects in BMP signaling that affect cartilage growth and development often result in skeletal defects. Enumerated in Table 1 are a selected number of congenital skeletal diseases and disorders, many of which are related to BMP signaling. One of these, Sox9, is a transcription factor that is the major regulator of chondrogenesis *(8)*. Haploinsufficiency of human SOX9 causes campomelic dysplasia, which presents multiple skeletal defects *(9,10)*. BMPs also regulate the osteogenic transcription factor Runx2/Cbfa1 *(11)*, Tbx5 *(12)*, Msx2 *(13)*, and Alx4 *(14)*. Regulation of type II, IV, and XI collagens by BMP is mediated by Sox9 *(8)*. Noggin is a BMP antagonist that is also regulated by Sox9 *(15)*. Other known genes that are associated with major skeletal dysmorphic syndromes and many syndromes with yet-to-be determined molecular origins (Table 2) could also be targets of faulty BMP signaling.

A number of mouse models have been produced to identify and characterize the functions of genes during cartilage formation (Table 1). Some of these models parallel homologous human mutations and associated human congenital disorders. Others may reflect only a subset of the phenotype observed in humans, suggesting that specific genetic modifiers are at work. Although these modifiers may appear to be species specific, it does not preclude that human genetic variations may also contain modifiers that augment or attenuate a particular mutation and its resultant deleterious outcome. In support, different groups in the human population have different susceptibility levels and prevalence to many dysmorphic syndromes. In addition, an environmental influence on genetic expression is a significant factor determining the outcome. Therefore, these mouse models prove to be invaluable for the understanding of the etiology of human genetic disorders, and additional genetic and environmental modifiers that may confer physiological susceptibility to the mutations.

BMP AND BMP SIGNALING

BMPs are a pleiotropic group of molecules first coined because of their ability to induce bone formation when injected into muscular compartments of animals *(16)*. BMP2 and BMP4 are mammalian homologs of the *Drosophila* prototype, decapentaplegic. This family of secreted molecules has at least 14 members to date, which in turn belongs to the transforming growth factor beta (TGF-β) superfamily of growth and differentiation factors *(17)*. BMPs are key regulators in embryogenesis and organogenesis of many systems, such as neurulation, limb patterning and outgrowth, mesoderm patterning, somatogenesis, oogenesis, development of eye, and kidney *(18–20)*. The pleiotropic functions of BMPs can be dependent on time, site, and concentration *(21)*. In tandem, BMPs are modulated by BMP-binding proteins and other growth and differentiation factors, resulting in combinatorial signaling and divergent outcomes depending on genetic or environmental modifiers *(22,23)*. One of

Table 1
Selected Genes Associated With Skeletal Diseases and Disorders

Human gene[a]	*Human diseases*[b]	*Brief description of skeletal defects*	*Animal models and citations*
Progressive ankylosis gene; ANKH, 5p15.2-p14.1 (605145)	Craniometaphyseal dysplasia, dysplasia, autosomal dominant (123000)	Cranial hyperostosis, wide nasal bridge, diaphyseal sclerosis, metaphyseal dysplasia, metaphyseal broadening	Autosomal-recessive ank mutation arose from animal stock. Mutation causes protein truncation. Animal is a model for arthritis. Decreased joint mobility in young mice that progresses rapidly with age. Animals die around 6 mo of age from complete rigidity. Histological evaluation reveals presence of hydroxyapatite crystals in joints, cartilage erosion, osteophyte formation and joint fusion *(166)*.
Aristaless-like 4; ALX4, 11p11.2 (605420)	Parietal foramina 2, autosomal dominant (168500)	Persistent wide fontanel, cleft lip/palate, symmetrical, oval defects in the parietal bone, medial frontal bone defect, cervical and lumbosacral spina bifida occulta	Targeted disruption. Decreased size of parietal plate of skull due to delayed ossification. Preaxial polydactyly associated with the formation of an ectopic anterior zone of polarizing activity in limb bud. Perinatal lethality due to gastroschesis *(167)*.
Cartilage oligomeric protein; COMP, 19p13.1 (600310)	Multiple epiphyseal dysplasia I, autosomal dominant (132400)	Mild-to-moderate short stature, mild short-limb dwarfism, ovoid vertebral bodies, mild irregularity of vertebral endplates, late ossifying epiphyses, small, irregular epiphyses, osteoarthritis, short femoral neck, metacarpals and phalanges	Targeted disruption. No detectable anatomical, histological, or ultrastructural abnormalities of skeletal development *(168)*.
	Pseudoachondroplastic dysplasia, autosomal dominant (177170)	Short-limb dwarfism identifiable during childhood	
Cathepsin K; CTSK, 1q21 (601105)	Pycnodysostosis, autosomal recessive (265800)	Short stature, frontal and occipital prominence, persistent open anterior fontanelle and delayed suture closure, micrognathia, hypoplasia of clavicle, osteosclerosis, susceptibility to fracture, wormian bone, dense skull, brachydactyly, acro-osteolysis of distal phalanges	Targeted disruption. Mice are osteoporotic with excessive trabeculation of the bone-marrow space. Osteoclasts are abnormally formed and their resorptive function severely impaired *(169)*.

Collagen, type I, alpha-1; COL1A1, 17q21.31-q22 (120150)	Osteogenesis imperfecta, Type I, (166200); Type II, (166210); Type III, (259420); Type IV, (166220)	Mainly characterized by multiple bone fracture, slightly smaller stature to short limb dwarfism, wormian bones, tibial and femoral bowing, subtypes vary in degree of severity in skeletal defects and the presence and absence of blue sclerae	(1) Transgenic expression of partially deleted Col1a1. A third of the animals exhibit extensive fractures, some are lethal. Femurs are significantly shorter and have decrease in mineral and collagen content. Biomechanical testing of femurs also shows increased brittleness *(170)*. (2) Knock-in of G349C Col1a1 mutation by Cre-lox recombination. Animals exhibit classical phenotype of osteogenesis imperfecta, including bone deformity, fragility, osteoporosis, and disorganized trabecular structure *(171)*.
Collagen, type II, alpha-1; COL2A1, 12q13.11-q13.2 (120140)	Spondyloepiphyseal dysplasia, autosomal dominant (183900)	Short-trunk dwarfism identifiable at birth, malar hypoplasia, cleft palate, kyphosis, scoliosis, lumbar lordosis, ovoid vertebral bodies, absent ossification in pubic, talus and calcaneal bones, flattened epiphyses, diminished joint mobility at elbows, knees, and hips	(1) Transgenic expression of an internally deleted COL2A1 gene. Phenotype resembles human chondrodysplasias, with 15% of animals presenting cleft palate. Older animals show osteoarthritis *(172)*. (2) Targeted disruption. The cartilage consists of disorganized chondrocytes with a complete lack of extracellular fibrils. There is no endochondral bone or epiphyseal growth plate in long bones. However, skeletal structures, such as the cranium and ribs were normally developed and mineralized *(173)*.
	Stickler syndrome, type I, autosomal dominant (108300)	Marfanoid habitus, flat midface, depressed nasal bridge, cleft palate, skeletal defects similar to spondyloepiphyseal dysplasia	(3) Heterozygous knockout of Col2a1. Animals are more susceptible to osteoarthritis *(174)*.
Collagen, type III, alpha-1; COL3A1, 2q31 (120180)	Ehlers-Danlos syndrome, type IV, autosomal dominant (130050)	Short stature, hypermobility of distal interphalangeal joints, acroosteolysis of hands and feet, club foot	Targeted disruption. Perinatal and early lethality due to yet unknown causes. Adult animals die of rupture blood vessels from lack of type 3 collagen fibers, disrupted fibrillogenesis and defective vessels *(175)*.
Collagen, type V, alpha-2; COL5A2, 2q31 very close to COL3A1, (120190)	Ehlers-Danlos syndrome, type I, autosomal dominant (130000)	Similar to type IV Ehlers-Danlos syndrome, with narrow maxilla, osteoarthritis	Insertional mutation. Perinatal and early lethality as a result of spinal abnormalities and consequential respiratory difficulties. Animals also show skin and eye abnormalities caused by disorganized collagen fibrils *(176)*.

(continued)

Table 1 (*Continued*)

Human gene[a]	*Human diseases*[b]	*Brief description of skeletal defects*	*Animal models and citations*
Collagen, type IX, alpha-1; COL9A1, 6q13 (120210)	Multiple epiphyseal dysplasia related to COL9A1, autosomal dominant (120210.0001)	Early osteoarthritis of knee leading to pain and stiffness, endplate irregularities, anterior osteophytes in the thoraco-lumbar vertebrae, including calcification of the intervertebral disc	(1) Transgenic expression of a truncated protein. Heterozygotes develop osteoarthritis of the knee, whereas homozygotes develop mild chondrodysplasia *(177)*. (2) Targeted disruption. Animals appear normal except for early onset osteoarthritis. After tooth extraction, there is significantly disturbed the restoration and remodeling of trabecular bone with minimal effects on the cortical bone *(178,179)*.
Collagen, type X, alpha-1; COL10A1, 6q21-q22.3 (120110)	Metaphyseal chondrodysplasia, Schmid type, autosomal dominant (156500)	Mild-to-moderate short stature, lower rib cage flared, anterior cupping and sclerosis of ribs, irregular acetabular roof, enlarged capital femoral epiphyses, femoral and tibial bowing, metaphyseal abnormalities of long bones	(1) Transgenic expression of mutant protein that functions as a dominant negative. Phenotype in animals is reminiscent of human pathological conditions, including compression of hypertrophic growth plate cartilage and decrease in newly formed bone *(180)*. (2) Targeted disruption. Appears normal *(181)*. However, additional analyses revealed a that subset of animals present perinatal lethality and growth plate compression within the proliferative zone *(182)*. (3) Targeted disruption. Phenotype resembles in part human syndrome, including abnormal trabecular bone architecture, coxa vara, reduction in thickness of growth plate resting zone and articular cartilage, altered bone content, and atypical distribution of matrix components within growth plate cartilage *(183)*.
Collagen, type XI, alpha-1; COL11A1, 1p21 (120280)	Marshall syndrome, autosomal dominant (154780)	Short stature, midface hypoplasia, micrognathia, cleft palate, calvarial thickening, absent frontal sinuses, meningeal calcifications, mild platyspondyly, small iliac bonesepiphyseal dysplasias, bowing of radius and ulnar	Autosomal-recessive chondrodysplasia (cho) mutation in Col11a1 gene in mice. Perinatal lethality. Abnormalities in cartilage of limbs, ribs, mandible, and trachea. Limb bones of newborn mice are wider at the metaphyses than normal and only about half the normal length *(184)*.
	Stickler syndrome, type 2, autosomal dominant (604841)	Similar to Marshall syndrome, with normal stature and mild spondyloepiphyseal dysplasia	

Fibrillin 1; FBN1, 15q21.1 (134797)	Marfan syndrome, autosomal dominant (154700)	Disproportionate tall stature, dolichocephaly, malar hypoplasia, high arched palate, narrow palate, micrognathia, retrognathia, premature arthritis, kyphoscoliosis, thoracic lordosis, spondylolisthesis, long bone overgrowth, joint hypermobility and contractures, arachnodactyly	Targeted mutation. Lethality around weaning because of defective elastic fiber formation leading to cardiovascular hemorrhages. Lung emphysema and bone overgrowth similar to patients with Marfan syndrome *(185,186)*.
Fibrillin 2; FBN2, 5q23-q31 (121050)	Congenital contractural arachnodactyly, autosomal dominant (121050)	Contractural arachnodactyly, severe kyphoscoliosis, generalized osteopenia, flexion contractures of fingers	(1) Radiation induced shaker-with-syndactylism (sy) mutation that affects fibrillin 2. Syndactylism of the middle digits that is more severe with the hindlimbs than forelimbs *(187)*. (2) Targeted disruption. Bilateral syndactyly caused by defective mesenchymal differentiation *(188)*.
Growth/differentiation factor 5; GDF5, 20q11.2 (601146)	Brachydactyly, type C, autosomal dominant (113100); Acromesomelic dysplasia, Hunter-Thompson type, autosomal recessive (201250); Chondrodysplasia, Grebe type, autosomal recessive (200700)	Syndromes are characterized by multiple limb defects that vary in severity, brachydactyly, short limb dwarfism, acromesomelia, severe malformations in distal limb skeleton.	(1) Spontaneous brachypodism (bp) mutation in mice. Length and number of bones in the limbs of mice are altered but spares the axial skeleton *(189)*. (2) Targeted disruption. Disruption in the formation of more than 30% of the synovial joints in the limb, leading to complete or partial fusions between skeletal elements, and changes in the patterns of repeating structures in the digits, wrists and ankles *(190)*.
Heparan sulfate proteoglycan of basement membrane; HSPG2, 1p36.1 q (142461)	Schwartz-Jample syndrome, type 1, autosomal recessive (255800)	Short stature, osteoporosis, delayed bone age, small mandible, kyphoscoliosis, lumbar lordosis, coronal cleft vertebrae, fragmentation and flattened femoral epiphyses, widened metaphyses, slender diaphysis, anterior bowing of long bones, limb contractures	Targeted disruption. Embryonic lethality in 40% of homozygotes from defective cephalic development. Perinatal lethality in others exhibiting skeletal dysplasia characterized by micromelia with broad and bowed long bones, narrow thorax and craniofacial abnormalities. Severe disorganization of the columnar structures of chondrocytes and defective endochondral ossification. Reduced and disorganized collagen fibrils and glycosaminoglycans. Proliferation of chondrocytes was reduced and the prehypertrophic zone was diminished *(191)*.

(continued)

Table 1 (*Continued*)

Human gene[a]	*Human diseases*[b]	*Brief description of skeletal defects*	*Animal models and citations*
	Dyssegmental dysplasia, Silverman-Handmaker type, autosomal recessive (224410)	Neonatal lethal, short-limbed dwarfism, occipital skull defect, micrognathia, chondroosseous morphology notable for short, irregular, chondrocyte columns, large, unfused calcospherites, perichondral bone overgrowth and patchy, mucoid degeneration of resting cartilage, dyssegmental dysplasia, anisospondyly, short, bent long bones	
Homeobox D13; HOXD13, 2q31-q32 (142989)	Syndactyly type II, autosomal dominant (186000)	Syndactyly, polydactyly, hypoplasia of middle phalanges of toes	(1) Spontaneous synpolydactyly homolog (spdh) mutation in mice. Severe malformations of all four feet, including polydactyly, syndactyly, and brachydactylia *(192)*. (2) Targeted disruption. Skeletal defects were restricted to distal parts of both autopods. Forelimbs show reduction in the size of the digits and deformation of the phalangeal and metacarpal bones, especially for digits II and V. Additional rudimentary digit present posteriorly. Similar alterations were seen in hindlimbs where all metatarsal bones were shortened and thicker *(193)*.
Indian hedgehog; IHH, 2q33-q35 (600726)	Brachydactyly, type A1, autosomal dominant (112500)	Short stature, brachydactyly, hypoplastic middle phalanges, occasional terminal symphalangism, short first digit proximal phalanges	(1) Targeted disruption. Reduced chondrocyte proliferation, maturation of chondrocytes at inappropriate position, and a failure of osteoblast development in endochondral bones *(194)*. (2) Targeted disruption. Ectopic branching of ventral pancreatic tissue resulting in an annular pancreas *(195)*.
Muscle segment homeobox 2; MSX2, 5q34-q35 (123101)	Craniosynostosis, type 2, autosomal dominant (604757)	Skull malformations, including craniosynostosis and cloverleaf anomaly	(1) Transgenic expression of wild-type or gain-of-function mutant. Mice exhibit precocious fusion of cranial bones and development of ectopic cranial bone *(196)*.
	Parietal foramina 1, autosomal dominant (168500)	Persistent wide fontanel with oval defects in parietal bone, cleft lip/palate, medial frontal bone defect, cervical and lumbosacral spina bifida occulta	(2) Transgenic expression of large human DNA fragment encompassing the gene. Perinatal lethality with multiple craniofacial malformations, including mandibular hypoplasia, cleft secondary palate, exencephaly, and median facial cleft *(197)*.

			(3) Targeted disruption. Mice are viable, but displayed pleiotropic defects of skeletal and ectodermal organs and appendages. The calvarium of adult mutants contains a large, midline foramen spanning the frontal bones. The interparietal and supraoccipital bones are small and abnormal in shape. Abnormal cartilage and endochondral bone formation is observed, resulting in axial and appendicular defects *(198)*.
Noggin; NOG, 17q22 (602991)	Symphalangism, (185800); multiple synostoses syndrome I (186500); Tarsal-carpal coalition syndrome (186570)	Autosomal-dominant syndromes, limb deformity, synostosis, absent, or accessory skeletal elements in the limb, syndromes vary in specific elements involved	Targeted disruption. Defective sclerotome formation. Axial skeletal defects that become more severe caudally; the skull and cervical vertebrae are relatively normal, but the thoracic vertebrae are fused and malformed, and the lumbar and tail vertebrae are missing. Joint fusion at the elbow, where the radius and humerus are joined by a continuous ossification. Digits have secondary fusions and occasional cartilaginous spurs, and lack joints *(199,200)*.
Parathyroid hormone receptor 1; PTHR1, 3p22-p21.1 (168468)	Metaphyseal chondrodysplasia, Jansen type, autosomal dominant (156400)	Severe short stature, brachycephaly, prominent supraorbital arches, mild frontonasal hyperplasia, micrognathia, short ribs, generalized osteopenia, fractures, thick skull base, bowing of long bones, especially lower limb, markedly expanded cup-shaped metaphyses, short, mildly broad diaphyses, short tubular bones, clinodactyly, short, clubbed fingers	Targeted disruption. Mostly embryonic lethal. Others are perinatal lethal resulting from respiratory failure. Mice that survived exhibit accelerated differentiation of chondrocytes in bone *(201)*.
	Chondrodysplasia, Blomstrand type, autosomal recessive (215045)	Severe midface hypoplasia, mandibular hypoplasia, short ribs, generalized sclerosis, advanced skeletal maturation, micromelia, marked metaphyseal flaring of long bones, die at birth or shortly after birth	

(continued)

Table 1 (*Continued*)

Human gene[a]	*Human diseases*[b]	*Brief description of skeletal defects*	*Animal models and citations*
Receptor tyrosine kinase-like orphan receptor 2; ROR2, 9q22 (602337)	Brachydactyly, type B1, autosomal dominant (113000)	Brachydactyly, hypoplastic middle and terminal phalanges, symphalangism, mild syndactyly, deformed thumbs and big toes	Targeted disruption. Perinatal lethality probably caused by cardiac spetla defects. Mice have shortened snout, limbs and tail, and cleft palate. All bones formed by endochondral ossification were foreshortened and misshapen, with a tendency toward greater abnormalities more distally. The digits were shortened and missing the middle phalanges *(202)*.
	Robinow syndrome, autosomal recessive (268310)	Short stature, macrocephaly, large anterior fontanel, frontal bossing, micrognathia, flat facial profile, rib fusion, absent ribs, delayed bone age, scoliosis, thoracic hemivertebrae, mesomelia, clinodactyly, broad thumbs and toes, bifid terminal phalanges	
Runt-related transcription factor 2; RUNX2, 6p21 (600211)	Cleidocranial dysplasia, autosomal dominant (119600)	Moderate-to-short stature, delayed fontanelle closure with metopic groove, frontal and parietal bossing, calvarial thickening, midface hypoplasia, micrognathia, cleft palate, hypoplastic clavicles, small scapula, short ribs, osteosclerosis, wormian bones, spondylolysis, scoliosis, kyphosis, delayed mineralization of pubic bone, broad femoral head with short femoral neck, hypoplastic iliac wing, brachydactyly	(1) Targeted disruption. Animals die just before birth. Skeleton exhibits complete lack of intramembraneous and endochondral ossification *(203)*. Tooth morphogenesis is also disrupted because of defects in ameloblast and odontoblast maturation *(204)*. (2) Radiation induced ccd mutation that is a Runx2 deletion. Phenotype is similar to that resulting from molecular gene targeting *(205,206)*. (3) Transgenic expression in osteoblasts. Animals have normal skeleton at birth and develop osteopenia later *(207)*.

SRY-related HMG-box gene 9; SOX9, 17q24.3-q25.1 (608160)	Campomelic dysplasia, autosomal dominant (114290)	Short limb dwarfism, large anterior fontanelle, macrocephaly, micrognathia, cleft palate, hypoplastic thoracic cage, missing twelfth pair of ribs, hypoplastic, poorly ossified cervical vertebrae, small iliac wings, short phalanges for both hands and feet, anterior bowing of tibia, short fibula, mildly bowed femur, absent ossification of proximal tibial, and distal femoral epiphysis	Targeted disruption. Perinatal lethality. Skeletal defects in all bones derived from endochondral ossification, include cleft secondary palate, hypoplasia and bending. Skeletal abnormalities similar to those found in campomelic dysplasia patients. Skeletal patterning was not affected. Premature mineralization of skeletal elements, including craniofacial region and vertebral column. Hypertrophic zone of growth plate was thicker *(208)*.
T-box 5; TBX5, 12q24.1 (601620)	Holt-Oram syndrome, autosomal dominant (142900)	Vertebral anomalies, thoracic scoliosis, absent or bifid thumb, triphalangeal thumb, carpal bone anomalies, upper extremity phocomelia, radial-ulnar anomalies	Conditional knockout. Embryonic lethality because of malformed heart tube. Elongated phalangeal segments of first forelimb digit and hypoplastic falciformis bones in the wrist were present in multiple heterozygous mutant mice *(209)*.
Transforming growth factor, beta-1; TGFB1, 19q13.1 (190180)	Camurati-Engelmann disease autosomal dominant (131300)	Sclerosis of skull base, mandible involvement, sclerosis of posterior part of vertebrae, scoliosis, progressive diaphyseal widening, thickened cortices, narrowing of medullary canal	Targeted disruption. Lethality around weaning due to massive inflammation lesions and tissue necrosis in many organs *(210,211)*.
Vitamin D3 receptor; VDR, 12q12-q14 (601769)	Vitamin D-resistant rickets, autosomal recessive (277440)	Rickets	Targeted disruption. Animals normal until after weaning. By 7 wk, null mice develop alopecia, flat face and short nose. Severe bone malformation leading to growth retardation and 40% loss of bone density. Early lethality around 15 wk *(212)*.

[a]Human gene description includes gene name, symbol, corresponding OMIM number, and locus.
[b]Human disease description includes disease name and corresponding OMIM number.

Table 2
Human Genetic Disorders with As-Yet No Known Genetic Associations

Disorder name	*OMIM number*	*Gene location*	*Brief description of skeletal defects*
Acrocallosal syndrome; ACLS	200990	12p13.3-p11.2	Macrocephaly, large anterior fontanel, prominent occiput and forehead, hypoplastic midface, cleft palate, tapered fingers, fifth finger clinodactyly, brachydactyly, postaxial polydactyly, bifid terminal phalanges of thumbs, toe syndactyly, duplicated halluces
Chondrocalcinosis 1; CCAL1	600668	8q (CCAL1)	CCAL1; chondrocalcinosis, severe degenerative osteoarthritis
Chondrocalcinosis 2; CCAL2	118600	5p15(CCAL2)	CCAL2; chondrocalcinosis, arthropathy, acute intermittent arthritis, ankylosis
Chondoma; CHDM	215400	7q33	Sacrococcygeal chordoma
Cohen syndrome; COH1	216550	8q22-q23	Microcephaly, maxillary hypoplasia, micrognathia, joint hyperextensibility, narrow hands and feet, mild shortening of metacarpals and metatarsals
Craniometaphyseal dysplasia; CMDR	218400	6q21-q22	Cranial hyperostosis, facial palsy, prominent supraorbital ridges and mandible, square profile, diaphyseal sclerosis, metaphyseal dysplasia, metaphyseal broadening
Otopalatodigital syndrome, type II; OPD2	304120	Xq28	Prominent forehead, severe micrognathia, midface hypoplasia, cleft palate, sclerotic skull base, bowing of long bones, small to absent fibula, subluxed elbow, wrist, and knee, flexed, overlapping fingers, short, broad thumbs, postaxial polydactyly, syndactyly, second finger clinodactyly, hypoplastic, irregular metacarpals
Craniosynostosis, Adelaide type; CRSA	600593	4p16	Craniosynostosis, coned epiphyses of hands and feet, distal and middle phalangeal hypoplasia, carpal bone malsegmentation, phalangeal, tarsonavicular and calcaneo-navicular foot fusions
FG syndrome; FGS1	305450	Xq12-q21.31	Macrocephaly, large anterior fontanel caused by delayed closure, plagiocephaly, micrognathia, cleft palate, joint contractures, broad thumbs, clinodactyly, syndactyly, broad halluces
Fibrodysplasia ossificans progressiva; FOP	135100	4q27-q31	Heterotopic ossification, especially of the neck, spine, and shoulder girdle, malformed cervical vertebrae, short broad femoral necks, malformed big toes, monophalangic big toes, short thumbs, fifth finger clinodactyly, severely restricted arm mobility
Larsen syndrome; LRS1	150250	3p21.1-p14.1	Cleft palate, flattened frontal bone, small skull base, shallow orbits, dysplastic epiphyseal centers, cervical vertebrae hypoplasia, scoliosis, spondylolysis, short metacarpals and metatarsals, multiple carpal and calcaneal ossification centers with delayed coalescence

Otopalatodigital syndrome, type I; OPD1	311300	Xq28	Prominent occiput and supraorbital ridges, cleft palate, absent frontal and sphenoid sinuses, thick frontal bone and skull base, delayed closure of anterior fontanel, steep clivus, dense middle-ear ossicles, short, broad distal phalanges, especially thumbs, short third, fourth, fifth metacarpals, supernumerary carpal bones, fusion of hamate and capitate, toe syndactyly, anomalous fifth metatarsal, extracalcaneal ossification center
Pituitary dwarfism II	262500	5p13-p12	Acrohypoplasia, short limbs, delayed bone age, markedly advanced osseous maturation for height and age
Russell-Silver syndrome; RSS	180860	7p11.2	Micrognathia, skeletal maturation retardation, craniofacial disproportion, delayed fontanel closure, asymmetry of arms and/or legs, fifth finger clinodactyly, fifth digit middle or distal phalangeal hypoplasia, syndactyly of second and third toes
Shwachman-diamond syndrome	260400		Costochondral thickening, irregular ossification at anterior rib ends, delayed skeletal maturation, slipped capital femoral epiphyses, metaphyseal chondrodysplasia of long bones
Sotos syndrome	117550	5q35	Macrocephaly, frontal bossing, prognathism, advanced bone age, large hands and feet, disharmonic maturation of phalanges and carpal bones
Spastic paraplegia 9; SPG9	601162	10q23.3-q24.1	Skeletal abnormalities, short fifth finger, clinodactyly, delayed bone age, shallow acetabulum, small carpal bones, dysplastic skull base
Syndactyly, type I	185900	2q34-q36	Syndactyly, complete or partial webbing between third and fourth fingers, fusion of third and fourth finger distal phalanges, complete or partial webbing between the second and third toes
Velocardiofacial syndrome	192430	22q11	Microcephaly, Pierre Robin syndrome, cleft palate

the many functions of BMPs is to induce cartilage, bone, and connective tissue formation in vertebrates *(24,25)*. This osteochondro-inductive capacity of BMPs is highly promising for orthopedic applications, such as skeletal repair and regeneration, and in dental applications, such as the treatment of periodontal diseases *(26–30)*. Since the discovery of BMPs over three decades ago, their ability to induce ectopic bone and cartilage formation remains a topic of intense investigation. In particular, the characterization of the molecular mechanisms of BMP functions was reignited after the cloning of the activin receptor, the first TGF-β type receptor, in 1991 *(31)*. Thereafter, the molecular pathways to differentiation have been meticulously dissected and exposed.

BMP signals through heterodimeric serine–threonine kinase receptor complexes, containing type I and type II receptors, each class having a number of subtypes *(32,33)*. Both type I and type II receptors are capable of low-affinity interaction with BMP but only when the ligand binds to both receptors can result in high-affinity heteromeric ligand–receptor complex formation capable of BMP-dependent signaling *(34,35)*. Therefore, it is likely that the presence and number of different BMP receptors determine the cellular responses to the many ligands. Evidence suggests that the subtype BMPR-IB is essential for chondrogenesis for the entire developing skeletal system *(36–39)*. However, target deletion studies of the BMPR-IB receptor suggest otherwise *(39,40)*. In these animals, the BMPR-IB does appear to have an essential role to play during limb bud morphogenesis because the abnormalities are located in the appendicular skeletal elements and not in the axial skeletal structures. Moreover, in vitro studies show that BMPR-IB does not possess exclusive chondrogenic potential, suggesting that other BMP type I receptors may exert redundant functions during chondrogenesis *(41–43)*. Taken together, the response to BMP signal is not solely defined by the identity of the type I receptor but additionally by elements in the signal transduction pathways that lie downstream of the receptor. These are the various cytoplasmic and nuclear transducers, both positive and negative.

Downstream from the receptors, Smads are the predominant effectors of TGF-β/BMP signaling *(44, 45)*. An important issue for BMP-dependent signaling is the type of Smad proteins involved in chondrogenic differentiation and whether the Smads alone are sufficient to direct differentiation. Smads function as dimeric complexes and belong to three classes: regulatory, inhibitory, and common. The receptor-regulated Smads (R-Smads) are further subdivided into two groups. Smad1, Smad5, and Smad8 are directly phosphorylated and activated by BMP type I receptors. Smad2 and Smad3 are mediators of activin or TGF-β type I receptor signaling. A series of in vitro studies have shown that Smad1, Smad5, and Smad8 may be involved in osteochondrogenic differentiation *(46–49)*. These findings suggest that different Smads or Smad combinations are engaged at different stages of mesenchymal cell differentiation into osteoblasts and chondrocytes. However, in vivo manipulations of Smads have not resulted in conclusive evidence because genetically engineered animal models targeted against Smads produce embryonic lethality *(50)*. Nevertheless, a glimpse of in vivo Smad function can be observed in Smad3 knockout animals, which manifest osteopenia and early onset osteoarthritis *(51)*. The class of inhibitory Smads (I-Smads) includes Smad6 and Smad7. They have been shown to inhibit the effect of R-Smads by competing for binding to activated type I receptors *(52–56)*. Indeed, I-Smads are potent inhibitors of skeletogenic differentiation *(48,57,58)*. The common Smad4 (Co-Smad) associates with activated R-Smad complex, which translocates into the nucleus and participates in the regulation of target genes *(59)*. Smad4 functions as a tumor suppressor gene, and mutations of the human SMAD4 lead to pancreatic carcinoma and juvenile intestinal polyposis, further illustrating the significance of TGF-β superfamily signaling and its regulation of cellular physiology *(60)*.

BMP signaling can be channeled through Smad-independent pathways, such as the extracellular signal-regulated kinase, Jun N-terminal kinase, Wnt, and p38 mitogen-activated protein kinase pathways *(61–65)*. Therefore, crosstalk between the signaling pathways during chondrogenic differentiation is inevitable. However, a detailed recount of these interactions is beyond the scope of this review. Finally, BMP and other growth factor signaling can coactivate chondrogenic differentiation. For example, fibroblast growth factor (FGF) signaling through mitogen-activated protein kinase promotes chondrogenesis by increasing the level of Sox9 expression as well as increases its binding affinity on the type II collagen promoter *(66)*. It is obvious that BMPs control of chondrogenesis is a highly regulated developmental process that involves multiple pathways and checkpoints. This combinatorial mode of signaling ensures fidelity in the patterning and timing of the cartilaginous template onto which most of the bony skeleton is produced.

CRANIOFACIAL MORPHOGENESIS AND CRANIAL NEURAL CREST CELLS (CNCCS)

CNCCs give rise to most of the craniofacial tissues *(67–69)*. Interestingly, this cell population is derived from the dorsal cephalic neural tube. During embryogenesis, the ectoderm at the midline overlying the notochord thickens to form the neural plate. Progressively, the flattened neural plate begins to bend, creating elevations, called the neural folds, with a central depression the neural groove. As neurulation proceeds, the bilateral neural folds oppose each other and fuse at the midline to form the closed neural tube. At the time of neural tube closure and at the junction of where the thickened neuroectoderm meets the non-thickened surface ectoderm, epithelial cells delaminate and emerge as mesenchymal cells into the underlying space. These are the neural crest cells *(70)*. Neural crest cells are formed along the entire length of the primary neural tube. CNCCs are formed from the neural tube at the level of the forebrain, midbrain, and hindbrain.

Neural crest cells are multipotential, and they give rise to a number of cell lineages *(71,72)*. Those arising from the cranial region have different sets of potentials when compared with those arising in the trunk. For example, trunk neural crest cells do not normally produce cartilage. However, recent evidence from lineage tracing and transplantation strategies suggest that some trunk crest cells are capable of differentiating into cranial cartilages when transplanted into the cranial region *(73,74)*. From a number of studies using various lineage tracing approaches, we have learned that neural crest cells from the forebrain and midbrain contribute to the frontonasal mesenchyme for the formation of the upper and midface structures, including part of the cranial base, nasal, and otic capsules *(75–77)*. CNCCs in the branchial arches are destined for skeletal, odontogenic, myogenic, neuronal, and connective tissue lineages of the lower face and neck regions. Following the cartilage lineage in particular, CNCCs in the first branchial arch contribute to form Meckel's cartilage and the temporomandibular joint cartilage. The hyoid is derived from CNCCs in both the second and third arches, and the fourth and sixth arches in combination give rise to the thyroid, cricoid, arytenoid, corniculate, and cuneiform cartilage *(68,72,75,78–80)*.

BMP REGULATION OF CRANIOFACIAL CARTILAGE DEVELOPMENT AND APOPTOSIS

The hindbrain is a segmented structure, each segment called a rhombomere (Fig. 1). In the vertebrate head, there are eight pairs of rhombomeres and each gives rise to segment-specific CNCCs. During the migratory phase of CNCC development, CNCCs converge into three major streams directed toward the branchial arches in an orderly and patterned manner *(81,82)*. Therefore, an early step in the regulation of craniofacial cartilage differentiation is CNCC production and patterning within the hindbrain. Similar to setting up the overall body plan, the hindbrain is patterned by a series of homeobox (Hox)- and homeobox-containing genes *(83)*. The production of CNCCs from these rhombomeres is in part regulated by their Hox genes. In addition, cell fate determination in the CNCCs is an orchestrated process *(84–86)*. CNCCs exert a "community effect" among themselves and cell–cell and/or cell–matrix signaling in the group can maintain their segmental identity *(87,88)*. In addition to this "community" effect, it is also discovered that the isthmus, a region between the midbrain and hindbrain, serves as a patterning center for the rhombomeres and the CNCC derivatives. The isthmus expresses high levels of FGF8 that regulates the expression of the Hox genes in the rhombomeres.

Transplantation experiments that include or exclude the isthmus yield different outcomes. The inclusion of the isthmus during grafting allows the rhombomeres and CNCCs to maintain their original identity, whereas the exclusion of the isthmus renders CNCCs responsive to environmental cues *(89)*. In addition to the isthmus, CNCCs can be patterned by signals from the endoderm to give rise to distinct pieces of craniofacial cartilages. Interestingly, this is only limited to CNCCs above the level of the second rhombomere, the so-called Hox-negative cells. CNCCs expressing *Hox* genes are not responsive to endodermal induction *(90)*.

Although each rhombomere can give rise to CNCCs, it is observed that those of rhombomeres 3 and 5 contribute to a minority of the population. A large number of CNCCs within the rhombomere undergo apoptosis, and only a small population migrate out. These cells join the major streams and, thus, lateral to rhombomeres 3 and 5, the area appears relatively free of CNCCs *(91–98)*. This may serve to gauge the number of CNCCs being produced and to better delimit the migratory streams and their eventual destination. Evidence suggests that CNCC apoptosis is regulated by BMP and Wnt signaling. BMP4 is expressed coincidentally within rhombomeres 3 and 5. BMP4 induces the expression of Msx2 in these rhombomeres, and ectopic expression of Msx2 increases the number of apoptotic CNCCs *(5,13,93,99)*. The lack of BMP signaling in even-numbered rhombomeres may be attributed to the presence of the BMP antagonist, noggin *(100)*. Taken together, these experiments suggest that CNCC apoptosis is regulated by signals from BMP4 and is mediated by Msx2. Wnt signaling is significant in this cascade because of the expression of cSFRP2 in rhombomeres that have limited apoptosis. cSFRP2 is an antagonist of the Wnt signaling and overexpression of cSFRP2 inhibits BMP4 expression and rescues CNCC from apoptotic elimination. Consistently, inhibition of cSFRP2 or overexpression of Wnt1 results in ectopic CNCC apoptosis *(101)*. However, another Wnt family member; Wnt6, has been recently shown to be necessary and sufficient for the induction of neural crest formation *(102)*. The use of different Wnt genes in combination that regulate CNCC formation is an elegant example of the complexity of the system.

As CNCCs migrate from the neural tube towards the forming face, they converge into major streams, migrating toward the respective branchial arches. Migration is largely governed by adhesive properties between cells and substrate, and a number of factors have defining roles in this developmental event *(103)*. During migration, the cells remain in an undifferentiated state such that they are allowed to reach their destination before they expand further and undergo overt differentiation. Localization studies reveal that premigratory CNCCs and a subpopulation of migrating CNCCs may already be partially committed to the cartilage lineage by virtue of their expression of the key cartilage transcription factor, Sox9 *(104,105)*. However, these cells do not differentiate yet. Differentiation of these cells may be suppressed by the coexpression of Msx2 in the Sox9-expressing cells. Msx2 may serve to maintain these cells in an undifferentiated state until migration is completed. Overexpression of dominant-negative forms of Msx2 in these migratory cells inhibits normal Msx2 functions and leads to precocious cartilage differentiation *(105)*.

The mandible and maxilla arise from the anterior and posterior processes of the first branchial arch, respectively. These structures receive extensive contributions of CNCCs from the posterior midbrain and rhombomeres 1 and 2 of the anterior hindbrain. In addition to the lineages found in the other branchial arches, CNCCs in the first arch also differentiate into tooth structures that are unique to this arch *(106,107)*.

Meckel's cartilage formed within the mandibular process has a unique pattern. It consists of an anterior, triangular piece at the midline, bilateral rod-shaped pieces that regress to form the sphenomandibular ligament, and posterior pieces that give rise to the malleus, incus, and temporomandibular joint cartilage. The formation of Meckel's cartilage is regulated by the mandibular epithelium through epithelial-mesenchymal interactions *(108,109)*. The instructive signal from the epithelium can be substituted by epidermal growth factor (EGF), which sustains mesenchymal proliferation and delays chondrocyte differentiation *(110,111)*. Removal of the epithelium results in increased but dysmorphic cartilage formation *(112,113)*. Indeed, EGF and EGF receptors are endogenous to the mandibular process *(114,115)*. Antisense oligonucleotide inhibition of EGF in the mandibular process results in ectopic cartilage formation. In contrast, exogenous EGF reduces and disrupts cartilage formation *(46,115)*. Furthermore, targeted disruption of EGF receptor in the mouse results in Meckel's cartilage deficiency as well *(116)*. These defects are attributed to changes in matrix metalloproteinases expression and its regulation of cartilage morphogenesis. Expression of matrix metalloproteinases is regulated by EGF, and they function in multiple tissue morphogenesis, including that of the anterior segment of the developing Meckel's cartilage *(117)*.

Within the mesenchyme, cartilage formation is further delimited by the expression of the transcription factor Msx2, which is excluded from regions with chondrogenic potential *(118)*. Antisense oligonucleotide inhibition of Msx2 expression in the mandible results in disruption of Meckel's cartilage formation *(119)*. Furthermore, adenoviral expression of ectopic Msx2 also abrogates cartilage formation *(120)*. Interestingly, endogenous Msx2 expression is regulated by BMP expression and that ectopic BMP signaling can alter Msx2 expression domain, leading to cartilage dysmorphogenesis *(120–122)*. Msx2 can also inhibit ectopic cartilage formation that is induced by BMP4 as a feedback reaction. However, the competence of the mesenchyme to respond to BMP4 is dependent on local signals and the key cartilage transcription factor Sox9, functions in antagonistic combination with Msx2 to regulate cartilage formation *(120)*.

LIMB MORPHOGENESIS AND LIMB MESENCHYME

The limb cartilage develops from paired primordial buds that appear on the embryo's lateral surface at specific levels along its anterior posterior body axis. At the early stages of limb development, the buds exhibit a paddle shape and consist of undifferentiated mesenchymal cells derived from the lateral plate and somitic mesoderm, and overlying ectoderm. At the distal tip of the bud, the ectoderm forms a specialized thickened epithelial structure, known as the apical ectodermal ridge (AER). Patterning along the proximal–distal axis depends in part on signaling molecules from the AER *(123, 124)*. Instrumental to this process is the family of FGFs *(125–130)*. The classic model of limb patterning involves the determination of positional values along the proximal–distal axis specified by instructive signaling from the AER to the subridge mesenchyme, known as the progress zone *(131)*. However, recent revolutionary interpretation of limb patterning describes the specification of distinct proximal–distal segments of the limb early in development, with subsequent development involving expansion of these mesenchymal progenitor before differentiation *(128,132)*. The anterior–posterior axis of the limb is patterned by the zone of polarizing activity (ZPA), which is located at the posterior margin of the limb *(124,133,134)*. The major morphogen from this organizing center is the sonic hedgehog (*Shh*) gene *(135)*, which maintains anterior–posterior patterning in conjunction with other gene products, such as the HoxD gene *(136)*, and participate in regulatory feedback signaling with the AER *(137)*. Dorsal–ventral patterning is governed by ectodermally expressed Wnt7a and engrailed-1 proteins and their coregulation of Lmx1b gene expression at the dorsal mesenchyme *(138,139)*. Therefore, patterning along the three axes is interlinked with each other.

The limb cartilage elements form in a temporal proximal-to-distal sequence but are initially contiguous *(36)*. Through the gradual recruitment of cells, the primary condensation of the stylopod (humorous/femur) forms first, the zeugopod (radius-ulna/tibia-fibula) forms second, and the autopod (carpals/tarsals and phalanges) forms last. There is considerable mixing of cells along the proximal–distal axis within each future segment but not between segments. Positional information is expressed by determinants of the Hox family of genes. The first part of the limb in which a subset of Hoxa and Hoxd genes are activated is the posterior limb *(140,141)*. Subsequently, the expression domains extend anteriorly, in the distal part. In the final stage of limb morphogenesis, the mesenchyme in the distal region of the limb bud (autopod) can have two different fates, chondrogenesis or apoptosis, depending on whether they are incorporated into the digital ray or into the interdigital regions. There is now considerable evidence to indicate that BMPs are essential mediators in specifying mesenchymal cells undergoing either apoptosis or chondrogenesis and in the determination of digit identity *(3,6,142–144)*. This point will be elaborated further in the next section. Finally, in regions of the mesenchymal condensation where joints from, condensed chondroprogenitors do not differentiate into chondrocytes but instead become tightly packed and adopt a fate of apoptosis as part of the normal program *(25,145,146)*. Therefore, the orchestration of the apoptotic and chondrogenic response results in the formation and delineation of the limb cartilaginous template. Failure of either process results in limb malformations such as syndactyly or polydactyly of soft or hard tissues.

BMP REGULATION OF LIMB CARTILAGE DEVELOPMENT AND APOPTOSIS

BMPs are instrumental to the formation of the limb and are intimately involved in multiple stages of limb development, including patterning, outgrowth, AER regression, digit formation, digit identity, and interdigital apoptosis. To function in multiple developmental events, BMPs engage in signaling networks during limb morphogenesis and operate in concert with other key morphoregulatory factors, such as FGFs and Shh. Furthermore, several BMPs are already present during early development. BMP2, BMP4, and BMP7 are expressed in the limb mesenchyme in overlapping patterns before the formation of precartilagenous condensation *(20)*. The specificity of BMPs for multistep action during limb morphogenesis is also reflected by different expression profile of the receptor subtypes transducing the BMP signal *(38)*. BMPs at an early stage regulate mesenchymal condensation into cartilage nodules, as well as the induction of the AER *(147)*. At later stages, BMPs are responsible for the maturation of limb cartilage and the regression of the AER *(148)*. In vitro evidence supports that exogenous BMP enhances chondrogenesis in limb mesenchyme after the condensation step *(149)*. Through their function in the maintenance of the AER and consequential regulation of limb outgrowth along the proximal–distal axis, BMPs also relay information and participate in interdependent developmental processes, such as patterning along the dorsal–ventral axis *(150)*. There is little genetic evidence to support the role of BMPs in limb development because target mutation in animal studies of BMPs and their receptors result in early lethality or lack of phenotype directly related to cartilage formation *(14,20,151)*. However, experiments using retroviral-mediated misexpression to simulate loss of function result in limbs that show a lack of Alcian blue stain cartilage elements *(37,42)*. However, infection of the chick limb with retrovirus encoding BMP2, BMP4, or constitutively active receptor type I to simulate BMP gain of function results in fusion and hyperplasia of the cartilage elements *(37,152)*. Mouse models show that BMP receptor type IB appears to be the necessary mediator of BMP-induced chondrogenesis *(39,40)*, although overexpression of the receptor or constitutive activation of the receptor can also cause apoptosis *(37,153)*.

In addition to driving chondrogenesis, BMPs are key regulators of interdigital apoptosis that leads to the delineation of the digits. Among them, BMP2, BMP4, and BMP7 are expressed in the interdigital regions before and during the occurrence of apoptosis, suggesting a role in cell death *(20)*. Implantation of BMP4-soaked beads in interdigital regions accelerates interdigital cell death. In addition, BMP4 can also cause ectopic cell death when applied at the tip of the developing digit pad *(154)*. The apoptotic effect of BMP4 can be antagonized by FGF2 *(155)*. Similarly, BMP2 and BMP7 are potent apoptotic signals for the undifferentiated limb mesenchyme but not for the ectoderm or the differentiating chondrogenic cells *(156)*. Perturbations of BMP signaling through manipulation of BMP receptors also result in aberrations in interdigital apoptosis. For example, overexpressing dominant-negative BMP receptors in chick leg bud via replication-competent retrovirus to block endogenous BMP signals results in inhibition of apoptosis in the interdigital mesenchyme, which leads to webbed chick feet *(37)*. Taken together, these results indicate that BMP signaling is necessary for the apoptotic cascade in the interdigital mesenchyme. Interestingly, in parallel with craniofacial apoptosis as described in previous sections, Msx2 is also a mediator of BMP-induced interdigital apoptosis

(157). However, it is still unclear as to how Msx2 expression is instructive or permissive to apoptosis. Therefore, the totality of limb development and the emergence of its intricate design are dependent in part on BMP signaling in the larger context of many other growth and transcription factor signaling networks.

Of particular interest are the role of retinoic acid and its interactions with BMP signaling and their coregulation of limb development. Retinoic acid is an endogenous morphogen at physiological levels and a teratogen in excess. Endogenous retinoids serve to pattern the hindbrain and the limb bud *(158)*. Excessive retinoids lead to retinoic acid embryopathy characterized by craniofacial abnormalities *(159)*. There are three distinct aspects of how retinoic acid modulates BMP signals. First, retinoic acid is well known for its ability to pattern the limb bud by virtue of its ability to substitute for the ZPA and for its upregulation of Shh that is endogenous to the ZPA *(160,161)*. In tandem, retinoic acid also upregulates BMP expression that is needed for anterior–posterior patterning event *(162,163)*. Second, retinoic acid regulates interdigital apoptosis by activating BMP expression and activities *(164)*. Third, retinoic acid can also enhance chondrogenesis mediated by both BMP-dependent and BMP-independent pathways *(164,165)*. Therefore, the regulation of chondrogenesis and apoptosis by BMP may rest on the ability of retinoic acid to divert BMP signaling to one pathway vs another, or the regulation by retinoic acid on distinct cofactors of BMP signaling for different pathways.

SUMMARY AND FUTURE CHALLENGES

Studies from classical developmental models suggest that cell fate determination is a progressive process that is dependent on combinatorial signaling of a repertoire of growth and differentiation factor networks. Signaling is modulated by restricted expression profiles of factors organized in precise temporal and spatial arrays. Signaling is gauged by checkpoints where rate-limiting factors determine the threshold for progression. Because BMPs are multifunctional factors, the challenge is to identify the molecular basis for chondrogenic differentiation of mesenchymal cells. Functional studies should establish the mechanisms of lineage commitment and diversification, and provide a platform for molecular manipulations with predictable lineage outcomes. This knowledge will provide the molecular basis for tissue engineering and biomimetics of mesenchymal cells.

ACKNOWLEDGMENTS

We are grateful to Dr. Rocky Tuan for his support and encouragement. We have benefited from a long-standing scientific partnership with Dr. Glen Nuckolls. We have been blessed with outstanding visiting and postdoctoral scientists who had contributed to our knowledge base. Finally, we are indebted to Dr. Harold Slavkin, who continues to be an inspiration. This work was supported by NIH funding Z01AR41114.

REFERENCES

1. Shum, L. and Nuckolls, G. (2002) The life cycle of chondrocytes in the developing skeleton. *Arthritis Res.* **4,** 14994–15106.
2. Lee, S., Christakos, S., and Small, M. B. (1993) Apoptosis and signal transduction: clues to a molecular mechanism. *Curr. Opin. Cell. Biol.* **5,** 286–291.
3. Chen, Y. and Zhao, X. (1998) Shaping limbs by apoptosis. *J. Exp. Zool.* **282,** 691–702.
4. Graham, A., Koentges, G., and Lumsden, A. (1996) Neural crest apoptosis and the establishment of craniofacial pattern: an honorable death. *Mol. Cell Neurosci.* **8,** 76–83.
5. Graham, A., Francis-West, P., Brickell, P., and Lumsden, A. (1994) The signalling molecule BMP4 mediates apoptosis in the rhombencephalic neural crest. *Nature* **372,** 684–686.
6. Tang, M. K., Leung, A. K., Kwong, W. H., Chow, P. H., Chan, J. Y., Ngo-Muller, V., Li, M., and Lee, K. K. (2000) Bmp-4 requires the presence of the digits to initiate programmed cell death in limb interdigital tissues. *Dev. Biol.* **218,** 89–98.
7. Ros, M. A., Piedra, M. E., Fallon, J. F., and Hurle, J. M. (1997) Morphogenetic potential of the chick leg interdigital mesoderm when diverted from the cell death program. *Dev. Dyn.* **208,** 406–419.

8. de Crombrugghe, B., Lefebvre, V., Behringer, R. R., Bi, W., Murakami, S., and Huang, W. (2000) Transcriptional mechanisms of chondrocyte differentiation. *Matrix Biol.* **19,** 389–394.
9. Wagner, T., Wirth, J., Meyer, J., Zabel, B., Held, M., Zimmer, J., et al. (1994) Autosomal sex reversal and campomelic dysplasia are caused by mutations in and around the SRY-related gene SOX9. *Cell* **79,** 1111–1120.
10. Foster, J. W., Dominguez-Steglich, M. A., Guioli, S., Kowk, G., Weller, P. A., Stevanovic, M., et al. (1994) Campomelic dysplasia and autosomal sex reversal caused by mutations in an SRY-related gene. *Nature* **372,** 525–530.
11. Ducy, P., Zhang, R., Geoffroy, V., Ridall, A. L., and Karsenty, G. (1997) Osf2/Cbfa1: a transcriptional activator of osteoblast differentiation. *Cell* **89,** 747–754.
12. Rodriguez-Esteban, C., Tsukui, T., Yonei, S., Magallon, J., Tamura, K., and Izpisua Belmonte, J. C. (1999) The T-box genes Tbx4 and Tbx5 regulate limb outgrowth and identity. *Nature* **398,** 814–818.
13. Takahashi, K., Nuckolls, G. H., Tanaka, O., Semba, I., Takahashi, I., Dashner, R., Shum, L., and Slavkin, H. C. (1998) Adenovirus-mediated ectopic expression of Msx2 in even-numbered rhombomeres induces apoptotic elimination of cranial neural crest cells in ovo. *Development* **125,** 1627–1635.
14. Dunn, N. R., Winnier, G. E., Hargett, L. K., Schrick, J. J., Fogo, A. B., and Hogan, B. L. (1997) Haploinsufficient phenotypes in Bmp4 heterozygous null mice and modification by mutations in Gli3 and Alx4. *Dev. Biol.* **188,** 235–247.
15. Zehentner, B. K., Haussmann, A., and Burtscher, H. (2002) The bone morphogenetic protein antagonist Noggin is regulated by Sox9 during endochondral differentiation. *Dev. Growth Differ.* **44,** 1–9.
16. Urist, M. R. (1965) Bone: formation by autoinduction. *Science* **150,** 893–899.
17. Ducy, P. and Karsenty, G. (2000) The family of bone morphogenetic proteins. *Kidney Int.* **57,** 2207–2214.
18. Wozney, J. M. (1998) The bone morphogenetic protein family: multifunctional cellular regulators in the embryo and adult. *Eur. J. Oral. Sci.* **106,** 160–166.
19. Graff, J. M. (1997) Embryonic patterning: to BMP or not to BMP, that is the question. *Cell* **89,** 171–174.
20. Hogan, B. L. (1996) Bone morphogenetic proteins in development. *Curr. Opin. Genet. Dev.* **6,** 432–438.
21. Mehler, M. F., Mabie, P. C., Zhu, G., Gokhan, S., and Kessler, J. A. (2000) Developmental changes in progenitor cell responsiveness to bone morphogenetic proteins differentially modulate progressive CNS lineage fate. *Dev. Neurosci.* **22,** 74–85.
22. Reddi, A. H. (2001) Interplay between bone morphogenetic proteins and cognate binding proteins in bone and cartilage development: noggin, chordin and DAN. *Arthritis Res.* **3,** 1–5.
23. Balemans, W. and Hul, W. V. (2002) Extracellular regulation of BMP signaling in vertebrates: a cocktail of modulators. *Dev. Biol.* **250,** 231–250.
24. Hoffmann, A. and Gross, G. (2001) BMP signaling pathways in cartilage and bone formation. *Crit. Rev. Eukaryot. Gene Exp.* **11,** 23–45.
25. Kingsley, D. M. (2001) Genetic control of bone and joint formation. *Novartis Found. Sympos.* **232,** 213–222; discussion 222–234, 272–282.
26. Yoon, S. T. and Boden, S. D. (2002) Osteoinductive molecules in orthopaedics: basic science and preclinical studies. *Clin. Orthop.* **Feb,** 33–43.
27. King, G. N. (2001) The importance of drug delivery to optimize the effects of bone morphogenetic proteins during periodontal regeneration. *Curr. Pharm. Biotechnol.* **2,** 131–142.
28. Li, R. H. and Wozney, J. M. (2001) Delivering on the promise of bone morphogenetic proteins. *Trends Biotechnol.* **19,** 255–265.
29. Wikesjo, U. M., Sorensen, R. G., and Wozney, J. M. (2001) Augmentation of alveolar bone and dental implant osseointegration: clinical implications of studies with rhBMP-2. *J. Bone Joint. Surg. Am.* **83-A Suppl 1,** S136–S145.
30. Reddi, A. H. (2001) Bone morphogenetic proteins: from basic science to clinical applications. *J. Bone Joint. Surg. Am.* **83-A Suppl 1,** S1–S6.
31. Mathews, L. S. and Vale, W. W. (1991) Expression cloning of an activin receptor, a predicted transmembrane serine kinase. *Cell* **65,** 973–982.
32. Miyazono, K., Kusanagi, K., and Inoue, H. (2001) Divergence and convergence of TGF-beta/BMP signaling. *J. Cell. Physiol.* **187,** 265–276.
33. Kawabata, M., Imamura, T., and Miyazono, K. (1998) Signal transduction by bone morphogenetic proteins. *Cytokine Growth Factor Rev.* **9,** 49–61.
34. Nohe, A., Hassel, S., Ehrlich, M., Neubauer, F., Sebald, W., Henis, Y. I., and Knaus, P. (2002) The mode of bone morphogenetic protein (BMP) receptor oligomerization determines different BMP-2 signaling pathways. *J. Biol. Chem.* **277,** 5330–5338.
35. Knaus, P. and Sebald, W. (2001) Cooperativity of binding epitopes and receptor chains in the BMP/TGFbeta superfamily. *J. Biol. Chem.* **382,** 1189–1195.
36. Sandell, L. J. and Adler, P. (1999) Developmental patterns of cartilage. *Front. Biosci.* **4,** D731–D742.
37. Zou, H., Wieser, R., Massague, J., and Niswander, L. (1997) Distinct roles of type I bone morphogenetic protein receptors in the formation and differentiation of cartilage. *Genes Dev.* **11,** 2191–2203.
38. Cheifetz, S. (1999) BMP receptors in limb and tooth formation. *Crit. Rev. Oral Biol. Med.* **10,** 182–198.
39. Yi, S. E., Daluiski, A., Pederson, R., Rosen, V., and Lyons, K. M. (2000) The type I BMP receptor BMPRIB is required for chondrogenesis in the mouse limb. *Development* **127,** 621–630.
40. Baur, S. T., Mai, J. J., and Dymecki, S. M. (2000) Combinatorial signaling through BMP receptor IB and GDF5: shaping of the distal mouse limb and the genetics of distal limb diversity. *Development* **127,** 605–619.

41. Akiyama, S., Katagiri, T., Namiki, M., Yamaji, N., Yamamoto, N., Miyama, K., et al. (1997) Constitutively active BMP type I receptors transduce BMP-2 signals without the ligand in C2C12 myoblasts. *Exp. Cell Res.* **235,** 362–369.
42. Kawakami, Y., Ishikawa, T., Shimabara, M., Tanda, N., Enomoto-Iwamoto, M., Iwamoto, M., et al. (1996) BMP signaling during bone pattern determination in the developing limb. *Development* **122,** 3557–3566.
43. Shukunami, C., Akiyama, H., Nakamura, T., and Hiraki, Y. (2000) Requirement of autocrine signaling by bone morphogenetic protein-4 for chondrogenic differentiation of ATDC5 cells. *FEBS Lett.* **469,** 83–87.
44. Moustakas, A., Souchelnytskyi, S., and Heldin, C. H. (2001) Smad regulation in TGF-beta signal transduction. *J. Cell. Sci.* **114,** 4359–4369.
45. Shi, Y. (2001) Structural insights on Smad function in TGFbeta signaling. *Bioessays* **23,** 223–232.
46. Nonaka, K., Shum, L., Takahashi, I., Takahashi, K., Ikura, T., Dashner, R., Nuckolls, G. H., and Slavkin, H. C. (1999) Convergence of the BMP and EGF signaling pathways on Smad1 in the regulation of chondrogenesis. *Int. J. Dev. Biol.* **43,** 795–807.
47. Ju, W., Hoffmann, A., Verschueren, K., Tylzanowski, P., Kaps, C., Gross, G., and Huylebroeck, D. (2000) The bone morphogenetic protein 2 signaling mediator Smad1 participates predominantly in osteogenic and not in chondrogenic differentiation in mesenchymal progenitors C3H10T1/2. *J. Bone Miner. Res.* **15,** 1889–1899.
48. Fujii, M., Takeda, K., Imamura, T., Aoki, H., Sampath, T. K., Enomoto, S., et al. (1999) Roles of bone morphogenetic protein type I receptors and Smad proteins in osteoblast and chondroblast differentiation. *Mol. Biol. Cell.* **10,** 3801–3813.
49. Nishimura, R., Kato, Y., Chen, D., Harris, S. E., Mundy, G. R., and Yoneda, T. (1998) Smad5 and DPC4 are key molecules in mediating BMP-2-induced osteoblastic differentiation of the pluripotent mesenchymal precursor cell line C2C12. *J. Biol. Chem.* **273,** 1872–1879.
50. Weinstein, M., Yang, X., and Deng, C. (2000) Functions of mammalian Smad genes as revealed by targeted gene disruption in mice. *Cytokine Growth Factor Rev.* **11,** 49–58.
51. Yang, X., Chen, L., Xu, X., Li, C., Huang, C., and Deng, C. X. (2001) TGF-beta/Smad3 signals repress chondrocyte hypertrophic differentiation and are required for maintaining articular cartilage. *J. Cell. Biol.* **153,** 35–46.
52. Hayashi, H., Abdollah, S., Qiu, Y., Cai, J., Xu, Y. Y., Grinnell, B. W., et al. (1997) The MAD-related protein Smad7 associates with the TGFbeta receptor and functions as an antagonist of TGFbeta signaling. *Cell* **89,** 1165–1173.
53. Nakao, A., Afrakhte, M., Moren, A., Nakayama, T., Christian, J. L., Heuchel, R., et al. (1997) Identification of Smad7, a TGFbeta-inducible antagonist of TGF-beta signalling. *Nature* **389,** 631–635.
54. Imamura, T., Takase, M., Nishihara, A., Oeda, E., Hanai, J., Kawabata, M., and Miyazono, K. (1997) Smad6 inhibits signalling by the TGF-beta superfamily. *Nature* **389,** 622–626.
55. Ishida, W., Hamamoto, T., Kusanagi, K., Yagi, K., Kawabata, M., Takehara, K., et al. (2000) Smad6 is a Smad1/5-induced smad inhibitor. Characterization of bone morphogenetic protein-responsive element in the mouse Smad6 promoter. *J. Biol. Chem.* **275,** 6075–6079.
56. Hata, A., Lagna, G., Massague, J., and Hemmati-Brivanlou, A. (1998) Smad6 inhibits BMP/Smad1 signaling by specifically competing with the Smad4 tumor suppressor. *Genes Dev.* **12,** 186–197.
57. Valcourt, U., Gouttenoire, J., Moustakas, A., Herbage, D., and Mallein-Gerin, F. (2002) Functions of transforming growth factor-beta family type i receptors and smad proteins in the hypertrophic maturation and osteoblastic differentiation of chondrocytes. *J. Biol. Chem.* **277,** 33545–33558.
58. Ito, Y., Bringas, P. Jr., Mogharei, A., Zhao, J., Deng, C., and Chai, Y. (2002) Receptor-regulated and inhibitory Smads are critical in regulating transforming growth factorbeta-mediated Meckel's cartilage development. *Dev. Dyn.* **224,** 69–78.
59. Attisano, L. and Wrana, J. L. (2000) Smads as transcriptional co-modulators. *Curr. Opin. Cell. Biol.* **12,** 235–243.
60. Schutte, M. (1999) DPC4/SMAD4 gene alterations in human cancer, and their functional implications. *Ann. Oncol.* **10,** 56–59.
61. Letamendia, A., Labbe, E., and Attisano, L. (2001) Transcriptional regulation by Smads: crosstalk between the TGF-beta and Wnt pathways. *J. Bone Joint. Surg. Am.* **83-A Suppl 1,** S31–S39.
62. Fischer, L., Boland, G., and Tuan, R. S. (2002) Wnt-3A enhances bone morphogenetic protein-2-mediated chondrogenesis of murine C3H10T1/2 mesenchymal cells. *J. Biol. Chem.* **277,** 30870–20878.
63. Mulder, K. M. (2000) Role of Ras and Mapks in TGFbeta signaling. *Cytokine Growth Factor Rev.* **11,** 23–35.
64. Williams, J. G. (2000) STAT signalling in cell proliferation and in development. *Curr. Opin. Genet. Dev.* **10,** 503–507.
65. Zhang, Y. and Derynck, R. (1999) Regulation of Smad signalling by protein associations and signalling crosstalk. *Trends Cell Biol.* **9,** 274–279.
66. Murakami, S., Kan, M., McKeehan, W. L., and de Crombrugghe, B. (2000) Up-regulation of the chondrogenic Sox9 gene by fibroblast growth factors is mediated by the mitogen-activated protein kinase pathway. *Proc. Natl. Acad. Sci. USA* **97,** 1113–1118.
67. Le Douarin, N. M. (1982) *The Neural Crest.* Cambridge University Press, Cambridge, UK.
68. Le Lievre, C. S. and Le Douarin, N. M. (1975) Mesenchymal derivatives of the neural crest: analysis of chimaeric quail and chick embryos. *J. Embryol. Exp. Morphol.* **34,** 125–154.
69. Noden, D. M. (1983) The role of the neural crest in patterning of avian cranial skeletal, connective, and muscle tissues. *Dev. Biol.* **96,** 144–165.
70. Tan, S. S. and Morriss-Kay, G. (1985) The development and distribution of the cranial neural crest in the rat embryo. *Cell Tissue Res.* **240,** 403–416.

71. Baker, C. V., Bronner-Fraser, M., Le Douarin, N. M., and Teillet, M. A. (1997) Early- and late-migrating cranial neural crest cell populations have equivalent developmental potential in vivo. *Development* **124,** 3077–3087.
72. Baroffio, A., Dupin, E., and Le Douarin, N. M. (1991) Common precursors for neural and mesectodermal derivatives in the cephalic neural crest. *Development* **112,** 301–305.
73. Epperlein, H., Meulemans, D., Bronner-Fraser, M., Steinbeisser, H., and Selleck, M. A. (2000) Analysis of cranial neural crest migratory pathways in axolotl using cell markers and transplantation. *Development* **127,** 2751–2761.
74. McGonnell, I. M. and Graham, A. (2002) Trunk neural crest has skeletogenic potential. *Curr. Biol.* **12,** 767–771.
75. Morriss-Kay, G., Ruberte, E., and Fukiishi, Y. (1993) Mammalian neural crest and neural crest derivatives. *Anat. Anz.* **175,** 501–507.
76. Chareonvit, S., Osumi-Yamashita, N., Ikeda, M., and Eto, K. (1997) Murine forebrain and midbrain crest cells generate different characteristic derivatives in vitro. *Dev. Growth Differ.* **39,** 493–503.
77. Osumi-Yamashita, N., Ninomiya, Y., Doi, H., and Eto, K. (1994) The contribution of both forebrain and midbrain crest cells to the mesenchyme in the frontonasal mass of mouse embryos. *Dev. Biol.* **164,** 409–419.
78. Wedden, S. E., Ralphs, J. R., and Tickle, C. (1988) Pattern formation in the facial primordia. *Development* **103,** 31–40.
79. Morriss-Kay, G. and Tucket, F. (1991) Early events in mammalian craniofacial morphogenesis. *J. Craniofac. Genet. Dev. Biol.* **11,** 181–191.
80. Serbedzija, G. N., Bronner-Fraser, M., and Fraser, S. E. (1992) Vital dye analysis of cranial neural crest cell migration in the mouse embryo. *Development* **116,** 297–307.
81. Lumsden, A. and Keynes, R. (1989) Segmental patterns of neuronal development in the chick hindbrain. *Nature* **337,** 424–428.
82. Trainor, P. A., Sobieszczuk, D., Wilkinson, D., and Krumlauf, R. (2002) Signalling between the hindbrain and paraxial tissues dictates neural crest migration pathways. *Development* **129,** 433–442.
83. Hunt, P., Wilkinson, D., and Krumlauf, R. (1991) Patterning the vertebrate head: murine Hox 2 genes mark distinct subpopulations of premigratory and migrating cranial neural crest. *Development* **112,** 43–50.
84. Vaglia, J. L. and Hall, B. K. (1999) Regulation of neural crest cell populations: occurrence, distribution and underlying mechanisms. *Int. J. Dev. Biol.* **43,** 95–110.
85. Trainor, P. A. and Krumlauf, R. (2000) Patterning the cranial neural crest: hindbrain segmentation and Hox gene plasticity. *Nat. Rev. Neurosci.* **1,** 116–124.
86. Grapin-Botton, A., Bonnin, M. A., and Le Douarin, N. M. (1997) Hox gene induction in the neural tube depends on three parameters: competence, signal supply and paralogue group. *Development* **124,** 849–859.
87. Schilling, T. F., Prince, V., and Ingham, P. W. (2001) Plasticity in zebrafish hox expression in the hindbrain and cranial neural crest. *Dev. Biol.* **231,** 201–216.
88. Trainor, P. and Krumlauf, R. (2000) Plasticity in mouse neural crest cells reveals a new patterning role for cranial mesoderm. *Nat. Cell Biol.* **2,** 96–102.
89. Trainor, P. A., Ariza-McNaughton, L., and Krumlauf, R. (2002) Role of the isthmus and FGFs in resolving the paradox of neural crest plasticity and prepatterning. *Science* **295,** 1288–1291.
90. Couly, G., Creuzet, S., Bennaceur, S., Vincent, C., and Le Douarin, N. M. (2002) Interactions between Hox-negative cephalic neural crest cells and the foregut endoderm in patterning the facial skeleton in the vertebrate head. *Development* **129,** 1061–1073.
91. Jeffs, P., Jaques, K., and Osmond, M. (1992) Cell death in cranial neural crest development. *Anat. Embryol. (Berl.)* **185,** 583–588.
92. Lumsden, A., Sprawson, N., and Graham, A. (1991) Segmental origin and migration of neural crest cells in the hindbrain region of the chick embryo. *Development* **113,** 1281–1291.
93. Graham, A., Heyman, I., and Lumsden, A. (1993) Even-numbered rhombomeres control the apoptotic elimination of neural crest cells from odd-numbered rhombomeres in the chick hindbrain. *Development* **119,** 233–245.
94. Sechrist, J., Scherson, T., and Bronner-Fraser, M. (1994) Rhombomere rotation reveals that multiple mechanisms contribute to the segmental pattern of hindbrain neural crest migration. *Development* **120,** 1777–1790.
95. Sechrist, J., Serbedzija, G. N., Scherson, T., Fraser, S. E., and Bronner-Fraser, M. (1993) Segmental migration of the hindbrain neural crest does not arise from its segmental generation. *Development* **118,** 691–703.
96. Birgbauer, E., Sechrist, J., Bronner-Fraser, M., and Fraser, S. (1995) Rhombomeric origin and rostrocaudal reassortment of neural crest cells revealed by intravital microscopy. *Development* **121,** 935–945.
97. Kontges, G. and Lumsden, A. (1996) Rhombencephalic neural crest segmentation is preserved throughout craniofacial ontogeny. *Development* **122,** 3229–3242.
98. Farlie, P. G., Kerr, R., Thomas, P., Symes, T., Minichiello, J., Hearn, C. J., et al. (1999) A paraxial exclusion zone creates patterned cranial neural crest cell outgrowth adjacent to rhombomeres 3 and 5. *Dev. Biol.* **213,** 70–84.
99. Graham, A. and Lumsden, A. (1996) Patterning the cranial neural crest. *Biochem. Soc. Sympos.* **62,** 77–83.
100. Smith, A. and Graham, A. (2001) Restricting Bmp-4 mediated apoptosis in hindbrain neural crest. *Dev. Dyn.* **220,** 276–283.
101. Ellies, D. L., Church, V., Francis-West, P., and Lumsden, A. (2000) The WNT antagonist cSFRP2 modulates programmed cell death in the developing hindbrain. *Development* **127,** 5285–5295.
102. Garcia-Castro, M. I., Marcelle, C., and Bronner-Fraser, M. (2002) Ectodermal Wnt Function As a Neural Crest Inducer. *Science* **297,** 848–851.
103. Lallier, T. E. (1991) Cell lineage and cell migration in the neural crest. *Ann. NY Acad. Sci.* **615,** 158–171.

104. Spokony, R. F., Aoki, Y., Saint-Germain, N., Magner-Fink, E., and Saint-Jeannet, J. P. (2002) The transcription factor Sox9 is required for cranial neural crest development in Xenopus. *Development* **129,** 421–432.
105. Takahashi, K., Nuckolls, G. H., Takahashi, I., Nonaka, K., Nagata, M., Ikura, T., Slavkin, H. C., and Shum, L. (2001) Msx2 is a repressor of chondrogenic differentiation in migratory cranial neural crest cells. *Dev. Dyn.* **222,** 252–262.
106. Le Lievre, C. S. (1978) Participation of neural crest-derived cells in the genesis of the skull in birds. *J. Embryol. Exp. Morphol.* **47,** 17–37.
107. Chai, Y., Jiang, X., Ito, Y., Bringas, P. Jr., Han, J., Rowitch, D. H., et al. (2000) Fate of the mammalian cranial neural crest during tooth and mandibular morphogenesis. *Development* **127,** 1671–1679.
108. Hall, B. K. (1980) Tissue interactions and the initiation of osteogenesis and chondrogenesis in the neural crest-derived mandibular skeleton of the embryonic mouse as seen in isolated murine tissues and in recombinations of murine and avian tissues. *J. Embryol. Exp. Morphol.* **58,** 251–264.
109. Tyler, M. S. and Hall, B. K. (1977) Epithelial influences on skeletogenesis in the mandible of the embryonic chick. *Anat. Rec.* **188,** 229–239.
110. Coffin-Collins, P. A. and Hall, B. K. (1989) Chondrogenesis of mandibular mesenchyme from the embryonic chick is inhibited by mandibular epithelium and by epidermal growth factor. *Int. J. Dev. Biol.* **33,** 297–311.
111. Hall, B. K. and Coffin-Collins, P. A. (1990) Reciprocal interactions between epithelium, mesenchyme, and epidermal growth factor (EGF) in the regulation of mandibular mitotic activity in the embryonic chick. *J. Craniofac. Genet. Dev. Biol.* **10,** 241–261.
112. Kollar, E. J. and Mina, M. (1991) Role of the early epithelium in the patterning of the teeth and Meckel's cartilage. *J. Craniofac. Genet. Dev. Biol.* **11,** 223–228.
113. Mina, M., Upholt, W. B., and Kollar, E. J. (1994) Enhancement of avian mandibular chondrogenesis in vitro in the absence of epithelium. *Arch. Oral Biol.* **39,** 551–562.
114. Kronmiller, J. E., Upholt, W. B., and Kollar, E. J. (1991) Expression of epidermal growth factor mRNA in the developing mouse mandibular process. *Arch. Oral. Biol.* **36,** 405–410.
115. Shum, L., Sakakura, Y., Bringas, P. Jr., Luo, W., Snead, M. L., Mayo, M., et al. (1993) EGF abrogation-induced fusilli-form dysmorphogenesis of Meckel's cartilage during embryonic mouse mandibular morphogenesis in vitro. *Development* **118,** 903–917.
116. Miettinen, P. J., Chin, J. R., Shum, L., Slavkin, H. C., Shuler, C. F., Derynck, R. et al. (1999) Epidermal growth factor receptor function is necessary for normal craniofacial development and palate closure. *Nat. Genet.* **22,** 69–73.
117. Chin, J. R. and Werb, Z. (1997) Matrix metalloproteinases regulate morphogenesis, migration and remodeling of epithelium, tongue skeletal muscle and cartilage in the mandibular arch. *Development* **124,** 1519–1530.
118. Mina, M., Gluhak, J., Upholt, W. B., Kollar, E. J., and Rogers, B. (1995) Experimental analysis of Msx-1 and Msx-2 gene expression during chick mandibular morphogenesis. *Dev. Dyn.* **202,** 195–214.
119. Mina, M., Gluhak, J., and Rodgers, B. (1996) Downregulation of Msx-2 expression results in chondrogenesis in the medial region of the avian mandible. *Connect. Tissue Res.* **35,** 79–84.
120. Semba, I., Nonaka, K., Takahashi, I., Takahashi, K., Dashner, R., Shum, L., et al. (2000) Positionally-dependent chondrogenesis induced by BMP4 is co-regulated by Sox9 and Msx2. *Dev. Dyn.* **217,** 401–414.
121. Ekanayake, S. and Hall, B. K. (1997) The in vivo and in vitro effects of bone morphogenetic protein-2 on the development of the chick mandible. *Int. J. Dev. Biol.* **41,** 67–81.
122. Barlow, A. J. and Francis-West, P. H. (1997) Ectopic application of recombinant BMP-2 and BMP-4 can change patterning of developing chick facial primordia. *Development* **124,** 391–398.
123. Capdevila, J. and Izpisua Belmonte, J. C. (2001) Patterning mechanisms controlling vertebrate limb development. *Annu. Rev. Cell Dev. Biol.* **17,** 87–132.
124. Ng, J. K., Tamura, K., Buscher, D., and Izpisua-Belmonte, J. C. (1999) Molecular and cellular basis of pattern formation during vertebrate limb development. *Curr. Top Dev. Biol.* **41,** 37–66.
125. Lewandoski, M., Sun, X., and Martin, G. R. (2000) Fgf8 signalling from the AER is essential for normal limb development. *Nat. Genet.* **26,** 460–463.
126. Sun, X., Lewandoski, M., Meyers, E. N., Liu, Y. H., Maxson, R. E. Jr., and Martin, G. R. (2000) Conditional inactivation of Fgf4 reveals complexity of signalling during limb bud development. *Nat. Genet.* **25,** 83–86.
127. Martin, G. R. (1998) The roles of FGFs in the early development of vertebrate limbs. *Genes Dev.* **12,** 1571–1586.
128. Sun, X., Mariani, F. V., and Martin, G. R. (2002) Functions of FGF signalling from the apical ectodermal ridge in limb development. *Nature* **418,** 501–508.
129. Xu, X., Weinstein, M., Li, C., and Deng, C. (1999) Fibroblast growth factor receptors (FGFRs) and their roles in limb development. *Cell Tissue Res.* **296,** 33–43.
130. Niswander, L. (1996) Growth factor interactions in limb development. *Ann. NY Acad. Sci.* **785,** 23–26.
131. Wolpert, L. (1969) Positional information and the spatial pattern of cellular differentiation. *J. Theor. Biol.* **25,** 1–47.
132. Dudley, A. T., Ros, M. A., and Tabin, C. J. (2002) A re-examination of proximodistal patterning during vertebrate limb development. *Nature* **418,** 539–544.
133. Johnson, R. L., Riddle, R. D., Laufer, E., and Tabin, C. (1994) Sonic hedgehog: a key mediator of anterior-posterior patterning of the limb and dorso-ventral patterning of axial embryonic structures. *Biochem. Soc. Trans.* **22,** 569–574.
134. Tickle, C. and Eichele, G. (1994) Vertebrate limb development. *Annu. Rev. Cell. Biol.* **10,** 121–152.
135. Riddle, R. D., Johnson, R. L., Laufer, E., and Tabin, C. (1993) Sonic hedgehog mediates the polarizing activity of the ZPA. *Cell* **75,** 1401–1416.

136. Duboule, D. (1992) The vertebrate limb: a model system to study the Hox/HOM gene network during development and evolution. *Bioessays* **14,** 375–384.
137. Pearse, R. V. II and Tabin, C. J. (1998) The molecular ZPA. *J. Exp. Zool.* **282,** 677–690.
138. Chen, H. and Johnson, R. L. (1999) Dorsoventral patterning of the vertebrate limb: a process governed by multiple events. *Cell Tissue Res.* **296,** 67–73.
139. Zeller, R. and Duboule, D. (1997) Dorso-ventral limb polarity and origin of the ridge: on the fringe of independence? *Bioessays* **19,** 541–546.
140. Yokouchi, Y., Sasaki, H., and Kuroiwa, A. (1991) Homeobox gene expression correlated with the bifurcation process of limb cartilage development. *Nature* **353,** 443–445.
141. Dolle P., Izpisua-Belmonte, J. C., Brown, J., Tickle, C., and Duboule, D. (1993) Hox genes and the morphogenesis of the vertebrate limb. *Prog. Clin. Biol. Res.* **383A,** 11–20.
142. Merino, R., Ganan, Y., Macias, D., Rodriguez-Leon, J., and Hurle, J. M. (1999) Bone morphogenetic proteins regulate interdigital cell death in the avian embryo. *Ann. NY Acad. Sci.* **887,** 120–132.
143. Macias, D., Ganan, Y., Rodriguez-Leon, J., Merino, R., and Hurle, J. M. (1999) Regulation by members of the transforming growth factor beta superfamily of the digital and interdigital fates of the autopodial limb mesoderm. *Cell Tissue Res.* **296,** 95–102.
144. Dahn, R. D. and Fallon, J. F. (2000) Interdigital regulation of digit identity and homeotic transformation by modulated BMP signaling. *Science* **289,** 438–441.
145. Rizgeliene, R. (1996) Skeleton pattern and joint formation in chorioallantoic grafts lacking the anterior or posterior necrotic zones. *J. Anat.* **189,** 601–608.
146. Nalin, A. M., Greenlee, T. K. Jr., and Sandell, L. J. (1995) Collagen gene expression during development of avian synovial joints: transient expression of types II and XI collagen genes in the joint capsule. *Dev. Dyn.* **203,** 352–362.
147. Pizette, S. and Niswander, L. (2000) BMPs are required at two steps of limb chondrogenesis: formation of prechondrogenic condensations and their differentiation into chondrocytes. *Dev. Biol.* **219,** 237–249.
148. Pizette, S. and Niswander, L. (1999) BMPs negatively regulate structure and function of the limb apical ectodermal ridge. *Development* **126,** 883–894.
149. Roark, E. F. and Greer, K. (1994) Transforming growth factor-beta and bone morphogenetic protein-2 act by distinct mechanisms to promote chick limb cartilage differentiation in vitro. *Dev. Dyn.* **200,** 103–116.
150. Pizette, S., Abate-Shen, C., and Niswander, L. (2001) BMP controls proximodistal outgrowth, via induction of the apical ectodermal ridge, and dorsoventral patterning in the vertebrate limb. *Development* **128,** 4463–4474.
151. Zhang, H. and Bradley, A. (1996) Mice deficient for BMP2 are nonviable and have defects in amnion/chorion and cardiac development. *Development* **122,** 2977–2986.
152. Duprez, D., Bell, E. J., Richardson, M. K., Archer, C. W., Wolpert, L., Brickell, P. M., et al. (1996) Overexpression of BMP-2 and BMP-4 alters the size and shape of developing skeletal elements in the chick limb. *Mech. Dev.* **57,** 145–157.
153. Zhang, Z., Yu, X., Zhang, Y., Geronimo, B., Lovlie, A., Fromm, S. H., and Chen, Y. (2000) Targeted misexpression of constitutively active BMP receptor-IB causes bifurcation, duplication, and posterior transformation of digit in mouse limb. *Dev. Biol.* **220,** 154–167.
154. Ganan, Y., Macias, D., Duterque-Coquillaud, M., Ros, M. A., and Hurle, J. M. (1996) Role of TGF beta s and BMPs as signals controlling the position of the digits and the areas of interdigital cell death in the developing chick limb autopod. *Development* **122,** 2349–2357.
155. Merino, R., Ganan, Y., Macias, D., Economides, A. N., Sampath, K. T., and Hurle, J. M. (1998) Morphogenesis of digits in the avian limb is controlled by FGFs, TGFbetas, and noggin through BMP signaling. *Dev. Biol.* **200,** 35–45.
156. Macias, D., Ganan, Y., Sampath, T. K., Piedra, M. E., Ros, M. A., and Hurle, J. M. (1997) Role of BMP-2 and OP-1 (BMP-7) in programmed cell death and skeletogenesis during chick limb development. *Development* **124,** 1109–1117.
157. Ferrari, D., Lichtler, A. C., Pan, Z. Z., Dealy, C. N., Upholt, W. B., and Kosher, R. A. (1998) Ectopic expression of Msx-2 in posterior limb bud mesoderm impairs limb morphogenesis while inducing BMP-4 expression, inhibiting cell proliferation, and promoting apoptosis. *Dev. Biol.* **197,** 12–24.
158. Dencker, L., Gustafson, A. L., Annerwall, E., Busch, C., and Eriksson, U. (1991) Retinoid-binding proteins in craniofacial development. *J. Craniofac. Genet. Dev. Biol.* **11,** 303–314.
159. Lammer, E. J., Chen, D. T., Hoar, R. M., Agnish, N. D., Benke, P. J., Braun, J. T., et al. (1985) Retinoic acid embryopathy. *N. Engl. J. Med.* **313,** 837–841.
160. Helms, J. A., Kim, C. H., Eichele, G., and Thaller, C. (1996) Retinoic acid signaling is required during early chick limb development. *Development* **122,** 1385–1394.
161. Helms, J., Thaller, C., and Eichele, G. (1994) Relationship between retinoic acid and sonic hedgehog, two polarizing signals in the chick wing bud. *Development* **120,** 3267–3274.
162. Heller, L. C., Li, Y., Abrams, K. L., and Rogers, M. B. (1999) Transcriptional regulation of the Bmp2 gene. Retinoic acid induction in F9 embryonal carcinoma cells and Saccharomyces cerevisiae. *J. Biol. Chem.* **274,** 1394–1400.
163. Francis, P. H., Richardson, M. K., Brickell, P. M., and Tickle, C. (1994) Bone morphogenetic proteins and a signalling pathway that controls patterning in the developing chick limb. *Development* **120,** 209–218.
164. Rodriguez-Leon, J., Merino, R., Macias, D., Ganan, Y., Santesteban, E., and Hurle, J. M. (1999) Retinoic acid regulates programmed cell death through BMP signalling. *Nat. Cell Biol.* **1,** 125–126.
165. Weston, A. D., Rosen, V., Chandraratna, R. A., and Underhill, T. M. (2000) Regulation of skeletal progenitor differentiation by the BMP and retinoid signaling pathways. *J. Cell Biol.* **148,** 679–690.

166. Ho, A. M., Johnson, M. D., and Kingsley, D. M. (2000) Role of the mouse ank gene in control of tissue calcification and arthritis. *Science* **289,** 265–270.
167. Qu, S., Tucker, S. C., Ehrlich, J. S., Levorse, J. M., Flaherty, L. A., Wisdom, R., et al. (1998) Mutations in mouse Aristaless-like4 cause Strong's luxoid polydactyly. *Development* **125,** 2711–2721.
168. Svensson, L., Aszodi, A., Heinegard, D., Hunziker, E. B., Reinholt, F. P., Fassler, R., et al. (2002) Cartilage oligomeric matrix protein-deficient mice have normal skeletal development. *Mol. Cell Biol.* **22,** 4366–4371.
169. Saftig, P., Hunziker, E., Wehmeyer, O., Jones, S., Boyde, A., Rommerskirch, W., et al. (1998) Impaired osteoclastic bone resorption leads to osteopetrosis in cathepsin-K-deficient mice. *Proc. Natl. Acad. Sci. USA* **95,** 13453–13458.
170. Pereira, R., Khillan, J. S., Helminen, H. J., Hume, E. L., and Prockop, D. J. (1993) Transgenic mice expressing a partially deleted gene for type I procollagen (COL1A1) A breeding line with a phenotype of spontaneous fractures and decreased bone collagen and mineral. *J. Clin. Invest.* **91,** 709–716.
171. Forlino, A., Porter, F. D., Lee, E. J., Westphal, H., and Marini, J. C. (1999) Use of the Cre/lox recombination system to develop a non-lethal knock- in murine model for osteogenesis imperfecta with an alpha1(I) G349C substitution. Variability in phenotype in BrtlIV mice. *J. Biol. Chem.* **274,** 37923–37931.
172. Helminen, H. J., Kiraly, K., Pelttari, A., Tammi, M. I., Vandenberg, P., Pereira, R., Dhulipala, R., Khillan, J. S., Ala-Kokko, L., Hume, E. L., et al. (1993) An inbred line of transgenic mice expressing an internally deleted gene for type II procollagen (COL2A1) Young mice have a variable phenotype of a chondrodysplasia and older mice have osteoarthritic changes in joints. *J. Clin. Invest.* **92,** 582–595.
173. Li, S. W., Prockop, D. J., Helminen, H., Fassler, R., Lapvetelainen, T., Kiraly, K., et al. (1995) Transgenic mice with targeted inactivation of the Col2 alpha 1 gene for collagen II develop a skeleton with membranous and periosteal bone but no endochondral bone. *Genes Dev.* **9,** 2821–2830.
174. Lapvetelainen, T., Hyttinen, M., Lindblom, J., Langsjo, T. K., Sironen, R., Li, S. W., et al. (2001) More knee joint osteoarthritis (OA) in mice after inactivation of one allele of type II procollagen gene but less OA after lifelong voluntary wheel running exercise. *Osteoarthritis Cartilage* **9,** 152–160.
175. Liu, X., Wu, H., Byrne, M., Krane, S., and Jaenisch, R. (1997) Type III collagen is crucial for collagen I fibrillogenesis and for normal cardiovascular development. *Proc. Natl. Acad. Sci. USA* **94,** 1852–1856.
176. Andrikopoulos, K., Liu, X., Keene, D. R., Jaenisch, R., and Ramirez, F. (1995) Targeted mutation in the col5a2 gene reveals a regulatory role for type V collagen during matrix assembly. *Nat. Genet.* **9,** 31–36.
177. Nakata, K., Ono, K., Miyazaki, J., Olsen, B. R., Muragaki, Y., Adachi, E., et al. (1993) Osteoarthritis associated with mild chondrodysplasia in transgenic mice expressing alpha 1(IX) collagen chains with a central deletion. *Proc. Natl. Acad. Sci. USA* **90,** 2870–2874.
178. Fassler, R., Schnegelsberg, P. N., Dausman, J., Shinya, T., Muragaki, Y., McCarthy M. T., et al. (1994) Mice lacking alpha 1 (IX) collagen develop noninflammatory degenerative joint disease. *Proc. Natl. Acad. Sci. USA* **91,** 5070–5074.
179. Ting, K., Ramachandran, H., Chung, K. S., Shah-Hosseini, N., Olsen, B. R., and Nishimura, I. (1999) A short isoform of Col9a1 supports alveolar bone repair. *Am. J. Pathol.* **155,** 1993–1999.
180. Jacenko, O., LuValle, P. A., and Olsen, B. R. (1993) Spondylometaphyseal dysplasia in mice carrying a dominant negative mutation in a matrix protein specific for cartilage-to-bone transition. *Nature* **365,** 56–61.
181. Rosati, R., Horan, G. S., Pinero, G. J., Garofalo, S., Keene, D. R., Horton, W. A., et al. (1994) Normal long bone growth and development in type X collagen-null mice. *Nat. Genet.* **8,** 129–135.
182. Gress, C. J. and Jacenko, O. (2000) Growth plate compressions and altered hematopoiesis in collagen X null mice. *J. Cell. Biol.* **149,** 983–993.
183. Kwan, K. M., Pang, M. K., Zhou, S., Cowan, S. K., Kong, R. Y., Pfordte, T., et al. (1997) Abnormal compartmentalization of cartilage matrix components in mice lacking collagen X: implications for function. *J. Cell. Biol.* **136,** 459–471.
184. Li, Y., Lacerda, D. A., Warman, M. L., Beier, D. R., Yoshioka, H., Ninomiya, Y., et al. (1995) A fibrillar collagen gene, Col11a1, is essential for skeletal morphogenesis. *Cell* **80,** 423–430.
185. Gayraud, B., Keene, D. R., Sakai, L. Y., and Ramirez, F. (2000) New insights into the assembly of extracellular microfibrils from the analysis of the fibrillin 1 mutation in the tight skin mouse. *J. Cell. Biol.* **150,** 667–680.
186. Pereira, L., Andrikopoulos, K., Tian, J., Lee, S. Y., Keene, D. R., Ono, R., et al. (1997) Targetting of the gene encoding fibrillin-1 recapitulates the vascular aspect of Marfan syndrome. *Nat. Genet.* **17,** 218–222.
187. Chaudhry, S. S., Gazzard, J., Baldock, C., Dixon, J., Rock, M. J., Skinner, G. C., et al. (2001) Mutation of the gene encoding fibrillin-2 results in syndactyly in mice. *Hum. Mol. Genet.* **10,** 835–843.
188. Arteaga-Solis, E., Gayraud, B., Lee, S. Y., Shum, L., Sakai, L., and Ramirez, F. (2001) Regulation of limb patterning by extracellular microfibrils. *J. Cell. Biol.* **154,** 275–281.
189. Storm, E. E., Huynh, T. V., Copeland, N. G., Jenkins, N. A., Kingsley, D. M., and Lee, S. J. (1994) Limb alterations in brachypodism mice due to mutations in a new member of the TGF beta-superfamily. *Nature* **368,** 639–643.
190. Storm, E. E. and Kingsley, D. M. (1996) Joint patterning defects caused by single and double mutations in members of the bone morphogenetic protein (BMP) family. *Development* **122,** 3969–3979.
191. Arikawa-Hirasawa, E., Watanabe, H., Takami, H., Hassell, J. R., and Yamada, Y. (1999) Perlecan is essential for cartilage and cephalic development. *Nat. Genet.* **23,** 354–358.
192. Johnson, K. R., Sweet, H. O., Donahue, L. R., Ward-Bailey, P., Bronson, R. T., and Davisson, M. T. (1998) A new spontaneous mouse mutation of Hoxd13 with a polyalanine expansion and phenotype similar to human synpolydactyly. *Hum. Mol. Genet.* **7,** 1033–1038.
193. Dolle, P., Dierich, A., LeMeur, M., Schimmang, T., Schuhbaur, B., Chambon, P., and Duboule, D. (1993) Disruption of the Hoxd-13 gene induces localized heterochrony leading to mice with neotenic limbs. *Cell* **75,** 431–441.

194. St-Jacques, B., Hammerschmidt, M., and McMahon, A. P. (1999) Indian hedgehog signaling regulates proliferation and differentiation of chondrocytes and is essential for bone formation. *Genes Dev.* **13,** 2072–2086.
195. Hebrok, M., Kim, S. K., St Jacques, B., McMahon, A. P., and Melton, D. A. (2000) Regulation of pancreas development by hedgehog signaling. *Development* **127,** 4905–4913.
196. Liu, Y. H., Kundu, R., Wu, L., Luo, W., Ignelzi, M. A. Jr., Snead, M. L., et al. (1995) Premature suture closure and ectopic cranial bone in mice expressing Msx2 transgenes in the developing skull. *Proc. Natl. Acad. Sci. USA* **92,** 6137–6141.
197. Winograd, J., Reilly, M. P., Roe, R., Lutz, J., Laughner, E., Xu, X., et al. (1997) Perinatal lethality and multiple craniofacial malformations in MSX2 transgenic mice. *Hum. Mol. Genet.* **6,** 369–379.
198. Satokata, I., Ma, L., Ohshima, H., Bei, M., Woo, I., Nishizawa, K., et al. (2000) Msx2 deficiency in mice causes pleiotropic defects in bone growth and ectodermal organ formation. *Nat. Genet.* **24,** 391–395.
199. McMahon, J. A., Takada, S., Zimmerman, L. B., Fan, C. M., Harland, R. M., and McMahon, A. P. (1998) Noggin-mediated antagonism of BMP signaling is required for growth and patterning of the neural tube and somite. *Genes Dev.* **12,** 1438–1452.
200. Brunet, L. J., McMahon, J. A., McMahon, A. P., and Harland, R. M. (1998) Noggin, cartilage morphogenesis, and joint formation in the mammalian skeleton. *Science* **280,** 1455–1457.
201. Lanske, B., Karaplis, A. C., Lee, K., Luz, A., Vortkamp, A., Pirro, A., et al. (1996) PTH/PTHrP receptor in early development and Indian hedgehog-regulated bone growth. *Science* **273,** 663–666.
202. Takeuchi, S., Takeda, K., Oishi, I., Nomi, M., Ikeya, M., Itoh, K., et al. (2000) Mouse Ror2 receptor tyrosine kinase is required for the heart development and limb formation. *Genes Cells* **5,** 71–78.
203. Komori, T., Yagi, H., Nomura, S., Yamaguchi, A., Sasaki, K., Deguchi, K., et al. (1997) Targeted disruption of Cbfa1 results in a complete lack of bone formation owing to maturational arrest of osteoblasts. *Cell* **89,** 755–764.
204. D'Souza, R. N., Aberg, T., Gaikwad, J., Cavender, A., Owen, M., Karsenty, G., et al. (1999) Cbfa1 is required for epithelial-mesenchymal interactions regulating tooth development in mice. *Development* **126,** 2911–2920.
205. Otto, F., Thornell, A. P., Crompton, T., Denzel, A., Gilmour, K. C., Rosewell, I. R., et al. (1997) Cbfa1, a candidate gene for cleidocranial dysplasia syndrome, is essential for osteoblast differentiation and bone development. *Cell* **89,** 765–771.
206. Selby, P. B. and Selby, P. R. (1978) Gamma-ray-induced dominant mutations that cause skeletal abnormalities in mice. II. Description of proved mutations. *Mutat. Res.* **51,** 199–236.
207. Ducy, P., Starbuck, M., Priemel, M., Shen, J., Pinero, G., Geoffroy, V., et al. (1999) A Cbfa1-dependent genetic pathway controls bone formation beyond embryonic development. *Genes Dev.* **13,** 1025–1036.
208. Bi, W., Huang, W., Whitworth, D. J., Deng, J. M., Zhang, Z., Behringer, R. R., et al. (2001) Haploinsufficiency of Sox9 results in defective cartilage primordia and premature skeletal mineralization. *Proc. Natl. Acad. Sci. USA* **98,** 6698–6703.
209. Bruneau, B. G., Nemer, G., Schmitt, J. P., Charron, F., Robitaille, L., Caron, S., et al. (2001) A murine model of Holt-Oram syndrome defines roles of the T-box transcription factor Tbx5 in cardiogenesis and disease. *Cell* **106,** 709–721.
210. Shull, M. M., Ormsby, I., Kier, A. B., Pawlowski, S., Diebold, R. J., Yin, M., et al. (1992) Targeted disruption of the mouse transforming growth factor-beta 1 gene results in multifocal inflammatory disease. *Nature* **359,** 693–699.
211. Kulkarni, A. B., Huh, C. G., Becker, D., Geiser, A., Lyght, M., Flanders, K. C., et al. (1993) Transforming growth factor beta 1 null mutation in mice causes excessive inflammatory response and early death. *Proc. Natl. Acad. Sci. USA* **90,** 770–774.
212. Yoshizawa, T., Handa, Y., Uematsu, Y., Takeda, S., Sekine, K., Yoshihara, Y., et al. (1997) Mice lacking the vitamin D receptor exhibit impaired bone formation, uterine hypoplasia and growth retardation after weaning. *Nat. Genet.* **16,** 391–396.

3
Regulation of Chondrocyte Differentiation

Andreia M. Ionescu, M. Hicham Drissi, and Regis J. O'Keefe

ENDOCHONDRAL OSSIFICATION: OVERVIEW

During the last decade, great progress has been made toward a better understanding of skeletal development, cartilage, and bone formation. In particular, many mechanisms underlying a variety of cellular and molecular processes that regulate growth and differentiation of chondrocytes, osteoblasts, and osteoclasts have been elucidated. This chapter will review some of the molecular and genetic pathways known to regulate cartilage development. Skeletal formation occurs through both endochondral and intramembraneous ossification. Flat bones and craniofacial bones are formed through intramembraneous ossification that relies on osteoblast differentiation directly from mesenchymal stem cells. The axial and appendicular skeleton form through endochondral ossification, which requires the formation of a cartilage intermediate that forms a template for osteoid deposition and bone formation. During endochondral bone formation, mesenchymal stem cells differentiate into both chondrocytes and osteoblasts. During development of the long bone, growth plates localize to either end of the skeletal element and the region of cartilage is surrounded by a perichondrium that is composed of undifferentiated mesenchymal cells. In the growth plates, chondrocytes undergo several stages of differentiation. One of the important transitions is from proliferation to hypertrophy, an event that precedes mineralization of the cartilage matrix (Fig. 1). Chondrocyte hypertrophy is characterized by profound physical and biochemical changes, including a 5- to 10-fold increase in volume and expression of alkaline phosphatase, type X collagen, and MMP-13 *(1,2)*. Type X collagen is a short-chain collagen found only in the hypertrophic zone of the growth plate. Although its exact function remains unclear, mutations in the *colX* gene have been found to cause Schmid metaphyseal chondrodysplasia *(3)*, and transgenic mice with disruption in the *colX* gene exhibit a mild alteration of the growth plate architecture *(4)*. Alkaline phosphatase is essential for calcification of the matrix and is present in high concentration in matrix vesicles, which are small membrane vesicles released by budding from the surfaces of hypertrophic chondrocytes into the surrounding matrix *(5)*. Matrix vesicles are the initial sites of mineralization in the hypertrophic region of the growth plate and are critical components of the calcification process. The calcified matrix subsequently serves as the template for primary bone formation. In parallel, the perichondrium flanking the cartilage element differentiates into osteoblast-forming periosteum.

Primary bone formation is initiated at the center of the cartilage template and results in the subsequent formation of two separate regions of endochondral bone that develop at either end of the long bone. The growth plate is responsible for longitudinal growth of bones. Both chondrocyte proliferation and

From: *The Skeleton: Biochemical, Genetic, and Molecular Interactions in Development and Homeostasis*
Edited by: E. J. Massaro and J. M. Rogers © Humana Press Inc., Totowa, NJ

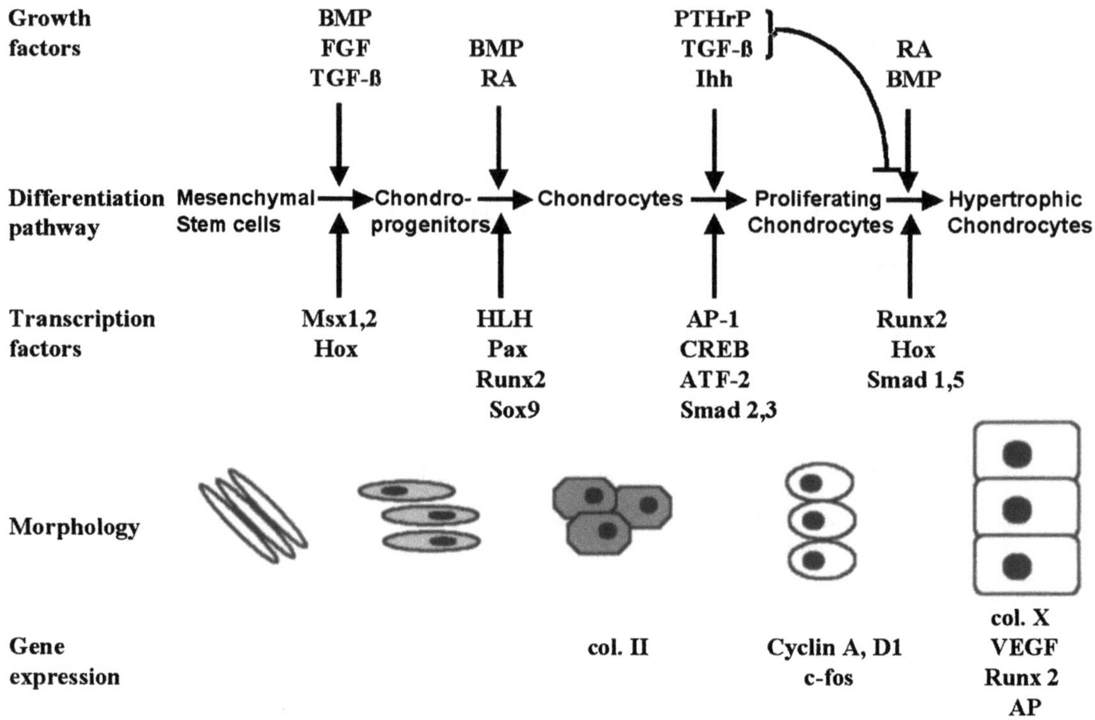

Fig. 1. Regulation of chondrocyte maturation. Multiple factors control cell differentiation from mesenchymal stem cells to hypertrophic chondrocytes, including members of the TGF-β superfamily and their downstream SMAD mediators, the homeodomain proteins and AP-1/CREB/ATF/Runx2 transcription factors. Phenotypic genes corresponding to each step of chondrocyte maturation are also indicated.

hypertrophy contribute to lengthening of the limb *(6,7)*. Because terminally differentiated hypertrophic cartilage is continuously replaced by bone, the tight regulation of the various steps of chondrocyte differentiation, particularly proliferation and hypertrophy, is critical for balancing the growth and ossification of the skeletal elements.

Both local and systemic signaling molecules regulate endochondral ossification. Here we review some of the factors that regulate chondrocyte maturation, including parathyroid hormone-related peptide (PTHrP), Indian hedgehog (Ihh), transforming growth factor-β (TGF-β), and bone morphogenetic proteins (BMPs). Although these factors are also involved in the early stages of endochondral ossification, such as chondrogenesis and differentiation of precursor mesenchymal cells in chondrocyte, we specifically address their role in the precise transition of chondrocytes from the proliferative phase to the hypertrophic phase (Fig. 1).

IHH/PTHRP SIGNALING LOOP: A CLASSIC MODEL FOR CHONDROCYTE DIFFERENTIATIONS

The paradigm for regulation of endochondral ossification involves the *Ihh* gene. *Ihh* expression delineates the zone of prehypertrophic chondrocytes. During limb development, secreted Ihh binds to receptors located on perichondrial cells and influences the expression of *PTHrP* by periarticular chondrocytes. PTHrP subsequently signals back to the growth plate and regulates the rate of chondrocyte differentiation (Fig. 2). It is still unclear whether Ihh controls *PTHrP* expression directly or indirectly through TGF-β superfamily members. Finally, it is possible that the role of Ihh in skeletal

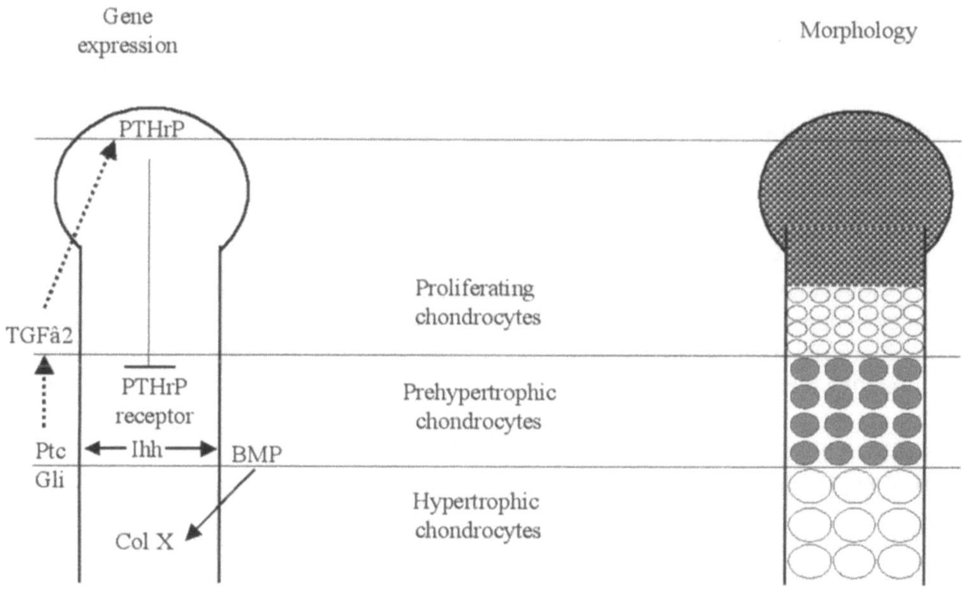

Fig. 2. The role of *Ihh/PTHrP* in endochondral ossification. Chondrocyte cell differentiation is associated with expression of specific genes involved in the regulation of chondrocyte maturation. *Ihh* is expressed in the prehypertrophic chondrocytes and signals through *TGF-β2* located in the perichondrium to enhance transcription of the *PTHrP* gene in the periarticular region.

development is primarily during embryonic growth and is less important postnatally, as we subsequently describe.

Hedgehog proteins are a conserved family of secreted molecules that provide key signals in embryonic patterning in many organisms. In vertebrates, there are three hedgehog genes: *sonic hedgehog* (*Shh*), *desert hedgehog* (*Dhh*), and the aforementioned *Ihh*. *Shh* functions in embryonic development by controlling the establishment of left–right and anterior–posterior limb axes, *Dhh* functions as a spermatocyte survival factor in the testes, whereas *Ihh* is involved in endochondral ossification *(8)*. Hedgehog proteins signal through a transmembrane receptor called Patched (Ptc) and a transcription factor called Gli. In vivo overexpression of *Ihh* in chicken limb bud through retrovirally mediated infection leads to shorter and broader skeletal elements with a continuous cartilage core that lacks hypertrophic chondrocytes *(9)*. In contrast, Ihh-deficient mice exhibit premature hypertrophic differentiation, reduced chondrocyte proliferation, and failure of osteoblast development *(10)*.

The phenotype of Ihh misexpression in either chicken limb bud or in transgenic mice is similar with the phenotype of PTHrP misexpression. Animals that overexpress PTHrP exhibit delay in chondrocyte terminal differentiation *(11)*. Humans with an activating mutation in the PTH/PTHrP receptor have Jansen's metaphyseal chondrodysplasia, characterized by disorganization of the growth plate and delayed chondrocyte terminal differentiation *(12)*. In contrast, mice null for either PTHrP *(13)* or its receptor *(14)* display accelerated chondrocyte differentiation and abnormal endochondral bone formation.

Several lines of evidence indicate that Ihh and PTHrP interact in a negative feedback loop regulating the onset of hypertrophic differentiation. Ihh overexpression in the chicken limb bud leads to induction of PTHrP expression in the periarticular region *(9)*, whereas lack of Ihh signaling in the Ihh-deficient mice leads to lack of PTHrP expression *(10)*. Additionally, limb explants of PTHrP knockout mice treated with hedgehog protein in culture demonstrate that intact PTHrP signaling is required to mediate the inhibitory effect of Ihh on chondrocyte differentiation *(9)*. These findings established the following mechanism for the Ihh/PTHrP regulation of chondrocyte differentiation: Ihh is produced by the prehypertrophic chondrocytes, signals through Ptc and Gli in the adjacent perichondrium, and induces expression of PTHrP in the periarticular region. In turn, PTHrP would diffuse across the growth plate, bind to its receptor, which is expressed in the prehypertrophic chondrocyte, and subsequently delay chondrocyte maturation.

One of the elusive aspects of this signaling pathway is the signals that are generated by Ihh-stimulated perichondrium to influence PTHrP expression in the periarticular cartilage. Indeed, removal of perichondrium causes inability of hedgehog signaling to delay chondrocyte hypertrophy *(15)*. Other studies have shown that removal of perichondrium results in an extended zone of cartilage expressing *colX* and an extended zone of cartilage incorporating BrdU, indicating that perichondrium negatively regulates both proliferation and hypertrophy of chondrocytes *(16)*. Possible candidates as Ihh secondary signals are the members of the TGF-β superfamily, namely the BMPs and TGF-β isoforms 1–3.

TGF-β SIGNALING: ROLE IN CHONDROCYTE DIFFERENTIATIONS

TGF-β family members are considered possible mediators of Ihh signaling on *PTHrP* expression. TGF-β enhances *PTHrP* expression in both mouse metatarsal explants *(17)* and isolated chondrocytes cultures *(18,19)*. Similarly, intact PTHrP signaling appears to be required for of TGF-β-mediated effects on chondrocyte hypertrophy *(17)*. Furthermore, transgenic mice overexpressing a dominant-negative TGF-β receptor exhibited a very similar phenotype to the PTHrP knockout mice. Both mouse models present an accelerated chondrocyte differentiation *(17,20)*. Finally, inhibition of TGF-β signaling in the perichondrium, with a dominant-negative type II receptor, also inhibits the effects of hedgehog on chondrocyte differentiation and on induction of PTHrP expression *(15)*. The dominant-negative type II receptor inhibits all three TGF-β isoforms.

Alvarez et al. recently showed that treatment of mouse metatarsals cultures with hedgehog protein leads to upregulation of *TGF-β2* and *TGF-β3* isoforms but not *TGF-β1* in the perichondrium. Furthermore, the effects of hedgehog protein signaling are specifically dependent on TGF-β2 because cultures from TGF-β3-null embryos respond to hedgehog protein signaling but cultures from TGF-β2-null embryos do not *(15)*. Altogether, the evidence suggests that TGF-β2 acts as a signal messenger between Ihh and PTHrP in the regulation of cartilage hypertrophic differentiation in embryonic development. Although the phenotype of the dominant-negative type II TGF-β receptor resembles the phenotypes of Ihh and PTHrP knockout mice, the skeletal malformations are still less severe, suggesting that, TGF-β may not be the only mediator of Ihh on PTHrP expression.

The role of Ihh/PTHrP signaling loop after embryonic development is not clearly established. It has been suggested that this pathway is not operational in neonatal mice because of low or absent levels of *Ihh* expression in the postnatal growth plate *(21)*. Also for postnatal development, the physical distance between the periarticular region and the growth plate increases dramatically, and the ability of PTHrP to diffuse to these tissues is questionable. A possible signaling scenario involving TGF-β and PTHrP in postnatal development has been defined by our group *(22)*. All of the necessary elements for a signaling pathway involving TGF-β and PTHrP are existent in the growth plate, eliminating the need for diffusion. The growth plate makes large amounts of TGF-β and PTHrP expression is induced up to 20-fold in chondrocytes stimulated with TGF-β *(18)*. Because TGF-β is secreted in an inactive complex, a possible source for TGF-β could be from hypertrophic cartilage during remodeling. Matrix metalloproteinase 13 (MMP-13) is highly expressed in the hypertrophic region and has been shown to activate latent TGF-β *(23)*. Another source is the zone of calcification as osteoclasts have been also been shown to activate TGF-β *(24)*. During matrix catabolism, TGF-β is activated from the latency-associated peptide (LAP) Activated TGF-β then acts in an autocrine/paracrine manner to stimulate the expression of PTHrP in the growth plate *(18)*. The elevated expression of PTHrP then slows the rate of chondrocyte differentiation. This leads to a decrease in the terminal differentiation and a fall in the activation of TGF-β, which results in a reacceleration in the rate of chondrocyte differentiation, with a subsequent increase in the release of active TGF-β from the matrix. This positive feedback loop between TGF-β and PTHrP in the growth plate results in a cycling of differentiation from an on or off state, similar to the effect of the Ihh/PTHrP signaling pathway during development. Interestingly, although animals overexpressing dominant-negative TGF-β receptors and the deletion of Smad3, a critical transcription factor downstream of TGF-β, both develop premature maturation, the phenotype only becomes evident postnatally *(25)*. This suggests that unique signals might be present during limb development and postnatal growth and that TGF-β might be particularly important in this latter process.

BMP REGULATION OF CHONDROCYTE DIFFERENTIATION

Similar to the TGF-β family, BMPs are key regulators of organogenesis in early embryonic development because they also play an active role in regulating cartilage formation and differentiation during later stages. *BMP-2*, *BMP-3*, *BMP-4*, *BMP-5*, and *BMP-7* all are expressed in the perichondrial cells *(26)*. Although *BMP-4* and *BMP-7* are expressed at low levels by chondrocytes undergoing maturation *(27)*, *BMP-6* and *BMP-7* are highly expressed by hypertrophic chondrocytes *(9)*. Finally, *BMP-2*, *BMP-4*, and *BMP-7* are expressed in the precartilaginous mesenchyme *(28)* and were shown to enhance chondrogenesis in vitro *(29)* and in vivo in chick limb buds *(30)*. Regulation of *BMP-2* and *BMP-4* expression by Ihh *(31)* further indicates that the interplay between these various signals in vivo increases the intricacy by which chondrocyte growth and differentiation is regulated.

The role of BMP signaling in chondrocyte differentiation has been somewhat controversial because of disparate effects that occur in vitro in isolated chondrocyte cell cultures and in in vivo in the chick limb bud model. Cell culture studies in various models all demonstrate an induction in chondrocyte maturation with gain of BMP signaling and a decrease in maturation with loss of function *(32,33)*. In contrast, in the chick limb bud, overexpression of activated type I BMP receptors inhibits chondrocyte maturation *(26)*. However, our laboratory has recently demonstrated that activated BMP signaling induces *Ihh* expression in chondrocytes, with a subsequent increase in PTHrP expression in the periarticular region *(34)*. This activation of the Ihh/PTHrP pathway likely explains the differential effects of BMP signaling on isolated chondrocytes compared with the developing limb. Whereas BMPs act to stimulate chondrocyte maturation directly, induction of Ihh/PTHrP signaling through paracrine-mediated events has the opposite effect and inhibits maturation. The findings suggest that BMP signaling is integrated into the Ihh/PTHrP signaling loop and that the ultimate effect is caused by a fine balance of BMP signaling.

INTEGRATION OF MULTIPLE SIGNALING PATHWAYS: COMBINATORIAL REGULATION OF CARTILAGE MATURATION

The growth factors and signaling molecules that control chondrocyte differentiation are interconnected and center on interactions between the Ihh/PTHrP loop and the TGF-β superfamily members. Although a significant amount of information about their role in skeletal development is available, less is known about the mechanisms by which their signaling pathways affect potential targets in the growth plate. Recently, we and others have characterized some of the transcriptional mechanisms downstream of these pathways *(35–38)*. It is indeed necessary to define how interactions between these signaling events result in progression toward the hypertrophic phenotype.

PTHrP Signaling

PTHrP signaling increases cAMP and calcium levels in chondrocytes, with subsequent activation of protein kinases A and C (PKA and PKC; refs. *39–41)*. Potential downstream targets of PKA/PKC signaling are the transcription factors cAMP response element binding protein (CREB) and activator protein 1 (AP-1) CREB is a member of the ATF/CREB family of transcription factors, which is activated in response to cAMP/PKA signals. CREB binds constitutively to DNA at a consensus cAMP response element primarily as a homodimer via a leucine zipper domain *(42)*. Activation occurs secondary to a phosphorylation event at Ser133. This results in the recruitment of the coactivator CBP (CREB-binding protein) and activation of the transcriptional machinery. The AP-1 complex is formed through dimerization between Fos and Jun family members. Subsequently, AP-1 binds DNA response elements known as TPA response elements.

Although PTHrP does not alter CREB protein levels or DNA binding, it stimulates kinases that activate CREB by stimulating phosphorylation at Ser133 *(35)*. In addition, PTHrP induces c-Fos protein production and enhances AP-1 binding to its consensus element. This stimulation of CREB and AP-1 signaling is associated with an increase in gene transcription while inhibition of their signaling leads to inhibition of PTHrP effects on both proliferation and maturation of chondrocytes *(35)*. Thus, the transcription factor CREB has a role in skeletal development through involvement in PTHrP signaling and direct regulation of chondrocyte differentiation.

In addition to PTHrP signaling through cAMP, several other growth factors, including insulin-like growth factor, epidermal growth factor, TGF-β, fibroblast growth factor, and platelet-derived growth factor have also been shown to promote the phosphorylation of CREB family members *(42,43)*, suggesting a potential role for these factors in cell proliferation. Therefore, it is possible that CREB can transduce signals of other signaling pathways and its role in skeletal development is more generalized than just PTHrP signaling. This idea is supported by transgenic animal models exhibiting disruptions in the CREB gene. CREB-null mice targeting all isoforms *(44)* have been generated and are smaller than their littermates and die immediately after birth from respiratory distress. This is similar to the fate of PTHrP knockout animals, which are runted and also die in the neonatal period of respiratory distress. Nevertheless, the skeleton of the CREB-null mice has not been analyzed and the causes for the observed dwarfism are not yet investigated. The function of CREB in skeletal formation also was assessed through the generation of transgenic mice in which a dominant-negative form of CREB (A-CREB; ref. *45*) was driven by the cartilage-specific collagen type II promoter/enhancer in the growth plate chondrocytes *(46)*. A-CREB transgenic mice show short-limb dwarfism and a markedly reduced rib cage that may underlie their perinatal lethality. Consistent with a pronounced defect in growth plate development, tibias from transgenic embryos were bowed and exhibited asymmetric deposition of cortical bone beneath perichondrium. The proposed cause for the severe dwarfism was inhibition of proliferation. In agreement with previous studies, the expression of the dominant-negative CREB inhibits proliferation, lowering the proportion of BrdU-positive cells in the growth plate and reducing the height of the proliferative zone in developing limbs. However, contrary to the initial hypothesis, the A-CREB transgenic mouse limbs exhibit delay of maturation accompanied by delay of vascularization and bone formation *(46)*. In contrast, in isolated chick chondrocytes cultures, the same dominant-negative CREB accelerates the process of maturation and inhibits PTHrP *(35)*. Similarly, inhibition of PTHrP signaling through disruption of the hormone, its receptor, or Gsα signaling leads to premature hypertrophy in the growth plate *(13,47,48)*. The discrepancy between the different studies may reside in the difference between the two systems used. Studies performed in a cell culture system allow perturbation of CREB signaling at later stages of chondrocyte development. In contrast, in the transgenic mice, Long et al. *(46)* used a system in which the transgene is overexpressed at very early embryonic stages. Therefore, the phenotype might reflect the effect of perturbation of CREB signaling at earlier stages of skeletal development, such as chondrogenesis, cell aggregation, and nodule formation or transition from precursor (mesenchymal) cells to chondrocytes. The alterations in these steps may have an overall negative impact on the normal progression of skeletal development by causing delay in the cartilage anlage formation.

TGF-β Signaling

TGF-β receptor binding results in activation of the TGF-β type I receptor with phosphorylation events that activate downstream signaling pathways, including the Smad family of transcription fac-

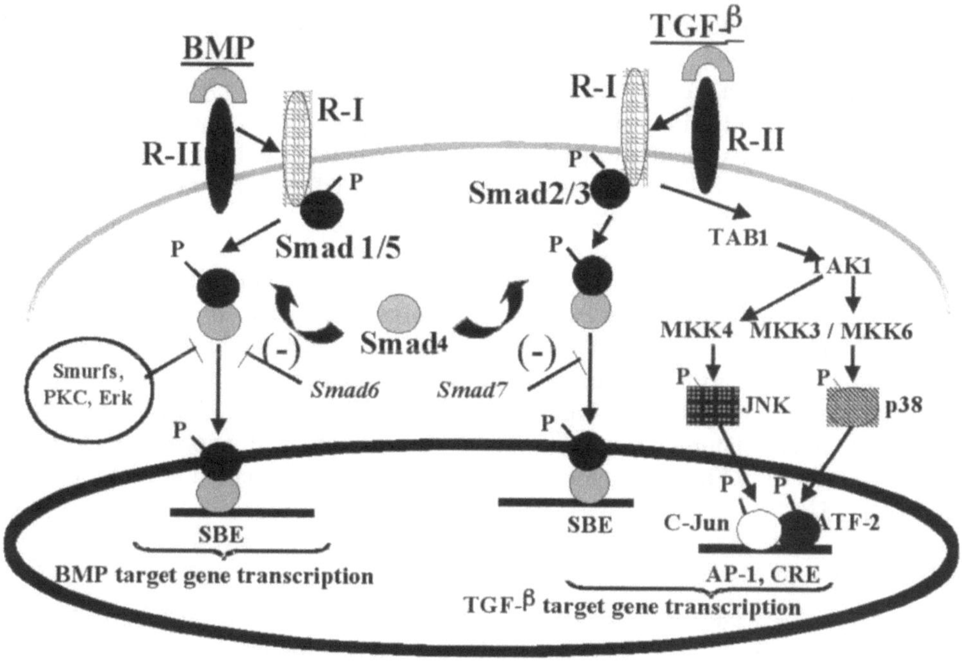

Fig. 3. Signal transduction pathway of TGF-β and BMP signaling. BMP signaling involves activation of Smad1, 5, and 8 and coupling with the coactivator Smad4, whereas negative regulators, such as Smad6, Smurfs, PKC, and ERK maintain a negative feedback loop. TGF-β signaling pathway involves activation of both Smad2 and 3 and the MAPK family members whereas Smad7 acts in an inhibitory manner.

tors *(49)* and the mitogen-activated protein kinase (MAPK) family (Fig. 3; ref. *50*) In chondrocytes, overexpression of either Smad2 or Smad3 mimics TGF-β treatment, whereas the dominant negatives are capable of diminishing TGF-β effects on cell differentiation *(51)*. Targeted disruption of the Smad3 gene in mice causes a skeletal phenotype consistent with inhibition of TGF-β signaling, with progressive loss of articular cartilage resembling osteoarthritis and enhanced terminal differentiation of epiphyseal chondrocytes *(25)*.

Activation of the MAPK family (the extracellular signal-regulated kinase, the c-Jun N-terminal kinase, and the p38 kinase) involves stimulation of transcription factors from the CREB/ATF and AP-1 family *(52–54)*. Not surprisingly, many promoters of the TGF-β-regulated genes contain either AP-1 sites, such as the PAI-1 *(55)*, TIMP-1 *(56)*, TGF-ββ1 *(57)*, c-Jun *(58)*, and α2(I) collagen *(59)* or CREB/ATF binding sites, such as fibronectin *(60)*, cyclinD1 *(37)*, and cyclin A *(38)*.

The presence of multiple DNA binding sites for different transcription factors allows for transcriptional crosstalk between Smads and the MAPKs during TGF-β-induced gene expression. Recent results from our group demonstrate that both Smad3 and ATF-2 contribute to TGF-β-mediated effects on chondrocyte differentiation, and both participate in the induction of PTHrP in chondrocytes *(36)*. TGF-β is capable of phosphorylating and activating transcription factor ATF-2 and, subsequently, ATF-2 cooperates with Smad3 to regulate TGF-β-regulated gene transcription. Either ATF-2 or Smad3 overexpressing chondrocytes exhibit delay of maturation with lower levels of *colX* but higher levels of *PTHrP*. Similarly, overexpression of the dominant negatives ATF-2 and Smad3 either alone or together block TGF-β inhibitory effects on chondrocyte maturation and *colX*. The role of ATF-2 seems to be restricted to TGF-β but not BMP because overexpression of either ATF-2 or its dominant-negative does not alter BMP signaling *(36)*.

Although the total disruption of TGF-β signaling in vivo accelerates chondrocyte maturation *(20)*, the relative contribution of ATF-2 as mediator of TGF-β effects is not entirely understood. Disruption of the ATF-2 gene results in a skeletal phenotype similar to hypochondrodysplasia *(61)*. Although the rate of survival is significantly diminished, the homozygotes reached adulthood and had a normal life span despite uniform dwarfism and disorganization of the growth plate. In vivo labeling of cartilage cells confirms that cartilage cell division is dramatically reduced, possibly as the result of reduced levels of cyclin D1 and cyclin A *(37,38)*.

However, further analysis of these mice demonstrated the presence of a mutant protein generated through alternative splicing that allowed residual ATF-2 signaling. Subsequently, Maekawa et al. designed a new ATF-2-null mouse that exhibits disruption in exon 10, corresponding to the DNA binding domain, which inactivates all the isoforms *(62)*. These mice die of meconium aspiration at the time of birth, therefore not allowing one to determine whether absence of ATF-2 function and signaling is associated with postnatal abnormalities in growth. Interestingly, however, these mice have no apparent skeletal abnormalities at the time of birth. A similar situation has been encountered for the Smad3 –/– mouse, whose phenotype (accelerated chondrocyte maturation) becomes apparent 3 wk after birth *(25)*.

BMP Signaling

BMP signaling involves direct transcriptional activation of receptor-regulated Smads 1, 5, and 8 with subsequent translocation to the nucleus and binding to specific DNA sequences (Fig. 3). This event has been shown to induce the differentiation of isolated chondrocytes and there are numerous points of control of these signaling events. Secreted extracellular molecules, including chordin, noggin, follistatin, and others, bind to BMPs and prevent their interaction with cell surface receptors. Our laboratory showed that chondrocytes express chordin and that overexpression of chordin in the chick limb bud results in a delay of maturation *(63)*. This suggests that BMP expression is necessary for chondrocyte maturation to proceed. Smad6 is an intracellular signaling molecule that acts as a negative regulator of BMP signaling. Smad6 blocks Smad1, 5, or 8 signaling by preventing receptor activation *(64,65)* as well as binding to the coactivator Smad4 *(66)*. Smad6 expression is induced by BMP-2 *(67)*, and we have shown that gain of Smad6 function inhibits chondrocyte maturation while loss of function induces maturation *(68)*.

Smad ubiquitination regulatory factor 1 (Smurf1), a member of the E3 class of ubiquitin ligases, is another inhibitor of BMP signaling that targets the Smads. Smurf1 specifically targets Smad1 and Smad5 for ubiquitination, leading to proteosomal degradation *(69)*. The degradation of Smad1 and 5 by Smurf1 occurs independent of BMP receptor activation, indicating that Smurf1 does not function downstream of activated Smads to turn off BMP signals, but may rather adjust the basal level of Smads available for BMP signaling *(69)*.

PTHrP blocks BMP effects on chondrocyte differentiation. Although work in our laboratory *(70)* has shown that PKA/CREB is responsible for this effect, this is likely not the sole mechanism. Other kinases, such as PKC and extracellular signal-regulated kinase, are activated by PTHrP and may directly alter Smad1 signaling through phosphorylation at residues important in DNA binding *(71)* or at residues involved in the translocation to the nucleus *(72)*. In addition, virtually nothing is known with respect to PTHrP interaction with Smurfs; therefore, future experiments will be needed for a complete elucidation of PTHrP/BMP antagonism in chondrocyte.

REFERENCES

1. Buckwalter, J. A., Mower, D., Ungar, R., Schaeffer, J., and Ginsberg, B. (1986) Morphometric analysis of chondrocyte hypertrophy. *J. Bone Joint. Surg. Am.* **68,** 243–255.
2. Linsenmayer, T. F., Chen, Q. A., Gibney, E., Gordon, M. K., Marchant, J. K., Mayne, R., et al. (1991) Collagen types IX and X in the developing chick tibiotarsus: analyses of mRNAs and proteins. *Development* **111,** 191–196.

3. Warman, M. L., Abbott, M., Apte, S. S., Hefferon, T., McIntosh, I., Cohn, D. H., et al. (1993) A type X collagen mutation causes Schmid metaphyseal chondrodysplasia. *Nat. Genet.* **5,** 79–82.
4. Gress, C. and Jacenko, O. (2000) Growth plate compressions and altered hematopoiesis in collagen X null mice. *J. Cell. Biol.* **149,** 983–993.
5. Anderson, H. C., Hsu, H. H., Morris, D. C., Fedde, K. N., and Whyte, M. P. (1997) Matrix vesicles in osteomalacic hypophosphatasia bone contain apatite-like mineral crystals. *Am. J. Pathol.* **15,** 1555–1561.
6. Erlebacher, A., Filvaroff, E. H., Gitelman, S. E., and Derynck, R. (1995) Toward a molecular understanding of skeletal development. *Cell* **80,** 371–378.
7. Baron, R. E. (1996) Anatomy and ultrastructure of the bone, in *Primer on the Metabolic Bone Diseases and Disorders of Mineral Metabolism,* (Favus, M. J., ed.), Lippencott-Raven, New York, pp. 3–10.
8. Ingham, P. W. (1998) Transducing hedgehog: the story so far. *EMBO J.* **17,** 3505–3511.
9. Vortkamp, A., Lee, K., Lanske, B., Segre, G. V., Kronenberg, H. M., and Tabin, C. J. (1996) Regulation of rate of cartilage differentiation by Indian hedgehog and PTH-related protein. *Science* **273,** 613–622.
10. St-Jacques, B., Hammerschmidt, M., and McMahon, A. P. (1999) Indian hedgehog signaling regulates proliferation and differentiation of chondrocytes and is essential for bone formation. *Genes Dev.* **13,** 2072–2086.
11. Weir, E. C., Philbrick, W. M., Amling, M., Neff, L. A., Baron, R., and Broadus, A. E. (1996) Targeted overexpression of parathyroid hormone-related peptide in chondrocytes causes chondrodysplasia and delayed endochondral bone formation. *Proc. Natl. Acad. Sci. USA* **93,** 10240–10245.
12. Schipani, E., Lanske, B., Hunzelman, J., Luz, A., Kovacs, C. S., Lee, K., et al. (1997) Targeted expression of con-stitutively active receptors for parathyroid hormone and parathyroid hormone-related peptide delays endochondral bone formation and rescues mice that lack parathyroid hormone-related peptide. *Proc. Natl. Acad. Sci. USA* **94,** 13689–13694.
13. Karaplis, A. C., Luz, A., Glowacki, J., Bronson, R. T., Tybulewicz, V. L., Kronenberg, H. M., et al. (1994) Lethal skeletal dysplasia from targeted disruption of the parathyroid hormone-related peptide gene. *Genes Dev.* **8,** 277–289.
14. Lanske, B., Karaplis, A. C., Lee, K., Luz, A., Vortkamp, A., Pirro, A., et al. (1996) PTH/PTHrP receptor in early development and Indian hedgehog-regulated bone growth (see comments). *Science* **273,** 663–666.
15. Alvarez, J., Sohn, P., Zeng, X., Doetschman, T., Robbins, D. J., and Serra, R. (2002) TGFβ2 mediates the effects of Hedgehog on hypertrophic differentiation and PTHrP expression. *Development* **129,** 1913–1924.
16. Long, F. and Linsenmayer, T. F. (1998) Regulation of growth region cartilage proliferation and differentiation by perichondrium. *Development* **125,** 1067–1073.
17. Serra, R., Karaplis, A., and Sohn, P. (1999) Parathyroid hormone-related peptide (PTHrP)-dependent and -independent effects of transforming growth factor beta (TGF-beta) on endochondral bone formation. *J. Cell Biol.* **145,** 783–794.
18. Pateder, D. B., Rosier, R. N., Schwarz, E. M., Reynolds, P. R., Puzas, J. E., D'Souza, M., et al. (2000) PTHrP expression in chondrocytes, regulation by TGF-beta, and interactions between epiphyseal and growth plate chondrocytes. *Exp. Cell Res.* **256,** 555–562.
19. Pateder, D., Ferguson, C., Ionescu, A., Schwarz, E., Rosier, R., Puzas, J., et al. (2001) PTHrP expression in chick sternal chondrocytes is regulated by TGF-beta through Smad-mediated signaling. *J. Cell. Physiol.* **188,** 343–351.
20. Serra, R., Johnson, M., Filvaroff, E., LaBorde, J., Sheehan, D., Derynck, R., et al. (1997) Expression of a truncated, kinase-defective TGF-beta type II receptor in mouse skeletal tissue promotes terminal chondrocyte differentiation and osteoarthritis. *J. Cell Biol.* **139,** 541–552.
21. Iwasaki, M., Le, A., and Helms, J. A. (1997) Expression of Indian Hedgehog, bone morphogenetic protein 6 and gli during skeletal morphogenesis. *Mech. Dev.* **69,** 197–202.
22. O'Keefe, R. J., Schwarz, E. M., Ionescu, A. M., Zuscik, M. J., Zhang, X., Puzas, J. E., et al. (2003) TGF-β and chondrocyte differentiation. *Mol. Biol. Orthopaed.* Section VI, pp. 289–301, edited by C. H. Evans and R. N. Rosier.
23. D'Angelo, M., Billings, P. C., Pacifici, M., Leboy, P. S., and Kirsch, T. (2001) Authentic matrix vesicles contain active metalloproteases (MMP) A role for matriz vesicle-associated MMP-13 in activation of transforming growth factor beta. *J. Biol. Chem.* **276,** 11347–11353.
24. Bonewald, L. F., Oreffo, R. O., Lee, C. H., Park-Snyder, S., Twardzik, D., and Mundy, G. R. (1997) Effects of retinol on activation of latent transforming growth factor beta by isolated chondrocytes. *Endocrinology* **138,** 657–666.
25. Yang, X., Chen, L., Xu, X., Li, C., Huang, C., and Deng, C. (2001) TGF-beta/Smad3 signals repress chondrocyte hypertrophic differentiation and are required for maintaining articular cartilage. *J. Cell Biol.* **153,** 35–46.
26. Zou, H., Wieser, R., Massague, J., and Niswander, L. (1997) Distinct roles of type I bone morphogenetic protein receptors in the formation and differentiation of cartilage. *Genes Dev.* **11,** 2191–2203.
27. Enomoto-Iwamoto, M., Iwamoto, M., Mukudai, Y., Kawakami, Y., Nohno, T., Higuchi, Y., et al. (1998) Bone morphogenetic signaling is required for maintenance of differentiated phenotype, control of proliferation, and hypertrophy in chondrocytes. *J. Cell Biol.* **140,** 409–418.
28. Lyons, K., Hogan, B., and Robertson, E. (1995) Colocalization of BMP7 and BMP2 RNAs suggests that these factors cooperatively mediate tissue interactions during murine development. *Mech. Dev.* **50,** 71–73.
29. Asahina, I., Sampath, T. K., and Hauschka, P. V. (1996) Human osteogenic protein-1 induces chondroblastic, osteoblastic, and/or adipocytic differentiation of clonal murine target cells. *Exp. Cell Res.* **222,** 38–47.
30. Duprez, D. M., Coltey, M., Amthor, H., Brickell, P. M., and Tickle, C. (1996) Bone morphogenetic protein-2 (BMP-2) inhibits muscle development and promotes cartilage formation in chick limb bud cultures. *Dev. Biol.* **174,** 448–452.
31. Pathi, S., Rutenberg, J., Johnson, R., and Vortkamp, A. (1999) Interaction of Ihh and BMP/Noggin signaling during cartilage differentiation. *Dev. Biol.* **209,** 239–253.

32. Grimsrud, C. D., Romano, P. R., D'Souza, M., Puzas, J. E., Reynolds, P. R., Rosier, R. N., and O'Keefe, R. J. (1999) BMP-6 is an autocrine stimulator of chondrocyte differentiation. *J. Bone Miner. Res.* **14,** 475–482.
33. Luca, F. D., Barnes, K. M., Uyeda, J. A., De-Levi, S., Abad, V., Palese, T., et al. (2001) Regulation of growth plate chondrogenesis by bone morphogenetic protein-2. *Endocrinology* **142,** 430–436.
34. Zhang, D., Schwarz, E. M., Puzas, J. E., Zuscik, M. J., Rosier, R. N., and O'Keefe, R. J. (2003) ALK2 functions as a BMP type I receptor and induces Indian Hedgehog in chondrocytes during skeletal development. *J. Bone Miner. Res.* **18,** 1593–1604.
35. Ionescu, A. M., Schwarz, E. M., Vinson, C., Puzas, J. E., Rosier, R., Reynolds, P. Ret al. (2001) PTHrP modulates chondrocyte differentiation through AP-1 and CREB signaling. *J. Biol. Chem.* **276,** 11639–11647.
36. Ionescu, A. M., Schwarz, E. M., Zuscik, M. J., Drissi, H., Puzas, J. E., Rosier, R. N., et al. (2003) ATF-2 cooperates with Smad3 to mediate TGF-β effects on chondrocyte maturation. *Exp. Cell Res.* **288,** 198–207.
37. Beier, F., Lee, R. J., Taylor, A. C., Pestell, R. G., and LuValle, P. (1999) Identification of the cyclin D1 gene as a target of activating transcription factor 2 in chondrocytes. *Proc. Natl. Acad. Sci. USA* **96,** 1433–1438.
38. Beier, F., Taylor, A., and LuValle, P. (2000) Activating transcription factor 2 is necessary for maximal activity and serum induction of the cyclin A promoter in chondrocytes. *J. Biol. Chem.* **275,** 12948–12953.
39. Zuscik, M. J., Puzas, J. E., Rosier, R. N., Gunter, K. K., and Gunter, T. E. (1994) Cyclic-AMP-dependent protein kinase activity is not required by parathyroid hormone to stimulate phosphoinositide signaling in chondrocytes but is required to transduce the hormone's proliferative effect. *Arch. Biochem. Biophys.* **315,** 352–361.
40. Zuscik, M. J., Gunter, T. E., Rosier, R. N., Gunter, K. K., and Puzas, J. E. (1994) Activation of phosphoinositide metabolism by parathyroid hormone in growth plate chondrocytes. *Cell Calcium* **16,** 112–122.
41. Abou-Samra, A. B., Juppner, H., Force, T., Freeman, M. W., Kong, X. F., Schipani, E., et al. (1992) Expression cloning of a common receptor for parathyroid hormone and parathyroid hormone-related peptide from rat osteoblast-like cells: a single receptor stimulates intracellular accumulation of both cAMP and inositol triphosphates and increases intracellular free calcium. *Proc. Natl. Acad. Sci. USA* **89,** 2732–2736.
42. Montminy, M. (1997) Transcriptional regulation by cyclic AMP. *Annu. Rev. Biochem.* **66,** 807–822.
43. Cesare, D. D., and Sassone-Corsi, P. (2000) Transcriptional regulation by cyclic AMP-responsive factors. *Prog. Nucleic Acid Res. Mol. Biol.* **64,** 343–369.
44. Rudolph, D., Tafuri, A., Gass, P., Hammerling, G. J., Arnold, B., and Schutz, G. (1998) Impaired fetal T cell development and perinatal lethality in mice lacking the cAMP response element binding protein. *Proc. Natl. Acad. Sci. USA* **95,** 4481–4486.
45. Ahn, S., Olive, M., Aggarwal, S., Krylov, D., Ginty, D. D., and Vinson, C. (1998) A dominant-negative inhibitor of CREB reveals that it is a general mediator of stimulus-dependent transcription of c-fos. *Mol. Cell Biol.* **18,** 967–977.
46. Long, F., Schipani, E., Asahara, H., Kronenberg, H., and Montminy, M. (2001) The CREB family of activators is required for endochondral bone development. *Development* **128,** 541–550.
47. Amizuka, N., Warshawsky, H., Henderson, J. E., Goltzman, D., and Karaplis, A. C. (1994) Parathyroid hormone-related peptide-depleted mice show abnormal epiphyseal cartilage development and altered endochondral bone formation. *J. Cell Biol.* **126,** 1611–1623.
48. Chung, U., Wei, W., Schipani, E., Hunzelman, J., Weinstein, L., and Kronenberg, H. (2000) In vivo function of stimulatory G protein (Gs) in the growth plate. *J. Bone Miner. Res.* **15,** S175.
49. Wrana, J., Attisano, L., Carcamo, J., Zentella, A., Doody, J., Laiho, M., Wang, X., and Massague, J. (1992) TGF beta signals through a heteromeric protein kinase receptor complex. *Cell* **71,** 1003–1014.
50. Mulder, K. (2000) Role of Ras and Mapks in TGFbeta signaling. *Cytokine & Growth Factor Rev.* **11,** 23–35.
51. Ferguson, C., Schwarz, E., Reynolds, P., Puzas, J., Rosier, R., and O'Keefe, R. (2000) Smad2 and 3 mediate transforming growth factor-beta1-induced inhibition of chondrocyte maturation. *Endocrinology* **141,** 4728–4735.
52. Xing, J., Ginty, D., and Greenberg, M. (1996) Coupling of the RAS-MAPK pathway to gene activation by RSK2, a growth factor-regulated CREB kinase. *Science* **273,** 959–963.
53. Jiang, Y., Chen, C., Li, Z., Guo, W., Gegner, J., Lin, S., and Han, J. (1996) Characterization of the structure and function of a new mitogen-activated protein kinase (p38beta). *J. Biol. Chem.* **271,** 17920–17926.
54. Derijard, B., Hibi, M., Wu, I., Barrett, T., Su, B., Deng, T., Karin, M., and Davis, R. (1994) JNK1: a protein kinase stimulated by UV light and Ha-Ras that binds and phosphorylates the c-Jun activation domain. *Cell* **76,** 1025–1037.
55. Keeton, M. R., Curriden, S. A., Zonneveld, A. J. V., and Loskutoff, D. J. (1991) Identification of regulatory sequences in the type 1 plasminogen activator inhibitor gene responsive to transforming growth factor beta. *J. Biol. Chem.* **266,** 23048–23052.
56. Campbell, C. E., Flenniken, A. M., Skup, D., and Williams, B. R. G. (1991) Identification of a serum- and phorbol ester-responsive element in the murine tissue inhibitor of metalloproteinase gene. *J. Biol. Chem.* **266,** 7199–7206.
57. Kim, S. J., Angel, P., Lafyatis, R., Hattori, K., Kim, K. Y., Sporn, M. B., et al. (1990) Autoinduction of transforming growth factor beta 1 is mediated by the AP-1 complex. *Mol. Cellular Biol.* **10,** 1492–1497.
58. Angel, P., Hattori, K., Smeal, T., and Karin, M. (1991) The *jun* proto-oncogene is positively autoregulated by its product, Jun/AP-1. *Cell* **55,** 875–885.
59. Chung, K. Y., Agarwal, A., Uitto, J., and Mauviel, A. (1996) An AP-1 binding sequence is essential for regulation of the human a2(I) collagen (COL1A2) promoter activity by transforming growth factor-β. *J. Biol. Chem.* **271,** 3272–3278.
60. Pesce, C., Nogues, G., Alonso, C., Baralle, F., and Kornblihtt, A. (1999) Interaction between the (-170) CRE and the (-150) CCAAT box is necessary for efficient activation of the fibronectin gene promoter by cAMP and ATF-2. *FEBS Lett.* **457,** 445–451.

61. Reimold, A. M., Grusby, M. J., Kosaras, B., Fries, J. W., Mori, R., Maniwa, S., et al. (1996) Chondrodysplasia and neurological abnormalities in ATF-2-deficient mice. *Nature* **379,** 262–265.
62. Maekawa, T., Bernier, F., Sato, M., Nomura, S., Singh, M., Inoue, Y., et al. (1999) Mouse ATF-2 null mutants display features of a severe type of Meconium Aspiration Syndrome. *J. Biol. Chem.* **274,** 17813–17819.
63. Zhang, D., Ferguson, C. M., O'Keefe, R. J., Puzas, J. E., Rosier, R. N., and Reynolds, P. R. (2002) A role for the BMP antagonist chordin in endochondral ossification. *J. Bone Miner. Res.* **17,** 293–300.
64. Imamura, T., Takase, M., Nishihara, A., Oeda, E., Hanai, J., Kawabata, M., and Miyazono, K. (1997) Smad6 inhibits signalling by the TGF-beta superfamily. *Nature* **389,** 622–626.
65. Lebrun, J. J., Takabe, K., Chen, Y., and Vale, W. (1999) Roles of pathway-specific and inhibitory Smads in activin receptor signaling. *Mol. Endocrinol.* **13,** 15–23.
66. Hata, A., Lagna, G., Massague, J., and Hemmati-Brivanlou, A. (1998) Smad6 inhibits BMP/Smad1 signaling by specifically competing with the Smad4 tumor suppressor. *Genes Dev.* **12,** 186–197.
67. Ishida, W., Hamamoto, T., Kusanagi, K., Yagi, K., Kawabata, M., Takehara, K., et al. (2000) Smad6 is a Smad1/5-induced smad inhibitor. Characterization of bone morphogenetic protein-responsive element in the mouse Smad6 promoter. *J. Biol. Chem.* **275,** 6075–6079.
68. Li, X., Ionescu, A. M., Schwarz, E. M., Zhang, X., Drissi, H., Puzas, J. E., et al. (2003) Smad6 is induced by BMP-2 and modulates chondrocyte differentiation. *J. Orthopaed. Res.* **21,** 908–913.
69. Zhu, H., Havsak, P., Abdollah, S., Wrana, J. L., and Thomsen, G. H. (1999) A Smad ubiquitin ligase targets the BMP pathway and affects embryonic pattern formation. *Nature* **400,** 687–693.
70. Ionescu, A. M., Drissi, A. M., Schwarz, E. M., Kato, M., Puzas, J. E., McCance, D. J., Rosier, R. N., Zuscik, M. J., and O'Keefe, R. J. (2003) CREB cooperates with BMP-stimulated Smad signaling to enhance transcription of the Smad6 promoter. *J. Cell. Physiol.*, in press.
71. Yakymovych, I., Ten Dijke, P., Heldin, C. H., and Souchelnytskyi, S. (2001) Regulation of Smad signaling by protein kinase C. *FASEB J.* **15,** 553–555.
72. Kretzschmar, M., Doody, J., and Massague, J. (1997) Opposing BMP and EGF signalling pathways converge on the TGF-beta family mediator Smad1. *Nature* **389,** 618–622.

4

Continuous Expression of *Cbfa1* in Nonhypertrophic Chondrocytes Uncovers Its Ability to Induce Hypertrophic Chondrocyte Differentiation and Partially Rescues Cbfa1-Deficient Mice

Shu Takeda, Jean-Pierre Bonnamy, Michael J. Owen, Patricia Ducy, and Gerard Karsenty

INTRODUCTION

Chondrocytes play critical roles at several stages of endochondral ossification. At the onset of skeletal development, in the areas of the skeleton that will undergo endochondral ossification, undifferentiated mesenchymal cells form condensations that have the shape of the future skeletal elements. Cells within these mesenchymal condensations differentiate into chondrocytes that express specific molecular markers, such as *α1(II) collagen*, whereas the remaining undifferentiated mesenchymal cells at the periphery of the condensations form the perichondrium (for review, *see* ref. *1*). Once these cartilaginous models have formed, chondrocytes in their centers further differentiate into hypertrophic chondrocytes. At the time chondrocyte hypertrophy occurs, the perichondrial cells differentiate into osteoblasts to form, around the cartilaginous core, the bone collar *(2)*.

Hypertrophic chondrocytes can be subdivided into two populations: the prehypertrophic chondrocytes that express *α1(II) collagen* predominantly and the hypertrophic chondrocytes proper that express *α1(X) collagen (3,4)* and become surrounded by a calcified extracellular matrix *(5)*. Through a vascular endothelium growth factor (VEGF)-dependent pathway, the extracellular matrix surrounding hypertrophic chondrocytes favors vascular invasion followed by degradation of the calcified cartilage matrix by chondroclasts *(6,7)*. The cartilaginous matrix is then replaced by a bone matrix made mostly of type I collagen secreted by invading osteoblasts coming from the bone collar. The ossification process proceeds centripetally, consuming much of the cartilage scaffold. As this cartilaginous front meets the distal ends of a future bone, distal chondrocytes proliferate before they hypertrophy. This zone of proliferating and hypertrophic chondrocytes becomes organized in columns forming the growth plate localized at each end of a bone (for review, *see* ref. *1*). The growth plates will be responsible for linear skeletal growth. This sequence of events illustrates the pivotal role of chondrocyte hypertrophy as a mandatory step between a cartilaginous scaffold and bona fide bone.

A complex network of regulatory molecules controls the proliferation and/or differentiation of various chondrocyte subpopulations. Early during development, the transcription factor Sox9 is required

From: *The Skeleton: Biochemical, Genetic, and Molecular Interactions in Development and Homeostasis*
Edited by: E. J. Massaro and J. M. Rogers © Humana Press Inc., Totowa, NJ

to form the mesenchymal condensations *(8)*. Genetic evidence in mouse and human show that FGF receptors play a critical role in the control of chondrocyte proliferation (for review, *see* ref. 9). Likewise, loss- and gain-of-function experiments have demonstrated that the growth factor parathyroid hormone-related peptide (PTHrP), secreted by cells of the periarticular perichondrium, acts on prehypertrophic chondrocytes to prevent their progression into a hypertrophic phenotype *(10–12)*. Indian hedgehog (Ihh), another growth factor secreted by the prehypertrophic chondrocytes, delays chondrocyte hypertrophy through a PTHrP-dependent and -independent pathway *(13,14)*. These studies have established that chondrocyte hypertrophy is under the control of genes expressed in prehypertrophic chondrocytes, yet, no transcriptional regulator of chondrocyte hypertrophy has been identified.

One transcription factor that may be involved in the control of chondrocyte hypertrophy is Cbfa1. Early during skeletal development and until 12.5 d postcoitum (dpc), *Cbfa1* is expressed at high level in the cells of the mesenchymal condensations *(15)*. Although *Cbfa1* continues to be expressed at low levels in some chondrocytes beyond 12.5 dpc *(16,17)* its expression is largely osteoblast specific and it is required for osteoblast differentiation in vivo *(18,19)*. Recent in-depth analyses of the Cbfa1-deficient mice have indicated that they also have a defective hypertrophic chondrocyte differentiation in some skeletal elements, raising the hypothesis that Cbfa1 may be one regulator of chondrocyte hypertrophy *(16,17)*. Beyond the control of chondrocyte hypertrophy itself, this is an important question because no transcription factor has been shown to govern the differentiation of both chondrocytes and osteoblasts, two skeletal-specific cell types that are thought to have a common progenitor *(20,21)*.

To assess the role that Cbfa1 may play during chondrocyte hypertrophy, we generated transgenic mice in which *Cbfa1* expression is maintained to a wild-type level in nonhypertrophic chondrocytes throughout development. We also restored *Cbfa1* expression in the mesenchymal condensations of the Cbfa1-deficient mice. Continuous *Cbfa1* expresssion in nonhypertrophic chondrocytes leads to ectopic as well as premature endochondral ossification throughout the skeleton. Using the Cbfa1-deficient mice, we show that this is the result of an ability of Cbfa1 to induce hypertrophic chondrocyte differentiation distinct from its osteoblast differentiation function. Thus, Cbfa1 is required for two critical stages of skeletogenesis: hypertrophic chondrocyte differentiation and osteoblast differentiation. To our knowledge, Cbfa1 is the first transcription factor identified that controls two distinct cellular processes during skeletal development.

RESULTS

Cbfa1 Expression in Prehypertrophic and Hypertrophic Chondrocytes During Skeletogenesis

To define the most appropriate experimental approach to study Cbfa1 function during chondrogenesis, we first analyzed its pattern of expression by *in situ* hybridization in proliferating, prehypertrophic, and hypertrophic chondrocytes between 14.5 dpc and birth. To properly define the identity of the *Cbfa1*-expressing cells, we also performed *in situ* hybridization using as probes *a1(II) collagen*; a marker of proliferating and prehypertrophic chondrocytes; *a1(X) collagen*, a marker of hypertrophic chondrocytes; and *a1(I) collagen*, a marker of osteoblasts *(4)*. In 14.5-dpc embryos *Cbfa1* was expressed in prehypertrophic chondrocytes of the scapula at a higher level than in hypertrophic chondrocytes (Fig. 1A). These cells were confirmed to be prehypertrophic chondrocyte because they expressed *α1(II) collagen* but not *α1(I) collagen* (Fig. 1B,C). In long bones of 16.5-dpc embryos, the overall level of *Cbfa1* expression in chondrocytes is markedly decreased, yet it appears to be slightly higher in prehypertrophic than in hypertrophic chondrocytes in all sections examined (Fig. 1D–G). At birth, *Cbfa1* expression in the growth plate was close to background level, so it was difficult to determine whether prehypertrophic or hypertrophic chondrocytes expressed it at a higher level (Fig. 1H–K). Although this analysis is in agreement overall with the results of Inada et al. *(16)* and Kim et al.

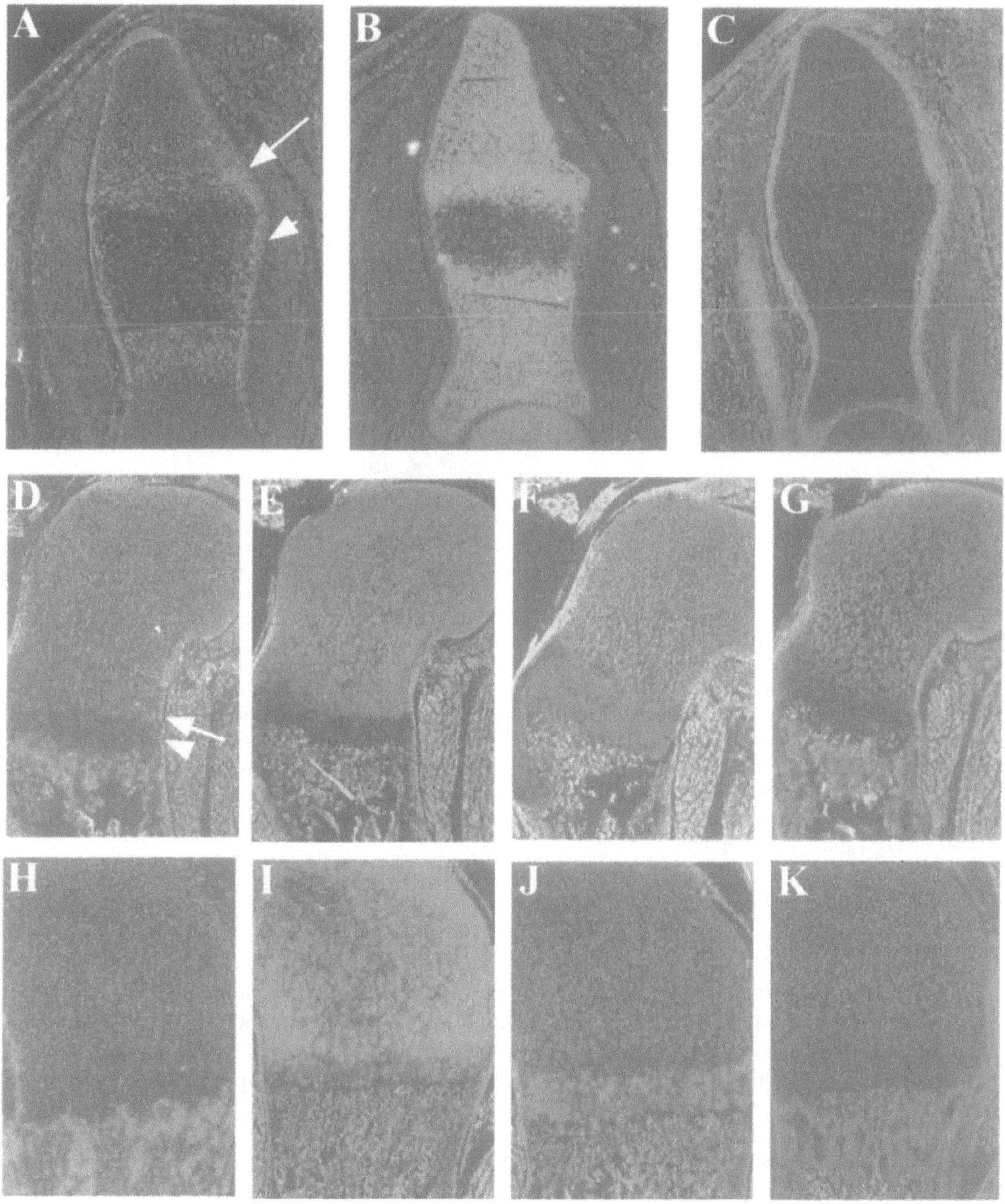

Fig. 1. Analysis of *Cbfa1* expression between 14.5 dpc and birth. Adjacent sections of 14.5 dpc (**A–C**), 16.5 dpc (**D–G**), or newborn (**H–K**) wild-type (wt) mouse embryos were hybridized with *Cbfa1* (**A,D,H**), *α1(II) collagen* (**B,E,I**), *α1(X) collagen* (**F,J**), and *α1(I) collagen* (**C,G,K**) probes. Note the decrease in *Cbfa1* expression in chondrocytes as development proceeds (**A,D,H**) and the stronger expression of *Cbfa1* in prehypertrophic chondrocytes (arrows) compared with hypertrophic chondrocytes in 14.5 and 16.5 dpc embryos (arrowheads; **A** and **D**).

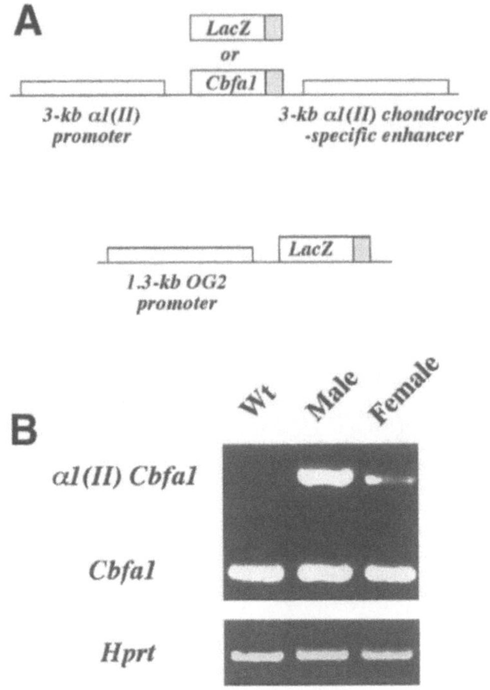

Fig. 2. Generation of α1(II) *Cbfa1* transgenic mice. **A**, Schematic representation of the constructs used. Transgenic mice contain either both the *Cbfa1* cDNA under the control of a chondrocyte-specific *α1(II) collagen* promoter/enhancer cassette and the *LacZ* gene driven by the *Osteocalcin* promoter or the chondrocyte-specific cassette driving *LacZ* alone. **B**, Comparison of endogenous *Cbfa1* expression and of the α1(II) Cbfa1 transgene expression in wt and male and female transgenic mice by reverse transcription. Transgene expression in male transgenic mice is similar to *Cbfa1* expression, whereas in female transgenic mice endogenous *Cbfa1* is expressed at a higher level than the transgene (top). *Hprt*t amplification was used as an internal control (bottom). Gray boxes indicate heterologous polyA regions.

(17), it differs from these two studies on two points. First, it demonstrates a progressive and nearly complete disappearance of *Cbfa1* expression in chondrocytes as skeletogenesis proceeds from 14.5 dpc to birth. Second and most importantly, it shows a higher expression of *Cbfa1* in prehypertrophic than in hypertrophic chondrocytes. This higher expression of *Cbfa1* in prehypertrophic chondrocytes is consistent with a role of Cbfa1 as an inducer of chondrocyte hypertrophy.

Generation of Transgenic Mice Expressing Cbfa1 in Nonhypertrophic Chondrocytes Throughout Development

In the absence of a transgenic mouse expressing, in a inducible manner, *cre* recombinase in proliferating and prehypertrophic chondrocytes, we hypothesized that maintaining *Cbfa1* expression in nonhypertrophic chondrocytes beyond 12.5 dpc would allow us to study its function during chondrocyte hypertrophy. We therefore constructed transgenic mice expressing *Cbfa1* under the control of a 3-kb fragment of the mouse α1(II) collagen promoter and its chondrocyte-specific enhancer (Fig. 2A; ref. *30*). Those mice were termed α1(II) Cbfa1 mice.

Two transgenic mouse lines were obtained. In a first line, male and female transgenic mice had different levels of expression of the transgene (Fig. 2B). In male transgenic mice, the level of expression of the transgene and of endogenous *Cbfa1* were nearly identical (Fig. 2B). These transgenic animals all died at birth. In female transgenic mice, the level of expression of the transgene was significantly lower than the one of endogenous *Cbfa1* (Fig. 2B) and progenies of this line survived several weeks. Male and female transgenic mice developed the same phenotypic abnormalities that only appeared postnatally in α1(II) Cbfa1 female mice. A second transgenic line was obtained. In this second line, the level of expression of the transgene was similar to the level of expression of endogenous *Cbfa1* in both sexes. All transgenic pups died perinatally with phenotypic abnormalities identical to the one observed in the male progenies of the first line.

Ectopic Hypertrophic Chondrocyte Differentiation in α1(II) Cbfa1 Mice

As an initial method to study skeletal cell differentiation, we used alcian blue/alizarin red staining of skeletal preparations *(31)*. Alcian blue stains unmineralized cartilaginous matrices whereas alizarin red stains mineralized cartilaginous and bony matrices. The most striking phenotypic abnormalities in the α1(II) Cbfa1 mice was the presence of extensive zones of mineralization in parts of the skeleton that never normally mineralize (Fig. 3A; ref. *32*). These included the chondrocostal cartilage, the trachea, and the spinous processes. Initially, we focused our analysis on the chondrocostal cartilage.

In the α1(II) Cbfa1 mice dying at birth, the existence of a mineralized and rigid rib cage prevented lung expansion (Fig. 3B). As a result, their lungs did not contain any air at birth (data not shown). In contrast, α1(II) Cbfa1 mice who survived had a normal-appearing rib cage at birth, their chondrocostal cartilage stained with alcian blue as they should until P7 (data not shown). In 14-d-old transgenic mice, however, small patches of mineralized tissues were visible (Fig. 3C). In 21-d-old and 28-d-old transgenic mice, there was a progressive extension of the area staining red (Fig. 3C). To monitor for osteoblast differentiation, the α1(II) Cbfa1 transgene was coinjected with a construct containing a 1.3-kb fragment of the mouse *Osteocalcin gene 2* (*OG2*) promoter driving the *LacZ* gene. This 1.3-kb *OG2* promoter fragment drives the expression of a reporter gene in differentiated osteoblasts in vivo *(33)*. As shown in Fig. 3D, the chondrocostal cartilage of α1(II) Cbfa1 mice stained blue after LacZ staining indicating that there were *Osteocalcin*-expressing cells, that is, differentiated osteoblasts, in this part of the ribs. Such staining was never observed in wild-type animals (Fig. 3D).

We performed a histological analysis of the chondrocostal cartilage at several points during development to monitor the progression of this phenotype. No hypertrophic chondrocytes were observed in wild-type animals at any stage analyzed (Fig. 3I). In contrast, hypertrophic chondrocytes were already present in the chondrocostal cartilage of 16.5-dpc α1(II) Cbfa1 embryos and at birth in female transgenic mice (Fig. 3E,F). In 14-d-old transgenic mice, there was a true growth plate cartilage with resting, proliferating, and hypertrophic chondrocytes (Fig. 3G). In 1-mo-old transgenic mice, there were, below the growth plate, bone trabeculae (Fig. 3H) containing alkaline phosphatase-positive osteoblasts and tartrate-resistant acid phosphatase (TRAP)-positive multinucleated osteoclasts (Fig. 3J,K).

Ectopic skeletal mineralization also was observed in the vertebral column of α1(II) Cbfa1 mice. At birth the atlas, the axis, the third cervical vertebrae, and the vertebrae between T10 and L3 were fused and their spinous processes mineralized (Fig. 3L,M). Histologic examination showed that these mineralized bridges between vertebrae contained both hypertrophic chondrocytes and bone trabecullae (Fig. 3N,O). Ectopic hypertrophic chondrocyte differentiation also affected the larynx: the cricoid and thyroid cartilage stained red in α1(II) Cbfa1 mice at birth (Fig. 3P) and at 2 mo of age, the tracheal rings of transgenic mice contained patches of mineralization that were never seen in wild-type littermates (Fig. 3Q). Histologic examination confirmed the presence of hypertrophic chondrocytes in the thyroid cartilage of newborn α1(II) Cbfal mice and in the tracheal rings of 2-mo-old transgenic mice (Fig. 3R,S). Taken together, these results indicate that continuous expression of *Cbfa1* in nonhypertrophic chondrocytes induces hypertrophic chondrocyte differentiation ectopically; this in turn leads to endochondral ossification.

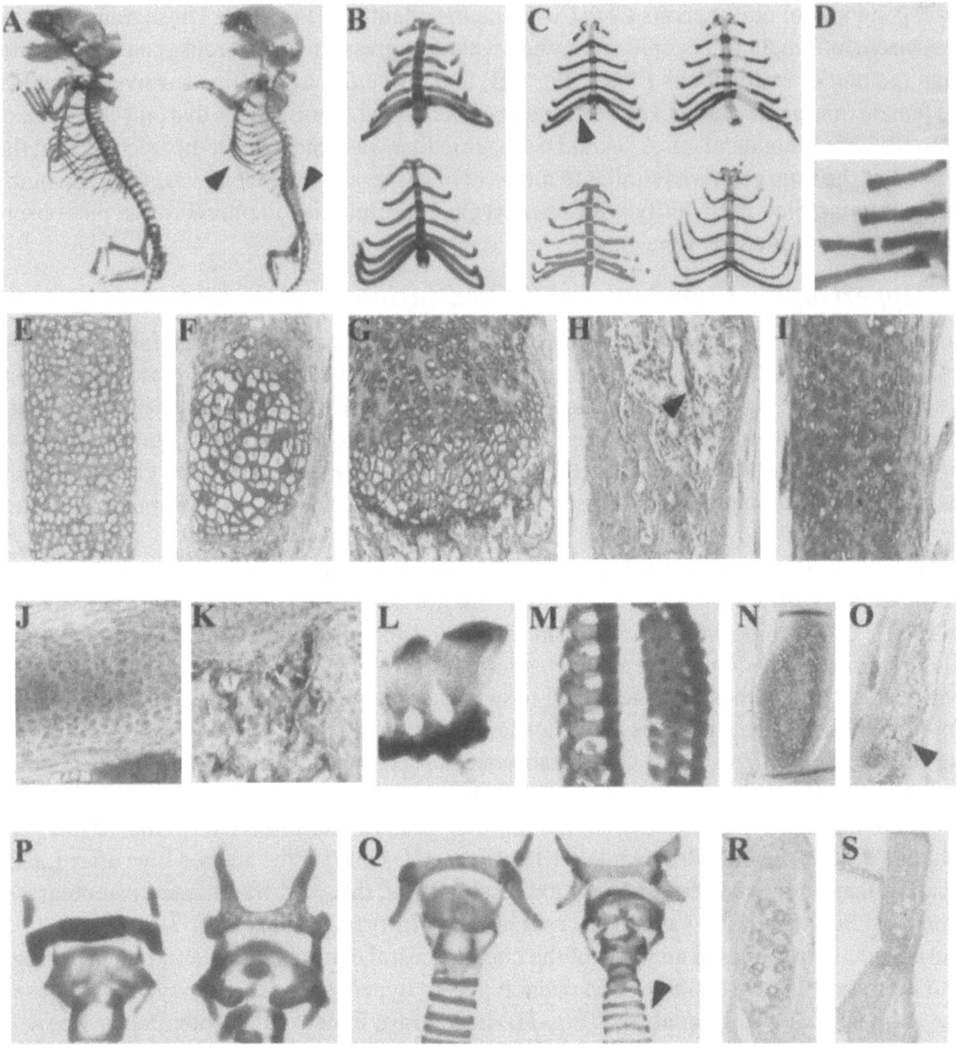

Fig. 3. Ectopic chondrocyte hypertrophy and endochondral ossification in α1(II) Cbfa1 mice. **A–C**, Alcian blue/alizarin red staining of skeletal preparations. **A**, Wt (left) and α1(II) Cbfa1 male (right) mice at birth (P0). Arrow point at sites of ectopic calcification in transgenic mice. **B**, Rib cages of wt (bottom) and α1(II) Cbfa1 male mice (top) at P0. **C**, Rib cages of α1(II) Cbfa1 female mice at P14 (top left), P21 (top right) and P28 (bottom left). Note the progressive appearance of mineralized areas (arrowhead) in the transgenic mice whereas the chondrocostal cartilage of wt mice remains unmineralized (bottom right, P28). **D**, LacZ staining showing *Osteocalcin* expression at P28 in the chondrocostal cartilage of the α1(II) Cbfa1 (bottom) but not of wt mice (top). **E–I**, Alcian blue/eosin staining of sections through the chondrocostal cartilage of α1(II) Cbfa1 males 16.5 dpc (**E**), α1(II) Cbfa1 females at P0 (**F**), P14 (**G**) and P28 (**H**), and wt mice at P28 (**I**). Hypertrophic chondrocytes (**E–G**), then bone trabeculae (**H**, arrowhead), are present in the transgenic but not in wt mice. **J** and **K**, Alkaline phosphatase/TRAP staining of chondrocostal cartilage sections of wt (**J**) and α1(II) Cbfa1 mice at P28 (**K**). **L** and **M**, Alcian blue/alizarin red staining of vertebrae from α1(II) Cbfa1 (**L,M** right) and wt (**M**, left) mice at P0. Fusion of the atlas, the axis and C3 (**L**) and of T10 to L3 in transgenic mice (**M**). **N** and **O**, Alcian blue/oesin staining of sections through the spinous process of vertebrae of wt (**N**) and α1(II) Cbfa1 line A male at P0 (**O**). The wt process is entirely cartilaginous, whereas the transgenic one shows hypertrophic chondrocytes (arrow) and bone matrix. **P** and **Q**, Alcian blue/alizarin red staining of the larynx from wt (left panel in **P** and **Q**) and transgenic mice at birth (right panel in **P**) and at 2 mo of age (right panel in **Q**). Note the mineralization of the tracheal rings in 2-mo-old transgenic mice (arrowhead). **R** and **S**, Alcian blue/eosin staining of tracheal ring sections of 2-mo-old wt (**R**) and α1(II) Cbfa1 (**S**) mice. Hypertrophic chondrocytes are present only in the transgenic mice.

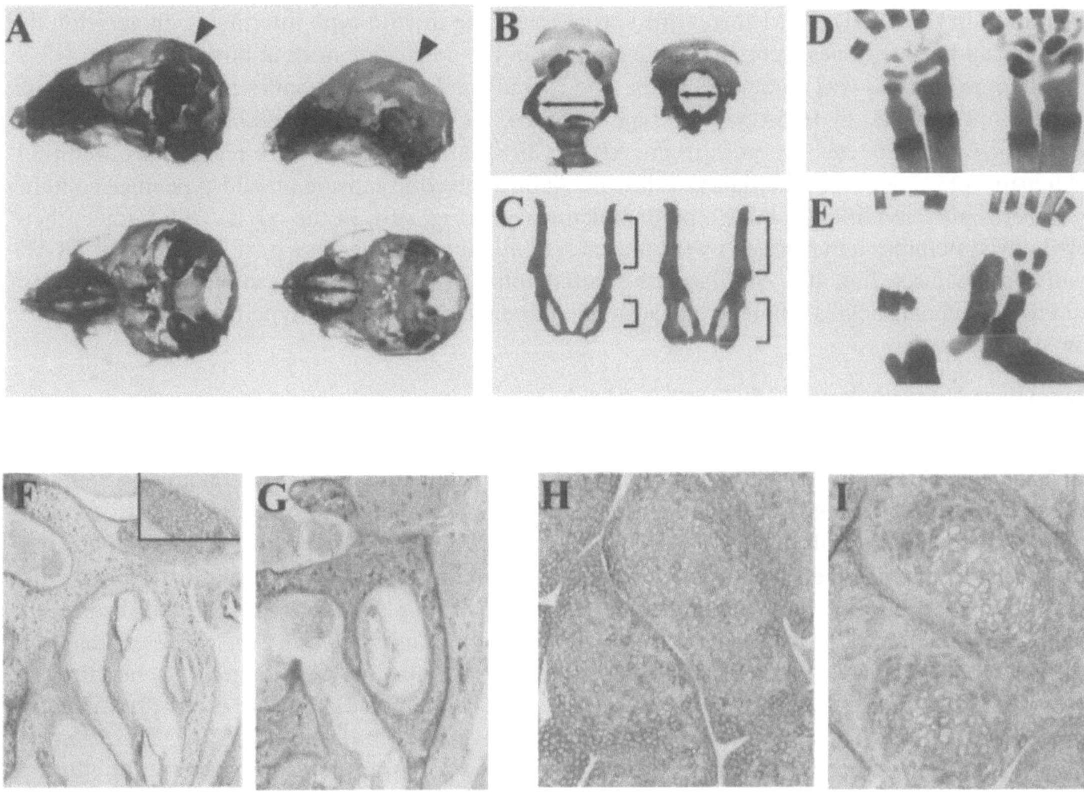

Fig. 4. Premature chondrocyte hypertrophy in α1(II) Cbfa1 mice. **A–E**, Alcian blue/alizarin red staining of skeletal elements. **A**, Premature mineralization of the skull of α1(II) Cbfa1 mice (right) compared with wt littermates (left) at P0 (arrowhead). All bones of the base of the skull are fused together (bottom white asterisk). **B**, Reduction of the size of the foramina magnum (double headed arrows) in transgenic (right) compared with wt mice (left). **C**, Enlarged areas of mineralization (brackets) of the pelvic bones in transgenic (right) compared with wt mice (left). **D** and **E**, Premature mineralization of carpal (**D**) and tarsal (**E**) bones in transgenic (right) compared to wt mice (left). **F** and **G**, Alkaline phosphatase/TRAP staining of sections through the otic capsule of wt (**F**) and α1(II) Cbfa1 mice at P0 (**G**). The wt structure contains only hypertrophic chondrocytes (inset in **F**, alcian blue/eosin staining) whereas the transgenic one contains already alkaline phosphatase positive osteoblasts and TRAP-positive osteoclasts. **H** and **I**, Alcian blue/eosin staining of carpal bones section of wt (**H**) and α1(II) Cbfa1 (**I**) mice at P0. Hypertrophic chondrocytes are present only in the transgenic mice.

Premature Hypertrophic Chondrocyte Differentiation in the α1(II) Cbfa1 Transgenic Mice

In areas of the skeleton normally undergoing endochondral ossification, premature mineralization and/or early ossification also was observed. For instance, the chondrocranium of the α1(II) Cbfa1 mice was fully mineralized at birth (Fig. 4A). All the bones of the base of the skull were fused together. The cartilaginous structures that separate in wild-type mice *(32)*, the basioccipital, exooccipital, supraoccipital, and pterygoid bones were mineralized, fusing them together and with the temporal bones and the otic capsule (Fig. 4A). There was also a marked reduction in the diameter of the foramina magnum in the α1(II) Cbfa1 mice compared with wild-type littermates (Fig. 4B). Premature mineralization was observed throughout the skeleton, although it was more marked in the pelvic, carpal, and tarsal bones (Fig. 4C–E). Among the carpal bones, the triangular and trapezoid bones were entirely mineralized in the α1(II) Cbfa1 mice, this was not the case in wild-type littermates. In addition the scaphoid and hamate bones were partly mineralized in the transgenic mice at birth (Fig. 4D).

Histologic analysis was conducted in the otic capsule and the carpal bones in 16.5-dpc embryos and newborn animals. In 16.5-dpc wild-type embryos, the otic capsule contained only resting and proliferating chondrocytes, whereas in the α1(II) Cbfa1 embryos there were resting, proliferating, and hypertrophic chondrocytes (data not shown). At birth, the otic capsule of wild-type mice containing hypertropic chondrocytes but no bony structures yet (Fig. 4F). In the α1(II) Cbfa1 mice, there were bony structures characterized by the presence of alkaline phosphatase-positive cells and TRAP-positive osteoclasts (Fig. 4G). Similarly, the carpal bones of wild-type mice at birth did not contain hypertrophic chondrocytes whereas in transgenic mice they did contain hypertrophic chondrocytes (Fig. 4H,I).

Abnormal Expression of Molecular Markers of Chondrocyte Hypertrophy in α1(II) Cbfa1 Mice

The presence in the α1(II) Cbfa1 mice of hypertrophic chondrocytes in skeletal areas where they normally are never observed indicated that chondrocyte hypertrophy may be controlled by *Cbfa1*. To demonstrate that this was the case, we also analyzed the expression of molecular markers of proliferating, prehypertrophic, and hypertrophic chondrocytes in chondrocostal cartilage. In 16.5-dpc wild-type embryos, chondrocytes only expressed *α1(II) collagen* (Fig. 5A). In the α1(II) Cbfa1 mice, the level of expression of *α1(II) collagen* was decreased in some ribs (Fig. 5A). *Ihh*, a gene expressed in prehypertrophic chondrocytes, was ectopically expressed revealing the prehypertrophic chondrocytes identity of some cells in the α1(II) Cbfa1 mice (Fig. 5A). There was also a large area of *α1(X) collagen*-expressing cells, that is, hypertrophic chondrocytes in α1(II) Cbfa1 mice (Fig. 5A). The pattern of expression of these molecular markers was the same in newborn transgenic mice except for a further decrease in α1(II) collagen expression and the presence of a small area of *α1(I) collagen*-expressing cells, indicating the beginning of osteogenesis (Fig. 5B).

We performed the same analysis in the scaphoid, a bone of the wrist where premature chondrocyte hypertrophy was noticed. At birth, *Ihh* and *α1(X) collagen* expressions were absent in the wild-type mice, whereas in α1(II) Cbfa1 mice *Ihh*-expressing cells were located at the periphery of the bone and *α1(X) collagen*-expressing cells in the center (Fig. 5C).

Cbfa1 Accelerates Chondrocyte Differentiation in Growth Plate Cartilage

No size difference could be observed at birth between wild-type and α1(II) Cbfa1 mice. However, transgenic mice become growth retarted over time (Fig. 6A). This led us to study their growth plates at 1 mo of age. As seen in Fig. 6B, the growth plate cartilage of α1(II) Cbfa1 mice was shorter than the one of wild-type littermates. The number of resting chondrocytes was decreased, and the columns of proliferating chondrocytes were shorter. In contrast, the size of the hypertrophic region was not altered in the α1(II) Cbfa1 mice. To test whether the reduction in size of the areas containing resting and proliferating chondrocytes was caused by an acceleration in chondrocyte differentiation, we performed BrdU labeling. In the transgenic mice, there were significantly fewer positive cells ($n = 56 \pm 4$) than wild-type mice ($n = 79 \pm 10$). This result demonstrates the acceleration of chondrocyte differentiation in α1(II) Cbfa1 mice (Fig. 6C).

The Transactivation Domain of Cbfa1 Is Required to Induce Chondrocyte Hypertrophy

Next, we asked whether the ectopic chondrocyte hypertrophy observed in these transgenic mice required the transactivation function of Cbfa1. We first generated lines of transgenic mice expressing a truncated form of Cbfa1 lacking the proline, serine, threonine-rich (PST) domain, one major transactivation domain of Cbfa1 (Fig. 7A; ref. 22). Offspring of two different founder lines had no morpho-

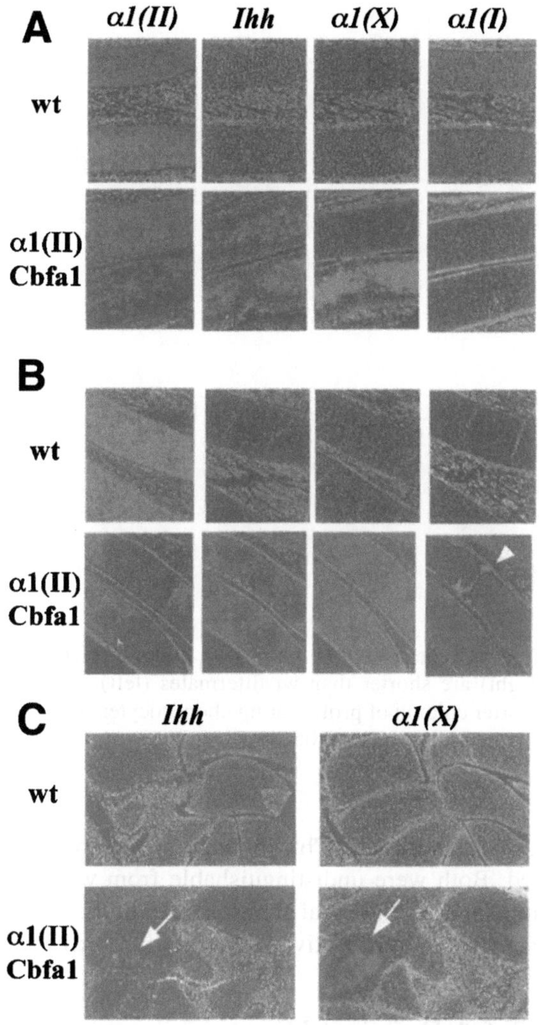

Fig. 5. Abnormal expression of molecular markers of chondrocyte hypertrophy in α1(II) Cbfa1 mice. *In situ* hybridization analysis of 16.5 dpc embryos (**A**) or newborn mice (**B** and **C**). **A** and **B**, Sections through the chondrocostal cartilage. *Alpha1(II) collagen* expression is decreased in transgenic mice compared with wt littermates. *Ihh* and *α1(X) collagen* are only expressed in transgenic mice. Note the *α1(I) collagen* expression in the transgenic cells (arrow in **B**). **C**, Sections through the carpal bones. Transgenic mice show premature expression of *Ihh* and *α1(X) collagen* in the scaphoid (arrows).

logical or histological abnormalities of bone and cartilage (Fig. 7C). We also used an alternative splice form of Cbfa1 that was isolated in the initial cloning effort for an osteoblast-specific transcription factor (Ducy and Karsenty, unpublished observation). This Cbfa1 isoform, temporarily called Cbfa1a, was also cloned as a site of proviral insertion *(34)*. The only difference between Cbfa1 and Cbfa1a is that exon 9, encoding most of the PST domain, has been replaced by another exon localized more 3' and encoding a different PST-rich domain (Fig. 7A and data not shown). Because the DNA-binding domain of Cbfa1 and Cbfa1a are identical, they bind equally well to their recognition sites (data now shown). However, in DNA cotransfection assays, Cbfa1a cannot transactivate a vector containing multiple copies of an oligonucleotide containing a consensus Cbfa1 binding site whereas Cbfa1 does

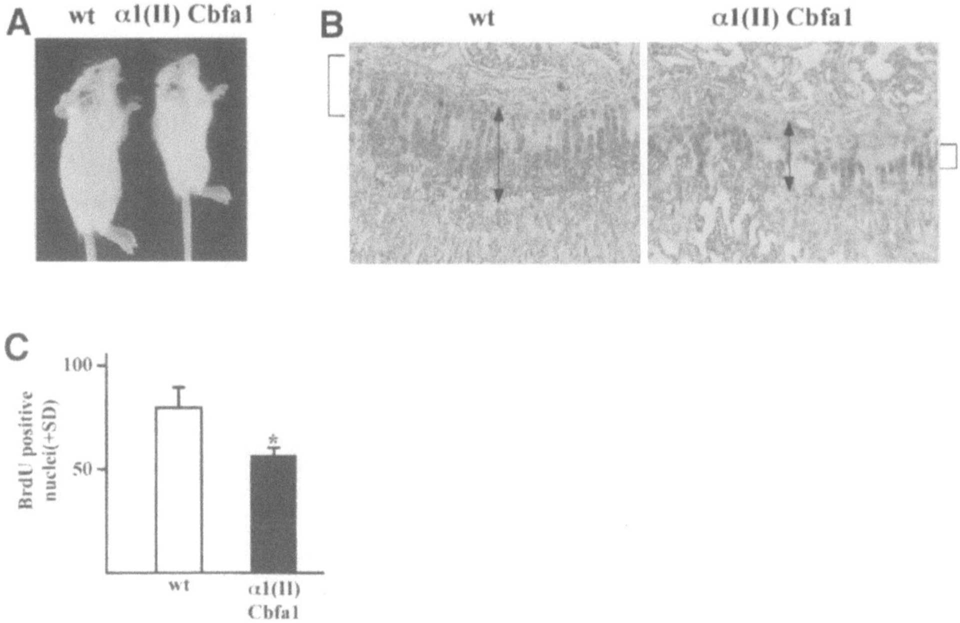

Fig. 6. Accelerated chondrocyte hypertrophy in the growth plate of α1(II) Cbfa1 mice. **A**, At 4 wk of age α1(II), Cbfa1 female mice (right) are shorter than wt littermates (left). Their growth plate is narrower (**B**, double-headed arrows) with shorter column of proliferating chondrocytes (brackets). **C**, Number of BrdU-positive nuclei per one section of growth plate. $*p < 0.05$.

(Fig. 7B). Two lines of mice overexpressing Cbfa1a under the control of the α1(II) collagen promoter/enhancer were generated. Both were undistinguishable from wild-type mice and in particular, they displayed no morphological or histological abnormalities of their skeleton (Fig. 7C and data not shown). These results indicate that the transactivation ability of Cbfa1 is required to induce chondrocyte hypertrophy.

Partial Rescue of the Cbfa1-Deficient Mice by Restoring Cbfa1 Expression in Mesenchymal Condensations

The existence of ectopic endochondral bone formation in the α1(II) Cbfa1 mice could be caused either by a distinct hypertrophic chondrocyte differentiation ability of Cbfa1 or to "transdifferentiation" of chondrocytes into osteoblasts secondary to the maintained expression of *Cbfa1* in nonhypertrophic chondrocytes. To address this question, we crossed the α1(II) Cbfa1 mice with heterozygote Cbfa1-deficient mice. By doing this, we simply restored Cbfa1 expression to its wild-type level.

Alcian blue/alizarin red staining of skeletal preparation of Cbfa1-deficient and α1(II) Cbfa1/Cbfa1-deficient mice in either 16.5-dpc embryos or newborn mice showed that the presence of the transgene rescued the absence of skeletal mineralization, one hallmark of Cbfa1-deficient mice (Fig. 8A). The shaft of all long bones, of the ribs, and the vertebrae were mineralized (Fig. 8A–C,F). As was the case with the α1(II) Cbfa1 mice, we observed ectopic mineralization in the chondrocostal cartilage, the base of the skull, the larynx, and the spinous processes of these "rescued" animals (Fig. 8C–F). This rescue was restricted to skeletal areas undergoing endochondral ossification and was never observed in skeletal areas undergoing intramembranous ossification. For instance, the α1(II) Cbfa1 transgene did not rescue the marked delay in clavicle development or the absence of fontanel closure observed in Cbfa1+/- mice (Fig. 9A; ref. *19*, and data not shown). To explain the restriction of this rescue, we studied the pattern of expression of the transgene using a α1(II) promoter/enhancer-LacZ transgene.

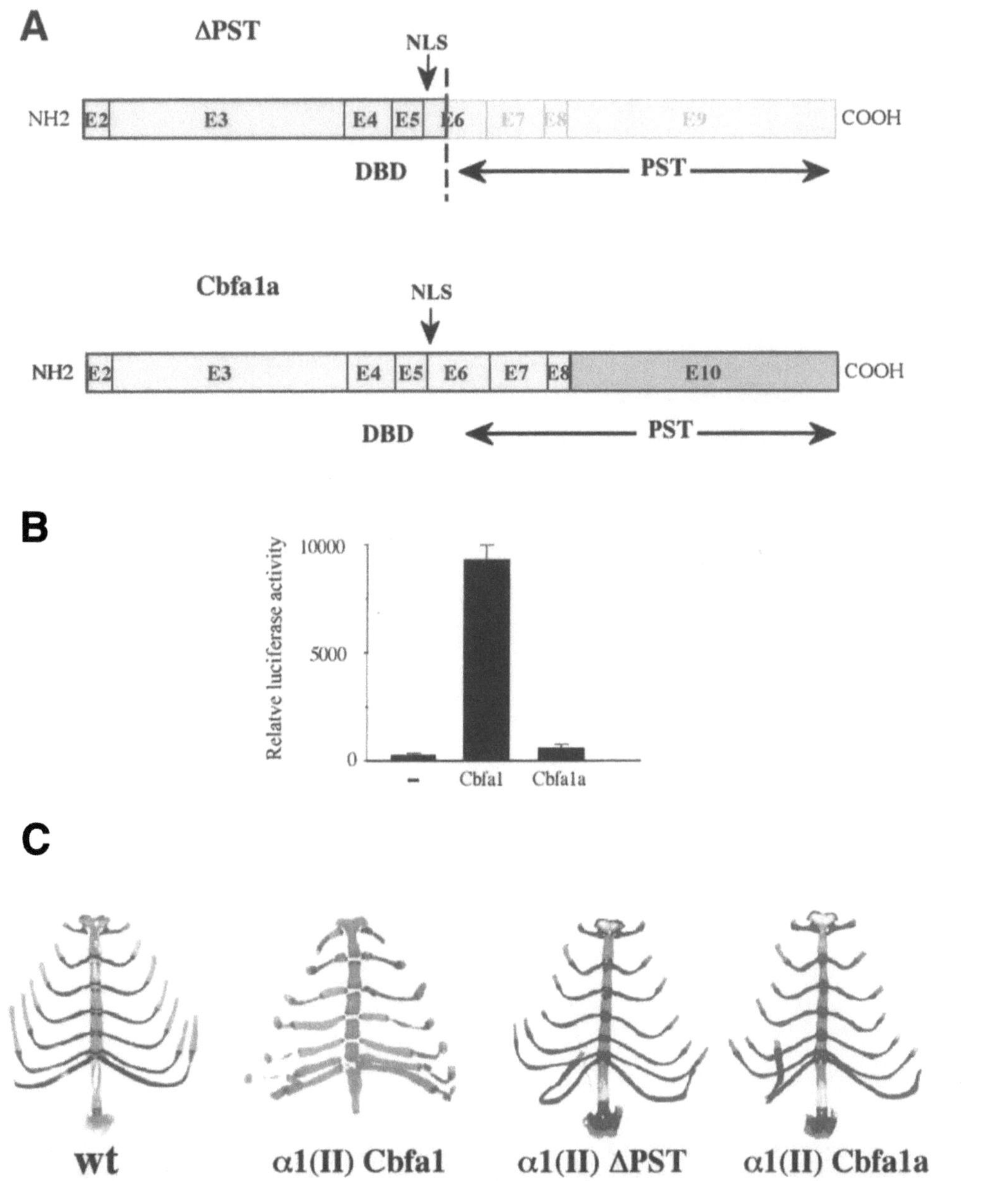

Fig. 7. Requirements of Cbfa2 transactivation function to induce chondrocyte hypertrophy. **A**, Schematic representation of the ΔPST (upper diagram) and Cbfa1a (lower diagram) forms of Cbfa1 used to generate transgenic mice. Boxes represent exons present and exons missing or replaced, respectively, in the mutated Cbfa1 cDNAs. **B**, Absence of transactivation of a reporter construct containing multimerized Cbfa1-binding sites upon cotransfection with a Cbfa1a expression vector. **C**, Absence of phenotypic abnormality in transgenic mice expressing either α1(II) ΔPST or α1(II) Cbfa1a. Skeletal preparations of rib cages from 1-mo-old animals. NLS, nuclear localization signal.

There was no staining in the calvaria, a skeletal area that was not rescued by the α1(II) Cbfa1 transgene and that ossifies through an intramembranous mechanism (Fig. 9B; ref. *32*). Thus, the fact that the rescue of the phenotype of the Cbfa1-deficient mice does not extend beyond the zone of expression of the transgene strongly suggests that this is occurring through a cell-autonomous mechanism.

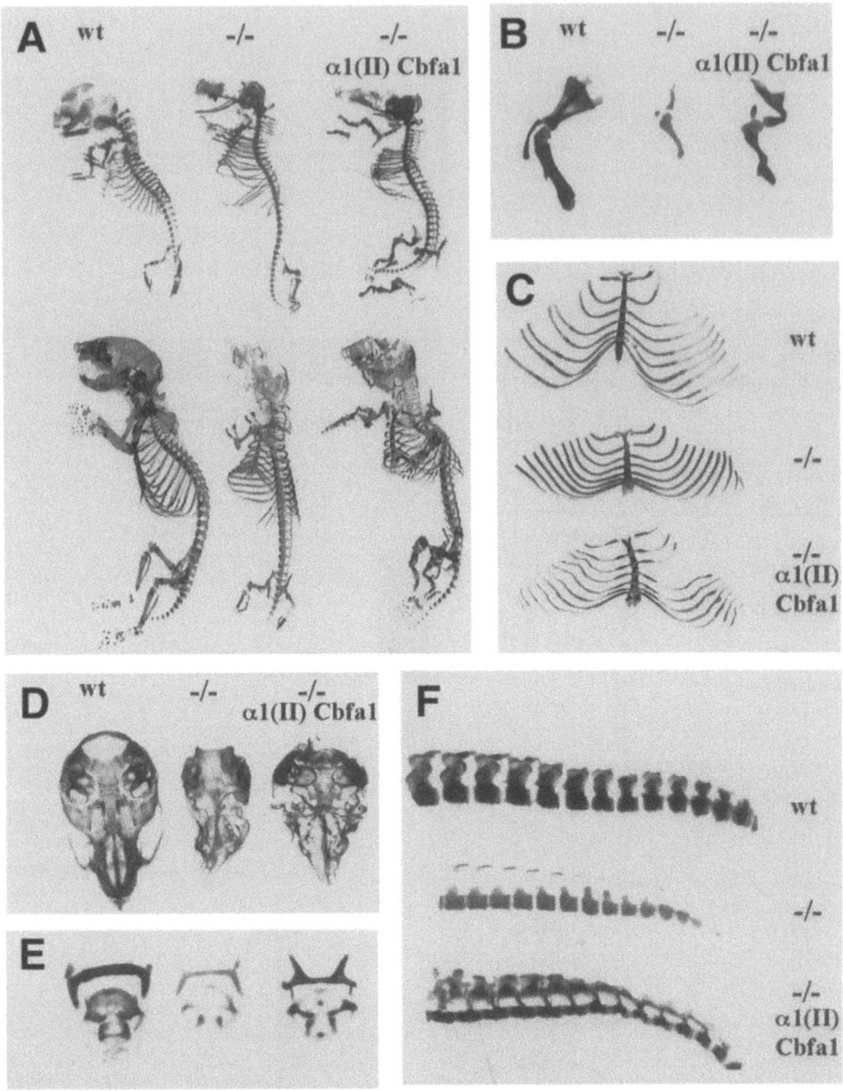

Fig. 8. Partial phenotypic rescue of the Cbfa1-deficient mice by the α1(II) Cbfa1 transgene. Alcian blue/alizarin red staining of skeletal preparations. **A**, Whole-mount preparations of 16.5-dpc (top) and 19.5-dpc (bottom) embryos. **B–F**, Embryos at 19.5 dpc. Forelimb (**B**), rib cage (**C**), skull (**D**), larynx (**E**), and lumbar vertebrae (**F**).

Hypertrophic Chondrocyte Differentiation, Vascular Invasion But No Osteoblast Differentiation in the α1(II) Cbfa1/Cbfa1-Deficient Mice

To determine whether the mineralized skeleton observed in the α1(II) Cbfa1/Cbfa1-deficient mice was caused by the presence of a calcified cartilaginous matrix only or to the presence of a bony matrix we performed a histological analysis in newborn mice. As shown in Fig. 9C,D, the α1(II) Cbfa1/Cbfa1a-deficient mice had hypertrophic chondrocytes in the femur, a bone where they cannot be found in Cbfa1-deficient mice as well as in all other bones examined (data not shown). In contrast, there was no bone trabeculae present in the femurs or any other skeletal elements analyzed in the α1(II) Cbfa1/Cbfa1-deficient mice.

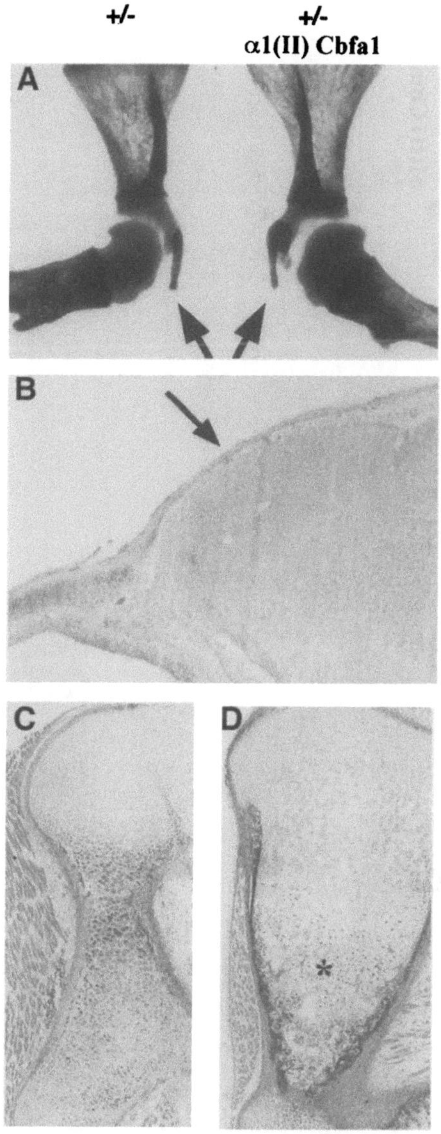

Fig. 9. Absence of rescue of intramembranous bone formation defects in the α1(II) Cbfa1/Cbfa1-deficient mice. **A**, Hypoplasia of the clavicle (arrows) in Cbfa1+/– mice harboring or not the α1(II) Cbfa1 transgene. **B**, Absence of LacZ staining in calvaria of an 18.5-dpc α1(II) LacZ transgenic embryo (arrow). **C** and **D**, LacZ/eosin staining of femurs from Cbfa1-deficient mice harboring (**D**) or not the α1(II) Cbfa1 transgene (**C**). Hypertrophic chondrocytes (asterisk) are observed only in the presence of the transgene.

To ascertain thoroughly the identity of these hypertrophic cells, we studied the expression of molecular markers in 18.5- and 19.5-dpc embryos. *Ihh*, a marker of prehypertrophic chondrocytes that is not expressed in the humerus or femur of the Cbfa1-deficient mice was expressed in the humerus and femurs of the α1(II) Cbfa1/Cbfa1-deficient mice at 18.5 dpc (Fig. 10A and data not shown). The same was true for *α1(X) collagen*, a marker of hypertrophic chondrocytes (Fig. 10A). The presence of Ihh-expressing cells induced the formation of a bone collar in the α1(II) Cbfa1-deficient skeleton (Fig. 9D).

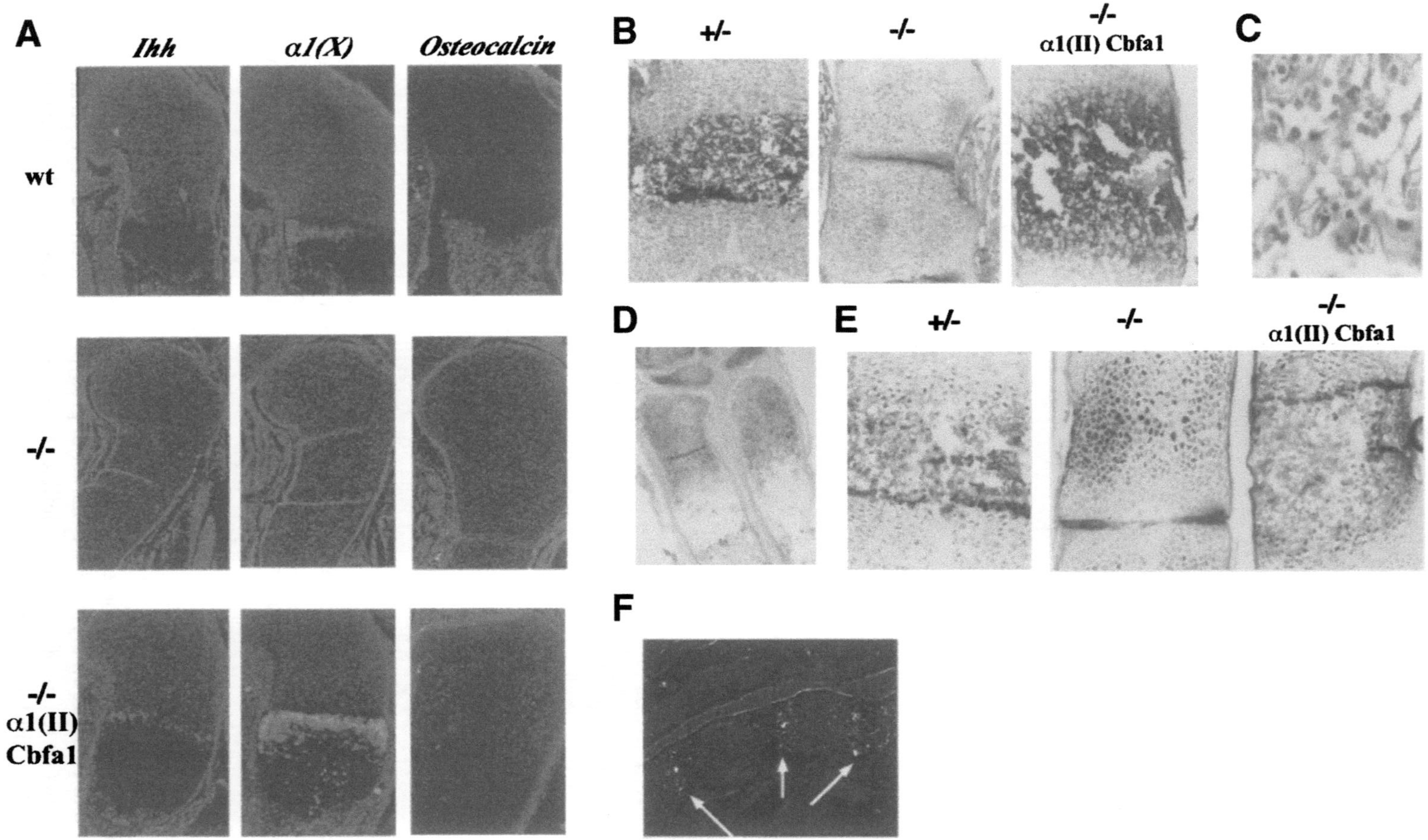

Fig. 10. Chondrocyte hypertrophy and vascular invasion in α1(II) Cbfa1/Cbfa1-deficient mice. **A**, *In situ* hybridization analysis of long bones of 18.5 (left and center panel) and 19.5 dpc (right panels) embryos. *Ihh*- and *α1(X) collagen*-expressing cells are present in wt and α1(II) Cbfa1/Cbfa1-deficient mice, indicating their hypertrophic chondrocytes nature. In Cbfa1-deficient background, no *Osteocalcin* expression is detectable whether the transgene is present or not, indicating the absence of osteoblasts. **B**, Immunohistochemistry showing VEGF synthesis in α1(II) Cbfa1/Cbfa1-deficient mice. **C**, Presence of erythrocytes indicative of vascular invasion in femurs of α1(II) Cbfa1/Cbfa1-deficient 19.5-dpc embryos. **D**, Absence of expression of the α1(II) LacZ transgene in cells of the bone collar of the femur of an 18.5-dpc embryo (arrowhead). **E**, TRAP-positive multinucleated cells in femurs of α1(II) Cbfa1/Cbfa1-deficient 19.5-dpc embryos. **F**, Gelatinase B activity (arrows) in femurs of α1(II) Cbfa1/Cbfa1-deficient 19.5-dpc embryos.

We also made use of the *LacZ* gene inserted in the *Cbfa1* locus of these Cbfa1-deficient mice *(19)*. LacZ staining showed the induction of expression of *Cbfa1* in the bone collar of the α1(II) Cbfa1/Cbfa1-deficient mice (Fig. 9C,D). This is consistent with the induction in these animals of *Ihh* expression (*see* below), a gene required for *Cbfa1* expression in cells of the bone collar *(14)*.

Immunohistochemistry analysis showed the presence of VEGF, a protein required for vascular invasion (Fig. 10B). The presence of VEGF hed to vascular invasion as illustrated by the presence of erythrocytes in the skeleton elements of the α1(II) Cbfa1/Cbfa1-deficient embryos (Fig. 10A). However, consistent with our histologic analysis, we could not detect any expression of *Osteocalcin*, a marker of osteoblasts in 19.5 dpc α1(II) Cbfa1/Cbfa1-deficient embryos whereas a positive signal could be detected in wild-type embryos (Fig. 10A). In conclusion, restored expression of *Cbfa1* in mesenchymal condensations of Cbfa1-deficient mice leads to hypertrophic chondrocyte differentiation. It does not lead to transdifferentiation of chondrocytes into osteoblasts.

The absence of osteoblasts in the α1(II) Cbfa1/Cbfa1-/- mice could only be explained if the transgene was not expressed in the bone collar. To test whether this was the case, we analyzed the pattern of expression of a α1(II) collagen-LacZ transgene. As shown in Fig. 10D, there was no LacZ staining in the bone collar of any long bones of 18.5-dpc embryos expressing the α1(II) LacZ transgene.

Cartilage Resorption in the α1(II) Cbfa1/Cbfa1-Deficient Mice

The α1(II) Cbfa1/Cbfa1-deficient mice had a second phenotypic abnormality. Most of their long bones were bent (Fig. 8A,B). This was surprising because the Cbfa1-deficient mice do not have abnormally shaped bones and raised the hypothesis that in the rescued animals, there was destruction of the cartilaginous matrices. Indeed, skeletal elements of the α1(II) Cbfa1/Cbfa1-deficient mice contained TRAP-positive, multinucleated cells (Fig. 10E). These cells also synthesized gelatinase B, an enzyme that degrades cartilaginous matrices (Fig. 10F; ref. *6*). The existence of these resorbing cells in a skeleton made only of cartilage suggests that they were similar to the chondroclasts modeling the cartilage described in another mouse mutant *(6)*. Thus, in absence of osteogenesis the destruction of cartilage by these cells led to the collapse of the shaft of the future bones and therefore explained their deformations.

DISCUSSION

To address the functional relevance of *Cbfa1* expression during chondrogenesis, we generated transgenic mice in which *Cbfa1* expression is maintained in proliferating and prehypertrophic chondrocytes beyond 12.5 dpc at the level observed at that stage of development. This approach also allowed us to restore *Cbfa1* expression to a wild-type level in the mesenchymal condensations of the future skeleton of Cbfa1-deficient mice. Together, our results provide evidence that *Cbfa1* expression in nonhypertrophic chondrocytes is required to induce chondrocyte hypertrophy during development, at least in some skeletal elements. This is best illustrated by the fact that skeletogenesis proceeds a step further in Cbfa1-deficient mice. This function is independent of the role of Cbfa1 as an osteoblast differentiation factor. Our analysis, together with previous studies *(18,19)*, demonstrates that Cbfa1 plays multiple roles in skeletogenesis.

Comparison of Cbfa1 Expression in Chondrocytes and Osteoblasts

Previous experiments have shown that *Cbfa1* is expressed at a high level until 12.5 dpc of development in cells expressing both *α1(I) collagen*, an osteoblast marker, and *α1(II) collagen*, a chondrocyte marker. On the basis of this coexpression of chondrocyte and osteoblast molecular markers, this cell type was termed osteochondroprogenitor, although evidence of an involvement of Cbfa1 in chondrogenesis was lacking at that time *(15)*. Beyond that stage of development, only osteoblast progenitor cells and differentiated osteoblasts maintain such a high level of *Cbfa1* expression. Nevertheless *Cbfa1* remains expressed at low levels in chondrocytes *(16,17)*. A systematic analysis of *Cbfa1* expression in chondrocytes between 14.5 dpc and birth shows that *Cbfa1* is expressed in prehypertrophic chondrocytes at a higher level than in hypertrophic chondrocytes between 14.5 dpc and birth. At birth, the level of *Cbfa1* expression in chondrocytes is close to background. These results are slightly different from those recently reported *(16,17)* by showing expression of *Cbfa1* predominantly in prehypertrophic chondrocytes and by detecting a major decline of *Cbfa1* expression in chondrocytes as skeletogenesis proceeds. Although the reasons for these discrepancies are not clear, taken together these studies and ours agree on one important observation: *Cbfa1* expression precedes chondrocyte hypertrophy. The fact that *Cbfa1* expression is predominant in nonhypertrophic chondrocytes and precedes chondrocyte hypertrophy during skeletogenesis is compatible with a role for Cbfa1 as an inducer of hypertrophic chondrocyte differentiation.

Cbfa1 Function During Chondrogenesis

To study the possible function of Cbfa1 as an inducer of chondrocyte hypertrophy, we used the *α1(II) collagen* promoter/enhancer-Cbfa1 transgene to prevent the decline of *Cbfa1* expression in nonhypertrophic chondrocytes beyond 12.5 dpc. This transgene also was able to restore *Cbfa1* expression in the skeletal mesenchymal condensations of the Cbfa1-deficient mice. The level of expression of enodgenous *Cbfa1* and of our transgene were nearly identical.

The analysis of the α1(II) Cbfa1 mice indicates the *Cbfa1* does have the ability to induce chondrocyte hypertrophy prematurely in areas where endochondral ossification will occur and ectopically in other skeletal areas. This latter phenotypic abnormality was particularly helpful to dissect the sequence of events leading to chondrocyte hypertrophy. Our analysis shows that *Cbfa1* expression in nonhypertrophic chondrocytes induced the appearance of prehypertrophic chondrocytes expressing *Ihh*. In turn, *Ihh* expression favors chondrocyte hypertrophy as shown by *α1(X) collagen* expression *(14)* but also induces *Cbfa1* expression in the bone collar *(14,35)*. This, along with the induction of *Vegf* expression in hypertrophic chondrocytes, initiates the cascade of ectopic endochondral ossification observed in these mice. We do not know yet whether *Cbfa1* induces *Ihh*, *Vegf*, and/or *α1(X) collagen* expression directly or indirectly. The identification of Cbfa1 binding sites in the promoter of the α1(X) collagen gene (B. Lee, personal communication) and the regulation of *Vegf* by *Cbfa1* (Zelzer et al., submitted) lend support to the former hypothesis.

Analysis of the α1(II) Cbfa1 mice could not determine whether *Cbfa1* was causing transdifferentiation of chondrocytes into osteoblasts as previously suggested *(17,36,37)* or rather if Cbfa1 induced chondrocyte hypertrophy independently of osteoblast differentiation. To address this question, we made use of the Cbfa1-deficient mice *(19)*. The α1(II) Cbfa1 transgene on a Cbfa1-deficient background induced, in skeletal elements where it is not observed, *Ihh* expression, chondrocyte hypertrophy, and expression of *Vegf*, a gene required for vascular invasion and osteogenesis *(7)*. However, the transgene could not rescue the absence of osteoblasts that is the hallmark of the Cbfa1-deficient mice. The absence of osteoblast differentiation in the Cbfa1-deficient mice expressing the α1(II) Cbfa1 transgene is explained by the expression pattern of our transgene, which is not expressed in cells of the bone collar. As noted above, *Ihh* normally induces *Cbfa1* expression in the bone collar, a mandatory step for osteoblast differentiation *(14)*. On a Cbfa1-deficient background, *Ihh* cannot induce *Cbfa1* expression and osteoblast differentiation in the bone collar; as a result, osteogenesis does not occur. The dissociation between the rescue of the chondrocyte hypertrophy differentiation defect by the α1(II) Cbfa1 transgene and the absence of rescue of the osteoblast-deficient phenotype demonstrates that *Cbfa1* regulates chondrocyte hypertrophy independently of its osteoblast differentiation function and argues against a transdifferentiation phenomenon.

At least three arguments suggest that the control of chondrocyte hypertrophy is a normal function of Cbfa1. First, Cbfa1-deficient mice lack hypertrophic chondrocytes in a few skeletal elements, such as humerus and femur that develop before other elements, like the tibia, where chondrocyte hypertrophy does occur normally. This indicates that chondrocyte hypertrophy, at least in these skeletal elements, is truly dependent on *Cbfa1* expression and not merely a delay of differentiation. Second, this function of Cbfa1 requires the presence of its transactivation domain. Third, the level of expression of the α1(II) Cbfa1 transgene is low and not higher than the one of endogenous *Cbfa1*, indicating that we are mimicking the function of *Cbfa1* rather than overexpressing it in nonhypertrophic chondrocytes. The fact that not all skeletal elements have delayed chondrocyte hypertrophy in the Cbfa1-deficient mice indicates that there are Cbfa1-independent pathways leading to chondrocyte hypertrophy elsewhere in the skeleton. The nature and numbers of these Cbfa1-independent pathways are so far unknown.

Cartilage Modeling in Absence of Bone

The partial rescue of the phenotype of the Cbfa1-deficient mice by the α1(II) Cbfa1 transgene also provides an opportunity to observe the fate of hypertrophic cartilage in an animal unable to produce bone. We observed multinucleated TRAP-positive cells, either osteoclasts or chondroclasts *(6)* in the "rescued" animals and not in the Cbfa1-deficient mice. This observation indicates that the presence of these cells is specific for the matrices produced by hypertrophic chondrocytes and is closely associated with vascular invasion. The expression of *Vegf* in the α1(II) Cbfa1/Cbfa1-deficient mice is consistent with this model *(7)*. The abnormal shape of the bones in α1(II) Cbfa1/Cbfa1-deficient mice reveals that the chondroclast-like cells do play an important role by removing the matrix produced by hypertrophic chondrocytes at the time of vascular invasion, Finally, the appearance of these cells in absence of any detectable osteoblast suggests either the existence of a differentiation pathway for chondroclasts, which is independent of osteoclast differentiation *(6)* or the existence of an osteoblast-independent pathway whereby clast cells are able to resorb both cartilaginous and bony matrices.

Toward a Genetic Understanding of Chondrocyte Hypertrophy

Our data together with those of others *(13,14,38)* begin to unravel a complex genetic network controlling chondrocyte hypertrophy. Our study suggests that *Cbfa1* is located upstream of *Ihh* during chondrogenesis, as shown by the induction of *Ihh* expression ectopically in the α(II) Cbfa1 transgenic and in the α1(II) Cbfa1/Cbfa1-deficient mice (Fig. 11). The absence of *Ihh* expression in some skeletal elements of the Cbfa1-deficient mice *(16,17)* also suggests that Cbfa1 is only one of several upstream regulators of *Ihh* expression. Once *Ihh*-expressing prehypertrophic chondrocytes have differentiated, *Cbfa1* may also be located downstream of *Ihh*. *Ihh* is likely to control, directly or indirectly, *Cbfa1* expression in the cells of the bone collar and thereby control osteoblast differentiation (Fig. 11). The importance of this function of Ihh is best illustrated by the absence of osteoblast differentiation in the bones developing through endochondral ossification in Ihh-deficient mice *(14)*.

In summary, this study provides evidence for a more important and complex role for Cbfa1 during skeletogenesis than originally anticipated. The ability of Cbfa1 to induce chondrocyte hypertrophy in wild-type and in Cbfa1-deficient mice indicates that Cbfa1 is one of the transcription factors required for this function. This along with its well-established role in osteoblast differentiation *(13,18)* identifies Cbfa1 as the first transcription factor regulating the differentiation of chondrocytes and osteoblasts, two cell types long thought to share a common progenitor *(20,21)*.

MATERIALS AND METHODS

DNA Constructions

α1(II) Cbfa1, α1(II) Cbfa1a, and α1(II) Cbfa1ΔPST transgenes were generated by subcloning full length Cbfa1 or full-length Cbfa1a cDNAs, or PST deletion mutant of Cbfa1 cDNA *(22)*, respectively, between a 3-kb fragment of the α1(II) promoter and its 3-kb chondrocyte-specific enhancer region. 1.3-kbOG2-LacZ construct was generated by subcloning 1.3-kb fragment of the mouse *OG2* promoter into pLacF *(24)*.

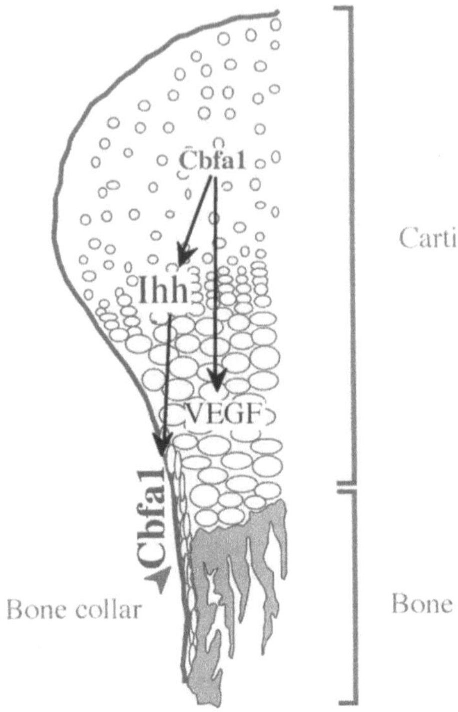

Fig. 11. Schematic representation of the roles of Cbfa1 in endochondral ossification. Cbfa1 favors chondrocyte hypertrophy via an Ihh-dependent pathway. In turn, Ihh induces differentiation of the cells of the bone collar through a Cbfa1-dependent pathway. Cbfa1 also favors *VEGF* expression.

Generation of Transgenic Mice

Plasmids were digested with appropriate restriction enzymes and inserts were purified by agarose gel electrophoresis. Linear DNA fragments were microinjected into pronuclei of fertilized C57BL/6SnJ mouse oocytes that were subsequently reimplanted into oviducts of pseudopregnant CD1 foster mothers (Jackson Laboratories). α1(II) Cbfa1, α1(II) Cbfa1a, and αI(II) Cbfa1ΔPST transgenes were respectively coinjected with the 1.3kb of OG2-LacZ construct to obtain transgenic mice coexpressing the two transgenes. Genotypes were determined by polymerase chain reaction (PCR) using the following as primers: 5'-GGCAGCACGCTATTAAATCCAA-3' and 5'-GGTTTCAGGGGGAGGTGTG GGAGG-3' for the α1(II) Cbfa1 mice; 5'-CTGGACATCATAGCAAAGGCCC-3' and 5'-GGTTTCAG GGGGAGGTGTGGGAGG-3' for the α1(II) Cbfa1a mice; and 5'-CGGAGCGGACGAGGCAAGA GTTTC-3' and 5'-GGTTTCAGGGGGAGGTGTGGGAGG-3' for the αI(II) Cbfa1ΔPST mice. Sex was determined by PCR using the *Sry*–specific primers 5'-CATGACCACCACCACCACCAA-3' and 5'-TC ATGAGACTGCCAACCACAG-3' *(25)*.

Reverse Transcription PCR Analysis

To monitor the transgene expression, total RNA was prepared from 12.5-dpc embryos. Three to four embryos were analyzed independently for each genotypes. RNA extraction, cDNA synthesis, and PCR amplification were performed using standard protocols *(26)*. Exon 2 amplification of the HPRT gene was used as internal control of the quantity and quality of the cDNAs. The following sets of the primers were used: transgene specific PCR, 5'-CCAGGCAGTTCCCAAGCATT-3' and 5'-AGAG CTATGACGTCGCATGCACAC-3'; endogenous *Cbfa1*, 5'-GGCAGCACGCTATTAAATCCAAA-3' and 5'-TGACTGCCCCCACCCTCTTAG-3'; and *Hprt*, 5'-GTTGAGAGATCATCTCCACC-3' and 5'-AGC GATGATGAACCAGGTTA-3'.

Skeletal Preparation

Mice were dissected, fixed in 100% ethanol overnight, then stained in alcian blue dye solution (0.015% alcian blue 8GX [Sigma], 20% acetic acid, 80% ethanol) overnight and transferred to 2% potassium hydroxide for 24 h or longer, dependent on the age of the mice. Subsequently, they were stained in alizarin red solution (0.005% Alizarin sodium sulfate [Sigma], 1% KOH) and cleared in 1% KOH/20% glycerol.

Histological Analyses and In Situ *Hybridization*

Tissues were fixed in 4% paraformaldehyde/phosphate-buffered saline overnight at 4°C and decalcified in 25% EDTA at 37°C for 3 d when older than newborn. Specimens were embedded in paraffin and sectioned at 6 μm. For histological analysis, sections were stained with alcian blue (1% alcian blue 8GX, 3% acetic acid) and counterstained with eosin. For alkaline phosphatase/TRAP staining, sections were first stained for alkaline phosphatase with Fast blue BB (Sigma) then for TRAP with pararosaniline (Sigma) following established conditions *(27)*. Gelatinase assay was performed as described *(28)*. *In situ* hybridization was performed using complementary ^{35}S-labeled riboprobes. *Cbfa1* and αI(II) collagen probes have been previously described *(15)*. The *Ihh* probe is a 540-bp fragment of *Ihh* 3' untranslated region. The *αI(X) collagen* probe was obtained from Dr. B.R. Olsen (Harvard Medical School, Boston, MA). Hybridizations were performed overnight at 55°C, and washes were performed at 63°C. Autoradiography and Hoechst 33528 staining were performed as described *(29)*.

LacZ Staining and Immunohistochemistry

Skinned and eviscerated animals were fixed in 1% paraformaldehyde, 0.2% glutalaldehyde in phosphate buffer (pH 7.3) for 45 min, and stained overnight with X-Gal (5-bromo-4-chloro-3indoyl β-D-galactosidase). Specimens were embedded in paraffin and sectioned at 6 μm. Sections were counterstained with eosin. Immunohistochemistry was performed according standard protocol *(26)*. Anti-VEGF antibody was purchased from Santa Cruz Biotechnology.

BrdU Labeling

Mice were injected intraperitoneally with 10^{-4} m*M* BrdU/g body weight 1 h before sacrifice. Tibiae were dissected, fixed, decalcified, and embedded in paraffin as previously. BrdU was detected using a Zymed kit following the manufacturer's protocol (Zymed). BrdU-positive cells present in the growth plate of at least five different sections were counted for both wt and αI(II) Cbfa1 mice. Statistical differences between groups were assessed by Student's *t*-test.

DNA Transfection Assays

F9 cells were transfected with 5 μg of empty or Cbfa1 or Cbfa1a expression vector *(15)*, 5 μg of p6OSE2-luc reporter vector *(23)*, and 2 μg of pSVβgal plasmid. Transfections, luciferase assays, and β-galactosidase assays were performed as described *(23)*. Data represent ratios of luciferase/β-galactosidase activities and values are means of six independent transfection experiments.

ACKNOWLEDGMENTS

The authors are indebted to J. Liu and J. Shen for their superb technical assistance and their commitment to this study. The authors also thank Dr. Chung, Kronenberg, McMahon, and Olsen for in situ hybridization probes. They are grateful to Dr. G. Friedrich and members of the Karsenty laboratory for critical reading of the manuscript. This work was supported by March of Dimes FY99-489 and NIH R01 AR45548, NIH P01 AR42919 and Eli Lilly grants to G.K.; Arthritis Foundation and March of Dimes FY99-761 grants to P.D.; and Arthritis Foundation Postdoctoral Fellowship to S.T.

REFERENCES

1. Horton, W. A. (1993) Morphology of connective tissue: Cartilage, in *Connective tissue heritable disorders,* Wiley-Liss, Inc., New York, pp. 73–84.
2. Caplan, A. I. and Pechak, D. G. (1987) The cellular and molecular embryology of bone formation, in *Bone and mineral research.* Vol. 5. (Peck, W. A., ed.), Elsevier, New York, pp. 117–183.
3. Linsenmayer, T. F., Chen, Q. A., Gibney, E., Gordon, M. K., Marchant, J. K., Mayne, R., et al. (1991) Collagen type IX and X in the developing chick tibiotarsus: analyses of mRNAs and proteins. *Development* **111,** 191–196.
4. Mundlos, S. (1994) Expression patterns of matrix genes during human skeletal development. *Prog. Histochem. Cytochem.* **28,** No. 3.
5. Poole, A. R. (1991) The growth plate: cellular physiology, cartilage assembly and mineralization, in *Cartilage: molecular aspects.* (Hall, B. K. and Newman, S. A., eds.), CRC Press, Boca Raton, FL.
6. Vu, T. H., Shipley, J. M., Bergers, G., Berger, J. E., Helms, J. A., Hanahan, D., et al. (1998) MMP-g/gelatinase B is a key regulator of growth plate angiogenesis and apoptosis of hypertrophic chondrocytes. *Cell* **93,** 411–422.
7. Gerber, H. P., Vu, T. H., Ryan, A. M., Kowalski, J., Werb, Z., and Ferrara, N. (1999) VEGF couples hypertrophic cartilage remodeling, ossification and angiogenesis during endochondral bone formation. *Nat. Med.* **5,** 623–628.
8. Bi, W., Deng, J. M., Zhang, Z., Behringer, R. R., and de Crombrugghe, B. (1999) Sox9 is required for cartilage formation. *Nat. Genet.* **22,** 85–89.
9. Ornitz, D. M. (2000) FGFs, heparan sulfate and FGFRs: complex interactions essential for development. *Bioessays* **22,** 108–112.
10. Karaplis, A. C., Luz, A., Glowacki, J., Bronson, R. T., Tybulewicz, V. L., Kronenberg, H. M., et al. (1994) Lethal skeletal dysplasia from targeted disruption of the parathyroid hormone-related peptide gene. *Genes Dev.* **8,** 277–289.
11. Lanske, B., Karaplis, A. C., Lee, K., Luz, A., Vortkamp, A., Pirro, A., et al. (1996) PTH/PTHrP receptor in early development and Indian hedgehog-regulated bone growth. *Science* **273,** 663–666.
12. Weir, E. C., Philbrick, W. M., Amling, M., Neff, L. A., Baron, R., and Broaduds, A. E. (1996) Targeted overexpression of parathyroid hormone-related peptide in chondrocytes causes chondrodysplasia and delayed endochondral bone formation. *Proc. Natl. Acad. Sci. USA* **93,** 10240–10245.
13. Vortkamp, A., Lee, K., Lanske, B., Segre, G. V., Kronenberg, H. M., and Tabin, C. J. (1996) Regulation of rate of cartilage differentiation by Indian hedgehog and PTH-related protein. *Science* **273,** 613–622.
14. St-Jacques, B., Hammerschmidt, M., and McMahon, A. P. (1999) Indian hedgehog signaling regulates proliferation and differentiation of chondrocytes and is essential for bone formation. *Genes Dev.* **13,** 2072–2086.
15. Ducy, P., Zhang, R., Geoffroy, V., Ridall, A. L., and Karsenty, G. (1997) Osf2/Cbfa1: a transcriptional activator of osteoblast differentiation. *Cell* **89,** 747–754.
16. Inada, M., Yasui, T., Nomura, S., Miyake, S., Deguchi, K., Himeno, M., et al. (1999) Maturational disturbance of chondrocytes in *Cbfa1*-deficient mice. *Dev. Dyn.* **214,** 279–290.
17. Kim, I. S., Otto, F., Abel, B., and Mundlos, S. (1999) Regulation of chondrocyte differentiation by *Cbfa1. Mech. Dev.* **809,** 159–170.
18. Komori, T., Yahi, H., Nomura, S., Yamaguchi, A., Sasaki, K., Deguchi, K., et al. (1997) Targeted disruption of Cbfa1 results in a complete lack of bone formation owing to maturational arrest of osteoblasts. *Cell* **89,** 755–764.
19. Otto, F., Thornell, A. P., Crompton, T., Denzel, A., Gilmour, K. C., Rosewell, I. R., et al. (1997) Cbfa1, a candidate gene for cleidocranial dysplasia syndrome, is essential for osteoblast differentiation and bone development. *Cell* **89,** 765–771.
20. Reddi, A. H. (1994) Bone and cartilage differentiation. *Curr. Opin. Genet. Dev.* **4,** 737–744.
21. Erlebacher, A., Filvaroff, E. H., Gitelman, S. E., and Derynck, R. (1995) Toward a molecular understanding of skeletal development. *Cell* **80,** 371–378.
22. Thirunavukkarasu, K., Mahajan, M., McLarren, K. W., Stifani, S., and Karsenty, G. (1998) Two domains unique to osteoblast-specific transcription factor Osf2/Cbfa1 contribute to its transactivation function and its inability to heterodimerize with CBFβ. *Mol. Cell. Biol.* **18,** 4197–4208.
23. Ducy, P. and Karsenty, G. (1995) Two distinct osteoblast-specific cis-acting elements control expression of a mouse osteocalcin gene. *Mol. Cell Biol.* **15,** 1858–1869.
24. Mercer, E. H., Hoyle, G. W., Kapur, R. P., Brinster, R. L., and Palmiter, R. D. (1991) The dopamine beta-hydroxylase gene promoter directs on of E. coli lacZ to sympathetic and other neurons in adult transgenic mice. *Neuron* **7,** 703–716.
25. Jeske, Y. W., Mishina, Y., Cohen, D. R., Behringer, R. R., and Koopman, P. (1996) Analysis of the role of Amh and Fra1 in Sry regulatory pathway. *Mol. Reprod. Dev.* **44,** 153–158.
26. Ausubel, F. M., Brent, R., Kingston, R. E., Moore, D. D., Seidman, J. G., Smith, J. A., et al. (1995) *Current protocols in molecular biology.* John Wiley & Sons, New York.
27. Bronckers, A. L. J. J., Goei, W., Luo, G., Karsenty, G., D'Souza, R. N., Lyaruu, D. M., et al. (1996) DNA fragmentation during bone formation in neonatal rodents assessed by transferase-mediated end labeling. *J. Bone Miner. Res.* **11,** 1281–1291.
28. Lee, E. R., Murphy, G., El-Alfy, M., Davoli, M. A., Lamplugh, L., Docherty, A. J., et al. (1999) Active gelatinase B is identified by histozymography in the cartilage resorption sites of developing long bones. *Dev. Dyn.* **215,** 190–205.
29. Sundin, O. H., Busse, H. G., Rogers, M. B., Gudas, L. J., and Eichele, G. (1990) Region-specific expression in early chick and mouse embryos of *Ghox-lab* and *Hox 1.6*, vertebrate homeobox-containing genes related to Drosophila *labial. Development* **108,** 47–58.

30. Zhou, G., Lefebvre, V., Zhang, Z., Eberspaecher, H., and de Crombrugghe, B. (1998) Three high mobility group-like sequences within a 48-base pair enhancer of the Col2a1 gene are required for cartilage-specific expression in vivo. *J. Biol. Chem.* **273,** 14989–14997.
31. Mcleod, M. J. (1980) Differential staining of cartilage and bone in whole mouse fetuses by alcian blue and alizarin red S. *Teratology* **22,** 299–301.
32. Kaufman, M. H. (1992) *The atlas of mouse development.* Academic Press, San Diego, CA.
33. Frendo, J.-L., Xiao, G., Franceschi, R., Karsenty, G., and Ducy, P. (1998) Functional hierarchy between two OSE2 elements in the control of osteocalcin gene expression in vivo. *J. Biol. Chem.* **273,** 30609–30516.
34. Stewart, M., Terry, A., Hu, M., O'Hara, M., Blyth, K., Baxter, E., Cameron, E., et al. (1997) Proviral insertions induce the expression of bone-specific isoforms of PEBP2alphaA (CBFA1): evidence for a new myc collaborating oncogene. *Proc. Natl. Acad. Sci. USA* **94,** 8646–8651.
35. Akiyama, H., Shigeno, C., Iyama, K., Ito, H., Hiraki, Y., Konoshi, J., et al. (1999) Indian hedgehog in the late-phase differentiation in mouse chondrogenic EC cells, ATDC5: upregulation of type X collagen and osteoprotegerin ligand mRNAs. *Biochem. Biophys. Res. Commun.* **257,** 814–820.
36. Kahn, A. J. and Simmons, D. J. (1977) Chondrocyte-to-osteocyte transformation in grafts of perichondrium-free epiphyseal cartilage. *Clin. Orthop.* **129,** 299–304.
37. Cancedda, R., Descalzi Cancedda, F., and Castagnola, P. (1995) Chondrocyte differentiation. *Int. Rev. Cytol.* **159,** 265–358.
38. Chung, U. I., Lanske, B., Lee, K., Li, E., and Kronenberg, H. (1998) The parathyroid hormone/parathyroid hormone-related peptide receptor coordinates endochondral bone development by directly controlling chondrocyte differentiation. *Proc. Natl. Acad. Sci. USA* **95,** 13030–13035.

5
Molecular Biology and Biosynthesis of Collagens

Johanna Myllyharju

INTRODUCTION

The collagens are a heterogeneous family of extracellular matrix proteins that have a major role in maintaining the structural integrity of various tissues and organs, although they also have many other important biological functions. Collagens are the most abundant proteins in the human body, with approx 30% of protein mass consisting of collagen. Tissues that are especially rich in collagens are bone, skin, tendon, cartilage, ligaments, and vascular walls. The extracellular matrix in bone and tendon consists of up to 90% of collagen and that of skin approx 50%. The collagen superfamily now includes at least 27 collagen types and more than 15 additional proteins that have collagen-like domains. Most collagens form polymeric assemblies, and the superfamily can be divided into several classes based on their supramolecular structures or other features. Biosynthesis of collagens is a complex process that requires eight specific post-translational enzymes. Collagens have an important role in the healing of wounds and fractures and, thus, inhibition of collagen synthesis will delay healing. However, excessive collagen formation can lead to fibrosis, thus impairing the normal functioning of the affected organ. The essential function of collagens is illustrated by the wide variety of disease phenotypes caused by mutations in their genes.

THE COLLAGEN SUPERFAMILY

At least 27 proteins with altogether 42 distinct polypeptide chains and corresponding genes are now known as collagens (refs. *1–8*; Table 1). Collagens are extracellular matrix proteins that consist of three polypeptide chains, called α chains, and contain at least one unique triple-helical domain with repeating -Gly-X-Y- sequences in each of the constituent chains. The presence of glycine, the smallest amino acid, in every third position in the triple-helical domain is critical because a larger amino acid does not fit into the restricted space in the centre of the triple helix. The X- and Y-position amino acids vary according to the collagen type and domain, but proline is frequently found in the X position and 4-hydroxyproline in the Y position. 4-Hydroxyproline residues have an important role in the thermal stability of the triple helix *(9)*. Depending on the collagen type, the α chains differ in length and in the number of possible interruptions in the triple helix (Fig. 1). In some collagen types, all the three α chains are identical, whereas in others the collagen molecule consists of two or three different α chains (Table 1). The collagen superfamily can be classified into eight groups based on their polymeric structures or other features (Fig. 1): A, fibril-forming collagens, types I–III, V, XI, XXIV, and XXVII; B, fibril-associated collagens with interrupted triple-helices (FACIT collagens), types IX, XII, XIV, XVI, XIX–XXII, and XXVI; C, collagens forming hexagonal networks, types VIII and X; D, the

From: *The Skeleton: Biochemical, Genetic, and Molecular Interactions in Development and Homeostasis*
Edited by: E. J. Massaro and J. M. Rogers © Humana Press Inc., Totowa, NJ

Table 1
Collagen Types, Their Constituent Polypeptide Chains, Genes, and Occurrence in Tissues[a]

Type	*Constituent*	*Gene*	*Occurrence*
I	α1(I)	*COL1A1*	Most connective tissues, especially in dermis, bone, tendon, ligament
	α2(I)	*COL1A2*	
II	α1(II)	*COL2A1*	Cartilage, intervertebrate disc, inner ear, vitreous humour, cornea
III	α1(III)	*COL3A1*	As type I collagen except absent in bone and tendon. Abundantly expressed in elastic tissues, such as skin, inner organs, and blood vessels
IV	α1(IV)	*COL4A1*	All basement membranes
	α2(IV)	*COL4A2*	
	α3(IV)	*COL4A3*	
	α4(IV)	*COL4A4*	
	α5(IV)	*COL4A5*	
	α6(IV)	*COL4A6*	
V	α1(V)	*COL5A1*	Tissues containing type I collagen
	α2(V)	*COL5A2*	
	α3(V)	*COL5A3*	
	α4(V)	*COL5A4*	Nervous system
VI	α1(VI)	*COL6A1*	Most connective tissues
	α2(VI)	*COL6A2*	
	α3(VI)	*COL6A3*	
VII	α1(VII)	*COL7A1*	Anchoring fibrils in skin, cornea, cervix, oral, and esophageal mucosa
VIII	α1(VIII)	*COL8A1*	Many tissues
	α2(VIII)	*COL8A2*	
IX	α1(IX)	*COL9A1*	Tissues containing type II collagen
	α2(IX)	*COL9A2*	
	α3(IX)	*COL9A3*	
X	α1(X)	*COL10A1*	Hypertrophic cartilage
XI	α1(XI)	*COL11A1*	Tissues containing type II collagen
	α2(XI)	*COL11A2*	
	α3(XI)[b]	*COL2A1*	
XII	α1(XII)	*COL12A1*	Tissues containing type I collagen
XIII	α1(XIII)	*COL13A1*	Many tissues
XIV	α1(XIV)	*COL14A1*	Tissues containing type I collagen
XV	α1(XV)	*COL15A1*	Many tissues in the basement membrane zone
XVI	α1(XVI)	*COL16A1*	Many tissues
XVII	α1(XVII)	*COL17A1*	Skin hemidesmosomes
XVIII	α1(XVIII)	*COL18A1*	Many tissues in the basement membrane zone
XIX	α1(XIX)	*COL19A1*	Many tissues in the basement membrane zone
XX	α1(XX)	*COL20A1*	Many tissues
XXI	α1(XXI)	*COL21A1*	Many tissues
XXII	α1(XXII)[c]	*COL22A1*	
XXIII	α1(XXIII)	*COL23A1*	Metastatic tumor cells
XXIV	α1(XXIV)	*COL24A1*	Developing bone and cornea
XXV	α1(XXV)	*COL25A1*	Neurons
XXVI	α1(XXVI)	*COL26A1*	Testis, ovary
XXVII	α1(XXVII)	*COL27A1*	Cartilage, eye, ear, and lung

[a] *See* refs. *1–8*.
[b] The α3(XI) is a post-translational variant of α1(II).
[c] Complete cDNA sequence characterized (M. Koch, M. Gordon, and R. E. Burgeson, personal communication).

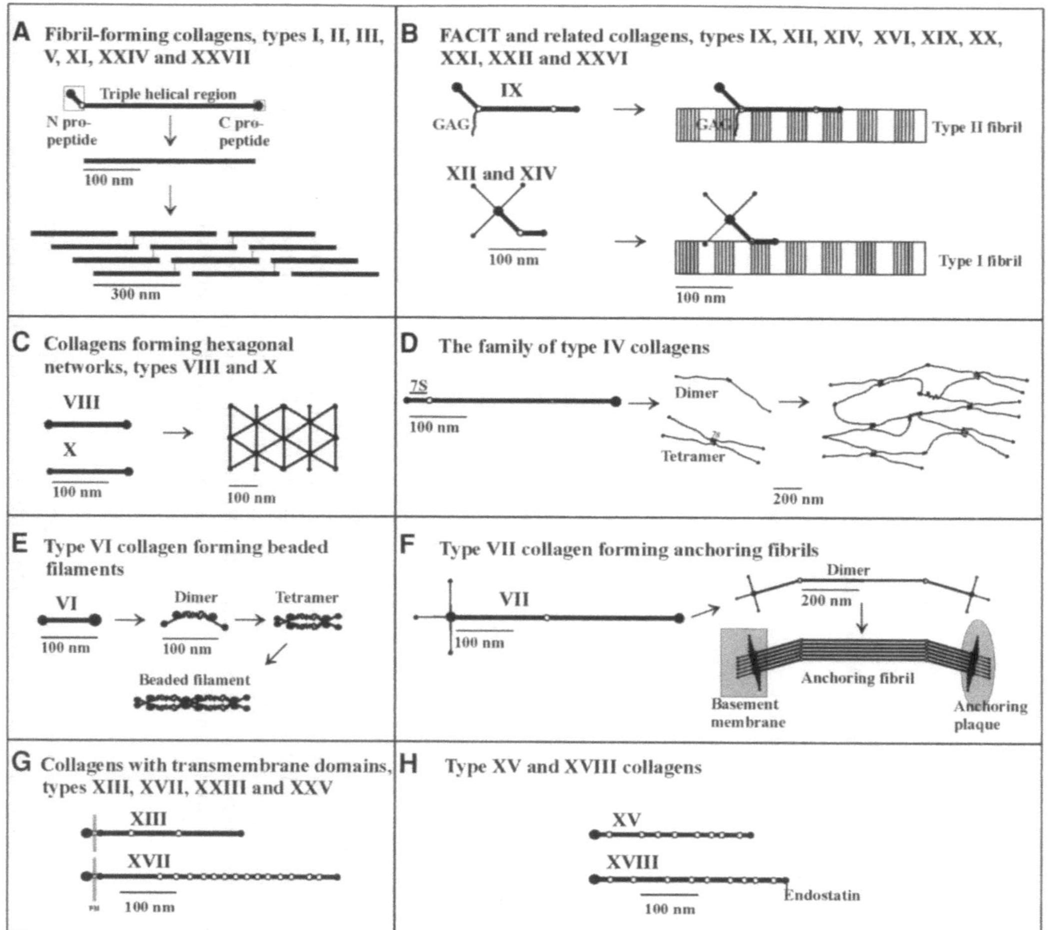

Fig. 1. Schematic representation of various members of the collagen superfamily and their known supramolecular assemblies. The letters refer to the families described in the text. The supramolecular assemblies of families G and H have not been elucidated and are hence not shown. The closed circles indicate N- and C-terminal noncollagenous domains, whereas open circles indicate noncollagenous domains interrupting the collagen triple helix. GAG, glycosaminoglycan; PM, plasma membrane. Modified from ref. *1* with permission.

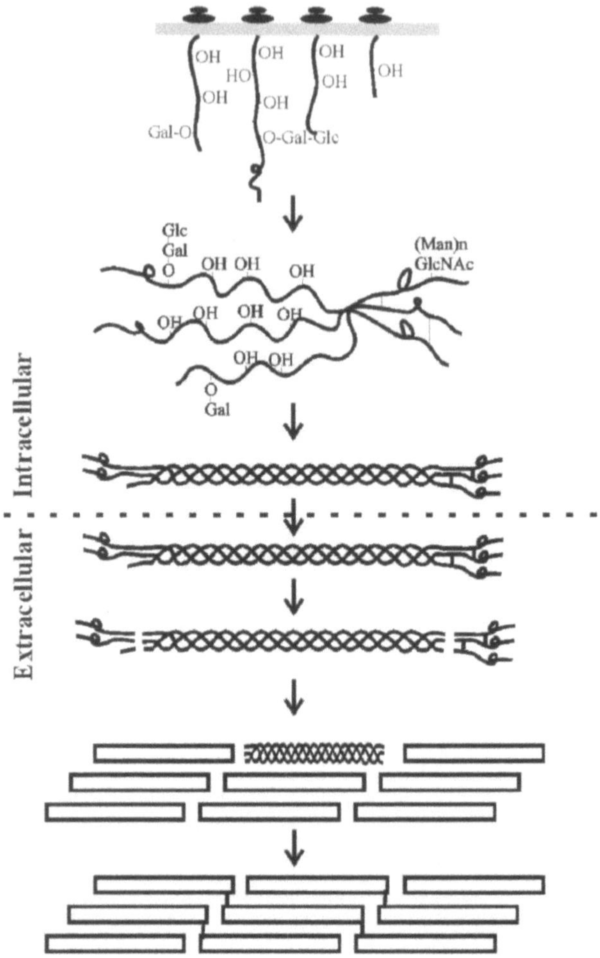

Fig. 2. Biosynthesis of a fibril-forming collagen. Procollagen polypeptide chains are synthesized on the ribosomes of the rough endoplasmic reticulum and secreted into the lumen, where the chains are modified by hydroxylation of certain proline and lysine residues and glycosylation before chain association and triple helix formation. The newly formed procollagen molecules are secreted into the extracellular space, where the N and C propeptides are cleaved by specific proteinases. The collagen molecules thus generated spontaneously assemble into fibrils, which are stabilized by the formation of covalent crosslinks. Reproduced from ref. *1* with permission.

family of type IV collagens found in basement membranes; E, type VI collagen that forms beaded filaments; F, type VII collagen that forms anchoring fibrils for basement membranes; G, collagens with transmembrane domains, types XIII, XVII, XXIII, and XXV; and H, the family of type XV and XVIII collagens *(1–3)*.

The most abundant type I–III collagens, in addition to type V and XI collagens, self-assemble into long quarter-staggered fibrils and are thus called fibril-forming collagens (Fig. 1; ref. *1*). The fibril-forming collagens contain large triple-helical domains of about 1000 amino acids with continuous -Gly-X-Y- repeats and short nontriple-helical N and C telopeptides at both ends. The telopeptides are the primary sites for intermolecular crosslinking, which is important for the stabilization of the collagen fibrils *(10)*. These collagens are first synthesized as larger precursors, procollagens, that have globular N and C propeptide domains, which are cleaved off from the mature collagen molecules (Figs. 1 and 2; ref. *1*).

Type I collagen is the major structural constituent of most connective tissues, including bone, whereas type II is the major component in cartilage (Table 1). Type III collagen is generally found in the same tissues as type I, but especially in elastic tissues (Table 1). Collagen fibrils are often heterogeneous, containing more than one collagen type. Type I collagen fibrils usually contain small amounts of type III, V, and XII, with type V being located in the core and types III and XII on the surface of the fibril *(1)*. The cartilage collagen fibrils have type II as their main component, with a core of type XI and a surface of type IX *(1)*. The type V and XI collagens have an important role in the regulation of the type I and type II fibril diameters, respectively *(11,12)*.

BIOSYNTHESIS OF COLLAGENS

Biosynthesis of collagens is a complex process that involves a number of intracellular and extracellular post-translational modifications *(1,13,14)*. The fibril-forming collagens are synthesized as larger precursors that have globular propeptide domains at both their N and C-terminal ends (Fig. 2). An N-terminal signal sequence targets the nascent proα chains into the endoplasmic reticulum (ER), where a series of modifications occur. The main intracellular modifications (Fig. 2) of the proα chains include the cleavage of the signal peptide; hydroxylation of specific proline and lysine residues to 4-hydroxyproline, 3-hydroxyproline, and hydroxylysine; *O*-linked glycosylation of some of the hydroxylysine residues to galactosylhydroxylysine and glucosyl galactosylhydroxylysine; *N*-linked glycosylation of one or both of the propeptides; and formation of intrachain and interchain disulfide bonds *(1,13,14)*. After the C propeptides have associated in a type-specific manner *(13)* and approx 100 proline residues in each chain have been hydroxylated, a nucleation site for triple helix formation is formed in the C-terminal end of the triple-helical domain and the triple helix is then propagated toward the N terminus.

The procollagen molecules are transported from the ER through the Golgi complex by progressive maturation of the Golgi cisternae rather than vesicular transport *(15)*. The extracellular steps *(1)* involve the conversion of procollagen molecules to collagen molecules by the cleavage of the N and C propeptides *(16)*, self-assembly of the collagen molecules into fibrils by nucleation and propagation, and formation of covalent crosslinks *(10)*.

The collagen synthesis described above is characteristic for fibril-forming collagens. The biosynthesis steps of nonfibrillar collagens are principally the same with certain exceptions *(1)*. Many collagens have globular N- and/or C-terminal domains that are not cleaved (Fig. 1), the triple helices of transmembrane collagens are probably propagated from the N to the C terminus *(17,18)*, and the triple helices of some collagens are modified by *N*-linked glycosylation or addition of glycosaminoglycan side chains.

The intracellular modifications require five specific enzymes: three collagen hydroxylases *(19–21)* and two collagen glycosyltransferases *(1)*, whereas the extracellular modifications require three specific enzymes: two proteinases that cleave the propeptides *(16)* and an oxidase *(22)* that converts certain lysine and hydroxylysine residues to reactive aldehyde derivatives required in the crosslink formation. The collagen hydroxylases, prolyl 4-hydroxylase, prolyl 3-hydroxylase, and lysyl hydroxylase, catalyze the formation of 4-hydroxyproline, 3-hydroxyproline, and hydroxylysine residues in -X-Pro-Gly, -Pro-4Hyp-Gly-, and -X-Lys-Gly- triplets, respectively *(19–21)*. 4-Hydroxyproline residues have an important role in stabilizing the collagen triple helix *(9)* and hydroxylysine residues serve as attachments sites for carbohydrate units and participate in the formation of intermolecular collagen crosslinks *(19)*. The function of 3-hydroxyproline residues is still unknown *(19)*.

The specific collagen-modifying enzymes were long assumed to be of one type only, with no isoenzymes, but this concept has changed recently. Vertebrate prolyl 4-hydroxylases are now known to have at least three isoenzymes *(19–21,23,24)*. Type I prolyl 4-hydroxylase is the main form in most cell types, whereas the type II enzyme is the major form in chondrocytes, osteoblasts, endothelial cells, and cells of epithelial structures *(25,26)*. Four lysyl hydroxylase isoenzymes *(19,27–30)* and three procollagen N proteinase isoenzymes *(16,31)* have been identified, whereas procollagen C proteinase has been found to belong to the family of tolloids, with other isoenzymes known as tolloid, tolloid-like 1, and tolloid-like 2, the last one lacking C proteinase activity *(18)*. Five lysyl oxidase isoenzymes have been cloned and characterized *(22,32–34)*. Knockout and transgenic mice are currently being generated to study the differences in functions and expression patterns of the multiple isoenzymes of the specific collagen-modifying enzymes. It has already been shown that transgenic mice with inactive procollagen N proteinase I develop fragile skin and surprisingly are also male sterile *(35)* and that homozygous knockout mice for the main lysyl oxidase isoenzyme are perinatal lethal and have severe dysfunction of the cardiovascular system *(36)*. The genes for prolyl 3-hydroxylase, collagen galactosyltransferase, and collagen glucosyltransferase have not been cloned yet. However, it has been reported that lysyl hydroxylase 3 has collagen glucosyltransferase and galactosyltransferase activities *(37–39)*, but the levels of these activities are so low that their biological significance remains to be established *(39)*. The functions of the hydroxylysine-linked carbohydrate units are not fully known, but their role in the regulation of fibril formation and fibril diameter has been confirmed using recombinant type II collagen with low and high levels of hydroxylysine and its glycosylated forms *(40)*.

In addition to the modifications catalyzed by the above specific enzymes, the signal peptides are cleaved as in other proteins, *N*-linked carbohydrate units are added to the propeptides of fibril-forming collagens and noncollagenous domains of some other collagen types, peptidyl proline cis-trans isomerases catalyze the isomerization of peptide bonds involving proline residues, and protein disulfide isomerase catalyzes the formation of intra- and interchain disulfide bonds *(1,13,14)*. Protein disulfide isomerase has at least two other distinct functions in the collagen biosynthesis: it acts as the β subunit in the prolyl 4-hydroxylase $\alpha_2\beta_2$ tetramer *(19–21)* and it retains unassembled procollagen chains within the ER *(41)*. Collagen synthesis also involves a specific chaperone, Hsp47 *(42,43)*, which is clearly required for normal development because homozygous Hsp47 knockout mice are embryonic lethal *(44)*. Hsp47 interacts with triple-helical procollagen molecules and probably functions early in the secretory pathway to prevent lateral aggregation of procollagen molecules *(45,46)*.

MUTATIONS IN COLLAGEN GENES

The essential function of collagens in providing structural integrity to tissues and organs is illustrated by the broad range of diseases caused by mutations in the human collagen genes (Table 2; ref. *1*). More than 1000 mutations have now been characterized for 13 of the 26 collagen types currently known *(1,47–50)*. A vast majority of these mutations are single base substitutions that alter a codon of an obligatory glycine in a -Gly-X-Y- triplet to a bulkier amino acid or lead to RNA splicing defects. Other amino acid substitutions and premature translational termination codons, as well as deletions, insertions, duplications, and complex rearrangements, have also been identified. The effects of the mutations vary depending on their nature and position in the collagen chain and thus mutations in the same gene can cause disease phenotypes ranging from relatively mild forms to severe and lethal forms or just confer a genetic risk factor for a certain disease. Glycine substitutions can either totally prevent the folding of the triple helix beyond the mutation point or cause an interruption in the triple helix. Because the triple helix of most collagens is propagated from the C terminus to the N terminus, a glycine mutation closer to its C terminus often produces a more severe phenotype than a corresponding mutation near the N terminus, but there are many exceptions to this rule *(1)*. Many of the collagen mutations have a procollagen suicide or dominant-negative effect because the mutant chains can still associate with normal chains, but folding of the triple helix is prevented, leading to the degradation of both normal and mutant chains. In other cases, the mutations may not interfere with the folding but result in a conformational change in the collagen molecule, possibly leading to its impaired function, or association of the mutant chains may be completely prevented, leading to degradation of only the mutant chains while the normal chains can still assemble into functional collagen molecules *(1)*.

Table 2
Diseases Caused by Mutations in Genes for Collagens[a]

Gene	*Disease[b]*
COL1A1; *COL1A2*	OI
	EDS type I, II, VIIA, VIIB
	Osteoporosis
COL2A1	Several chondrodysplasias
	Osteoarthrosis
COL3A1	EDS type IV
	Arterial aneurysms
COL4A3; *COL4A4*; *COL4A5*	Alport syndrome
COL4A5 and *COL4A6*	Alport syndrome with diffuse esophageal leiomyomatosis
COL5A1; *COL5A2*	EDS types I and II
COL6A1; *COL6A2*; *COL6A3*	Bethlem myopathy
COL7A1	EB, dystrophic forms
COL8A2	Corneal endothelial dystrophy
COL9A1; *COL9A2*; *COL9A3*	Multiple epiphyseal dysplasia
	Lumbar disc disease
	Osteoarthrosis
COL10A1	Schmid metaphyseal chondrodysplasia
COL11A1; *COL11A2*	Several mild chondrodysplasias
	Nonsyndromic hearing loss
	Osteoarthrosis
COL17A1	Generalized atrophic benign EB
COL18A1	Knobloch syndrome

[a]Refs. *1,47–51,58–78*.
[b]OI, osteogenesis imperfecta; EDS, Ehlers-Danlos syndrome; EB, epidermolysis bullosa.

Collagen Mutations in Diseases Affecting Skeletogenesis

Collagens have a critical role in the development and proper function of the skeleton, as illustrated by the numerous collagen mutations identified in osteochondrodysplasias *(1,47,49–52)*. Several mouse models with skeletal defects caused by collagen mutations are now available and have proven very valuable in understanding of the corresponding human diseases *(1,51,53–56)*.

Osteogenesis Imperfecta (OI) and Osteoporosis (Collagen I)

Over 300 mutations have now been identified in the two genes encoding the proα1(I) and proα2(I) chains of the type I procollagen heterotrimer, $[\text{pro}\alpha1(\text{I})]_2\text{pro}\alpha2(\text{I})$ *(49,50)*, a vast majority of them being found in patients with OI (Table 2; refs. *1,47,49–51*). OI is characterized by a generalized decrease in bone mass that leads to brittle bones, but also other tissues rich in type I collagen are affected and, therefore, OI patients frequently have blue sclerae, dental abnormalities, thin skin, weak tendons, and progressive hearing loss *(1,47,51)*. OI is clinically highly heterogeneous and is divided into four main types. Type II OI is the most severe form, leading to perinatal death, whereas the types I and IV are the mildest *(51)*. The types of mutation and their consequences are similar to those described above, with approx 85% of the identified OI mutations being glycine substitutions in the triple-helical domain and approx 12% of them causing exon skipping *(51)*. The mildest OI forms are usually caused by mutations that inactivate one gene allele because of a premature translation termination codon *(1,47)*.

Because OI is a highly heterogeneous disorder, it is in some cases difficult to distinguish patients with milder forms of OI from familial osteoporosis, which result in fractures *(1)*. Therefore, type I collagen mutations have also been found in some patients who show little evidence of OI but have osteopenia and fractures *(1,47)*. However, type I collagen mutations are not likely to be common causes of osteoporosis *(1,47)*.

Chondrodysplasias, Osteoarthrosis, and Lumbar Disc Disease

Type II collagen constitutes 80–85% of the total collagen content of cartilage and forms fibrils that contain small amounts of type IX and XI collagens, their quantities ranging between 3% and 10%, depending on the cartilage source and age *(57)*. Type X collagen is expressed in the hypertrophic zone of calcifying cartilage during skeletal development and bone growth *(57)*.

Type II collagen mutations produce a spectrum of chondrodysplasias (Table 2) that range in severity from perinatal lethality to mildly affected individuals *(1)*. Over 50 mutations in the *COL2A1* gene have now been reported in patients with achondrogenesis II/hypochondrogenesis, spondyloepiphyseal dysplasia, spondyloepimetaphyseal dysplasia, and the Kniest, Wagner and Stickler syndromes *(49)*. All the main types of collagen mutations described above have been found in the *COL2A1* gene *(1)*.

Mutations have also been identified in the two minor components of cartilage collagen fibrils, the type IX and XI collagens (Table 2). Type IX collagen mutations have been shown to cause multiple epiphyseal dysplasia, a clinically and genetically heterogeneous disorder characterized by early-onset osteoarthrosis and mildly short stature *(58–65)*. Mutations in type IX collagen genes have also been found in the two most common musculoskeletal disorders, osteoarthrosis and lumbar disc disease *(66–70)*. Type XI collagen mutations have been identified in Stickler and Marshall syndromes, otospondylomegaepiphyseal dysplasia, and Weissenbacher-Zweymüller syndrome *(71–77)*. About 30 type X collagen mutations have been characterized in patients with Schmid metaphyseal chondrodysplasia *(49,78)*.

REFERENCES

1. Myllyharju, J. and Kivirikko, K. I. (2001) Collagens and collagen-related diseases. *Ann. Med.* **33,** 7–21.
2. Koch, M., Foley, J. E., Hahn, R., Zhou, P., Burgeson, R. E., Gerecke, D. R., and Gordon, M. K. (2001) α1(XX) collagen, a new member of the collagen subfamily, fibril-associated collagens with interrupted triple helices. *J. Biol. Chem.* **276,** 23120–23126.
3. Fitzgerald, J. and Bateman, J. F. (2001) A new FACIT of the collagen family: COL21A1. *FEBS Lett.* **505,** 275–280.
4. Banyard, J., Bao, L., and Zetter, B. R. (2003) Type XXIII collagen, a new transmembrane collagen identified in metastatic tumor cells. *J. Biol. Chem.* **278,** 20989–20994.
5. Koch, M., Laub, F., Zhou, P., Hahn, R. A., Tanaka, S., Burgeson, R. E., et al. (2003) Collagen XXIV, a vertebrate fibrillar collagen with structural features of invertebrate collagens: selective expression in developing cornea and bone. *J. Biol. Chem.* **278,** 43236–43244.
6. Hashimoto, T., Wakabayashi, T., Watanabe, A., Kowa, H., Hosoda, R., Nakamura, A., et al. (2002) CLAC: a novel Alzheimer amyloid plaque component derived from a transmembrane precursor, CLAC-P/collagen type XXV. *EMBO J.* **21,** 1524–1534.
7. Sato, K., Yomogida, K., Wada, T., Yorihuzi, T., Nishimune, Y., Hosokawa, N., et al. (2002) Type XXVI collagen, a new member of the collagen family, is specifically expressed in the testis and ovary. *J. Biol. Chem.* **277,** 37678–37684.
8. Pace, J. M., Corrado, M., Missero, C., and Byers, P. H. (2003) Identification, characterization and expression analysis of a new fibrillar collagen gene, *COL27A1*. *Matrix Biol.* **22,** 3–14.
9. Jenkins, C. L. and Raines, R. T. (2002) Insights on the conformational stability of collagen. *Nat. Prod. Rep.* **19,** 49–59.
10. Knott, L. and Bailey, A. J. (1998) Collagen cross-links in mineralizing tissues: a review of their chemistry, function and clinical relevance. *Bone* **22,** 181–187.
11. Birk, D. E. (2001) Type V collagen: heterotypic type I/V collagen interactions in the regulation of fibril assembly. *Micron* **32,** 223–237.
12. Blaschke, U. K., Eikenberry, E. F., Hulmes, D. J., Galla, H. J., and Bruckner, P. (2000) Collagen XI nucleates self-assembly and limits lateral growth of cartilage fibrils. *J. Biol. Chem.* **275,** 10370–10378.
13. McLaughlin, S. H. and Bulleid, N. J. (1998) Molecular recognition in procollagen chain assembly. *Matrix Biol.* **16,** 369–377.
14. Lamandé, S. R. and Bateman, J. F. (1999) Procollagen folding and assembly: the role of endoplasmic reticulum enzymes and molecular chaperones. *Semin. Cell Dev. Biol.* **10,** 455–464.
15. Bonfanti, L., Mironov, A. A. Jr., Martinez-Menárguez, J. A., Martella, O., Fusella, A., Baldassarre, M., Buccione, R., et al. (1998) Procollagen traverses the Golgi stack without leaving the lumen of cisternae. *Cell* **95,** 993–1023.

16. Prockop, D. J., Sieron, A. L., and Li, S.-W. (1998) Procollagen N-proteinase and procollagen C-proteinase. Two unusual metalloproteinases that are essential for procollagen processing probably have important roles in development and cell signaling. *Matrix Biol.* **16,** 399–408.
17. Snellman, A., Tu, H., Väisänen, T., Kvist, A.-P., Huhtala, P., and Pihlajaniemi, T. (2000) A short sequence in the N-terminal region is required for the trimerization of type XIII collagen and is conserved in other collagenous transmembrane proteins. *EMBO J.* **19,** 1–10.
18. Areida, S. K., Reinhardt, D. P., Müller, P. K., Fietzek, P. P., Köwitz, J., Marinkovich, M. P., et al. (2001) Properties of the collagen type XVII ectodomain. Evidence for N- to C-terminal triple helix folding. *J. Biol. Chem.* **276,** 1594–1601.
19. Kivirikko, K. I. and Pihlajaniemi, T. (1998) Hydroxylation of proline and lysine residues in collagens and other animal and plant proteins. *Adv. Enzymol. Rel. Areas Mol. Biol.* **72,** 325–399.
20. Kivirikko, K. I. and Myllyharju, J. (1998) Prolyl 4-hydroxylases and their protein disulfide isomerase subunit. *Matrix Biol.* **16,** 357–368.
21. Myllyharju, J. (2002) Prolyl 4-hydroxylases, the key enzymes of collagen biosynthesis. *Matrix Biol.* **22,** 15–24.
22. Csiszar, K. (2001) Lysyl oxidases: a novel multifunctional amine oxidase family. *Prog. Nucleic Acid Res. Mol. Biol.* **70,** 1–32.
23. Kukkola, L., Hieta, R., Kivirikko, K. I., and Myllyharju, J. (2003) Identification and characterization of a third human, rat and mouse collagen prolyl 4-hydroxylase isoenzyme. *J. Biol. Chem.* **278,** 47685–47693.
24. Van Den Diepstraten, C., Papay, K., Bolender, Z., Brown, A., and Pickering, J. G. (2003) Cloning of a novel prolyl 4-hydroxylase subunit expressed in the fibrous cap of human atherosclerotic plaque. *Circulation* **108,** 508–511.
25. Annunen, P., Autio-Harmainen, H., and Kivirikko, K. I. (1998) The novel type II prolyl 4-hydroxylase is the main enzyme form in chondrocytes and capillary endothelial cells, whereas the type I enzyme predominates in most cells. *J. Biol. Chem.* **273,** 5989–5992.
26. Nissi, R., Autio-Harmainen, H., Marttila, P., Sormunen, R., and Kivirikko, K. I. (2001) Prolyl 4-hydroxylase isoenzymes I and II have different expression patterns in several human tissues. *J. Histochem. Cytochem.* **49,** 1143–1153.
27. Valtavaara, M., Papponen, H., Pirttilä, A.-M., Hiltunen, K., Helander, H., and Myllylä, R. (1997) Cloning and characterization of a novel human lysyl hydroxylase isoform highly expressed in pancreas and muscle. *J. Biol. Chem.* **272,** 6831–6834.
28. Passoja, K., Rautavuoma, K., Ala-Kokko, L., Kosonen, T., and Kivirikko, K. I. (1998) Cloning and characterization of a third human lysyl hydroxylase isoform. *Proc. Natl. Acad. Sci. USA* **95,** 10482–10486.
29. Valtavaara, M., Szpirer, C., Szpirer, J., and Myllylä, R. (1998) Primary structure, tissue distribution, and chromosomal localization of a novel isoform of lysyl hydroxylase (lysyl hydroxylase 3). *J. Biol. Chem.* **273,** 12881–12886.
30. Bank, R. A., Robins, S. P., Wijmenga, C., Breslau-Siderius, L. J., Bardoel, A. F. J., Van der Sluijs, H. A., et al. (1999) Defective collagen crosslinking in bone, but not in ligament or cartilage, in Bruck syndrome: indications for a bone-specific telopeptide lysyl hydroxylase on chromosome 17. *Proc. Natl. Acad. Sci. USA* **96,** 1054–1058.
31. Colige, A., Vandenberghe, I., Thiry, M., Lambert, C. A., Van Beeumen, J., Li, S.-W., et al. (2002) Cloning and characterization of ADAMTS-14, a novel ADAMTS displaying high homology with ADAMTS-2 and ADAMTS-3. *J. Biol. Chem.* **277,** 5756–5766.
32. Mäki, J. M., Tikkanen, H., and Kivirikko, K. I. (2001) Cloning and characterization of a fifth human lysyl oxidase isoenzyme: the third member of the lysyl oxidase-related subfamily with four scavenger receptor cysteine-rich domains. *Matrix Biol.* **20,** 493–496.
33. Ito, H., Akiyama, H., Iguchi, H., Iyama, K., Miyamoto, M., Ohsawa, K., and Nakamura, T. (2001) Molecular cloning and biological activity of a novel lysyl oxidase-related gene expressed in cartilage. *J. Biol. Chem.* **276,** 24023–24029.
34. Asuncion, L., Fogelgren, B., Fong, K. S., Fong, S. F., Kim, Y., and Csiszar, K. (2001) A novel human lysyl oxidase-like gene (LOXL4) on chromosome 10q24 has an altered scavenger receptor cysteine rich domain. *Matrix Biol.* **20,** 487–491.
35. Li, S.-W., Arita, M., Fertala, A., Bao, Y., Kopen, G. C., Långsjö, T. K., et al. (2001) Transgenic mice with inactive alleles for procollagen N-proteinase (ADAMTS-2) develop fragile skin and male sterility. *Biochem. J.* **355,** 271–278.
36. Mäki, J. M., Räsänen, J., Tikkanen, H., Sormunen, R., Mäkikallio, K., Kivirikko, K. I., and Soininen, R. (2002) Inactivation of the lysyl oxidase gene leads to aortic aneurysms, cardiovascular dysfunction and perinatal death in mice. *Circulation* **106,** 2503–2509.
37. Heikkinen, J., Risteli, M., Wang, C., Latvala, J., Rossi, M., Valtavaara, M., and Myllylä, R. (2000) Lysyl hydroxylase 3 is a multifunctional protein possessing collagen glucosyltransferase activity. *J. Biol. Chem.* **275,** 36158–36163.
38. Wang, C., Risteli, M., Heikkinen, J., Hussa, A.-K., Uitto, L., and Myllylä, R. (2002) Identification of amino acids important for the catalytic activity of the collagen glucosyltransferase associated with the multifunctional lysyl hydroxylase 3 (LH3). *J. Biol. Chem.* **277,** 18568–18573.
39. Rautavuoma, K., Takaluoma, K., Passoja, K., Pirskanen, A., Kvist, A.-P., Kivirikko, K. I., et al. (2002) Characterization of three fragments that constitute the monomers of the human lysyl hydroxylase isoenzymes 1–3. The 30-kDa N-terminal fragment is not required for lysyl hydroxylase activity. *J. Biol. Chem.* **277,** 23084–23091.
40. Notbohm, H., Nokelainen, M., Myllyharju, J., Fietzek, P. P., Müller, P. K., and Kivirikko, K. I. (1999) Recombinant human type II collagens with low and high levels of hydroxylysine and its glycosylated forms show marked differences in fibrillogenesis *in vitro*. *J. Biol. Chem.* **274,** 8988–8992.
41. Bottomley, M. J., Batten, M. R., Lumb, R. A., and Bulleid, N. J. (2001) Quality control in the endoplasmic reticulum: PDI mediates the ER retention of unassembled procollagen C-propeptides. *Curr. Biol.* **11,** 1114–1118.
42. Nagata, K. (1998) Expression and function of heat shock protein 47: a collagen-specific molecular chaperone in the endoplasmic reticulum. *Matrix Biol.* **16,** 379–386.

43. Hendershot, L. M. and Bulleid, N. J. (2000) Protein-specific chaperones: the role of hsp47 begins to gel. *Curr. Biol.* **10,** R912–R915.
44. Nagai, N., Hosokawa, M., Itohara, S., Adachi, E., Matsushita, T., Hosokawa, N., and Nagata, K. (2000) Embryonic lethality of molecular chaperone Hsp47 knockout mice is associated with defects in collagen biosynthesis. *J. Cell Biol.* **150,** 1499–1505.
45. Koide, T., Takahara, Y., Asada, S., and Nagata, K. (2002) Xaa-Arg-Gly triplets in the collagen triple helix are dominant binding sites for the molecular chaperone HSP47. *J. Biol. Chem.* **277,** 6178–6182.
46. Tasab, M., Jenkinson, L., and Bulleid, N. J. (2002) Sequence-specific recognition of collagen triple helices by the collagen-specific molecular chaperone HSP47. *J. Biol. Chem.* **277,** 35007–35012.
47. Kuivaniemi, H., Tromp, G., and Prockop, D. J. (1997) Mutations in fibrillar collagens (types I, II, III and XI), fibril-associated collagen (type IX), and network-forming collagen (type X) cause a spectrum of diseases of bone, cartilage, and blood vessels. *Hum. Mutat.* **9,** 300–315.
48. Biswas, S., Munier, F. L., Yardley, J., Hart-Holden, N., Perveen, R., Cousin, P., et al. (2001) Missense mutations in *COL8A2*, the gene encoding the α2 chain of type VIII collagen, cause two forms of corneal endothelial dystrophy. *Hum. Mol. Genet.* **10,** 2415–2423.
49. Krawczak, M. and Cooper, D. N. (1997) The human gene mutation database. *Trends Genet.* **13,** 121–122.
50. Dalgleish, R. (1997) The human type I collagen mutation database. *Nucleic Acids Res.* **25,** 181–187.
51. Forlino, A. and Marini, J. C. (2000) Osteogenesis imperfecta: prospects for molecular therapeutics. *Mol. Genet. Metab.* **71,** 225–232.
52. Olsen, B. R., Reginato, A. M., and Wang, W. (2000) Bone development. *Annu. Rev. Cell Dev. Biol.* **16,** 191–220.
53. Aszódi, A., Bateman, J. F., Gustafsson, E., Booth-Handford, R., and Fässler, R. (2000) Mammalian skeletogenesis and extracellular matrix: what can we learn from knockout mice? *Cell Struct. Funct.* **25,** 73–84.
54. Gustafsson, E. and Fässler, R. (2000) Insights into extracellular matrix functions from mutant mouse models. *Exp. Cell Res.* **261,** 52–68.
55. McLean, W. and Olsen, B. R. (2001) Mouse models of abnormal skeletal development and homeostasis. *Trends Genet.* **10,** S38–S43.
56. Helminen, H. J., Säämänen, A.-M., Salminen, H., and Hyttinen, M. M. (2002) Transgenic mouse models for studying the role of cartilage macromolecules in osteoarthritis. *Rheumatology* **41,** 848–856.
57. Cremer, M. A., Rosloniec, E. F., and Kang, A. H. (1998) The cartilage collagens: a review of their structure, organization, and role in the pathogenesis of experimental arthritis in animals and in human rheumatic disease. *J. Mol. Med.* **76,** 275–288.
58. Muragaki, Y., Mariman, E. C. M., van Beersum, S. E. C., Perälä, M., van Mourik, J. B. A., Warman, M. L., et al. (1996) A mutation in the gene encoding the α2 chain of the fibril-associated collagen IX, *COL9A2*, causes multiple epiphyseal dysplasia (EDM2). *Nat. Genet.* **12,** 103–105.
59. Holden, P., Canty, E. G., Mortier, G. R., Zabel, B., Spranger, J., Carr, A., et al. (1999) Identification of novel pro-α2(IX) collagen gene mutations in two families with distinctive oligo-epiphyseal forms of multiple epiphyseal dysplasia. *Am. J. Hum. Genet.* **65,** 31–38.
60. Paassilta, P., Lohiniva, J., Annunen, S., Bonaventure, J., Le Merrer, M., Pai, L., et al. (1999) *COL9A3*: a third locus for multiple epiphyseal dysplasia. *Am. J. Hum. Genet.* **64,** 1036–1044.
61. Bönnemann, C. G., Cox, G. F., Shapiro, F., Wu, J. J., Feener, C. A., Thompson, T. G., et al. (2000) A mutation in the (3 chain of type IX collagen causes autosomal dominant multiple epiphyseal dysplasia with mild myopathy. *Proc. Natl. Acad. Sci. USA* **97,** 1212–1217.
62. Lohiniva, J., Paassilta, P., Seppänen, U., Vierimaa, O., Kivirikko, S., and Ala-Kokko, L. (2000) Splicing mutations in the COL3 domain of collagen IX cause multiple epiphyseal dysplasia. *Am. J. Med. Genet.* **90,** 216–222.
63. Spayde, E. C., Joshi, A. P., Wilcox, W. R., Briggs, M., Cohn, D. H., and Olsen, B. R. (2000) Exon skipping mutation in the *COL9A2* gene in a family with multiple epiphyseal dysplasia. *Matrix Biol.* **19,** 121–128.
64. Czarny-Ratajczak, M., Lohiniva, J., Rogala, P., Kozlowski, K., Perälä, M., Carter, L., et al. (2001) A mutation in *COL9A1* causes multiple epiphyseal dysplasia: further evidence for locus heterogeneity. *Am. J. Hum. Genet.* **69,** 969–980.
65. Briggs, M. D. and Chapman, K. L. (2002) Pseudoachondroplasia and multiple epiphyseal dysplasia: mutation review, molecular interactions, and genotype to phenotype correlations. *Hum. Mutat.* **19,** 465–478.
66. Mustafa, Z., Chapman, K., Irven, C., Carr, A. J., Clipsham, K., Chitnavis, J., et al. (2000) Linkage analysis of candidate genes as susceptibility loci for osteoarthritis suggestive linkage of *COL9A1* to female hip osteoarthritis. *Rheumatology* **39,** 299–306.
67. Loughlin, J., Mustafa, Z., Dowling, B., Southam, L., Marcelline, L., Räinä, S. S., et al. (2002) Finer linkage mapping of a primary hip osteoarthritis susceptibility locus on chromosome 6. *Eur. J. Hum. Genet.* **10,** 562–568.
68. Annunen, S., Paassilta, P., Lohiniva, J., Perälä, M., Pihlajamaa, T., Karppinen, J., et al. (1999) An allele of *COL9A2* associated with intervertebral disc disease. *Science* **285,** 409–412.
69. Paassilta, P., Lohiniva, J., Göring, H. H. H., Perälä, M., Räinä, S. S., Karppinen, J., et al. (2001) Identification of a novel common genetic risk factor for lumbar disc disease. *JAMA* **285,** 1843–1849.
70. Ala-Kokko, L. (2002) Genetic risk factors for lumbar disc disease. *Ann. Med.* **34,** 42–47.
71. Vikkula, M., Mariman, E. C. M., Lui, V. C. H., Zhidkova, N. I., Tiller, G. E., Goldring, M. B., et al. (1995) Autosomal dominant and recessive osteochondrodysplasias associated with the *COL11A2* locus. *Cell* **80,** 431–437.

72 Richards, A. J., Yates, J. R. W., Williams, R., Payne, S. J., Pope, F. M., Scott, J. D., and Snead, M. P. (1996) A family with Stickler syndrome type 2 has a mutation in the *COL11A1* gene resulting in the substitution of glycine 97 by valine in α1(XI) collagen. *Hum. Mol. Genet.* **5,** 1339–1343.

73. Sirko-Osadsa, D. A., Murray, M. A., Scott, J. A., Lavery, M. A., Warman, M. L., and Robin, N. H. (1998) Stickler syndrome without eye involvement is caused by mutations in *COL11A2,* the gene encoding the (2(XI) chain of type XI collagen. *J. Pediatr.* **132,** 368–371.

74. Griffith, A. J., Sprunger, L. K., Sirko-Osadsa, D. A., Tiller, G. E., Meisler, M. H., and Warman, M. L. (1998) Marshall syndrome associated with a splicing defect at the *COL11A1* locus. *Am. J. Hum. Genet.* **62,** 816–823.

75. Annunen, S., Körkkö, J., Czarny, M., Warman, M. L., Brunner, H. G., Kääriäinen, H., et al. (1999) Splicing mutations of 54-bp exons in the *COL11A1* gene cause Marshall syndrome, but other mutations cause overlapping Marshall/Stickler phenotypes. *Am. J. Hum. Genet.* **65,** 974–983.

76. Pihlajamaa, T., Prockop, D. J., Faber, J., Winterpacht, A., Zabel, B., Giedion, A., Wiesbauer, P., Spranger, J., and Ala-Kokko, L. (1998) Heterozygous glycine substitution in the *COL11A2* gene in the original patient with the Weissenbacher-Zweymüller syndrome demonstrates its identity with heterozygous OSMED (nonocular Stickler syndrome). *Am. J. Med. Genet.* **80,** 115–120.

77. Melkoniemi, M., Brunner, H. G., Manouvrier, S., Hennekam, R., Superti-Furga, A., Kääriäinen, H., et al. (2000) Autosomal recessive disorder otospondylomegaepiphyseal dysplasia is associated with loss-of-function mutations in thc *COL11A2* gene. *Am. J. Hum. Genet.* **66,** 368–377.

78. Chan, D. and Jacenko, O. (1998) Phenotypic and biochemical consequences of collagen X mutations in mice and humans. *Matrix Biol.* **17,** 169–184.

6
Mechanotransduction Pathways in Cartilage

Qian Chen

SIGNIFICANCE

It is known that cartilage homeostasis is regulated by mechanical signals during limb development, fracture repair, and skeletal remodeling. The dramatic effect of mechanical stimulation of bone growth is best illustrated by distraction osteogenesis, in which distraction forces are applied to a healing limb to stimulate bone formation *(1,2)*. When distraction stress is applied at certain amplitude and frequency, new bone formation is sustained, thereby achieving limb lengthening. In recent years, great progress has been made in understanding how new bone formation is activated by mechanical stimulation and the cellular signal transduction pathway to receive and convert mechanical signals into tissue growth and regeneration. In this chapter, we will summarize recent studies elucidating the molecular mechanism of biophysical regulation of cartilage growth, an important step during endochondral bone formation and fracture healing.

The mechanical effects on cartilage growth were proposed in the classical model, the Hueter-Volkmann Law, which states that "while compression forces inhibit growth, tensile forces stimulate growth" *(3,4)*. Although the general theme of this model has been supported by clinical treatment outcomes and laboratory tests *(5–7)*, the relationship between mechanical stimulation and cartilage growth lacks quantification and mechanistic analysis. A detailed analysis of the differential effects of mechanical factors on every stage of cartilage growth is needed to understand how chondrocytes sense and convert biophysical signals into a biochemical process—growth. One hypothesis is that matrix deformation, as a result of mechanical loading, stimulates not only chondrocyte proliferation but also subsequent differentiation events. Furthermore, there are specific extracellular and intracellular molecules involved in transducing mechanical signals in cartilage. Some of these molecules have been identified. These molecules will be described here. Cartilage growth and differentiation may occur in endochondral bone formation, osteoarthritis development, and fracture healing. These three processes are described in the following.

Endochondral Bone Formation

The process of cartilage growth during endochondral bone formation is a complex one that consists of multiple stages, as delineated by studies from our laboratory and many other laboratories (Fig. 1; refs. *8–10*). In the first stage, a resting chondrocyte is activated and enters into a dividing cycle. The increase of cell numbers results in growth of cartilage at this stage. The molecular markers for proliferating chondrocytes include type II collagen (IIb), aggrecan, and link protein. In the second stage, chondrocytes cease proliferation, start the maturation process, and increase their matrix production.

From: *The Skeleton: Biochemical, Genetic, and Molecular Interactions in Development and Homeostasis*
Edited by: E. J. Massaro and J. M. Rogers © Humana Press Inc., Totowa, NJ

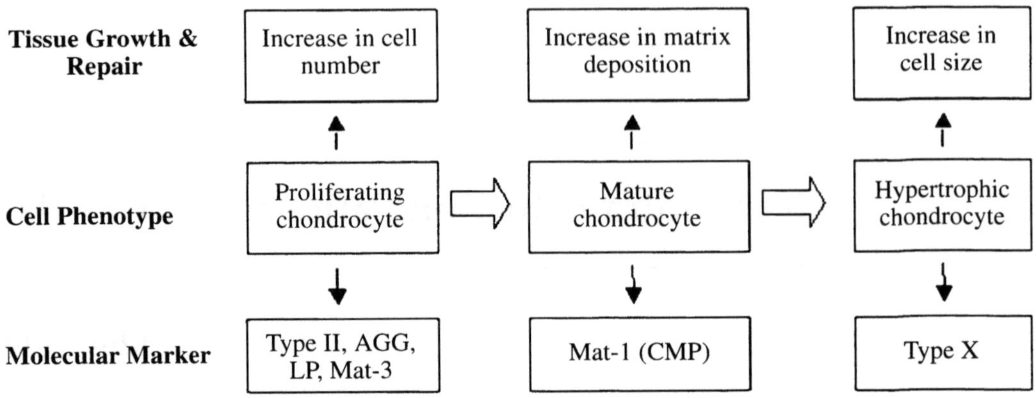

Fig. 1. Diagram depicting chondrocyte differentiation process. Type II, type II collagen; AGG, aggrecan; LP, link protein; Mat-3, matrilin-3; Mat-1, matrilin-1; CMP, cartilage matrix protein; Type X, type X collagen.

The increase of matrix deposition will also lead to growth of cartilage tissue. We identified matrilin-1, also called cartilage matrix protein (CMP), as a molecular marker for this stage. In the third stage, chondrocytes become hypertrophic and synthesize type X collagen. The enlarged cell size also contributes to the increase of cartilage volume. Finally, calcification of matrix takes place, cells undergo apoptosis (programmed cell death), and cartilage is removed and replaced by bone. Therefore, growth of cartilage can be attributed not only to proliferation of chondrocytes, but also to the differentiation process of chondrocytes, that is, maturation and hypertrophy. Conversely, apoptosis and degradation of cartilage matrix can also inhibit the growth process. Mechanical factors may regulate cartilage growth by affecting proliferation, maturation, hypertrophy, apoptosis, or all of these biological events. This question can be answered by measuring the proliferation of cells, and by quantifying gene expression of molecular markers from different chondrocyte differentiation stages, during mechanical stimulation of chondrocytes.

Cartilage Homeostasis and Osteoarthritis

This series of events (Fig. 1), which include chondrocyte proliferation, maturation, and differentiation, are recapitulated during cartilage repair and regeneration. This concept is supported by our recent discovery that matrilin-1, a molecule that is present in developing cartilage but absent from adult articular cartilage, is up-regulated (more than sixfold in this amount of protein) in osteoarthritic (OA) cartilage from adult metacarpal joints. Other molecular markers during chondrocyte differentiation, such as collagen IIa, cartilage oligomeric matrix protein, and collagen X, are also upregulated *(11)*.

Interestingly, in OA articular cartilage, CMP is detected in the middle zone and type X collagen is in the deep zone adjacent to subchondral bone. This distribution pattern mimics the one in a growth plate. These data suggest an apparent attempt by articular chondrocytes to repair their matrix networks, possibly after cells have detected the destruction and deformation of matrix during the OA process. It will be important to understand how chondrocytes sense the micromechanical environment, including the deformation of matrix, and how chondrocytes respond to the deformation signals by activating expression of matrix genes. Therefore, such study will help us not only to better understand the mechanical signal transduction pathways during cartilage growth, but also the regeneration process in a pathological condition as OA.

Fracture Healing

Bone formation during fracture healing may undergo through two pathways: intramembraneous or endochondral. Interestingly, biomechanical environment may determine which bone formation pathway a skeletal precursor cell would go through. The endochondral pathway is prevalent under unstable mechanical conditions, whereas the intramembraneous pathway is preferred under stable mechanical conditions *(12,13)*. It is not clear how mechanical environment influences cell lineage determination of an osteochondral precursor cell. Although this interesting observation is first made in vivo, analysis of the underlying mechanism may rely on experiments performed systematically in vitro. Some of these in vitro model systems are described in the next section.

IN VITRO MODEL SYSTEMS

It is well accepted that cartilage matrix deformation, as a result of mechanical loading, regulates matrix synthesis and chondrocyte behavior. To achieve this regulation, mechanical signals are transduced from outside of the cell to inside of the nucleus in a multistep process. In the first step, mechanical loading results in matrix deformation, which leads to a complex biophysical environment within the tissue, including direct mechanical strain on chondrocytes, electrokinetic effects, and fluid flow *(14–16)*. All of these factors may be important to mechanotransduction. Furthermore, in cartilage, chondrocytes are completely surrounded by extracellular matrix networks, thus they receive biomechanical signals from a 360° environment. These complexities make it difficult to study the biophysical effects of matrix deformation on chondrocytes. To address this question, different model systems have been developed. Each model system has its pros and cons. Three major types of model systems are described in the following, with emphasis on a model that was developed in our laboratory.

Cartilage Compression

This is one of the most well-developed systems to test the effect of mechanical loading on cartilage. A cartilage plug, either attached to underlying bone or not, is subject to mechanical compression. The effects on biosynthesis are then quantified. The advantage of such a system is that chondrocytes maintain their extracellular matrix environment in vivo, and that test condition may mimic mechanical load to joint articular cartilage. Such cartilage compression studies have provided important insight into the effect of compressive load on chondrocyte biosynthesis. It was revealed that although static compression of cartilage inhibits biosynthesis of extracellular matrix *(17–20)*, cyclic mechanical strain, hydrostatic pressure, and dynamic compression at certain frequencies and amplitudes increase biosynthesis *(21–24)*. Thus, static and dynamic compression system may exert opposite effects on chondrocyte biosynthesis. However, cartilage compression system may have disadvantages as well. The cartilage plug under testing may contain different zones of chondrocytes, whose properties may vary between each other. In addition, it is difficult to test the effect of tensile forces on chondrocytes with this system.

Manipulation of Single Chondrocyte or Monolayer

Many current studies of mechanical effects on cells have used monolayer cultures. The advantage of such a monolayer system includes the ease of growing large number of cells for testing and the simplicity of imaging the cells. One popular monolayer system is the "flexcel" system, in which cells are cultured on a flexible membrane that is deformed cyclically by a vacuum pump. Monolayer cells are also suitable for studying the effect of shear stress induced by fluid flow *(25)*.

Recently, studies have been conducted to examine the mechanical effect on single chondrocytes. It was found that mechanical deformation of plasma membrane causes deformation of chondrocyte nucleus, implicating the involvement of cytoskeletal network in transducing mechanical signals to the nucleus *(15)*. However, chondrocytes in vivo do not exist in monolayer or as single cells. Instead, they are surrounded by extracellular matrix in a three-dimensional (3D) network. The surrounding 3D matrix network may be critical in transducing mechanical signals to chondrocytes. Therefore, cell culture in one dimension or two dimensions may not reflect the mechanical microenvironment in cartilage. To overcome these difficulties, we adapted a novel 3D culture system that has been used to study mechanical effects on other types of cells *(26,27)*.

Stretch-Induced Matrix Deformation

In this system, chondrocytes are cultured in a sponge of collagen scaffolds. The collagen scaffolds can be stretched with precision by a computer-controlled "Bio-Stretcher." Matrix deformation, as a result of mechanical stretch, will transduce mechanical signals to chondrocytes, which are adhered to the collagen scaffolding. Therefore, in this culture system, chondrocytes receive matrix deformation signals from surrounding matrix, simulating what occurs within the tissue. Using this system, we observed a dramatic increase of chondrocyte proliferation in response to a 5% cyclic matrix deformation. To our knowledge, this is the first time that this new device is used for biophysical stimulation of chondrocytes. A Bio-Stretch device consists of a Bio-Stretch controller, a Bio-Stretch manager software running under Windows in a PC, and solenoid (magnet) boards, on which a 3D collagen sponge is stretched. One end of the sponge is affixed to the bottom of the culture dish by a special clamp, and the other end is clipped with a metal bar. The stretch (elongation) of the sponge is achieved by the movement of the metal bar, which is driven by the magnetic force and recoil property of the sponge.

The 3D collagen sponge is Gelfoam, prepared sterilely from purified pork skin collagen and commercially available from Upjohn. From our experience of using Gelfoam to culture chondrocytes, we have observed several excellent features of this culture system. First, Gelfoam is capable to absorb and hold within its interstices 45 times its weight in fluid. Therefore, it is used clinically to arrest bleeding by producing a mechanical matrix that facilitates clotting. With these mechanical properties, this spongy matrix is capable of holding hundreds of millions of cells. These seeded chondrocytes attach to the collagen scaffolding within 24 h and start to proliferate and produce their own matrix to connect to the collagen network, and to each other.

Second, the collagen scaffolding can be easily dissolved by collagenase digestion before the cell number is counted and intracellular proteins are extracted for analysis from cultured chondrocytes. Thus, characterization of cells in this 3D culture is convenient. Clinically, Gelfoam becomes liquefied within a week in a body, and is completely absorbed in 4 to 6 wk without inducing excessive scar formation *(28)*. Therefore, this 3D culture system may have potentials as matrix scaffolds for tissue engineering of cartilage repair. Third, the collagen sponge becomes transparent and light permeable after it is immersed in medium. Therefore, living cells cultured in the sponge can be observed and analyzed in real time with conventional microscope (confocal microscope is not necessary).

We performed experiments to examine whether cultured cells maintain chondrocyte phenotype in this collagenous sponge. This is out of the concern that skin collagen, which composes the Gelfoam, consists mainly of collagen types I and III, whereas the major fibrillar collagen in cartilage is type II. To determine the phenotype of cultured cells, we examined the expression of molecular markers of cartilage during the culture period by western blot. We found that primary cells cultured in this 3D matrix network maintain their chondrocyte phenotype. Furthermore, these cells proliferate and form cartilage-like nodules supported by the collagen lattice when the incubation progresses. These chondrocytes secrete and deposit cartilage-specific aggrecan in the matrix, which are stained by Alcian blue. Thus, cells form organotypic structures in this 3D culture system. The biggest advantage of this system, however, is that cyclic deformation can be applied to the collagen network, and the cellular responses can be characterized. Some of the responses to matrix deformation are described in the following.

Mechanical Effects on Cells

Cell Proliferation

We performed cyclic deformation of collagen sponge with cultured chondrocytes with an intermittent stretch pattern (5% elongation, 60 stretch/min, 15 min/h; Fig. 2). This pattern is applied because (1)

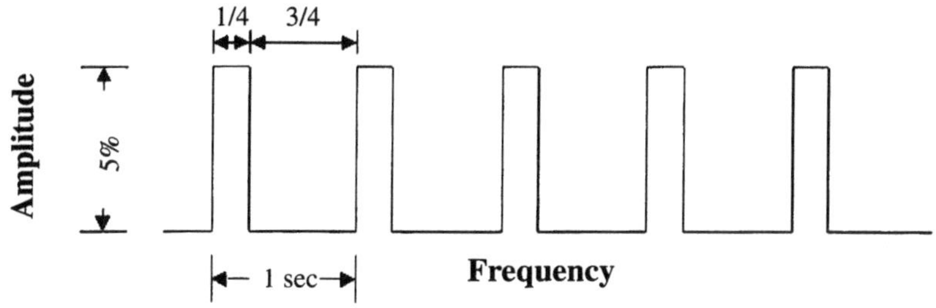

Fig. 2. Stretch pattern exerted by "Biostretch" system.

this extent of matrix deformation may be comparable to that experienced in vivo *(24)*, (2) this extent of matrix deformation does not induce cytotoxicity of cells cultured in this system *(26,29)*, and (3) other types of cells, such as fetal rat lung cells, increase proliferation in respond to this stretch pattern *(26,27)*. Under this stretch pattern, proliferation of chondrocytes was greatly stimulated. Cell number relative to nonstretched cells increased 85% after 48 h and 101% after 72 h. Cell doubling time is reduced from 72 to 43 h. With the same stretch pattern, lung cell number increased only 10% after 48 h. Thus, chondrocytes have much more dynamic responses to matrix deformation than lung cells. Although cyclic matrix deformation greatly stimulated proliferation of immature chondrocytes, it did not stimulate proliferation of hypertrophic chondrocytes. This indicates that mechanical stimulation of chondrocyte proliferation is specific to developmental stage *(30)*.

Cell Differentiation

With this 3D chondrocyte system, we found that synthesis of matrilin-1, a mature chondrocyte marker, and type X collagen, a hypertrophic chondrocyte marker, was upregulated by stretch induced matrix deformation. Therefore, genes of matrilin-1 and type X collagen are responsive to mechanical stress. Mechanical stimulation of the mRNA levels of matrilin-1 and type X collagen occurred exactly at the same points when these markers were synthesized by nonloading cells. This indicates that cyclic matrix deformation does not alter the speed of differentiation, but affects the extent of differentiation. The addition of a stretch-activated channel blocker gadolinium during loading abolished mechanical stimulation of chondrocyte proliferation, but did not affect the upregulation of matrilin-1 mRNA by mechanical stretch. In contrast, a calcium channel blocker nifedipine inhibited both the stretch-induced proliferation and the increase of matrilin-1 mRNA. This suggests that stretch-induced matrix deformation regulated chondrocyte proliferation and differentiation via two signal transduction pathways, with stretch-activated channels involved in transducing the proliferative signals, and calcium channels involved in transducing the signals for both proliferation and differentiation *(30)*.

Mechanotransduction Pathways

Extracellular Transducers

The matrix deformation signals are transduced to the cell membrane by extracellular matrix, in particular the pericellular matrix molecules. Extracellular matrix in cartilage consists of collagen fibrils, the hyaluronan–aggrecan-link protein complex, and noncollagenous matrix proteins. Although not all of the matrix molecules are involved in mechnotransduction, genetic analysis of a mechnotransducing complex in *Caenorhabditis elegans* has indicated a collagen and a noncollagenous matrix protein that contains epidermal growth factor repeats as extracellular components of the complex *(31)*. Our experimental evidences suggest that matrilin-1, a non-collagenous protein that contains epidermal growth factor repeats, is a prime candidate to transduce matrix deformation signal to the cell. Matrilin-1 is located around the cells and form "suspension bridge-like" filaments to connect different colonies of cells *(8)*. Furthermore, matrilin-1 forms pericellular filaments, which are connected to type II collagen fibrils to form an integrated matrix network *(8)*. Matrilin-1 also interacts with aggrecan in cartilage matrix *(32,33)*. Thus matrilin-1 could potentially transmit a mechanical deformation signal from interstitial collagen fibers and aggrecan complcx to chondrocytes.

Intracellular Pathways

When biophysical signals reach to the chondrocyte membrane, they are transduced within the cell and ultimately to the nucleus. Intracellular signaling molecules include cytosolic Ca^{2+}, cAMP, and various kinases *(34–38)*. Our recent studies focus on mitogen-activated protein (MAP) kinase pathways in mechanical transduction in chondrocytes based on the following evidence. First, MAP kinases are activated by mechanical stimulation in a variety of cell types, including cardiac myocytes and endothelial cells *(39,40)*. MAP kinases are activated by phosphorylation on their threonine and tyrosine residues by upstream MAP kinase kinases. The activated MAP kinases then translocate into the nucleus to phosphorylate transcriptional factors *(41,42)*. As a result, biosynthesis may be stimulated and cell proliferation and differentiation altered *(43,44)*. Second, MAP kinase activation is dependent on integrins, which connect extracellular matrix to cytoskeletons *(39,40)*. Thus, a matrix deformation signal may activate MAP kinases through integrins. Third, chondrocytes including articular chondrocytes possess MAP kinases *(45,46)*. These kinases are activated by extracellular stress signals, such as oxidation *(46)*, and tumor necrosis factor alpha treatment *(45)*. Finally, two of the three major MAP kinase pathways are activated by cyclic matrix deformation in our model system. There are three major MAP kinase pathways. The ERK pathway (extracellular signal-regulated protein kinase) is mainly involved in transmitting signals to induce proliferation or enhance differentiation *(41,44)*. The other two MAP kinase pathways, Jun-N-terminal kinase and p38, are not activated primarily by mitogens but by cellular stress and inflammatory cytokines *(42,43)*. We have obtained direct evidence that ERK and p38 are greatly activated by matrix deformation in our 3D culture system, whereas Jun-N-terminal kinase is only minimally activated. The activation of ERK and p38 accompanies the stimulation of chondrocyte proliferation by cyclic matrix deformation.

Interestingly, our results have shown that ERK and p38 were also activated in chondrocytes by treatment of 0.1 μM human parathyroid hormone (PTH) (1-24). Their respective activation time course and amplitude were remarkably similar to those from biophysical stimulation by matrix deformation. ERK was activated more than twofold after 15 min of treatment and p38 was activated more than fivefold after 60 min of treatment. At any time point tested, the activities of ERK and p38 remained at the basal level from chondrocytes cultured without either matrix deformation or PTH stimulation. Future studies will focus on whether activation of MAP kinases and stimulation of cell proliferation are coupled, and whether PTH can enhance the stimulation of chondrocyte proliferation during cyclic matrix deformation.

Mechanotransduction Mechanisms

Indian Hedgehog as a Central Mediator

Indian hedgehog (Ihh) is a member of the vertebrate hedgehog family that consists of sonic, Indian, and desert. Ihh is expressed not only in cartilaginous growth plate during limb development *(47)* but also during fracture healing in bone callus *(48,49)*. Recent studies have shown that Ihh is a key molecule that regulates chondrocyte proliferation and differentiation during endochondral bone formation *(47,48,50)*. Ihh achieves these functions by inducing a series of downstream factors, including its receptor patched (Ptc), a 12-pass transmembrane protein *(51)*, parathyroid hormone-related peptide *(47)*, and bone morphogenetic proteins (BMPs; refs. *52*, *53*). Recently, we have shown a novel function of Ihh, namely, that it acts as an essential mediator of mechanotransduction in cartilage *(54)*. Cyclic mechanical stress greatly induces the expression of Ihh by chondrocytes. This induction is abolished by gadolinium, an inhibitor of stretch-activated channels. This suggests that the Ihh gene is mechanoresponsive. The mechanoinduction of Ihh is essential for stimulating chondrocyte proliferation by mechanical loading. The presence of an Ihh functional blocking antibody during loading completely abolishes the stimulatory effect of mechanical load on proliferation. Our data suggest that Ihh may transduce mechanical signals during cartilage growth and repair processes.

This newly discovered function of Ihh might be important not only for skeleton formation during development but also for fracture healing in the adult. First, during endochondral bone formation, Ihh is expressed exclusively by prehypertropic mature chondrocytes that separate proliferating cells from hypertrophic cells in a growth plate. It was shown previously that Ihh inhibited neighboring chondrocytes undergoing hypertrophy at the distal end of the growth plate. Out study shows Ihh may also promote proliferation of the neighboring cells at the proximal end of the growth plate. This is also supported by the phenotype of Ihh knockout mouse in which chondrocyte proliferation is severely retarded *(50)*. Second, although Ihh mRNA expression is ceased when a growth plate is closed, its expression is reactivated during fracture healing in adult *(48,49)*. Our data suggest that Ihh is an essential mediator that connects mechanical stress to chondrocyte proliferation. Thus, Ihh may play an important role in sustaining and amplifying mechanical signals to promote cartilage and bone remodeling in adult as well. This hypothesis remains to be tested.

Every Road Leads to BMP

BMPs are another family of secreted proteins that regulate cartilage growth and differentiation *(55)*. BMPs are found to be downstream of the Ihh pathway in vertebrate *(52,49)*. Furthermore, the equivalent of BMP in *Drosophila*, DPP, is induced by hedgehog *(56,57)*. The actions of BMP can be inhibited by it antagonists, such as noggin. Noggin knockout mice exhibits fused and malformed joints, a consequence from overproliferation and defective differentiation of chondrocytes *(58)*.

Recently, we identified BMP 2/4 as the molecules that were upregulated by mechanical stress in an Ihh-dependent manner *(54)*. Thus, Ihh mediates the mechanotransduction process in a BMP-dependent and parathyroid hormone-related peptide-independent manner. BMP 2/4 are upregulated by mechanical stress through the induction of Ihh, and BMP antagonist noggin inhibits mechanical stimulation of chondrocyte proliferation. This suggests BMP lies downstream of Ihh in mechanotransduction pathway. In support of our data, previous studies have shown that (1) BMP 2/4 are the closest homologues of DPP, which lies downstream of Hh in the Drosophila signaling pathway *(56,57)*, (2) BMP 2/4 have the highest affinity for the BMP antagonist noggin *(58)*, which abolished the mechanical stimulatory effect in our study, and (3) BMP 2/4 have been identified to be upregulated by mechanical loading in vivo *(59)*. BMPs have been shown previously to have proliferative effects on chondrocytes *(60)*. Conversely, it has also been shown that expression of a dominant-negative BMP receptor actually increased chondrocyte proliferation *(61)*. Thus, BMP pathways may stimulate or inhibit cell proliferation depending on cellular context, that is, whether other BMP-independent pathways are also activated by extracellular signals *(55)*. Thus, the Ihh-BMP 2/4 pathway and other pathways may act together to regulate chondrocyte proliferation. The complete elucidation of these different mechanotransduction pathways awaits further experimentation, such as microarray analysis.

Based on our data, we suggest that the mechanotranduction process can be divided into two stages (Fig. 3). In the first stage, mechanical signals resulting from cyclic matrix deformation induce the gene expression of Ihh by chondrocytes, among activation of other genes. During this stage, mechanical stress signals are converted to chemical signals. In the second stage, Ihh may induce BMPs that participate in stimulation of cartilage growth under permissive environment. During this stage, chemical signals are converted to biological responses. Thus, Ihh may serve as a critical link to a pathway that connects mechanical signals and the activity of cells in response to those signals.

QUESTIONS AND FUTURE DIRECTION

In summary, our study have provided some answers to the mechanisms of mechanotransduction in cartilage: (1) mechanical to chemical conversion is important for sustaining and amplifying mechanical

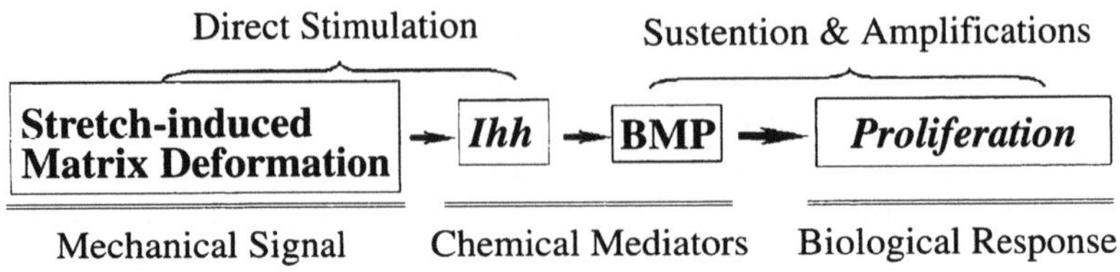

Fig. 3. Diagram depicting Ihh-dependent mechanotransduction pathway in cartilage. Ihh, indian hedgehog; BMP, bone morphogenic proteins.

effects to surrounding cells and tissues, (2) many mechanoresponsive genes are mechanotransducers themselves, thereby providing and important feedback mechanism for regulation, and (3) the structure of extracellular matrix that transduces mechanical signals is modified by mechanical load, thereby achieving mechanical adaptation.

There are still questions remaining to be answered in the future studies. For example, there are at least three types of pathways to transduce mechanical signals: electrical, chemical, and biological. Although the speed of electrical transmission is fast (seconds), the speed of chemical transmission is medium (minutes to hours), and the speed of biological transmission that involves gene expression is slow (hours to days). Which type(s) is important for mechanotransduction in cartilage? Second, how is the mechanoregulatory effect achieved? Does it involve one cell, a population of cells, or a population of cells plus surrounding extracellular matrix and tissues? Third, how is mechanical adaptation achieved by cartilage? The extent of adaptation varies by site, age, and gender. Why are some cells responsive and other cells are unresponsive? Why do some cells have positive responses whereas other cells have negative responses? Is there any feedback mechanism? Finally, what are the molecules that are involved in mechanotransduction? Is there any overlap between mechanoresponsive genes and mechanotransducing genes? If so, what is the significance of this overlap?

REFERENCES

1. Einhorn, T. A. (1998) One of nature's best kept secrets (editorial; comment). *J. Bone Miner. Res.* **13,** 10–12.
2. Welch, R. D., Birch, J. G., Makarov, M. R., and Samchukov, M. L. (1998) Histomorphometry of distraction osteogenesis in a caprine tibial lengthening model [see comments]. *J. Bone Miner. Res.* **13,** 1–9.
3. Morscher, E. (1968) Strength and morphology of growth cartilage under hormonal influence of puberty: animal experiements and clinical study on the etiology of local growth disorders during puberty. *Reconstr. Surg. Traumatol.* **10,** 3–104.
4. Smith, W. S. and Cunningham, J. B. (1957) The effect of alternating distracting forces on the epiphyseal plates of calves: a preliminary report. *Clin. Orthopaedics* **10,** 125–130.
5. Carter, D. R. and Wong. M. (1988) Mechanical stresses and endochondral ossification in the chondroepiphysis. *J. Orthopaed. Res.* **6,** 148–154.
6. Cohen, B., Chorney, G. S., and Phillips, D. P. (1992) The microstructural tensile properties and biochemcial composition of the bovine distal femoral growth plate. *J. Orthopaed. Res.* **10,** 263–275.
7. Haas, S. L. (1973) The localization of the growing point in the epiphyseal cartilage plate of bones. *Am. J. Orthopaed. Surg.* **15,** 563–586.
8. Chen, Q., Johnson, D. M., Haudenschild, D. R., Tondravi, M. M., and Goetinck, P. F. (1995) Cartilage matrix protein forms a type II collagen-independent filamentous network: analysis in primary cell cultures with a retrovirus expression system. *Mol. Biol. Cell.* **6,** 1743–1753.
9. Castagnola, P., Dozin, B., Moro, G., and Cancedda, R. (1988) Changes in the expression of collagen genes show two stages in chondrocyte differentiation in vitro. *J. Cell Biol.* **106,** 461–467.
10. Oohira, A., Kimata, K., Suzuki, S., Takata, K., Suzuki, I., and Hoshino, M. (1974) A correlation between synthetic activities for matrix macromolecules and specific stages of cytodifferentiation in developing cartilage. *J. Biol. Chem.* **249,** 1637–1645.
11. von der Mark, K., Kirsch, T., Nerlich, A., Kuss, A., Weseloh, G., Gluckert, K., and Stoss, H. (1992) Type X collagen synthesis in human osteoarthritic cartilage. Indication of chondrocyte hypertrophy. *Arthritis Rheumatism* **35,** 806–811.
12. Hiltunen, A., Aro, H. T., and Vuorio, E. (1993) Regulation of extracellular matrix genes during fracture healing in mice. *Clin. Orthopaed. Rel. Res.* **297,** 23–27.

13. Scammell, B. E., and Roach, H. (1996) A new role for the chondrocyte in fracture repair: Endochondral ossification includes direct bone formation by former chondrocytes. *J. Bone Miner. Res.* **11,** 737–745.
14. Frank, E. H. and Grodzinsky, A. J. (1987) Cartilage electromechanics-I. Electrokinetic transduction and the effects of electrolyte pH and ionic strength. *J. Biomechanics* **20,** 615–627.
15. Guilak, F., Ratcliffe, A., and Mow, V. C. (1995) Chondrocyte deformation and local tissue strain in articular cartilage: a confocal microscopy study. *J. Orthopaed. Res.* **13,** 410–421.
16. Lai, W. M., Hou, J. S., and Mow, V. C. (1991) A triphasic theory for the swelling and deformation behaviors of articular cartilage. *J. Biomechanical Eng.* **113,** 245–258.
17. Jones, I. L., Klamfeldt, A., and Sandstrom, T. (1982) The effect of continuous mechanical pressure upon the turnover of articular cartilage proteoglycans in vitro. *Clin. Orthopaed. Rel. Res.* **165,** 283–289.
18. Kim, Y. J., Sah, R. L., Grodzinsky, A. J., Plaas, A. H., and Sandy, J. D. (1994) Mechanical regulation of cartilage biosynthetic behavior: physical stimuli. *Arch. Biochem. Biophys.* **311,** 1–12.
19. Sah, R. L., Kim, Y. J., Doong, J. Y., Grodzinsky, A. J., Plaas, A. H., and Sandy, J. D. (1989) Biosynthetic response to cartilage explants to dynamic compression. *J. Orthopaed Res.* **7,** 619–636.
20. Schneiderman, R., Keret, D., and Maroudas, A. (1986) Effects of mechanical and osmotic pressure on the rate of glycosaminoglycan synthesis in the human adult femoral head cartilage: an in vitro study. *J. Orthopaed. Res.* **4,** 393–408.
21. Lee, R. C., Rich, J. B., Kelley, K. M., Weiman, D. S., and Mathews, M. B. (1982) A comparison of in vitro cellular responses to mechanical and electrical stimulation. *Am. Surg.* **48,** 567–574.
22. Smith, R. L., Rusk, S. F., Ellison, B. E., Wessells, P., Tsuchiya, K., Carter, D. R., et al. (1996) In vitro stimulation of articular chondrocyte mRNA and extracellular matrix synthesis by hydrostatic pressure. *J. Orthop. Res.* **14,** 53–60.
23. Buschmann, M. D., Gluzband, Y. A., Grodzinsky, A. J., and Hunziker, E. B. (1995) Mechanical compression modulates matrix biosynthesis in chondrocyte/agarose culture. *J. Cell Sci.* **108,** 1497–1508.
24. Sah, R. L., Grodzinsky, A. J., Plaas, A. H., and Sandy, J. D. (1990) Effects of tissue compression on the hyaluronate-binding properties of newly synthesized proteoglycans in cartilage explants. *Biochem. J.* **267,** 803–808.
25. Yellowley, C. E., Jacobs, C. R., Li, Z., Zhou, Z., and Donahue, H. J. (1997) Effects of fluid flow on intracellular calcium in bovine articular chondrocytes. *Am. J. Physiol.* **273,** C30–C36.
26. Liu, M., Skinner, S. J., Xu, J., Han, R. N., Tanswell, A. K., and Post, M. (1992) Stimulation of fetal rat lung cell proliferation in vitro by mechanical stretch. *Am. J. Physiol.* **263,** L376–L383.
27. Xu, J., Liu, M., Liu, J., Caniggia, I., and Post, M. (1996) Mechanical strain induces constitutive and regulated secretion of glycosaminoglycans and proteoglycans in fetal lung cells. *J. Cell Sci.* **109,** 1605–1613.
28. Centra, M., Ratych, R. E., Cao, G. L., Li, J., Williams, E., Taylor, R. M., et al. (1992) Culture of bovine pulmonary artery endothelial cells on Gelfoam blocks. *FASEB J.* **6,** 3117–3121.
29. Liu, M., Xu, J. Souza, P., Tanswell, B., Tanswell, A. K., and Post M. (1995) The effect of mechanical strain on fetal rat lung cell proliferation: comparison of two- and three-dimensional culture systems. *In Vitro Cell. Dev. Biol. Animal* **31,** 858–866.
30. Wu, Q. and Chen, Q. (2000) Mechanoregulation of chondrocyte proliferation, maturation and hypertrophy: ion-channel dependent transduction of matrix deformation signals. *Exp. Cell Res.* **256,** 383–391.
31. Tavernarakis, N. and Driscoll, M. (1997) Molecular modeling of mechanotransduction in the nematode Caenorhabditis elegans. *Annu. Rev. Physiol.* **59,** 659–689.
32. Hauser, N., Paulsson, M., Heinegard, D., and Morgelin, M. (1996) Interaction of cartilage matrix protein with aggrecan-increased covalent cross-linking with tissue maturation. *J. Biol. Chem.* **271,** 32247–32252.
33. Paulsson, M. and Heinegard, D. (1979) Matrix proteins bound to associatively prepared proteoglycans from bovine cartilage. *Biochem. J.* **183,** 539–545.
34. Ando, J., Ohtsuka, A., Korenaga, R., Kawamura, T., and Kamiya, A. (1993) Wall shear stress rather than shear rate regulated cytoplasmic Ca++ responses to flow in vascular endothelial cells. *Biochem. Biophys. Res. Commun.* **190,** 716–723.
35. Beit-Or, A., Nevo, Z., Kalina, M., and Eilam, Y. (1990) Decrease in the basal levels of cytosolic free calcium in chondrocytes during aging in culture: possible role as differentiation-signal. *J. Cell. Physiol.* **144,** 197–203.
36. Eilam, Y., Beit-Or, A., and Nevo, Z. (1985) Decrease in cytosolic free Ca2+ and enhanced proteoglycan synthesis induced by cartilage derived growth factors in cultured chondrocytes. *Biochem. Biophys. Res. Commun.* **132,** 770–779.
37. Hung, C. T., Pollack, S. R., Reilly, T. M., and Brighton, C. T. (1995) Real-time calcium response of cultured bone cells to fluid flow. *Clin. Orthop. Rel. Res.* **313,** 256–269.
38. Reich, K. M. and Frangos, J. A. (1991) Effect of flow on prostaglandin E2 and inositol trisphosphate levels in osetoblasts. *Am. J. Physiol.* **261,** C428–C432.
39. Shyy, J. Y. and Chien, S. (1997) Role of integrins in cellular responses to mechanical stress and adhesion. *Curr. Opin. Cell Biol.* **9,** 707–713.
40. MacKenna, D. A., Dolfi, F., Vuori, K., and Ruoslahti, E. (1998) Extracellular signal-regulated kinase and c-Jun NH2-terminal kinase activation by mechanical stretch is integrin-dependent and matrix-specific in rat cardiac fibroblasts. *J. Clin. Invest.* **101,** 301–310.
41. Cobb, M. H. and Goldsmith, E. J. (1995) How MAP kinases are regulated. *J. Biol. Chem.* **270,** 14843–14846.
42. Kyriakis, J. M. and Avruch, J. (1996) Sounding the alarm: protein kinase cascades activated by stress and inflammation. *J. Biol. Chem.* **271,** 24313–24316.
43. Kummer, J. L., Rao, P. K., and Heidenreich, K. A. (1997) Apoptosis induced by withdrawal of trophic factors in mediated by p38 mitogen-activated protein kinase. *J. Biol. Chem.* **272,** 20490–20494.

44. Karin, M. (1996) The regulation of AP-1 activity by mitogen-activated protein kinases. *Philos. Trans. Royal Soc. London* **351,** 127–134.
45. Geng, Y., Valbracht, J., and Lotz, M. (1996) Selective activation of the mitogen-activated protein kinase subgroups c-Jun NH2 terminal kinasc and p38 by IL-1 and TNF in human articular chondrocytes. *J. Clin. Invest.* **98,** 2425–2430.
46. Lo, Y. Y. C., Wong, J. M. S., and Cruz, T. F. (1996) Reactive oxygen species mediate cytokine activation of c-Jun NH2-terminal kinases. *J. Biol. Chem.* **271,** 15703–15707.
47. Vortkamp, A., Lee, K., Lanske, B., Segre, G. V., Kronenberg, H. M., and Tabin, C. J. (1996) Regulation of rate of cartilage differentiation by Indian hedgehog and PTH-related protein (see comments). *Science* **273,** 613–622.
48. Vortkamp, A., Pathi, S., Peretti, G. M., Caruso, E. M., Zaleske, D. J., and Tabin, C. J. (1998) Recapitulation of signals regulating embryonic bone formation during postnatal growth and in fracture repair. *Mech. Dev.* **71,** 65–76.
49. Ferguson, C., Alpern, E., Miclau, T., and Helm, J. A. (1999) Does adult fracture repair recapitulate embryonic skeletal formation? *Mech. Dev.* **87,** 57–66.
50. St-Jacques, B., Hammerschmidt, M., and McMahon, A. P. (1999) Indian hedgehog signaling regulates proliferation and differentiation of chondrocytes and is essential for bone formation (published erratum appears in Genes Dev. **13,** 2617, 1999). *Genes Dev.* **13,** 2072–2086.
51. McMahon, A. P. (2000) More surprised in the Hedgehog signaling pathway. *Cell* **100,** 185–188.
52. Pathi, S., Rutenberg, J. B., Johnson, R. L., and Vortkamp, A. (1999) Interaction of Ihh and BMP Noggin signaling during cartilage differentiation. *Dev. Biol.* **209,** 239–253.
53. Zou, H., Wieser, R., Massague, J., and Niswander, L. (1997) Distinct roles of type I bone morphogenetic protein receptors in the formation and differentiation of cartilage. *Genes Dev.* **11,** 2191–2203.
54. Wu, Q., Zhang, Y., and Chen, Q. (2001) Indian hedgehog is an essential component of mechanotransduction complex to stimulate chondrocyte proliferation. *J. Biol. Chem.* **276,** 35290–35296.
55. Hogan, B. L.M. (1996) Bone Morphogenetic Proteins In Development. *Curr. Opin. Genet. Dev.* **6,** 432–438.
56. Fietz, M. J., Concordet, J. P., Barbosa, R., Johnson, R., Krauss, S., McMahon, A. P., et al. (1994) The hedgehog gene family in Drosophila and vertebrate development. *Development Suppl.,* 43–51.
57. Tanimoto, H., Itoh, S., ten Dijke, P., and Tabata, T. (2000) Hedgehog creates a gradient of DPP activity in Drosophila wing imaginal discs. *Mol. Cell.* **5,** 59–71.
58. Brunet, L. J., McMahon, J. A., McMahon, A. P., and Harland, R. M. (1998) Noggin, cartilage morphogenesis, and joint formation is the mammalian skeleton (see comments). *Science* **280,** 1455–1457.
59. Sata, M., Ochi, T., Nakase, T., Hirota, S., Kitamura Y., Nomura, S., and Yasui, N. (1999) Mechanical tension-stress induces expression of bone morphogenetic protein (BMP)-2 and BMP-4, but not BMP-6, BMP-7, and GDF-5 mRNA, during distraction osteogenesis. *J. Bone Miner. Res.* **14,** 1084–1095.
60. Suzuki, F. (1992) Effects of various growth factors on a chondrocyte differentiation model. *Adv. Exp. Med. Biol.* **324,** 101–106.
61. Enomotoiwamoto, M., Iwamoto, M., Mukudai, Y., Kawakami, Y., Nohno, T., Higuchi, Y., et al. (1998) Bone morphogenetic protein signaling is required for maintanance of differentiated phenotype, control of proliferation, and hypertrophy in chondrocytes. *J. Cell Biol.* **140,** 409–418.

II
Control of Skeletal Development

7

Molecular Genetic Analysis of the Role of the *HoxD* Complex in Skeletal Development

Impact of the loxP/*Cre System in Targeted Mutagenesis of the Mouse* HoxD *Complex*

Marie Kmita, Denis Duboule, and József Zákány

INTRODUCTION

There is an ever-growing list of human and mouse genes with implications in skeletal development. Among them, *Hox* genes represent a particular class for at least two reasons: first, in absence of *Hox* gene products, skeletal development becomes altered in many respects, including variation in spatial anatomical pattern and temporal tissue-maturation sequence. Second, *Hox* genes show clustered genomic organization, which in itself is expected to exert profound, as yet poorly understood, influences in executing their function through influencing gene expression control. Therefore, analyzing the role of *Hox* genes in skeletal development must involve large-scale manipulations at the level of gene complexes. In this chapter, we give a brief overview of our experimental strategies that involve site-specific recombination at the *HoxD* gene cluster. These are experimental manipulations of the mouse genome applying the *loxP*/Cre recombination system (Fig. 1). The most important aspect of this system for targeted mutagenesis is that it allows sequential modifications of the genome at predefined positions as a result of the specificity of recognition and polarity of recombination induced by the Cre enzyme between loxP sites *(1)*. This 35-nucleotide long recombination target site, the *loxP* site, does not normally occur in the mammalian genome but can be introduced to selected genomic positions by homologous recombination thanks to embryonic stem (ES) cell technology. When two *loxP* sites and the Cre recombinase are present in a cell, the recombination reaction can occur either in vitro or in vivo in individuals derived from such modified ES cells. A large number of alleles can be generated in this way, facilitating the genetic analysis of complex loci, like the *Hox* gene clusters (Fig. 2).

HOXD GENES IN SKELETAL PATTERNING

Hox genes are developmental control genes. They code for transcription factors that are related to the products of the homeotic genes of *Drosophila*. Like in *Drosophila*, *Hox* genes are clustered and together determine morphological specification along the anterior–posterior body axis. Vertebrate *Hox* genes are essential for the proper organization of the body plan during development. Inactivation of

From: *The Skeleton: Biochemical, Genetic, and Molecular Interactions in Development and Homeostasis*
Edited by: E. J. Massaro and J. M. Rogers © Humana Press Inc., Totowa, NJ

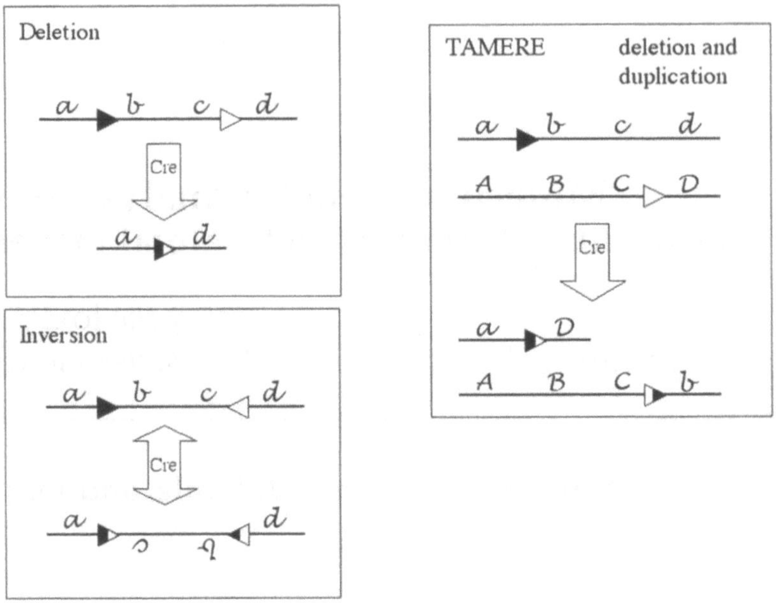

Fig. 1. Site-specific targeted recombination strategies. Depending on the orientation and relative position of *loxP* sites, genetic loci can be rearranged as a result of Cre-mediated site-specific recombination acting on those *loxP* sites. Three recombination reactions, giving rise to four different recombinant chromosomes, are schematized. **A**, A model chromosome segment, containing loci a, b, c, and d, is depicted. Arrowheads represent *loxP* sites. Their left or right polarity reflects the polarity of the *loxP* sites. Two identically oriented sites located on the same chromosome (in *cis*) when recombined lead to the loss of the intervening loci resulting in a deletion. **B**, Recombination between two inversely oriented *loxP* sites located in *cis* results in the inversion of the intervening loci. **C**, When one *loxP* site is located on one chromosome while a second is on the homologous chromosome (i.e., in *trans*), with both *loxP* sites being identically oriented, Cre-mediated recombination induces targeted chromosomal exchanges. In this example, the result is a deletion on one hand and a reciprocal duplication on the other hand of the DNA fragment located in between the relative position of the two *loxP* sites. This reaction occurs with high frequency during meiotic pairing of homologous chromosomes during spermatogenesis (targeted meiotic recombination, or TAMERE for short).

these genes usually leads to important alterations, or transformations, in the identities of the affected developing structures. The structural and functional organization of the four vertebrate *Hox* gene clusters (*HoxA*, *B*, *C*, and *D*) are very similar. All four are composed of up to 11 genes, each of which belongs to one of 13 paralogy groups. Paralogous genes follow one another in the same order in all four clusters, and this gene order is colinear with their functional domains along the body axis (spatial colinearity). The gene order also determines the activation sequence in time during ontogenesis *(2,3)*. *Hox* genes, which are functional in anterior body regions, turn on early, whereas progressively more posterior genes get active gradually (temporal colinearity). The transcriptional 5' to 3' polarity of the genes in all four complexes is invariant. It is believed that the correct timing of activation of this gene family is necessary to properly establish the various gene specific expression domains. Slight modifications in the respective times of gene activation (heterochronies) may shift expression domains along the rostrocaudal axis and thus induce concurrent changes in morphologies *(3)*. This strict structural and functional organization is the molecular basis of anterior to posterior specification, but it lends itself to determine polarity along other axes, like, for example, the proximodistal limb axis. Genes that control the development of digits are located at the posterior, 5' end of the *HoxA* and *HoxD* clusters.

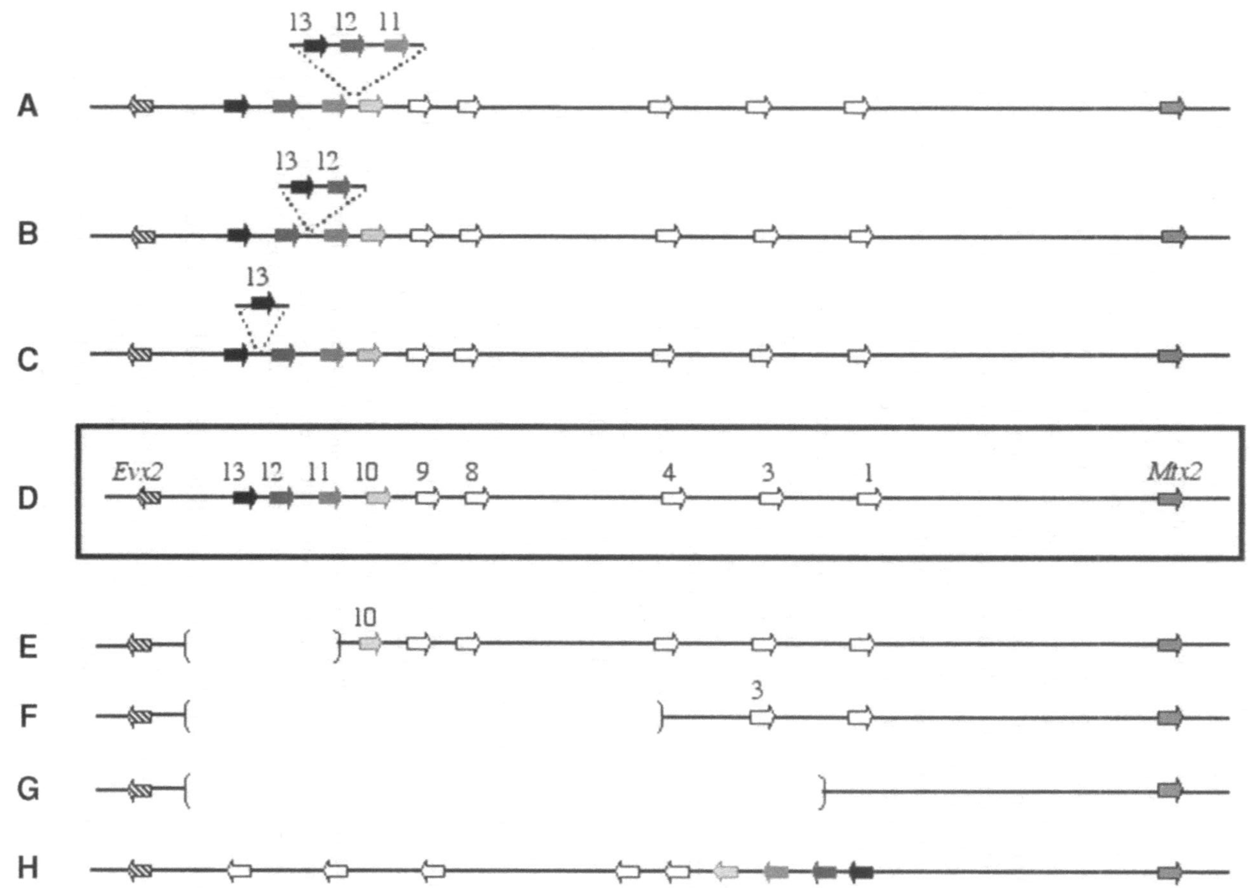

Fig. 2. Schemes of some selected variants of the murine *HoxD* cluster produced by site-specific targeted recombination. Horizontal block arrows represent individual genes, and their orientation shows the direction of transcription of each gene along the chromosome. *Evx2* and *Mtx2* are the two neighbor genes of the *HoxD* cluster. The wild-type chromosome is depicted by scheme **D**. It contains the normal set of nine *Hoxd* genes: *Hoxd1*, *Hoxd3*, *Hoxd4*, *Hoxd8*, *Hoxd9*, *Hoxd10*, *Hoxd11*, *Hoxd12*, and *Hoxd13*, identified here by gene number only. Darker shadows indicate the contiguous set of four *Hoxd* genes involved in digit development. Schemes **A**, **B**, and **C** show recombinant chromosomes obtained by targeted meiotic recombination that all contain parts of the *HoxD* cluster duplicated, all including *Hoxd13*. Schemes **E**, **F**, and **G** depict a nested deletion series, including *Hoxd13*, and progressively larger chromosomal segments. Scheme **G** represents a full cluster deletion. Scheme **H** depicts a targeted inversion of the entire *HoxD* cluster.

A major aim of our laboratory during the past few years has been to find out about the molecular mechanisms that control *Hox* gene expression. The posterior end of the *HoxD* cluster was the point of departure and the study of its role in digit development proved to be a complex task *(3)*. We now know that several genes are involved in digit development because mice homozygous for a simultaneous deficiency of *Hoxd13*, *12*, and *11*, in particular, showed small-digit primordia, a disorganized cartilage pattern and reduced skeletal mass. Although loss of any one of these genes' functions alone produced digit defects, the combined loss proved more severe than any single gene loss. The anatomical alterations were similar to the defects seen in a human synpolydactyly, suggesting that this syndrome, which is associated with a subtle mutation in HOXD13, may involve the loss of function of several *Hoxd* genes. These results illustrated the existence and pathological relevance of a functional hierarchy among these genes, and provided an animal model to study a human digit syndrome *(4)*.

Besides digits, homeobox genes located in the 5' part of the *HoxA* and *HoxD* complexes are required for proliferation of skeletal progenitor cells in broader domains of the limb. Specific combinations of gene products determine the length of the upper arm (genes belonging to groups 9 and 10), the lower arm (groups 10, 11, and 12), and the digits (groups 11, 12, and 13). In these different domains, individual gene products appear to quantitatively contribute to an overall protein dose with predominant roles for group 11 in the lower arm *(5)* and 13 in the digits *(6)*. Quantitative reduction in the gene dose in each set results in truncations of the corresponding anatomical regions.

Although the skeletal patterns of the upper and lower arm are relatively stable throughout the tetrapods, more variation is seen in the digits. In genetic analyses using multiple loss-of-function alleles, a simple picture arises. A progressive reduction in the dose of *Hox* gene products leads first to ectrodactyly and then to oligodactyly and adactyly. Interestingly, this transition between the pentadactyl to the adactyl formula goes through a step of polydactyly. This suggests that in the distal appendage of polydactylous short-digited ancestral tetrapods, such as Acanthostega, the *HoxA* complex may be predominantly active. Subsequent recruitment of the *HoxD* complex might contribute to both reductions in digit number and increase in digit length. Thus, transition through a polydactylous limb before reaching and stabilizing the pentadactyl pattern may rely, at least in part, on asynchronous and independent changes in the regulation of *HoxA* and *HoxD* gene complexes *(7,8)*.

In mechanistic terms, the physical order of the genes in the *HoxA* and *HoxD* complexes, as well as a unidirectional sequence in gene activation, emerged as decisive players for completion of the process in a precise order, which in turn makes possible the sequential outgrowth of the respective primordia. Molecular analysis of the underlying regulatory processes promised further exciting insights into the genetic control of development, pathology, and the course of evolution. In the next section, an account is given of the various targeted alleles that were established and analyzed in an effort to understand the functional organization of the *HoxD* gene cluster, with special emphasis given to skeletal development along the main, anterior–posterior body axis or the vertebral column, and the appendicular or limb axis.

ANALYSIS OF LOCALLY ACTING GENE REGULATORY SEQUENCES

Identification and experimental manipulations of gene proximal regulatory regions in the *HoxD* complex in mice have given insight into coordinate gene regulation along the main body axis. Targeted mutagenesis of small regulatory regions, and in some cases targeted base substitutions, required that the alleles be created free of selection cassettes and associated exogenous promoters and regulatory elements. In all the alleles summarized below, the *loxP*/Cre system was used to eliminate such artifactual inserts in and around the *HoxD* cluster. As a consequence, a single copy of a *loxP* site was left behind. Up to date, there has been no report of any activity of this short 35-basepair long sequence motif that could introduce interference.

The relationship between the clustered organization of vertebrate *Hox* genes and their coordinate transcription in space and time is still lacking a convincing mechanistic explanation. Recent work on the regulatory interactions within *Hox* complexes suggests some reasons why these genes have remained clustered. Although these results did not address the puzzling issue of colinearity directly, they nevertheless added novel important input to the debate.

It is worth considering the case of the *Hoxd11* locus. *Hoxd11* and *Hoxa11* are paralogous genes that are required for proper development of the vertebral column, the limbs, and the urogenital system. When, for example, a *Hoxd11*-expressing transgene is introduced into *Hoxa11/Hoxd11* mutant genetic backgrounds, the functional equivalence between these gene products can be revealed in patterning the lumbosacral transition zone of the vertebral column (Fig. 3). A range of phenotypes is observed, with transgenic mice displaying as few as four lumbar vertebrae, whereas double-null mutant mice have as many as eight instead of the normal number of six, whereas transgenic, double-null mutant animals show six lumbar vertebrae, that is, the normal set, instead of the eight usually observed *(9)*. This result showed that *Hoxd11* and *Hoxa11* proteins are functionally equivalent in patterning the vertebral column and that regulatory sequences located in the proximity of the *Hoxd11* gene are sufficient to control its expression at the lumbosacral transition zone, even when located outside of the *HoxD* cluster.

A considerable amount of molecular genetic evidence was gathered to explain how expression of *Hoxd11* is regulated in the lumbosacral transition zone. This gene is expressed in the posterior part of the embryo, up to the level of prevertebra 27, and its expression boundary is mimicked by a *Hoxd11/lac* transgene. Expression of this transgene anterior to prevertebra 27 is prevented by the silencing activity of a *cis*-acting element. This repression of *Hoxd11* is necessary to position the sacrum properly. This silencing activity depends on phylogenetically conserved sequences able to bind in vitro retinoic acid receptors and COUP-TFs. ES cell technology was used to generate mice carrying a subtle mutation involving the substitution of seven nucleotides that abolished binding of nuclear receptors at this regulatory region. Mutant mice displayed an anterior shift of their lumbosacral transition inherited as a codominant trait. In mutant embryos, the expression of both *Hoxd11* and *Hoxd10* mRNAs in the prevertebral column was anteriorized. These results illustrate the sharing, in *cis*, of a single regulatory element to establish the expression boundaries of two neighboring *Hoxd* genes *(10)*.

In a parallel set of experiments, a phylogenetically conserved transcriptional enhancer necessary for the activation of *Hoxd11* was deleted from the endogenous *HoxD* complex of mice. Although genetic and expression analyses demonstrated the role of this regulatory element in the activation of *Hoxd11* during early somitogenesis, the function of this gene in developing limbs and the urogenital system was not affected, suggesting that *Hox* transcriptional controls are different in different axial structures. In the trunk of mutant embryos, transcriptional activation of *Hoxd11* and *Hoxd10* was severely delayed but subsequently resumed with appropriate spatial distributions. The resulting caudal transposition of the sacrum indicated that proper vertebral specification requires a precise temporal control of *Hox* gene expression, in addition to spatial regulation. A slight time delay in expression (transcriptional heterochrony) cannot be compensated for at a later developmental stage and, in turn, eventually lead to morphological alterations *(11)*. The reciprocal temporal modulation was achieved also by bringing forward the expression of the *Hoxd10* and *Hoxd11* genes. The same evolutionary conserved *Hox* regulatory sequence was replaced by its fish counterpart in the *HoxD* complex of mice. Fetuses carrying this replacement activated *Hoxd11* transcription prematurely, which led to a rostral shift of its expression boundary and a consequent anterior transposition of the sacrum *(12)*.

Looking further into the *HoxD* cluster, extensive sequencing in several vertebrate species has revealed many conserved DNA sequences interspersed between neighboring *Hox* genes. Their high degree of conservation strongly suggests that they serve regulatory purposes. However, this was not always easy to establish. The deletion of the most tightly conserved regulatory sequence located in the *HoxD* complex gave different results, depending on the transgenic approach used. In "conventional" transgenesis, it was necessary for proper expression in a subdomain of the developing limb, but no effect was seen, when the element was deleted from its endogenous genomic context, that is the *HoxD* cluster. This ambiguity could illustrate a redundancy in regulatory circuits and, thus, justify the combination of parallel experimental strategies *(13)*.

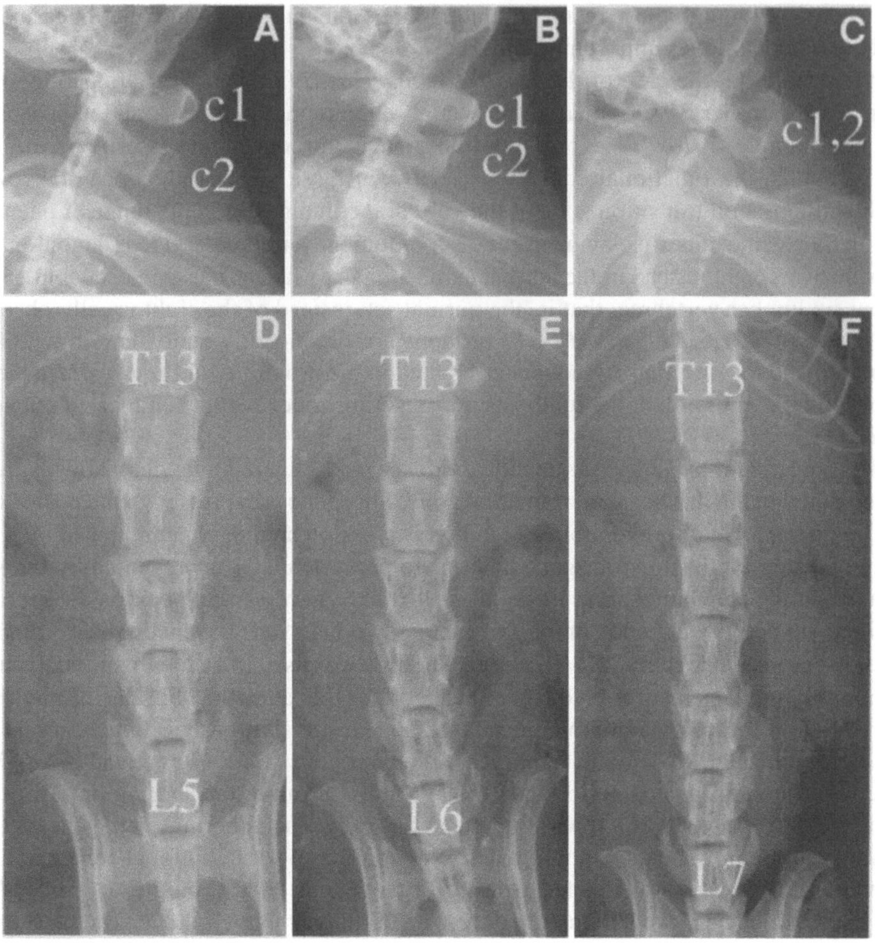

Fig. 3. Vertebral column defects due to *HoxD* cluster mutations. **A–C**, Lateral views of the cervical region of adult mice as revealed by X-ray analysis. **A**, Normal mouse. **B**, Targeted inactivation of the *Hoxd1* gene induces malformations of the atlas and axis, the first two cervical vertebrae (c1 and c2, respectively). **C**, Targeted deletion of the entire *HoxD* cluster induces a severe reduction of both atlas and axis that most often form a single fused structure (c1,2). Malformations of the atlas-axis complex arise from genetic constitutions involving loss of function of *Hoxd1*, *Hoxd3*, and *Hoxd4*. Such severe vertebral fusions, depicted in panel C, are common in simultaneous absence of all three gene products. **D–F**, Frontal views of the lumbar region of adult mice. The last thoracic vertebra is marked T13, and the last lumbar vertebra is marked L5, L6, or L7. **D**, In stocks, where the *Hoxd11* gene is expressed ectopically in slightly more anterior regions, involving the primordia of the sixth lumbar vertebra, the latter is often transformed into the form of the first sacral vertebra giving the L5 formula. In mice with a strong ectopic expression of *Hoxd11* in the primordia of both the fifth and the sixth lumbar vertebrae, an L4 formula also occurs as a result of the transformation of both these two structures. **E**, Normal anatomy characterized by six lumbar vertebrae, an L6 type. **F**, In stocks, where the *Hoxd11* gene is inactivated transition from lumbar to sacral character becomes delayed by one vertebra, resulting in the vertebral formula L7. The same transformation occurs in absence of the *Hoxa11* gene. In compound mutant *Hoxd11;Hoxa11* double homozygous animals the vertebral formula is L8.

Another regulatory element located in the vicinity of the *Hoxd12* gene is well conserved in tetrapods, but little sequence similarity was scored when compared with the cognate fish DNA. Analyses of animals homozygous for the mutant allele of this regulatory region revealed its function in controlling *Hoxd12* expression in the presumptive posterior lower arm, where it genetically interacts with *Hoxa11*.

Downregulation of *Hoxd12* expression was also detected in the trunk, suggesting that this element may mediate a rather general function in gene activation. This is evidence that locally active elements are necessary to build up the complex expression patterns of *Hoxd* genes during limb development, and some of the regions may serve both in the vertebral column and limb regulatory circuits *(14)*.

An engineered fusion of the 5' exon of *Hoxd13* with the 3' exon of *Hoxd12* was also studied in this respect. This hybrid transcription unit was regulated like *Hoxd11*, with expression limits in the trunk, limbs, intestinal, and urogenital systems more anterior than those expected for either *Hoxd13* or *Hoxd12*. This suggested the presence of a regulatory element between *Hoxd13* and *Hoxd12* that may contribute to the establishment, early on, of a repressive state over these two genes *(15)*.

A reverse approach corroborated most of the above findings but also brought the importance of global regulatory influences into focus. During development, the functional domains of individual *Hox* genes are colinear with their genomic positions within the *HoxD* cluster such that *Hoxd13* and *Hoxd12* are necessary for digit and lower sacral vertebral column development, whereas *Hoxd11* and *Hoxd10* are involved in making lower arms, and the lumbosacral transition region. To study the nature of this control, the posterior part of the *HoxD* complex was scanned with a targeted reporter transgene. The response of this foreign promoter to limb regulatory influences suggested that this regulation was achieved through the opposite effects of two enhancer elements. The physical position of a given gene within this genomic interval of opposite regulations might thus determine its final expression pattern *(16)*.

Previous work has suggested that *Hox* genes are made progressively available for transcription in the course of gastrulation, implying the existence of an element capable of initiating a repressive conformation and later allowing this repression to be relieved sequentially according to the order of the genes along the clusters. By combining a genomic walk with successive transgene insertions upstream of the *HoxD* complex, followed by a series of deletions, evidence was found for the position of such a regulatory region. The largest deficiency induced posterior homeotic transformations coincidentally with an earlier activation of *Hoxd* genes. These data suggest that a regulatory element located upstream of the complex is necessary for setting up the early pattern of *Hox* gene colinear activation along the main body axis *(17)*. This is in agreement with transposition of *Hoxd* genes to a more posterior 5' location within the *HoxD* complex. These studies reinforced the hypothesis that colinearity in the expression of these genes was caused, in part, by the existence of a silencing mechanism originating at the 5' end of the cluster and extending towards the 3' direction.

Both the strength and specificity of this repression was tested by inserting a *Hoxb1/lac* transgene near *Hoxd13*. This recombinant cluster thus contained a copy of the most anterior gene (group 1) inserted at the most posterior position, that is, near group 13. A complex interference was obtained. Although the anterior-specific activity of the transgene in the hindbrain was lost, early and anterior transgene expression in the mesoderm was unexpectedly not suppressed. Rather, the transgene induced a transient ectopic activation of the neighboring *Hoxd13* gene without affecting other genes of the complex. Such a local and transient break in colinearity was also observed after transposition of the *Hoxd9/lac* reporter gene, indicating that it may be a general property of these transgenes when transposed at an ectopic location *(18)*.

Taken together, the mutagenesis of short DNA fragments and transgene relocations followed by subsequent internal modifications point to the combined importance of local and global distantly acting regulatory regions in the regulation of multigenic complexes, such as *Hox* clusters.

A SERIES OF NESTED TARGETED DELETIONS IN THE *HOXD* CLUSTER

The interplay of the various regulatory strategies was clearly seen in the series of alleles based on the *Hoxd11*/lac transgene. *Hoxd11* is one of the digit genes; yet, when a conventional transgene is introduced into transgenic mice, that is, inserted at heterologous genomic loci, it mimics aspects of regulation only along the main body axis. It gives a posterior expression domain but it is never expressed in the digit primordia. To get expression in digits, the transgene must be re-introduced into the *HoxD* cluster *(19)*. Site-specific transgene insertion is achieved by homologous recombination in ES cells. Depending on the immediate neighborhood, the *Hoxd11/lac* transgene expression pattern shows modulations: expression could be more or less restricted both along the main body axis and along the limb axis. The first of the *Hoxd11/lac* alleles was made by introducing this transgene, flanked by a *loxP* site at the 5' end of the *HoxD* cluster, just upstream of *Hoxd13*. In later rounds of homologous recombination, an identically oriented *loxP* site was introduced to one of various positions of interest, one between *Hoxd11* and *Hoxd10*, one between *Hoxd4* and *Hoxd3*, and one into *Hoxd1*. The last step was the application of Cre to bring along the excision reaction between two *loxP* sites, either in ES cells, or in mice, thus eliminating the intervening genes. In the first case we deleted several digit genes, *Hoxd13*, *12*, and *11 (4)*; in another case, the *Hoxd13* to *Hoxd4* region *(20)*, and finally the entire cluster *(21)*. The first manipulation induced a deficiency, eliminating the products of the *Hoxd13*, *Hoxd12*, and *Hoxd11* genes simultaneously. The *Hoxd11/lac* reporter gene replaced the deleted region and allowed monitoring the effect of this triple inactivation at the cellular level. Indeed, the same reporter was maintained after each deletion event.

From detailed analysis of early and late phases of limb development by using the *Hoxd11lac* marker and other histological markers, *Hox* gene dependence of a broad spectrum of developmental features becomes apparent (Fig. 4). Deficits are seen first in early limb bud size; later in the size of the distal limb, which includes the digit primordia, and the pattern of the emerging prechondrogenic condensations; even later in the sequence of appearance of ossification centers; and last in the progression and completion of endochondral ossification *(4)*.

Deleting the whole complex was interesting from the regulatory perspective *(22)* because even in the absence of all digit *Hoxd* genes, reporter gene expression in the digit domain was maintained. Deletion of the entire complex was a good way to show that the shared digit regulatory element was outside of the complex. We have collected thus far a set of five mouse strains that contain the *Hoxd11/lac* reporter gene all in the identical 5' environment. This is a valuable resource, not only for studying the function of the *HoxD* complex but also its underlying regulation. Progressive deficiencies toward the inside of the cluster signal the presence of regulatory regions interspersed with the genes. *HoxD*-type regulation observed in the absence of the entire cluster suggests regulatory influences coming from the outside. Simply using the X-gal assay on similarly staged embryos, one can monitor differences in reporter gene expression and thus make a number of interesting observations.

At a relatively early stage, the main influence of the internal part of the cluster is to suppress early/anterior activation of a posterior gene. When close to early acting anterior element, the posterior gene-derived reporter can be expressed in anterior, early forming structures, like the hindbrain, or the cervical spinal column. The next endpoint can localize such elements, in this case near the *Hoxd3* gene. Although such anterior elements cannot access the posterior genes, it appears to access the nearby anterior promoter easily. The full deficiency suggested that the digit element is located outside of the cluster *(21,22)*.

This latter claim needed independent support because the reporter gene was derived from a proper digit gene. To show formally that a digit enhancer was located outside of the cluster, a reporter gene replacement was necessary. An allele raised with the *Hoxb1/lac* gene was used for this purpose, in the TAMERE protocol (*see Trans*-Allelic Targeted Meiotic Recombination section). By crossing mice containing the *Hoxb1/lac* allele relocated to the posterior *Hoxd* cluster and a *Hoxd11*/lac reporter with a

Fig. 4. (*opposite page*) Limb defects caused by *HoxD* cluster mutations. Limb skeletons of adult (**A–F**) and juvenile mice (**G** and **H**) illustrate the involvement of several *Hoxd* genes in digit development. **A** and **D** shows part of the forelimb and hindlimb skeleton, respectively, of hemizygous animals, with one complete set of *HoxD* genes, and a deficient chromosome that lacks *Hoxd13*, *Hoxd12*, and *Hoxd11*, produced as a result of targeted deletion. The anatomical pattern is almost completely normal, except for slight reductions of the second phalanges of digits II and IV in the forelimb. **B** and **E** show forepaw and hindpaw of an animal homozygous for a mutation

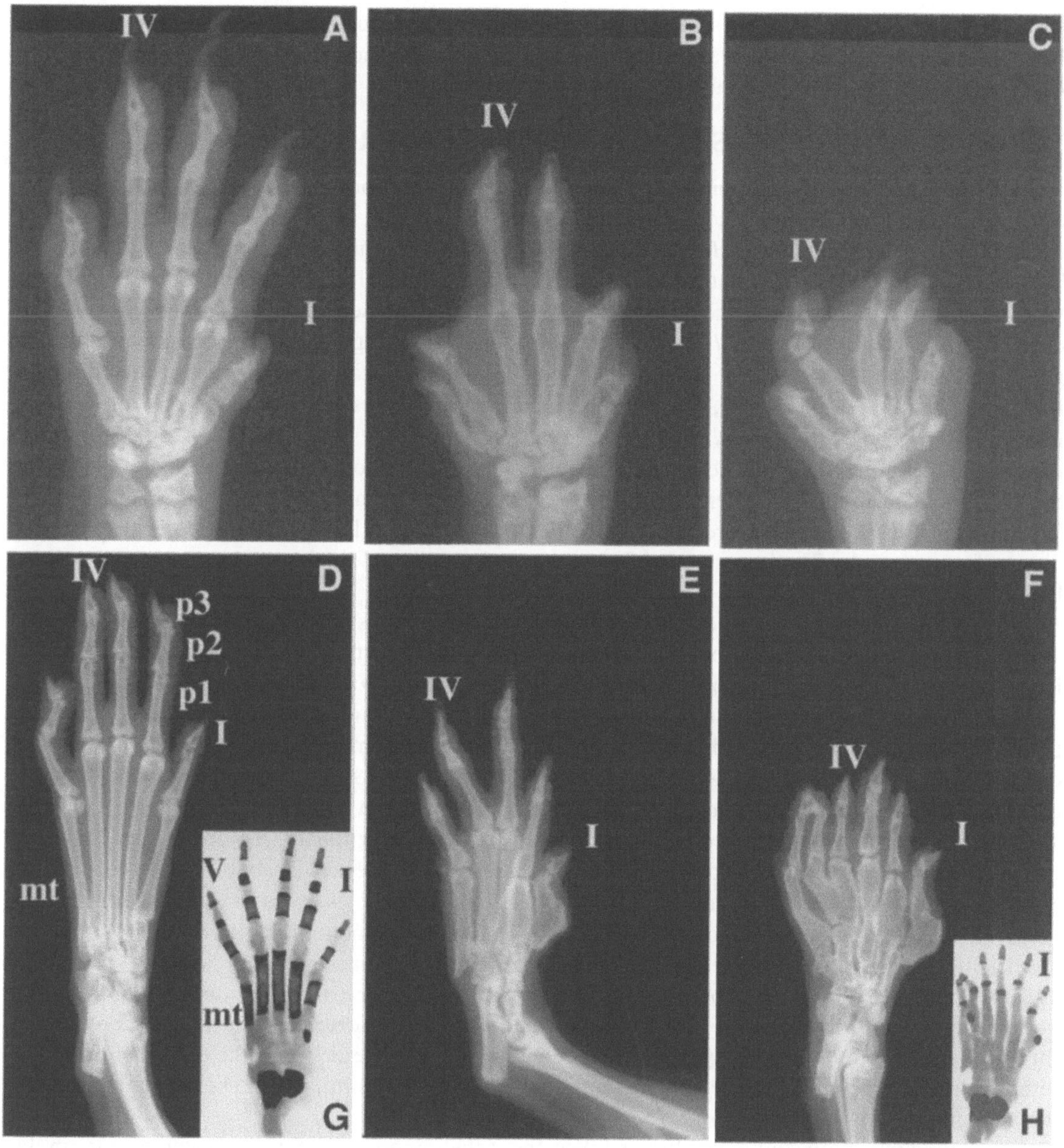

of *Hoxd13*. The gene is present, but no functional HOXD13 protein is produced because of a targeted insertion of *lacZ* sequence into the homeodomain. Digit defects are present in essentially the same structures but to a less severe degree as compared with the simultaneous loss of *Hoxd13*, *Hoxd12*, and *Hoxd11* (see next panels). **C** and **F** show the corresponding parts of the skeleton of a homozygous mutant of the *Hoxd13*-, *Hoxd12*-, and *Hoxd11*-deficient chromosome. In homozygous individuals, all digits are shorter (ectrodactyly), lack well-formed articulations between the phalanges (p2, p3, etc., in panel **C**), and a diagnostic pattern of synpolydactyly is observed in the hindlimb, which involves the fourth digit (IV in panel **F**). In addition to these patterning defects, skeletons of mice 1 wk after birth show ossification deficiency. Ossification centers of the different skeletal elements were visualized by alizarin red staining, and here appear in dark grey in panels **G** and **H**. When comparing **G** and **H**, the absence of the longest metatarsal ossification centres signals a delay of approx 10 d in endochondral ossification. Similar heterochrony is seen in all mutants that involve a loss of the *Hoxd13* gene product, but the full extent of the defect can be seen only when both *Hoxd12* and *Hoxd11* are inactivated in addition to *Hoxd13* (*see* scheme **E** in Fig. 2).

large *HoxD* cluster deficiency, the same deficiency was established, but this time with the novel reporter. *Hoxb1/lac* expression in digits was strong evidence of the independence of the digit enhancer from *Hoxd11* proximal sequences (Kmita et al., unpublished results).

TARGETED INVERSIONS IN THE *HOXD* CLUSTER

After these sections of describing experiments involving short or longer *loxP*/Cre mediated deletions, we should touch upon a second kind of *cis* manipulation, that involving inversions. Two major functional involvements of the *HoxD* cluster were linked to multiple gene regulatory domains. In both of these cases, distant regulatory elements that appeared to be located outside of the cluster provide for gene dose-dependent mechanism by regulating contiguous sets of genes. As discussed earlier, doses of *Hoxd13*, *Hoxd12*, *Hoxd11*, and *Hoxd10* are involved in digits and coexpression of all these genes seems to be a result of the activity of a shared enhancer located 5'. The rest of the complex, including *Hoxd9*, *Hoxd8*, *Hoxd4*, *Hoxd3*, and *Hoxd1*, is not expressed in digits to any appreciable level. However, genes from *Hoxd11* to *Hoxd1* were all found expressed at the transition of the small intestine to the large bowel, the so-called ileo-cecal valve. We hypothesized that the coregulation of this contiguous set of the first seven genes reflects the activity of a shared gut enhancer located in the 3'. When five of the seven genes were deleted together, a smooth muscle organ, the ileo-cecal sphincter, did not form properly. The importance of gene dose was indicated by the need to inactivate at least five genes simultaneously *(20)*.

When taken together, it became apparent that the *HoxD* cluster is subdivided into two overlapping domains of regulation. *Hoxd12* belongs to the digit domain, but it and the more posterior *Hoxd13* is excluded from the gut regulatory domain. At the same time, *Hoxd11* and *Hoxd10* belong to both domains. Because of the multiple polarities involved, it seemed to be a good approach to reverse polarity of the region that included the limit of the gut expression domain. First a *Hoxd13/lac* locus was created, ending with a *loxP* site. A second inversely oriented *loxP* site was then introduced between the *Hoxd11* and *Hoxd10* genes in *cis*. This allele was established as a mouse line. To achieve the inversion, these mice were then crossed with mice expressing Cre ubiquitously. As long as the Cre transgene was present both direct and inverse configurations were present in about equal proportions. After segregating out this transgene in the next generation, both alleles could be established independently. Mice carrying the inversion showed a reciprocal re-assignment of the limb vs gut regulatory specificities, suggesting the presence of a silencer element with a unidirectional property. This polar silencer appears to limit the number of genes that respond to one type of regulation and thus indicates how separate regulatory domains may be implemented within intricate gene clusters. A corollary of this mechanism is that the activity of the unidirectional silencer element and the enhancer promoter interactions do not involve tissue specific components, but work similarly in skeletogenic progenitors and gut mesoderm *(23)*.

In a second inversion study, we obtained data about the importance of gene cluster polarity in the control of spatial and temporal colinearity at earlier stages of the development of the main body axis, and in limb buds. The entire *HoxD* cluster was inverted in ES cells by *loxP*/Cre manipulations (Fig. 2H). Using this allele, we can test further the hypothesis about unidirectional silencer elements. This will also provide a means to test if functional domains can be redefined in an even broader context.

TRANS-ALLELIC TARGETED MEIOTIC RECOMBINATION

Functional studies of large transcription units, clustered genes, and chromosomal loci required the design of novel experimental tools to engineer genomic macro-rearrangements. We established a novel strategy to produce deficiencies or duplications directly in vivo by crossing mice carrying a *loxP* site on homologous chromosomes. When a *loxP* site is present in both parental chromosomes, during meiotic pairing, at a stage crossing over normally occurs, targeted recombination between these two sites located in *trans* could be used to generate unequal interchromosomal exchanges. These give rise to rearrangements, such as deletion and reciprocal duplication of the DNA fragment located between the relative position of the two *loxP* sites (Fig. 1C). This was successfully achieved with the use of a transgene in which the *Cre* coding sequences are under the control of the *Synaptonemal complex protein 1* promoter that recapitulates the expression profile in pachytene spermatocytes of the *Synaptonemal complex protein 1* gene that is involved in meiotic chromosome pairing.

This *trans*-allelic targeted meiotic recombination protocol, through the combination of various alleles within a particular locus, allows the production of a variety of novel genetic configurations without multiple targeting and selection steps in embryonic stem cells. Application of this genetic protocol is limited by the availability of *loxP* inserts but the high frequency of such targeted exchanges in vivo makes the *trans*-allelic targeted meiotic recombination a powerful genetic tool *(24)*.

The first time, we used a set of sites inserted near the digit genes *Hoxd13*, *12*, *11*, and *10*. These *loxP* sites were offset by one, two, or three genes *(4,10,13,14,16)*. By crossing any pair of them and bringing the two alleles in the same "transloxer" male, deletions and reciprocal duplications of one, two or three digit genes could be established (schemes A, B, and C in Fig. 2). We embarked on such systematic deletion and duplication approach with the aim of dissecting the function of these posterior *Hoxd* genes in an unambiguous manner as well as to investigate the mechanism underlying colinearity in limbs. Such systematic modifications either in the presence or in the absence, in the respective positions, or in the total number of genes helped elucidate the underlying processes. Indeed, comparative analysis of this allelic series revealed that modifications of either the topology or number of 5' *Hoxd* genes induce regulatory reallocations that give rise to abnormal number and morphology of the digits. Such digit phenotypes are seen only when the *Hoxd13* gene is altered, as expected from the prevalent role of HOXD13 protein in digit morphogenesis. Interestingly, 5' *Hoxd* genes are expressed in the presumptive digit domain after a gradual decrease in transcriptional efficiency with the 5'-most gene in the cluster, *Hoxd13*, being the most widely activated. This phenomenon, referred to as quantitative colinearity *(25)*, could be related to the special importance of *Hoxd13* in making digits. The regulatory reallocations observed, as a result of the rearrangements we produced, prove that actually 5' *Hoxd* genes compete for the activity of the digit enhancer. However, competition between 5' *Hoxd* promoters is not related to a distance effect toward the enhancer and does not primarily rely on promoter identity. Instead, comparative analysis of our allelic series clearly suggested that the preference of the digit enhancer for the 5'-most *Hoxd* gene depends mostly, although not entirely, upon regulatory sequences located at the 5' extremity of the *HoxD* cluster *(26)*. As a consequence, the enhancer would gradually loose the capacity of activating genes located further 3', thus explaining why only the four most 5' genes are activated in the digit domain. Such mechanism could have been established to secure high level of HOXD13 protein in distal limb because of its particular importance in making the distal part of our limb, that is, hands and feet.

PERSPECTIVES

In ongoing experiments, we are extending the scope of our analysis beyond the bounds of the *HoxD* cluster, into the flanking regions, both in the 5' and the 3' direction, in an attempt to establish long-range chromosomal rearrangements. We also are trying to establish alleles of *Hoxd* genes, marked with molecular markers, that could be used in isolating purified native cells representing early stages of skeletogenic patterning. Targeted deletions, inversions, and duplications will no doubt stay with us for some time and will facilitate the analysis of complex genetic loci. We are also considering the availability of future tools, such as variant *loxP* sites, Flip recombinase target sequence (FRTs), and *flip*-ases and the zoo of Cre-expressing mice, to increase the potential of this molecular genetic approach. Together. these studies will help to find answers to some of the many unresolved questions concerning the role of *Hox* genes in limb development, evolution and human dysmorphogenesis *(27,28)*.

ACKNOWLEDGMENTS

We are grateful to P. Chambon, F. Cusin, R. Krumlauf, S. Potter, and K. Rajewsky for generous shearing of reagents and mice. We thank many past and present colleagues from the laboratory for their help. Our laboratory is supported by funds from the Canton de Genève, the Swiss National Research Fund, the Claraz, Latsis, Cloetta and Jeantet foundations, as well as the NCCR "Frontiers in Genetics."

REFERENCES

1. Sauer, B. and Henderson, N. (1989) Cre-stimulated recombination at loxP-containing DNA sequences placed into the mammalian genome. *Nucleic Acids Res.* **17,** 147–161.
2. Duboule, D. (1994) Temporal colinearity and the phylotypic progression: a basis for the stability of a vertebrate Bauplan and the evolution of morphologies through heterochrony. *Development* **Suppl,** 135–142.
3. Duboule, D. (1995) Vertebrate *Hox* genes and proliferation: an alternative pathway to homeosis? *Curr. Opin. Genet. Dev.* **5,** 25–28.
4. Zakany, J. and Duboule, D. (1996) Synpolydactyly in mice with a targeted deficiency in the *HoxD* complex. *Nature* **384,** 69–71.
5. Davis, A. P., Witte, D. P., Hsieh-Li, H. M., Potter, S. S., and Capecchi, M. R. (1995) Absence of radius and ulna in mice lacking hoxa-11 and hoxd-11. *Nature* **375,** 791–795.
6. Dolle, P., Dierich, A., LeMeur, M., Schimmang, T., Schuhbaur, B., Chambon, P., et al. (1993) Disruption of the Hoxd-13 gene induces localized heterochrony leading to mice with neotenic limbs. *Cell* **75,** 431–441.
7. Zakany, J., Fromental-Ramain, C., Warot, X., and Duboule, D. (1997) Regulation of number and size of digits by posterior *Hox* genes: a dose-dependent mechanism with potential evolutionary implications. *Proc. Natl. Acad. Sci. USA* **94,** 13695–13700.
8. Kondo, T., Zakany, J., Innis, J. W., and Duboule, D. (1997) Of fingers, toes and penises. *Nature* **390,** 29.
9. Zakany, J., Gerard, M., Favier, B., Potter, S. S., and Duboule, D. (1996) Functional equivalence and rescue among group 11 *Hox* gene products in vertebral patterning. *Dev. Biol.* **176,** 325–328.
10. Gerard, M., Chen, J. Y., Gronemeyer, H., Chambon, P., Duboule, D., and Zakany, J. (1996) In vivo targeted mutagenesis of a regulatory element required for positioning the Hoxd-11 and Hoxd-10 expression boundaries. *Genes Dev.* **10,** 2326–2334.
11. Zakany, J., Gerard, M., Favier, B., and Duboule, D. (1997) Deletion of a *HoxD* enhancer induces transcriptional heterochrony leading to transposition of the sacrum. *EMBO J.* **16,** 4393–4402.
12. Gerard, M., Zakany, J., and Duboule, D. (1997) Interspecies exchange of a Hoxd enhancer in vivo induces premature transcription and anterior shift of the sacrum. *Dev. Biol.* **190,** 32–40.
13. Beckers, J. and Duboule D. (1998) Genetic analysis of a conserved sequence in the *HoxD* complex: regulatory redundancy or limitations of the transgenic approach? *Dev. Dyn.* **213,** 1–11.
14. Herault, Y., Beckers, J., Kondo, T., Fraudeau, N., and Duboule, D. (1998) Genetic analysis of a Hoxd-12 regulatory element reveals global versus local modes of controls in the *HoxD* complex. *Development* **125,** 1669–1677.
15. Kondo, T., Zakany, J., and Duboule, D. (1998) Control of colinearity in AbdB genes of the mouse *HoxD* complex. *Mol. Cell* **1,** 289–300.
16. Herault, Y., Beckers, J., Gerard, M., and Duboule, D. (1999) *Hox* gene expression in limbs: colinearity by opposite regulatory controls. *Dev. Biol.* **208,** 157–165.
17. Kondo, T. and Duboule, D. (1999) Breaking colinearity in the mouse *HoxD* complex. *Cell* **97,** 407–417.
18. Kmita, M., van Der Hoeven, F., Zakany, J., Krumlauf, R., and Duboule, D. (2000) Mechanisms of *Hox* gene colinearity: transposition of the anterior Hoxb1 gene into the posterior *HoxD* complex. *Genes Dev.* **14,** 198–211.
19. van der Hoeven, F., Zakany, J., and Duboule, D. (1996) Gene transpositions in the *HoxD* complex reveal a hierarchy of regulatory controls. *Cell* **85,** 1025–1035.
20. Zakany, J. and Duboule, D. (1999) *Hox* genes and the making of sphincters. *Nature* **401,** 761–762.
21. Zakany, J., Kmita, M., Alarcon, P., de la Pompa, J. L., and Duboule, D. (2001) Localized and transient transcription of *Hox* genes suggests a link between patterning and the segmentation clock. *Cell* **106,** 207–217.
22. Spitz, F., Gonzalez, F., Peichel, C., Vogt, T. F., Duboule, D., and Zakany, J. (2001) Large scale transgenic and cluster deletion analysis of the *HoxD* complex separate an ancestral regulatory module from evolutionary innovations. *Genes Dev.* **15,** 2209–2214.
23. Kmita, M., Kondo, T., and Duboule, D. (2000) Targeted inversion of a polar silencer within the *HoxD* complex re-allocates domains of enhancer sharing. *Nat. Genet.* **26,** 451–454.
24. Herault, Y., Rassoulzadegan, M., Cuzin, F., and Duboule, D. (1998) Engineering chromosomes in mice through targeted meiotic recombination (TAMERE). *Nat. Genet.* **4,** 381–384.
25. Dolle, P., Izpisua-Belmonte, J. C., Brown, J. M., Tickle, C., and Duboule, D. (1991) HOX-4 genes and the morphogenesis of mammalian genitalia. *Genes Dev.* **5,** 1767–1776.
26. Kmita, M., Fraudeau, N., Hérault, Y., and Duboule, D. (2002) Serial deletions and duplications suggest a mechanism for the colinearity of *Hoxd* genes in limbs. *Nature* **420,** 145–150.
27. Zakany, J. and Duboule, D. (1999) *Hox* genes in digit development and evolution. *Cell Tissue Res.* **296,** 19–25.
28. Goodman, F. R. (2002) Limb malformations and the human HOX genes. *Am. J. Med. Genet.* **112,** 256–265.

8

Control of Development and Homeostasis Via Regulation of BMP, Wnt, and Hedgehog Signaling

Renee Hackenmiller, Catherine Degnin, and Jan Christian

INTRODUCTION

Secreted signaling proteins play fundamental roles in the embryonic patterning of multicellular organisms from insects to humans. Three protein families, bone morphogenetic proteins (BMPs), Wnts, and hedgehog (Hh) are secreted cell–cell signaling molecules that have been shown to be important regulators of a wide variety of normal and pathological developmental processes. BMPs, Wnts, and Hh can all be termed as morphogens in that they act directly at a distance and induce distinct differentiation programs at different concentrations. Signaling by BMPs, Wnts, and Hh is regulated in both positive and negative fashions at the extracellular, membrane, cytoplasmic, and nuclear levels. The range of molecular strategies involved in regulating the signaling activities of these proteins in a developing embryo highlights the crucial importance of maintaining tight spatial and temporal control of morphogens during development.

BMPs comprise a subclass of the transforming growth factor-β (TGF-β) superfamily, which also includes TGF-βs, activins, inhibins, and Mullerian inhibiting substance. The first BMPs were identified by their ability to induce ectopic bone formation when implanted under the skin of rodents *(1)*. Molecular cloning has subsequently identified a family of structurally related proteins, including BMP-2 through -8, *Xenopus* Vg1, Nodals, GDFs, and the *Drosophila* proteins Decapentaplegic (Dpp), Screw and 60A. BMP ligand dimers bind to a heteromeric complex of type I and type II transmembrane serine/threonine kinase receptors. Ligand binding to a receptor complex results in the phosphorylation of cytoplasmic proteins Smad1, 5, or 8, which then translocate to the nucleus and regulate BMP target gene expression (Fig. 1A).

Wnt-1, the first Wnt family member to be discovered, was originally identified as an oncogene leading to mouse mammary tumors when activated by viral integration *(2)*. It was later shown to be the vertebrate ortholog of the *Drosophila* segment polarity gene, *wingless* (*wg*; ref. *3*). In vertebrates, the Wnt family of proteins encodes more than a dozen structurally related secreted glycoproteins. There are several Wnt signaling pathways, but the canonical Wnt pathway describes the salient signaling events and introduces the important players. In the absence of Wnt signal, the constitutively active serine–threonine kinase GSK3 phosphorylates β-catenin, targeting it for ubiquitination and proteasome-mediated degradation. Upon Wnt stimulation by binding of ligand to its receptor, Frizzled, GSK3, no longer phosphorylates β-catenin, and β-catenin becomes enriched in the cytosol and nucleus, where it binds to T-cell/lymphoid-enhancing transcription factors to derepress transcription of Wnt target genes (Fig. 1B).

From: *The Skeleton: Biochemical, Genetic, and Molecular Interactions in Development and Homeostasis*
Edited by: E. J. Massaro and J. M. Rogers © Humana Press Inc., Totowa, NJ

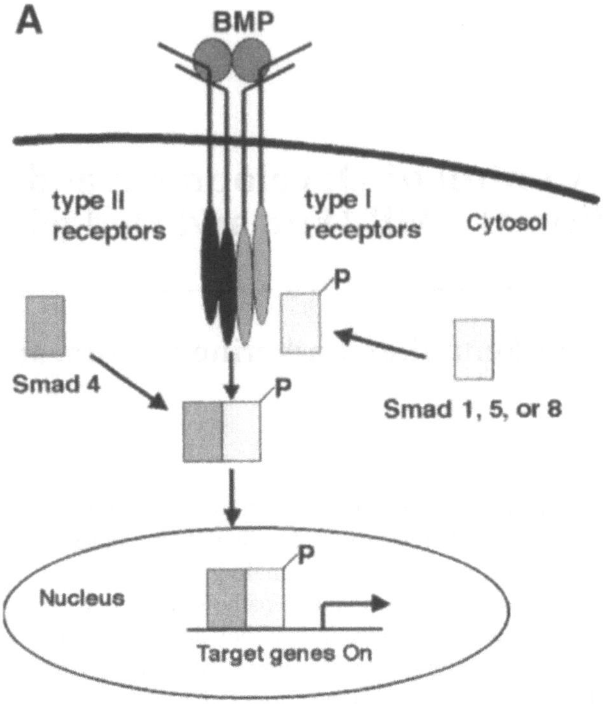

Fig. 1. Schematic representation of BMP, Wnt, and Hh signaling pathways (*see* text for details). **A**, The BMP signaling pathway.

Hedgehog (*hh*) was identified in the Nusslein–Volhard and Wieschaus screen looking for genes that are required for segmentation of the *Drosophila* embryo *(4)*. Three mouse homologs have been identified: Indian Hedgehog, Desert Hedgehog, and Sonic Hedgehog. The Hh signal is transduced when Hh ligands bind to the multipass membrane protein Patched (Ptc), antagonizing Ptc activity. Binding of Hh to Ptc relieves inhibition of Smoothened (Smo), a transmembrane protein related to the secretin G protein-coupled receptor. Uninhibited Smo transmits the Hh signal intracellularly through several cytoplasmic steps, leading to the nuclear action of the Ci/Gli proteins, which regulate Hh target genes. In the absence of Hh signaling, Ci is constitutively cleaved, generating a repressor form that binds to and inactivates Hh target genes. When Smo transmits the Hh signal, Ci is no longer cleaved and the full-length Ci protein activates Hh target genes (Fig. 1C). The exact mechanism through which Smo transduces the Hh signal remains unclear, but it most likely involves a conformational change in the receptor complex or a cellular redistribution of the Smo and/or Ptc protein. Although this is the generally accepted view of basic Hh signaling, the specifics are still being debated.

The finding that BMPs, Wnts, and Hh function as long-range signals in some tissues, but only signal to neighboring cells in others suggest complex regulatory mechanisms that control the actions of these proteins. Dpp, for example, acts over long range to specify cell fate in the *Drosophila* wing disc but signals only at short range between germ layers of the gut *(5)*. Wnt also shows both short- and long-range activities, with both activities even being observed within a single tissue. In the embryonic epidermis, for example, Wnt protein can be detected in vesicles three to four cells anterior, but only one cell posterior, to where the gene is transcribed *(6)*. Similarly, Hh signals at short range to induce floor plate within the neural tube but at long range in patterning the limb *(7)*. How the range of action of a signaling molecule can be restricted in one tissue or cell type but not another is a complex problem in trying to understand the actions of these morphogens.

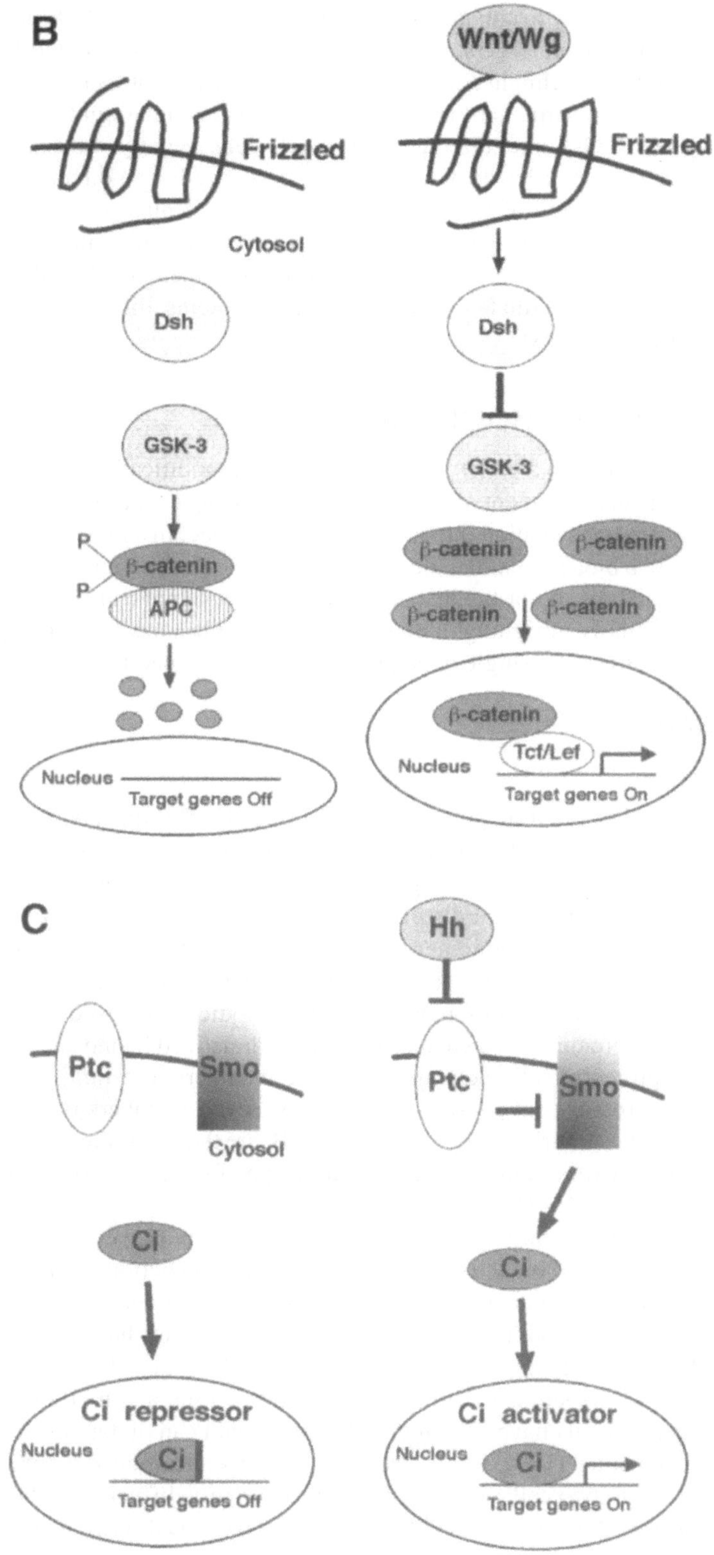

Fig. 1. B, The Wnt signaling pathway. **C**, The hedgehog signaling pathway.

Here, we focus on regulatory events that occur after translation of BMP, Wnt, and Hh but before receptor-mediated signaling events. First, we discuss how posttranslational modifications can lead to activity changes. Second, we highlight some of the extracellular regulators that impact on BMP, Wnt, and Hh activity and action, in particular the role of secreted extracellular binding proteins and heparan sulfate proteoglycans (HSPGs) in regulating these morphogens. Finally, we examine autoregulatory feedback loops that alter receptor levels or activation on target cells as a direct result of BMP-, Wnt-, or Hh-mediated regulation. Each of these signaling pathways is also regulated at the intracellular level after receptor activation, and readers are referred to several recent reviews that include coverage of these intracellular mechanisms *(8–10)*. It is important to remember that although we discuss a variety of mechanisms used to regulate the actions of these proteins, different strategies may be used in different developmental context.

POSTTRANSLATIONAL MODIFICATION

BMPs, Wnts, and Hh undergo a variety of posttranslational modifications, including cleavage, glycosylation, and/or covalent attachment of lipids. These processing events occur during transit through the secretory pathway or after secretion into the extracellular space. In some cases, these modifications are required to generate a bioactive molecule; in others, they are not essential for activity but instead modify the level of signaling and/or the distance over which a signal can spread. The latter types of modifications are particularly intriguing in that they may provide a mechanism to posttranslationally alter the signaling properties of a single gene product in a tissue-specific fashion.

Processing of BMPs

Proteolytic Activation

BMPs are synthesized as prepropeptides consisting of a signal sequence, a minimally conserved amino (N)-terminal prodomain and a more highly conserved carboxy (C)-terminal mature domain *(11)*. After cotranslational cleavage of the signal peptide, BMPs form homo- or heterodimers that are covalently linked via an intermolecular disulfide bond between a conserved cysteine residue located within the mature domain of each monomer (reviewed in ref. *12*). An additional six conserved cysteines in the mature domain form intramolecular bonds that help fold each monomer into a characteristic cystine knot motif. After dimerization, BMPs are proteolytically cleaved immediately C-terminal to a RXXR-motif and the prodomain fragments and mature dimerized ligand are secreted from the cell.

The enzymes that proteolytically activate BMPs are members of a family of higher eukaryotic endoproteases, the proprotein convertases. In mammals, seven members of this family have been characterized. Three of these, furin, PACE-4, and PC5/6B, are the most likely candidates for processing BMPs based on their expression patterns, substrate specificity, in vivo inhibitor studies, and/or mutational analysis in mice (*13–18*).

The prodomains of TGF-β family members lack signaling activity, yet the presence of this region is essential for the generation of bioactive dimers in most cases. Deletion of the prodomain of activin A or TGF-β, for example, prevents dimerization and secretion of the mature ligand, but activity can be rescued by addition of the prodomain *in trans (19)*. These findings have led to the suggestion that the prodomain of TFG-β family members, like that of several prokaryotic and eukaryotic proteases, acts as an intramolecular chaperone to direct proper folding of the mature domain (reviewed in ref. *20*). Domain swap experiments have shown that the prodomain can dictate the half-life, bioactivity, and signaling range of mature TGF-β family members. BMP-4 and nodals, for example, normally act over a range of only one to two cells, whereas activinβB is freely diffusible. When the prodomain of activinβB is fused to the mature domain of either BMP-4 *(21)* or Nodals *(22)*, ligand cleaved from these precursors is more readily released from the cell and can signal over many cell diameters. Furthermore, mature Nodal cleaved from its native precursor protein is highly unstable whereas that cleaved from a chimeric precursor containing the BMP-4 prodomain is stable *(16)*.

The requirement for proteolytic removal of the prodomain for activity is supported by the finding that cleavage mutant forms of BMPs in which the -RXXR- motif has been disrupted are inactive and can dimerize with and inhibit the cleavage, secretion and bioactivity of native BMPs *(23)*. A few exceptions to this rule do exist, however, in that precursor forms of inhibin A *(24)*, lefty *(25)*, and *Xenopus* nodal related-2 *(26)* possess some bioactivity.

The mechanism(s) by which the prodomain regulates the activity of mature BMPs is unknown and is likely to vary between individual family members. In the case of TGF-β, which has been better studied than BMPs, the prodomain remains noncovalently associated with the mature ligand, forming an inactive, latent complex that is stored in the extracellular matrix (ECM) in association with the latent TGF-β binding protein. The major regulatory step controlling TGF-β activity takes place outside of the cell when proteases or other agents either release the prodomain or induce a conformational change that exposes the receptor binding sites on TGF-β *(27)*. Analogous to TGF-β, the prodomain of BMP-7 remains noncovalently associated with the mature region after cleavage but, unlike TGF-β, this complex can bind to and activate BMP receptors without further processing or alteration *(28)*. Recent genetic data support a functional interaction between BMP-7 and the latent TGF-β binding protein family member Fibrillin-2 and suggest that the bioactivity or availability of BMP-7, like that of TGF-β, may be regulated by interactions with the ECM *(29)*. Processing of BMP-4 is more complex than that of BMP-7 in that the precursor is sequentially cleaved by furin at two sites and this ordered proteolysis regulates the activity and signaling range of mature BMP-4 *(14,15)*. Specifically, proBMP-4 is initially cleaved at a consensus furin motif adjacent to the mature ligand domain and this allows for subsequent cleavage at an upstream nonconsensus furin motif within the prodomain. Failure to cleave at the upstream site generates a ligand that is targeted for rapid degradation, leading to lower bioactivity and signaling distance in vivo. Conversely, a mutant form of the precursor that is rapidly cleaved at both sites generates ligand that is more active and signals over a greater range. An intriguing possibility is that the upstream site is cleaved in a tissue-specific fashion, thereby providing a mechanism to spatially regulate the levels and distance of BMP signaling in vivo. This same mechanism may operate for the closely related family member BMP-2 because the two cleavage sites are conserved in BMP-4 and BMP-2 from all species, but not in other family members.

Role of Homo- vs Heterodimerization

Closely related members of the BMP family, for example BMP-2-4 and/or -7, BMP-2 and GDF-6, or different nodal-related proteins, can form heterodimers within the secretory pathway before proteolytic processing and in some cases the heterodimers are more potent signaling molecules than are homodimers *(30–33)*. Recent studies have shown that more distantly related family members can also heterodimerize. BMP-4, for example, forms heterodimers with *Xenopus* derriere or nodal-related proteins *(26)* and BMP-7 forms heterodimers with nodal *(34)*. BMP-4 and -7 bind to a distinct class of receptors and activate a different intracellular signal transduction pathway than do derriere or nodals, raising the questions of whether these heterodimers are active and, if so, which class of receptors and signaling pathways are activated. An alternate possibility is that this class of heterodimer blocks activation of both signaling pathways as has been suggested for BMP-7/nodal heterodimers *(34)*.

Processing of Wnts

Regulated Glycosylation

Unlike Hh and BMPs, Wnts are subject only to regulated glycosylation and not cleavage. In transfected tissue culture cells, most Wnt protein is retained as an unglyosylated form in the endoplasmic reticulum associated with an HSP70 protein *(35)*. This inefficient processing suggests that generation of active Wnt protein is a complex process and may require tissue specific accessory proteins. Consistent with this, genetic studies identified Porcupine (Porc) as a member of an evolutionarily conserved family of multipass transmembrane ER proteins, which is required for processing the *Drosophila* Wnt family member, Wg *(36,37)*. Porc was recently shown to bind an N-terminal region of Wg that is highly conserved among all Wnts and to stimulate glycosylation of nearby sites. In addition, Porc was shown to be dispensable for *N*-glycosylation in the presence of dithiothreitol (DTT), suggesting that the cotranslational formation of intramolecular disulfide bonds in Wnt proteins normally inhibits efficient glycosylation. Based on these studies, a model has been proposed in which Porc tethers Wg to the ER membrane bringing it into close proximity with the oligosaccharyl transferase complex, thereby accelerating glycosylation and minimizing competition with cotranslational disulfide bond formation. Porc shares homology with a family of acetyltransferases, raising the possibility that it may anchor Wg to the ER membrane via acetylation *(38)*.

Processing of Hedgehog

Autoproteolysis and Cholesterol Attachment

Hh is synthesized as a 45-kDa precursor that is autoprocessed to generate a 20-kDa N-terminal fragment (Hh-N) that possesses all known signaling activity and a 25-kDa C-terminal domain (Hh-C) that catalzyes intramolecular cleavage of the precursor *(39–41)*. Cleavage occurs through the formation of a thioester intermediate that undergoes nucleophilic attack by cholesterol, resulting in the covalent attachment of cholesterol to the C-terminus of Hh-N *(42)*. This yields the mature signaling form of Hh, which is denoted Hh-Np.

The addition of cholesterol to Hh-N initially was thought to be essential for ligand function, possibly by mediating binding to the Hh receptor, Ptc (reviewed in ref. *43*), but is now known to be dispensable for activity and receptor binding. This was demonstrated with a truncated form of Hh lacking the cholesterol modification, which retains full signaling activity both in vitro and in vivo *(41,44)* and binds to Ptc with similar affinity as does Hh-Np *(45)*.

In *Drosophila*, the cholesterol adduct can limit the range over which Hh signals, as evidenced by the finding that overexpressed Hh-N signals over a much greater distance than does Hh-Np. This restriction is caused by the ability of Ptc to sequester and thereby limit the travels of Hh-Np, but not Hh-N. This presents an unresolved paradox, however, because earlier studies have shown that Ptc binds to Hh-N and Hh-Np with equal affinity. The difference in receptor interactions in vivo may be mediated by differential association of Hh-N and Hh-Np with HSPGs, as described in the Activity Regulation by HSPGs section.

Curiously, the cholesterol moiety not only restricts the range over which Hh can signal but also enables Hh to signal beyond producing cells. Hh-Np can signal across several cell diameters whereas a membrane tethered form of Hh can signal only to adjacent cells, thereby demonstrating that cholesterol does not function as a simple membrane anchor. Release of Hh-Np from producing cells is dependent on the function of yet-to-be identified HSPGs, which is discussed in the next section on extracellular regulation of activity, and a novel transmembrane protein, Dispatched (Disp).

Disp is a 12 pass transmembrane protein with a sterol sensing group that was identified by genetic studies as being required in Hh-producing cells for release of Hh-Np but not Hh-N *(46)*. In the absence of functional Disp, Hh-Np is synthesized, processed, reaches the cell surface, and can signal *(47)* but is not released from the cell. The mechanism by which Disp regulates Hh release is unknown.

Most of what is known about the role of cholesterol in modulating the range of Hh signaling has come from genetic studies in *Drosophila*. Recent studies in mice led to the surprising conclusions that, unlike in the fly, addition of cholesterol to vertebrate Hh is essential for long range activity but is dispensable for short-range signaling and sequestration by Ptc *(48)*. Specifically, mice were generated in which a stop codon was introduced into the Sonic Hh (Shh) gene such that only a truncated form of Shh analogous to Hh-N was expressed. This unprocessed, unmodified form of Shh protein was expressed at normal levels, interacted genetically with Ptc, and was able to signal to nearby cells but was not distributed to distal cells that normally receive Shh. The observed differences in the signaling range of Hh-N in the fly vs the mouse may be caused by the use of overexpression approaches in *Drosophila* vs knock-in mutations in the mouse, the use of different accessory proteins to regulate Hh signaling in each species (e.g., Disp in flies, HIP in mouse, *see* below), or differences in cellular context.

Palmitoylation

In addition to cholesterol modification, Hh undergoes an additional posttranslational lipid modification, the palmitoylation of its most N-terminal cysteine via an acylation intermediate *(45)*. Studies in tissue culture suggest that palmitoylation, like cholesterol coupling, can anchor Hh to the membrane *(45)*, but a variety of indirect evidence suggests that acylation alone is not sufficient to restrict the range of action of Hh in vivo. This issue remains to be resolved, but what is clear is that palmitoylation is essential to generate a fully active ligand. In *Drosophila*, acylation is catalyzed by a transmembrane acyltransferase encoded by the *skinny hedgehog* (*ski*) gene *(49)*, also referred to as *sightless* (*sit*; ref. *50)*, *central missing* (*cmn*; ref. *47*), or *Rasp (51)*. The activity of Hh-N and Hh-Np is abolished in embryos mutant for this gene. Further evidence that acylation is required to generate functional Hh is provided by studies in which the N-terminal cysteine to which palmitate is attached was mutated. This mutation inactivates the protein and generates a dominant mutant form that interferes with endogenous Hh activity *(52)*. In vertebrates, palmitoylation is not absolutely essential for Hh activity but generates a more potent signaling molecule in cell culture *(45)* and tissue assays. Specifically, although unacylated recombinant Shh can induce formation of ventral cell types in chick forebrain explant cultures, it is much less potent on mouse forebrain explants than is acylated protein *(53)*. In addition, mutation of the N-terminal cysteine residue to serine generates a signaling molecule with reduced patterning activity in a mouse limb bud assay relative to the wild-type Shh *(52)*.

The mechanism by which acylation potentiates the signaling activity of Hh is unclear. Addition of hydrophobic amino acids or other hydrophobic moieties to the N-terminus of Shh enhances the potency of the ligand but does not alter binding affinity for Ptc and has no apparent effect on structure *(54)*. Although these modifications do not appear to restrict the range of Hh, they may localize the protein to specific membrane domains and/or alter its affinity for cofactors or other proteins involved in signaling and transport.

ACTIVITY REGULATION BY EXTRACELLULAR MODES

In addition to the posttranslational modifications that impact on the action of BMP, Wnt, and Hh, there are a large number of extracellular proteins that regulate ligand activity and/or availability. In this section we focus on two extracellular regulatory mechanisms: secreted extracellular binding proteins and cell surface HSPGs. These diverse extracellular modulators either facilitate or inhibit the signaling activities of BMP, Wnt, and Hh by a variety of molecular mechanisms.

Sequestration of BMPs and Wnts by Secreted Extracellular Binding Proteins

In general, the soluble extracellular binding proteins described below affect the concentrations of BMPs and Wnts (no secreted extracellular regulators have been identified for Hh) that signal at the surface of responding cells. These interactions serve to regulate the amount of a particular ligand that a cell "sees," thus indicating its position within the morphogen gradient. Most of these extracellular regulators are high-affinity secreted binding proteins that prevent receptor activation by binding to the ligand, thereby acting as antagonists. Interestingly, there is little or no sequence similarity between the different classes discussed below.

BMP-Secreted Extracellular Regulators

Noggin

Noggin is a small glycoprotein (32 kDa) that was originally identified as a molecular component of Spemann's organizer, a specialized signaling center located on the dorsal side of gastrulating *Xenopus* embryos. Noggin functions as a homodimer that binds specifically to BMPs secreted by ventral cells and antagonizes BMP signaling by blocking interaction with its receptors *(55)*. These interactions are critical for normal dorsoventral patterning in *Xenopus* embryos. Noggin can also bind to and inhibit *Xenopus* GDF-6 (a TGF-β family member), preventing its ability to induce epidermis and blocking neural tissue formation *(56)*. Additional biochemical studies have shown that noggin binds to BMP-2, BMP-4 and GDF-6 with high affinity, but to BMP-7 with low affinity *(55,56)*.

Noggin-null mice demonstrate that antagonism of BMP activity by noggin is critical for proper skeletal development. In addition to defects in neural tube and somite development noggin-null mice have excess cartilage and fail to initiate joint formation *(57)*. Two human genetic disorders, proximal symphalangism and multiple synostoses syndrome, which are characterized by bony fusions of joints, have been shown to be caused by dominant mutations in noggin *(58)*, further underscoring the importance of noggin in joint development.

Chordin/Short Gastrulation (Sog)

Chordin is a 120-kDa protein secreted from the Spemann's organizer. In the same manner as noggin, chordin, and its *Drosophila* ortholog, short gastrulation (Sog) antagonizes BMP signaling by binding the ligand and preventing it from interacting with its receptor *(59)*. Because it is much larger than other BMP antagonists, chordin may diffuse less efficiently in tissues, altering its ability to function as a BMP inhibitor.

In both vertebrates and invertebrates, the activity of chordin orthologs is negatively regulated by a family of secreted zinc metalloproteases, including *Drosophila* Tolloid, *Xenopus* Xolloid, and human BMP-1. Biochemical studies have shown that Tolloid cleaves chordin and decreases its affinity for BMP ligands, thus functioning as a BMP agonist *(60–62)*. The activity of *Drosophila* Tolloid appears to be different than that of the other Tolloid orthologs. *Drosophila* Tolloid cleavage activity is dependent on the formation of the Dpp–Sog complex, whereas in *Xenopus* and zebrafish, chordin cleavage is independent of BMP binding *(60,61,63)*. Nonetheless, Tolloid orthologs can regulate the availability of BMP signals by regulating the amount of BMP bound by chordin.

Paradoxically, in *Drosophila*, whereas Dpp is inhibited by high levels of Sog, it appears to be enhanced by low levels of Sog, and this process requires Tolloid *(64)*. Sog may facilitate diffusion of Dpp, allowing the inactive complex to accumulate and then be activated by tolloid-mediated cleavage at sites distant from the Sog source.

Adding complexity, it has recently been shown that the secreted protein Twisted gastrulation (Tsg) acts as a BMP antagonist when complexed with chordin and BMP *(65–68)*. Tsg promotes the binding of chordin to BMP and together the three form a ternary complex that inactivates BMP signaling more efficiently than chordin alone. Additionally, Tsg enhances tolloid cleavage of chordin. It is not clear whether this generates "supersog-like molecules," that can inhibit additional members of the BMP family not inhibited by unprocessed Sog *(69)* or whether it inactivates chordin, freeing BMP to signal *(70)*. One possibility is that the chordin/Tsg/BMP complex helps BMP diffuse through the embryo, in part by preventing its association with cell surface receptors along the way. This would allow for high levels of BMP signaling at a distance from the chordin source (*see* above and ref. *71*).

Follistatin

Follistatin is a soluble secreted glycoprotein with cysteine-rich modules originally identified as a protein that binds and inhibits activin *(72)*. When follistatin is overexpressed in ventral blastomeres of a *Xenopus* embryo, it can induce a secondary body axis *(73)* and when overexpressed in *Xenopus* ectoderm, it can induce neural tissue *(74)*. These results suggest that follistatin might inhibit the action of proteins in addition to activin, namely BMPs. Additionally, follistatin has been shown to co-immunoprecipitate with BMP-4 in tissue culture *(75)*, indicating a direct interaction between BMPs and follistatin. In contrast to the mode of action of noggin and chordin, follistatin does not compete with the type I receptor for BMP-4 binding. Instead, it forms a tetrameric complex with BMP and the type I and type II BMP receptor to block receptor activation *(73)*.

DAN Family

DAN, Cerberus, Gremlin, Caronte, and other structurally related proteins are collectively called the DAN family *(76)*. All members of this family characterized to date have been shown to antagonize BMP signaling by preventing BMP–receptor interaction. Unrelated to other BMP antagonists, all DAN family members have a conserved 90 amino-acid cystine-knot motif that at least in Cerberus and Caronte includes the BMP-binding region *(77,78)*.

DAN

DAN, originally isolated as a putative zinc-finger protein that has tumor-suppressor activity *(79,80)* was later shown to be a secreted factor that like other BMP antagonist can neutralize ectodermal explants from *Xenopus* embryos and convert ventral mesoderm to more dorsal fates *(76)*. DAN directly binds to BMP-2 in vitro *(76)* but experimental evidence suggests it may be a more potent inhibitor of the GDF class of BMPs in vivo *(81)*. The exact role of DAN in developmental processes is unclear because DAN mutant mice have no obvious abnormalities *(81)*. In developing mouse neurons *dan* mRNA is localized to axons, suggesting a potential role for DAN in axonal outgrowth or guidance.

Cerberus

The *Xenopus* cerberus gene was identified as a Spemann organizer-associated transcript that encodes a secreted protein able to induce ectopic heads when injected into *Xenopus* embryos *(82)*. Cerberus is a multidimensional antagonist: it has been shown to bind and inhibit BMPs, Wnts, Nodals, and Activin, but the binding sites are independent *(77)*. BMP-4 and Xnr1 (nodal family member) bind in the cystine-knot region, whereas *Xenopus* wnt-8 (Xwnt-8) binds to the unique amino terminal half of cerberus. Cerberus appears to restrict trunk formation to the posterior part of the body by coordinately antagonizing three trunk-forming pathways—the BMP, Nodal, and Wnt pathways—in the anterior part of the developing embryo.

Gremlin

Gremlin was isolated in studies to identify dorsalizing factors that can induce a secondary axis in the *Xenopus* embryo *(76)*. In addition to antagonizing BMP activity, Gremlin also blocks signaling of Activin and Nodal-like members of TGF-β superfamily. Gremlin is expressed in cells of the neural crest lineage, suggesting it may have a role in neural crest induction and later patterning events. Gremlin has also been shown to be a central player in the outgrowth and patterning of the vertebrate limb *(83)*.

Wnt-Secreted Extracellular Regulators

The sFRP Family

The Wnt antagonists known as secreted frizzled-related proteins (sFRP) are a large family of secreted proteins that share homology to the putative Wnt-binding region of the Frizzled (Fz) family of transmembrane receptors *(84,85)*. Frzb-1 is the founding family member, and it was identified by researchers two ways: in a screen while looking for cDNAs enriched in the *Xenopus* Spemann's organizer *(84,85)* and in articular cartilage extracts while looking for in vivo chondrogenic activity *(86)*. Frzb-1 coimmunopreciptates with Xwnt-8, showing a direct interaction between Frzb and Wnts *(84)*, and Frzb blocks the axis-inducing activity of Xwnt-8 and mouse Wnt-1 when coinjected on the ventral side of cleaving embryos, demonstrating that Frzb is an antagonist of Wnt signaling. Additional experiments have demonstrated that the antagonistic effects of Frzb and Wnt take place in the extracellular space where the two proteins are secreted *(87)*, preventing productive interactions between Wnt and the Fz receptor.

All sFRP family members have been shown to have dorsalizing activities in *Xenopus* whole embryo assays, but the various family members have diverse expression patterns and different affinities for specific Wnts *(88)*. This suggests that particular sFRPs are required at specific times and in specific tissues to antagonize signaling of specific Wnts. Biochemical data regarding the target Wnt protein for the various sFRPs has been inconclusive. For example, Frzb1 can bind to Xwnt-3a, Xwnt-5, and Xwnt-8 in vitro but only interacts with Xwnt-8 in the embryo *(89)*. Similar results have been obtained for Frzb2 and Sizzled 2 *(90)*, making the in vivo requirement for the different sFRPs unclear.

A simple interaction between sFRP and Wnt proteins may not be able to fully explain the mechanism by which FRPs act. Recent data have demonstrated that sFRPs interact not only with Wnt proteins but also with other FRPs and with Fz receptors *(91)*, leaving open an alternative mode of action for sFRP-mediated antagonism of Wnt signaling.

Wnt Inhibitory Factor-1

Wnt inhibitory factor-1 (WIF-1) is another secreted Wnt antagonist that binds to Wnt proteins and blocks their interaction with the Fz receptors *(92)*. Its earliest expression is seen at neurula stages in the somitic mesoderm and anterior forebrain of mice *(92)*, and WIF-1 has been shown to bind to Xwnt-8 and Wg in vitro. WIF-1 has an N-terminal signal sequence, a domain of approx 150 amino acids termed the WIF domain that binds to Wnt/Wg, five epidermal growth factor-like repeats, and a hydrophobic domain of approx 45 amino acids at the C-terminus. The WIF domain partially overlaps with the Wnt binding domain in Fz-2.

Xenopus studies demonstrate that the action of WIF-1 is different than that of the Frzb family members. Coinjection of the BMP antagonist chordin with Frzb leads to a low frequency of secondary axis formation and when formed, the ectopic heads are always cyclopic. By contrast, co-injection of WIF-1 and chordin promotes complete secondary axes and no cyclopic eyes. The WIF domain alone is able to synergize with chordin to give secondary axes, but the heads are always cyclopic, suggesting that the epidermal growth factor-like repeats are necessary for full activity of WIF-1 *(92)*.

Cerberus

As discussed above, cerberus is a multivalent inhibitor that can block BMP, Wnt, Nodal, and Activin signaling. Cerberus directly binds to Xwnt-8, inhibiting its interaction with the Fz receptors. It is expressed in the *Xenopus* Spemann's organizer and is thought to have a role in head induction, a process inhibited by ectopic Xwnt-8 signaling in the gastrula dorsal mesoderm *(93)*.

Dickkopf

Dickkopf (Dkk-1) encodes a member of a novel protein family of secreted Wnt antagonists. Dkk-1 is expressed in the anterior mesentoderm and is proposed to function in head induction *(94)*. Dickkopf's mode of antagonism is different than previously described antagonistic proteins. Dkk-1 antagonizes Wnt signaling by binding to and inactivating the Wnt co-receptor LRP (arrow in *Drosophila*; refs. *95–98*) but does not directly bind to Wnt. Dkk regulates coreceptor availability rather than ligand availability. It has recently been demonstrated that the membrane-anchored molecule Kremen binds to Dkk and triggers internalization and clearing of the Dkk-LRP complex from the cell surface *(99)*. This renders Wnt unable to activate the intracellular pathway necessary for target gene expression. It remains to be determined how Kremen triggers internalization of the Dkk-LRP complex.

Activity Regulation by HSPGs

HSPGs are large macromolecules found abundantly on the cell surface that modulate the function of intracellular signaling molecules in many ways *(100)*. BMPs, Wnts, and Hh have been shown to interact with components of the ECM, such as HSPGs, and it is becoming clear that these interactions play an important role in modulating the levels, facilitating the movement, and/or acting as coreceptors for these ligands *(101)*.

BMP

In *Drosophila*, genetic analysis of a mutation in the glypican gene *dally* (division abnormally delayed) has implicated this protein in both Wg (discussed below) and Dpp signaling *(102,103)*. Reducing Dpp levels in a *dally* mutant background enhances defects in the eye, antenna and genitalia, and overexpression of Dpp can rescue the defects in these tissues *(104)*. Interestingly, although these genetic interactions indicate that Dally regulates Dpp activity *(103)*, the requirement for Dally in Dpp signaling appears to be restricted to the imaginal disks.

Several studies on mouse *glypican-3* (*gpc-3*) knockouts have provided evidence that BMP/HSPG interactions are important in mouse embryogenesis. When *gpc-3*-deficient animals are mated to BMP-4 haploinsufficient mice, the offspring display a high penetrance of postaxial polydactyly and rib malformations not seen in either parent strain *(105)*. Additional studies show that Gpc-3 modulates BMP-7 activity during embryogenic kidney morphogenesis *(106)*.

Work in Xenopus has identified a basic core of amino acids in the N-terminal region of BMP-4 necessary for BMP binding to HSPGs *(107)*. Mutating these three amino acids does not alter receptor binding or induction of target genes but does increase the effective range of BMP signaling, indicating that HSPGs restrict the diffusion of BMPs in vivo. Together, these results demonstrate that HSPGs are important regulators of BMP function and signaling range during both *Drosophila* and vertebrate development.

Wnt/Wg

Genetic studies in *Drosophila* confirm a role for HSPGs in Wg signaling. *Sugarless* (*sgl/kiwi*) encodes an uridine diphosphate (UDP)-glucuronate involved in the biosynthesis of heparin, heparan sulfate (HS), chondroitin sulfate, and hyaluronic acid. Mutations of *sgl* demonstrate a noncell autonomous defect in Wg-receiving cells *(102,108)*, which is mediated by loss of HS. Exogenous HS can rescue *sgl* mutants whereas overexpression of HS in wild-type embryos gives rise to excess Wg signaling *(102)*. Wg signaling is also impaired in *sulfateless* (*slf*) mutants, which lack an enzyme involved in the modification of HS. Together, these studies suggest that proteoglycans and specifically HSPGs interact with Wg in receiving cells either to stabilize the ligand, limit its diffusion, increase the effective local concentration of the ligand *(102)*, or to act as a low-affinity co-receptor *(108)*.

As discussed above, Dally is a GPI-linked glypican that is modified by Sfl. Dally protein is expressed in the same cells as the Wg receptor, Dfz2 where it may act as a co-receptor with Dfz2 to generate a high-affinity binding site for Wg *(103,109)*.

A second glypican molecule involved in reception of Wg signaling is Dally-like (Dly). Overexpression of Dly leads to an accumulation of extracellular Wg and generates a *wg* phenotype. This suggests Dly acts to sequester Wg and acts as an antagonist, preventing access to or activation of Dfz2 *(110)*. In contrast to the apical localization of Wg mRNA, association of Wg with glycosylphosphatidylinositol (GPI)-linked HSPG targets it to the basolateral surface of cells *(111)*, contributing to the posterior spread of Wg signaling.

QSulf1, a sulfatase family member, is another genetically linked enzyme in the Wg pathway *(112)* necessary for the degradation of HSPGs *(113)*. Disruption of *QSulf1* specifically inhibits expression of *MyoD*, a Wnt-responsive gene, suggesting that breakdown of HSPGs is integral to Wnt signaling. In transient transfection assays, addition of QSulf1 enhances Wnt signaling, whereas addition of heparin or chlorate antagonizes QSulf1, abrogating Wnt signaling *(112)*. One explanation for how Qsulf1 alters Wnt signaling is that QSulf1 desulfates HS to locally release Wnt-bound HSPG, enabling the ligand to bind its cognate receptor and initiate signaling.

Hh

Genetic evidence that HSPGs are essential for trafficking of Hh was provided by the identification of *tout velu* (*ttv*) as a gene that is required for movement of Hh-Np, but not Hh-N, in *Drosophila (114, 115). Ttv* is a homolog of the human EXT genes that were identified through their association with the bone disorder multiple exostoses *(116)*. These genes encode enzymes essential for heparan sulfate glycosaminoglycan biosynthesis *(117)*. Glycosaminoglycan have also been shown to be important for movement of vertebrate Hh away from its source *(118)*. Several models have been proposed for the role of HSPGs in Hh-Np movement or receptor binding. It is possible, for example, that association of Hh-Np, but not Hh-N, with HSPGs increases its local concentration, thereby enabling it to bind to and be sequestered by Ptc. Alternatively, or in addition, binding to a specific class of HSPGs, such as the GPI-linked glypicans, might enable transport of Hh from cell to cell directly *(119)* or via transcytosis *(120)* as has been observed for other GPI-linked proteins. Association with glypicans might also function to promote localization of Hh-Np to lipid raft microdomains within the membrane through which transport can occur. Rafts are microdomains rich in cholesterol, sphingolipids, and GPI-anchored proteins and Hh-Np is associated with this membrane fraction, either by virtue of its sterol modification alone, or perhaps by association with a glypican molecule *(121)*.

REGULATION OF RECEPTOR ACTIVATION: FEEDBACK LOOPS

Research in recent years has shown that the BMP-, Wnt-, and Hh-signaling pathways are often subjected to regulation by autofeedback loops in addition to the action of extracellular regulators. Most of these feedback loops consist of transcriptional targets of the pathways that once activated turn off or downregulate BMP, Wnt, or Hh activity by interfering with future signaling events. Intracellular targets, such as inhibitory SMADs, which block intracellular events in the BMP pathway, are not discussed, although these are an important component of feedback loops that are further described in several recent reviews *(8–10)*. Instead, we highlight feedback loops that alter receptor activation or accessibility.

BMP Feedback Loops

BAMBI

BMP and activin membrane-bound inhibitor) (Bambi; ref. *122*) is a transmembrane protein related to TGF-β-family type I receptors that lacks an intracellular kinase domain. In all species examined, embryonic expression of Bambi overlaps that of BMPs and is induced by BMP ligands. Bambi acts as a pseudoreceptor by intercalating in the TGF-β complex and disrupting receptor signaling, thus functioning as a naturally occurring dominant mutant of BMP signaling.

Tkv

In the developing wing disk of *Drosophila*, Dpp negatively regulates expression of its own type I receptor thickveins (Tkv; ref. *123*). This results in Tkv levels being lowest in Dpp-expressing cells and highest in cells furthest from the source of Dpp *(123,124)*. Low levels of Tkv enable Dpp to spread over long distances, in part generating the Dpp morphogen gradient. High levels of Tkv presumably limit the spread of Dpp. Hh also represses *tkv* expression in dpp-expressing cells *(125)*, adding an additional level of regulation.

Noggin

Noggin expression in chondrocyte and osteoblast cultures is increased by BMP signaling and noggin in turn abolishes the bioactivity of BMPs (*see* Regulation of Receptor Activation: Feedback Loops section and refs. *126,127)*. This suggests that noggin may participate in a BMP-negative feedback loop.

Wnt Feedback Loops

Binding of Wg to its receptor, Dfz2, has been shown to stabilize Wg in the wing imaginal disk *(128)*. This stabilization allows Wg to diffuse further from its source at the dorsoventral boundary of the imaginal disk. Wg signaling represses *dfz2* transcription, resulting in *dfz2* expression being low near secreting cells and increasing distally. This sets up an inverted gradient of *wg/dfz2* expression, which promotes ligand stability at a distance *(129)*. Conversely, early in embryogenesis, overexpression of Dfz2 acts to restrict distribution of Wg, suggesting the receptor can also act to sequester ligand *(87)*.

Hedgehog Feedback Loops

ptc *Upregulation*

The *ptc* gene is a transcriptional target of the Hh-signaling pathway. In *Drosophila* and mouse, *ptc* upregulation in response to Hh signaling is responsible for the sequestration of Hh and restriction of Hh movement *(130,131)*. Hh upregulation of ptc is a self-limiting mechanism by which Hh attenuates its own movement through responsive tissues. In addition, high levels of Ptc block the intrinsic activity of Smo. As discussed above, Ptc-mediated sequestration of Hh is dependent on cholesterol modification of Hh.

HIP

Hedgehog-interacting protein (HIP) is a membrane glycoprotein that binds to all three mammalian Hh proteins with an affinity similar to Ptc *(132)*. HIP was the only protein identified in an expression screen for Hh-interacting proteins that promoted cell surface binding of Hh. Binding of Hh to HIP most likely regulates the availability of ligand, resulting in signal attenuation *(10)*. An example of HIP-negative regulation of Hh signaling is seen in cartilage where Indian hedgehog (Ihh) controls growth, and overexpression of HIP leads to a shortened skeleton similar to that observed in *ihh* knockout mice *(132)*. *Hip*, like *ptc*, is a transcriptional target of Hh signaling. HIP expression is induced by ectopic Hh expression and is absent in Hh-responsive cells in Hh mutants. Interestingly, no HIP othologs have been identified in *Drosophila*, providing a possible molecular mechanism to explain the different actions of Hh in the mouse vs the fly.

CONCLUSION

mRNA expression patterns alone do not describe the activities and interactions of BMPs, Wnt, and Hh as mediators of many fundamental processes in embryonic development. As we have described, these proteins are regulated at multiple levels beyond transcription. They are regulated posttranslationally via covalent modifications, proteolytic processing, and regulated secretion; within the extracellular space by secreted binding proteins and HSPGs; and via autoregulartory feedback loops. These modifications and interactions result in a complex pattern of ligand activity that cannot be achieved by transcriptional regulation alone.

Although we have tried to highlight some of the modes of regulating the activity of BMP, Wnt, and Hh signaling, there has been a large amount of recent work on how ligands move from cell to cell. Passive diffusion, long thought to be the way morphogen gradients were generated, is now viewed as only one of a handful of ways that a tissue/organism traffics its morphogens. Movement by carrier molecules, endocytosis, argosomes (vesicle-mediated transport), transcytosis (sequential endocytosis and exocytosis), and cytonemes (threads of cytoplasm connecting distant cells) are additional mechanisms used to generate morphogens gradients (for recent reviews, *see* refs. *133–136*). It is becoming apparent that depending on the time in development the tissue, and even the organism, many different tools can be used establish the necessary distribution of particular morphogens. Future studies will likely show that differently modified forms of the ligands have different affinities for antagonistic proteins and HSPG molecules and that these associations in turn regulate how, when, and where the ligand is transported. Although many of the specifics of the BMP, Wnt, and Hh pathways have been worked out, understanding how these pathways (and others) are integrated to form complex organisms remains a critical problem in developmental biology.

REFERENCES

1. Wozney, J. M., Rosen, V., Celeste, A., et al. (1988) Novel regulators of bone formation: molecular clones and activities. *Science* **242,** 1528–1534.
2. Nusse, R. and Varmus, H. E. (1982) Many tumors induced by the mouse mammary tumor virus contain a provirus integrated in the same region of the host genome. *Cell* **31,** 99–109.
3. Rijsewijk, F., Schuermann, M., Wagenaar, E., et al. (1987) The Drosophila homolog of the mouse mammary oncogene int-1 is identical to the segment polarity gene wingless. *Cell* **50,** 649–657.
4. Nusslein-Volhard, C. and Wieschaus, E. (1980) Mutations affecting segment number and polarity in Drosophila. *Nature* **287,** 795–801.
5. Neumann, C. and Cohen, S. (1997) Morphogens and pattern formation. *Bioessays* **19,** 721–729.
6. Gonzalez, F., Swales, L., Bejsovec, A., et al. (1991) Secretion and movement of wingless protein in the epidermis of the Drosophila embryo. *Mech. Dev.* **35,** 43–54.
7. Johnson, R. L. and Tabin, C. (1995) The long and short of hedgehog signaling. *Cell* **81,** 313–316.
8. Nakayama, T., Cui, Y., and Christian, J. L. (2000) Regulation of BMP/Dpp signaling during embryonic development. *Cell Mol. Life Sci.* **57,** 943–956.
9. Huelsken, J. and Birchmeier, W. (2001) New aspects of Wnt signaling pathways in higher vertebrates. *Curr. Opin. Genet. Dev.* **11,** 547–553.
10. Ingham, W. and McMahon, A. (2001) Hedgehog signaling in animal development: paradigms and principles. *Genes Dev.* **15,** 3059–3087.
11. Hammonds, R. G. Jr., Schwall, R., Dudley, A., et al. (1991) Bone-inducing activity of mature BMP-2b produced from a hybrid BMP-2a/2b precursor. *Mol. Endocrinol* **5,** 149–155.
12. Massague, J. (1990) The transforming growth factor-beta family. *Annu. Rev. Cell Biol.* **6,** 597–641.
13. Steiner, D. F. (1998) The proprotein convertases. *Curr. Opin. Chem. Biol.* **2,** 31–39.
14. Cui, Y., Jean, F., Thomas, G., et al. (1998) BMP-4 is proteolytically activated by furin and/or PC6 during vertebrate embryonic development. *EMBO J.* **17,** 4735–4743.
15. Cui, Y., Hackenmiller, R., Berg, L., et al. (2001) The activity and signaling range of mature BMP-4 is regulated by sequential cleavage at two sites within the prodomain of the precursor. *Genes Dev.* **15,** 2797–2802.
16. Constam, D. B. and Robertson, E. J. (1999) Regulation of bone morphogenetic protein activity by pro domains and proprotein convertases. *J. Cell Biol.* **144,** 139–149.
17. Constam, D. B. and Robertson, E. J. (2000) SPC4/PACE4 regulates a TGFbeta signaling network during axis formation. *Genes Dev.* **14,** 1146–1155.
18. Roebroek, A. J., Umans, L., Pauli, I. G., et al. (1998) Failure of ventral closure and axial rotation in embryos lacking the proprotein convertase Furin. *Development* **125,** 4863–4876.
19. Gray, A. M. and Mason, A. J. (1990) Requirement for activin A and transforming growth factor—beta 1 pro-regions in homodimer assembly. *Science* **247,** 1328–1330.
20. Shinde, U. and Inouye, M. (2000) Intramolecular chaperones: polypeptide extensions that modulate protein folding. *Semin. Cell Dev. Biol.* **11,** 35–44.
21. Kessler, D. S. and Melton, D. A. (1995) Induction of dorsal mesoderm by soluble, mature Vg1 protein. *Development* **121,** 2155–2164.
22. Jones, C. M., Armes, N., and Smith, J. C. (1996) Signalling by TGF-beta family members: short-range effects of Xnr-2 and BMP-4 contrast with the long-range effects of activin. *Curr. Biol.* **6,** 1468–1475.
23. Hawley, S. H., et al. (1995) Disruption of BMP signals in embryonic Xenopus ectoderm leads to direct neural induction. *Genes Dev.* **9,** 2923–2935.
24. Mason, A. J., Farnworth, G., and Sullivan, J. (1996) Characterization and determination of the biological activities of noncleavable high molecular weight forms of inhibin A and activin A. *Mol. Endocrinol* **10,** 1055–1065.
25. Ulloa, L. and Tabibzadeh, S. (2001) Lefty inhibits receptor-regulated Smad phosphorylation induced by the activated transforming growth factor-beta receptor. *J. Biol. Chem.* **276,** 21397–2404.
26. Eimon, M. and Harland, R. M. (2002) Effects of heterodimerization and proteolytic processing on Derriere and Nodal activity: implications for mesoderm induction in Xenopus. *Development* **129,** 3089–3103.
27. Khalil, N. (2001) Post translational activation of latent transforming growth factor beta (L-TGF-beta): clinical implications. *Histol. Histopathol.* **16,** 541–551.
28. Jones, W. K., Richmond, E. A., White, K., et al. (1994) Osteogenic protein-1 (OP-1) expression and processing in Chinese hamster ovary cells: isolation of a soluble complex containing the mature and pro-domains of OP-1. *Growth Factors* **11,** 215–225.
29. Arteaga-Solis, E., Gayraud, B., Lee, S. Y., et al. (2001) Regulation of limb patterning by extracellular microfibrils. *J. Cell Biol.* **154,** 275–281.
30. Aono, A., Hazama, M., Notoya, K., et al. (1995) Potent ectopic bone-inducing activity of bone morphogenetic protein-4/7 heterodimer. *Biochem. Biophys. Res. Commun.* **210,** 670–677.

31. Hazama, M., Aono, A., Ueno, N., et al. (1995) Efficient expression of a heterodimer of bone morphogenetic protein subunits using a baculo-virus expression system. *Biochem. Biophys. Res. Commun.* **209,** 859–866.
32. Suzuki, A., Kaneko, E., Maeda, J., et al. (1997) Mesoderm induction by BMP-4 and -7 heterodimers. *Biochem. Biophys. Res. Commun.* **232,** 153–156.
33. Nishimatsu, S. and Thomsen, G. H. (1998) Ventral mesoderm induction and patterning by bone morphogenetic protein heterodimers in Xenopus embryos. *Mech. Dev.* **74,** 75–88.
34. Yeo, C. and Whitman, M. (2001) Nodal signals to Smads through Cripto-dependent and Cripto-independent mechanisms. *Mol. Cell* **7,** 949–957.
35. Kitajewski, J., Mason, J. O., and Varmus, H. E. (1992) Interaction of Wnt-1 proteins with the binding protein Bi. *Mol. Cell Biol.* **12,** 784–790.
36. Kadowaki, T., Wilder, E., Klingensmith, J., et al. (1996) The segment polarity gene porcupine encodes a putative multitransmembrane protein involved in Wingless processing. *Genes Dev.* **10,** 3116–3128.
37. Tanaka, K., Okabayashi, K., Asashima, M., et al. (2000) The evolutionarily conserved porcupine gene family is involved in the processing of the Wnt family. *Eur. J. Biochem.* **267,** 4300–4311.
38. Tanaka, K., Kitagawa, Y., and Kadowaki, T. (2002) Drosophila segment polarity gene product porcupine stimulates the posttranslational N-glycosylation of wingless in the endoplasmic reticulum. *J. Biol. Chem.* **277,** 12816–12823.
39. Bumcrot, D. A., Takada, R., and McMahon, A. (1995) Proteolytic processing yields two secreted forms of sonic hedgehog. *Mol. Cell Biol.* **15,** 2294–2303.
40. Lee, J. J., Ekker, S. C., von Kessler, D. P., et al. (1994) Autoproteolysis in hedgehog protein biogenesis. *Science* **266,** 1528–1537.
41. Porter, J. A., von Kessler, D. P., Ekker, S. C., et al. (1995) The product of hedgehog autoproteolytic cleavage active in local and long-range signalling. *Nature* **374,** 363–366.
42. Porter, J. A., Young, K. E., and Beachy, A. (1996) Cholesterol modification of hedgehog signaling proteins in animal development. *Science* **274,** 255–259.
43. Osborne, T. F. and Rosenfeld, J. M. (1998) Related membrane domains in proteins of sterol sensing and cell signaling provide a glimpse of treasures still buried within the dynamic realm of intracellular metabolic regulation. *Curr. Opin. Lipidol.* **9,** 137–140.
44. Marti, E., Bumcrot, D. A., Takada, R., et al. (1995) Requirement of 19K form of Sonic hedgehog for induction of distinct ventral cell types in CNS explants. *Nature* **375,** 322–325.
45. Pepinsky, R. B., Zeng, C., Wen, D., et al. (1998) Identification of a palmitic acid-modified form of human Sonic hedgehog. *J. Biol. Chem.* **273,** 14037–14045.
46. Burke, R., Nellen, D., Bellotto, M., et al. (1999) Dispatched, a novel sterol-sensing domain protein dedicated to the release of cholesterol-modified hedgehog from signaling cells. *Cell* **99,** 803–815.
47. Amanai, K. and Jiang, J. (2001) Distinct roles of central missing and dispatched in sending the Hedgehog signal. *Development* **128,** 5119–5127.
48. Lewis, M., Dunn, M. P., McMahon, J. A., et al. (2001) Cholesterol modification of sonic hedgehog is required for long-range signaling activity and effective modulation of signaling by Ptc1. *Cell* **105,** 599–612.
49. Chamoun, Z., Mann, R. K., Nellen, D., et al. (2001) Skinny hedgehog, an acyltransferase required for palmitoylation and activity of the hedgehog signal. *Science* **293,** 2080–2084.
50. Lee, J. D. and Treisman, J. E. (2001) Sightless has homology to transmembrane acyltransferases and is required to generate active Hedgehog protein. *Curr. Biol.* **11,** 1147–1152.
51. Micchelli, C. A., The, I., Selva, E., et al. (2002) Rasp, a putative transmembrane acyltransferase, is required for Hedgehog signaling. *Development* **129,** 843–851.
52. Lee, J. D., Kraus, P., Gaiano, N., et al. (2001) An acylatable residue of Hedgehog is differentially required in Drosophila and mouse limb development. *Dev. Biol.* **233,** 122–136.
53. Kohtz, J. D., Lee, H. Y., Gaiano, N., et al. (2001) N-terminal fatty-acylation of sonic hedgehog enhances the induction of rodent ventral forebrain neurons. *Development* **128,** 2351–2363.
54. Taylor, F. R., Wen, D., Garber, E. A., et al. (2001) Enhanced potency of human Sonic hedgehog by hydrophobic modification. *Biochemistry* **40,** 4359–4371.
55. Zimmerman, L. B., De Jesus-Escobar, J. M., and Harland, R. M. (1996) The Spemann organizer signal noggin binds and inactivates bone morphogenetic protein 4. *Cell* **86,** 599–606.
56. Chang, C. and Hemmati-Brivanlou, A. (1998) Neural crest induction by Xwnt7B in Xenopus. *Dev. Biol.* **194,** 129–134.
57. Brunet, L. J., McMahon, J. A., McMahon, A. P., et al. (1998) Noggin, cartilage morphogenesis, and joint formation in the mammalian skeleton. *Science* **280,** 1455–1457.
58. Gong, Y., Krakow, D., Marcelino, J., et al. (1999) Heterozygous mutations in the gene encoding noggin affect human joint morphogenesis. *Nat. Genet.* **21,** 302–304.
59. Piccolo, S., Sasai, Y., Lu, B., et al. (1996) Dorsoventral patterning in Xenopus: inhibition of ventral signals by direct binding of chordin to BMP-4. *Cell* **86,** 589–598.
60. Piccolo, S., Agius, E., Lu, B., et al. (1997), Cleavage of chordin by Xolloid metalloprotease suggests a role for proteolytic processing in the regulation of Spemann organizer activity. *Cell* **91,** 407–416.
61. Marques, G., Musacchio, M., Shimell, M. J., et al. (1997) Production of a DPP activity gradient in the early Drosophila embryo through the opposing actions of the SOG and TLD proteins. *Cell* **91,** 417–426.
62. Larrain, J., Bachiller, D., Lu, B., et al. (2000) BMP-binding modules in chordin: a model for signalling regulation in the extracellular space. *Development* **127,** 821–830.

63. Blader, P, Rastegar, S., Fischer, N., et al. (1997) Cleavage of the BMP-4 antagonist chordin by zebrafish tolloid. *Science* **278,** 1937–1940.
64. Ashe, H. L. and Levine, M. (1999) Local inhibition and long-range enhancement of Dpp signal transduction by Sog [see comments]. *Nature* **398,** 427–431.
65. Scott, I. C., Blitz, I. L., Pappano, W. N., et al. (2001) Homologues of Twisted gastrulation are extracellular cofactors in antagonism of BMP signalling. *Nature* **410,** 475–478.
66. Ross, J. J., Shimmi, O., Vilmos, P., et al. (2001) Twisted gastrulation is a conserved extracellular BMP antagonist. *Nature* **410,** 479–483.
67. Chang, C., Holtzman, D. A., Chau, S., et al. (2001) Twisted gastrulation can function as a BMP antagonist. *Nature* **410,** 483–487.
68. Ray, R. and Wharton, K. A. (2001) Twisted perspective: new insights into extracellular modulation of BMP signaling during development. *Cell* **104,** 801–804.
69. Yu, K., Srinivasan, S., Shimmi, O., et al. (2000) Processing of the Drosophila Sog protein creates a novel BMP inhibitory activity. *Development* **127,** 2143–2154.
70. Oelgeschlager, M., Larrain, J., Geissert, D., et al. (2000) The evolutionarily conserved BMP-binding protein Twisted gastrulation promotes BMP signalling. *Nature* **405,** 757–763.
71. Harland, R. M. (2001) Developmental biology. A twist on embryonic signalling. *Nature* **410,** 423–424.
72. de Winter, J., ten Dijke, P., de Vries, C. J., et al. (1996) Follistatins neutralize activin bioactivity by inhibition of activin binding to its type II receptors. *Mol. Cell Endocrinol.* **116,** 105–114.
73. Iemura S, Y. T., Takagi, C., Uchiyama, H., Natsume, T., Shimasaki, S., Sugino, H., et al. (1998) Direct binding of follistatin to a complex of bone-morphogenetic protein and its receptor inhibits ventral and epidermal cell fates in early Xenopus embryo. *Proc. Natl. Acad. Sci. USA* **95,** 9337–9342.
74. Hemmati-Brivanlou, A., Kelly, O. G., and Melton, D. A. (1994) Follistatin, an antagonist of activin, is expressed in the Spemann organizer and displays direct neuralizing activity. *Cell* **77,** 283–295.
75. Fainsod, A., Deissler, K., Yelin, R., et al. (1997) The dorsalizing and neural inducing gene follistatin is an antagonist of BMP-4. *Mech. Dev.* **63,** 39–50.
76. Hsu, D.R., Economides, A. N., Wang, X., et al. (1998) The Xenopus dorsalizing factor Gremlin identifies a novel family of secreted proteins that antagonize BMP activities. *Mol. Cell* **1,** 673–683.
77. Piccolo, S., Agius, E., Leyns, L., et al. (1999) The head inducer Cerberus is a multifunctional antagonist of Nodal, BMP and Wnt signals. *Nature* **397,** 707–710.
78. Yokouchi, Y., Vogan, K. J., Pearse, R. V., 2nd, et al. (1999) Antagonistic signaling by Caronte, a novel Cerberus-related gene, establishes left-right asymmetric gene expression. *Cell* **98,** 573–583.
79. Ozaki, T. and Sakiyama, S. (1993) Molecular cloning and characterization of a cDNA showing negative regulation in v-src-transformed 3Y1 rat fibroblasts. *Proc. Natl. Acad. Sci. USA* **90,** 2593–2597.
80. Ozaki, T. and Sakiyama, S. (1994) Tumor-suppressive activity of N03 gene product in v-src-transformed rat 3Y1 fibroblasts. *Cancer Res.* **54,** 646–648.
81. Dionne, M. S., Skarnes, W. C., and Harland, R. M. (2001) Mutation and analysis of Dan, the founding member of the Dan family of transforming growth factor beta antagonists. *Mol. Cell Biol.* **21,** 636–643.
82. Bouwmeester, T., Kim, S., Sasai, Y., et al. (1996) Cerberus is a head-inducing secreted factor expressed in the anterior endoderm of Spemann's organizer. *Nature* **382,** 595–601.
83. Zuniga, A., Haramis, A. P., McMahon, A. P., et al. (1999) Signal relay by BMP antagonism controls the SHH/FGF4 feedback loop in vertebrate limb buds. *Nature* **401,** 598–602.
84. Wang, S., Krinks, M., Lin, K., et al. (1997) Frzb, a secreted protein expressed in the Spemann organizer, binds and inhibits Wnt-8. *Cell* **88,** 757–766.
85. Leyns, L., Bouwmeester, T., Kim, S. H., et al. (1997) Frzb-1 is a secreted antagonist of Wnt signaling expressed in the Spemann organizer. *Cell* **88,** 747–756.
86. Hoang, B., Moos, M., Jr., Vukicevic, S., et al. (1996) Primary structure and tissue distribution of FRZB, a novel protein related to Drosophila frizzled, suggest a role in skeletal morphogenesis. *J. Biol. Chem.* **271,** 26131–26137.
87. Reichsman, F., Smith, L., and Cumberledge, S. (1996) Glycosaminoglycans can modulate extracellular localization of the wingless protein and promote signal transduction. *J. Cell Biol.* **135,** 819–827.
88. Wang, S., Krinks, M., and Moos, M. Jr. (1997) Frzb-1, an antagonist of Wnt-1 and Wnt-8, does not block signaling by Wnts -3A, -5A, or -11. *Biochem. Biophys. Res. Commun.* **236,** 502–504.
89. Lin, K., Wang, S., Julius, M. A., et al. (1997) The cysteine-rich frizzled domain of Frzb-1 is required and sufficient for modulation of Wnt signaling. *Proc. Natl. Acad. Sci. USA* **94,** 11196–11200.
90. Bradley, L., Sun, B., Collins-Racie, L., et al. (2000) Different activities of the frizzled-related proteins frzb2 and sizzled2 during Xenopus anteroposterior patterning. *Dev. Biol.* **227,** 118–132.
91. Bafico, A., Gazit, A., Pramila, T., et al. (1999) Interaction of frizzled related protein (FRP) with Wnt ligands and the frizzled receptor suggests alternative mechanisms for FRP inhibition of Wnt signaling. *J. Biol. Chem.* **274,** 16180–16187.
92. Hsieh, J. C., Kodjabachian, L., Rebbert, M. L., et al. (1999) A new secreted protein that binds to Wnt proteins and inhibits their activities. *Nature* **398,** 431–436.
93. Christian, J. L. and Moon, R. T. (1993) Interactions between Xwnt-8 and Spemann organizer signaling pathways generate dorsoventral pattern in the embryonic mesoderm of Xenopus. *Genes Dev.* **7,** 13–28.
94. Glinka, A., Wu, W., Delius, H., et al. (1998) Dickkopf-1 is a member of a new family of secreted proteins and functions in head induction. *Nature* **391,** 357–362.

95. Wehrli, M., Dougan, S. T., Caldwell, K., et al. (2000) arrow encodes an LDL-receptor-related protein essential for Wingless signalling. *Nature* **407,** 527–530.
96. Mao, B., Wu, W., Li, Y., et al. (2001) LDL-receptor-related protein 6 is a receptor for Dickkopf proteins. *Nature* **411,** 321–325.
97. Semenov, M. V., Tamai, K., Brott, B. K., et al. (2001) Head inducer Dickkopf-1 is a ligand for Wnt coreceptor LRP6. *Curr. Biol.* **11,** 951–961.
98. Bafico, A., Liu, G., Yaniv, A., et al. (2001) Novel mechanism of Wnt signalling inhibition mediated by Dickkopf-1 interaction with LRP6/Arrow. *Nat. Cell Biol.* **3,** 683–686.
99. Mao, B., Wu, W., Davidson, G., et al. (2002) Kremen proteins are Dickkopf receptors that regulate Wnt/beta-catenin signalling. *Nature* **417,** 664–667.
100. Selleck, S. B. (1999) Overgrowth syndromes and the regulation of signaling complexes by proteoglycans. *Am. J. Hum. Genet.* **64,** 372–377.
101. Perrimon, N. and Bernfield, M. (2000) Specificities of heparan sulphate proteoglycans in developmental processes. *Nature* **404,** 725–728.
102. Binari, R. C., Staveley, B. E., Johnson, W.A., et al. (1997) Genetic evidence that heparin-like glycosaminoglycans are involved in wingless signaling. *Development* **124,** 2623–2632.
103. Tsuda, M., Kamimura, K., Nakato, H., et al. (1999) The cell-surface proteoglycan Dally regulates Wingless signalling in Drosophila. *Nature* **400,** 276–280.
104. Jackson, S. M., Nakato, H., Sugiura, M., et al. (1997) Dally, a Drosophila glypican, controls cellular responses to the TGF-beta-related morphogen, Dp. *Development* **124,** 4113–4120.
105. Paine-Saunders, S., Viviano, B. L., Zupicich, J., et al. (2000) glypican-3 controls cellular responses to Bmp4 in limb patterning and skeletal development. *Dev. Biol.* **225,** 179–187.
106. Grisaru, S., Cano-Gauci, D., Tee, J., et al. (2001) Glypican-3 modulates BMP- and FGF-mediated effects during renal branching morphogenesis. *Dev. Biol.* **231,** 31–46.
107. Ohkawara, B., Iemura, S., ten Dijke, P., et al. (2002) Action range of BMP is defined by its N-terminal basic amino acid core. *Curr. Biol.* **12,** 205–209.
108. Haerry, T. E., Heslip, T. R., Marsh, J. L., et al. (1997) Defects in glucuronate biosynthesis disrupt Wingless signaling in Drosophila. *Development* **124,** 3055–3064.
109. Lin, X. and Perrimon, N. (1999) Dally cooperates with Drosophila Frizzled 2 to transduce Wingless signalling. *Nature* **400,** 281–284.
110. Baeg, G. H., Lin, X., Khare, N., et al. (2001) Heparan sulfate proteoglycans are critical for the organization of the extracellular distribution of Wingless. *Development* **128,** 87–94.
111. Strigini, M. and Cohen, S. M. (2000) Wingless gradient formation in the Drosophila wing. *Curr. Biol.* **10,** 293–300.
112. Dhoot, G. K., Gustafsson, M. K., Ai, X., et al. (2001) Regulation of Wnt signaling and embryo patterning by an extracellular sulfatase. *Science* **293,** 1663–1666.
113. Robertson, D. A., Freeman, C., Morris, C. P., et al. (1992) A cDNA clone for human glucosamine-6-sulphatase reveals differences between arylsulphatases and non-arylsulphatases. *Biochem. J.* **288,** 539–544.
114. Bellaiche, Y., The, I., and Perrimon, N. (1998) Tout-velu is a Drosophila homologue of the putative tumour suppressor EXT-1 and is needed for Hh diffusion. *Nature* **394,** 85–88.
115. The, I., Bellaiche, Y., and Perrimon, N. (1999) Hedgehog movement is regulated through tout velu-dependent synthesis of a heparan sulfate proteoglycan. *Mol. Cell.* **4,** 633–639.
116. Stickens, D., Clines, G., Burbee, D., et al. (1996) The EXT2 multiple exostoses gene defines a family of putative tumour suppressor genes. *Nat. Genet.* **14,** 25–32.
117. Lind, T., Tufaro, F., McCormick, C., et al. (1998) The putative tumor suppressors EXT1 and EXT2 are glycosyltransferases required for the biosynthesis of heparan sulfate. *J. Biol. Chem.* **273,** 26265–26268.
118. Gritli-Linde, A., Lewis, P., McMahon, A. P., et al. (2001) The whereabouts of a morphogen: direct evidence for short- and graded long-range activity of hedgehog signaling peptides. *Dev. Biol.* **236,** 364–386.
119. Kooyman, D. L., Byrne, G. W., McClellan, S., et al. (1995) In vivo transfer of GPI-linked complement restriction factors from erythrocytes to the endothelium. *Science* **269,** 89–92.
120. Dierick, H. and Bejsovec, A. (1999) Cellular mechanisms of wingless/Wnt signal transduction. *Curr. Top. Dev. Biol.* **43,** 153–190.
121. Rietveld, A., Neutz, S., Simons, K., et al. (1999) Association of sterol- and glycosylphosphatidylinositol-linked proteins with Drosophila raft lipid microdomains. *J. Biol. Chem.* **274,** 12049–12054.
122. Onichtchouk, D., Chen, Y.-G., Dosch, R., et al. (1999) Silencing of TGF-β signalling by the pseudoreceptor BAMBI. *Nature* **401,** 480–485.
123. Lecuit, T. and Cohen, S. M. (1998) Dpp receptor levels contribute to shaping the Dpp morphogen gradient in the Drosophila wing imaginal disc. *Development* **125,** 4901–4907.
124. Haerry, T. E., Khalsa, O., O'Connor, M. B., et al. (1998) Synergistic signaling by two BMP ligands through the SAX and TKV receptors controls wing growth and patterning in Drosophila. *Development* **125,** 3977–3987.
125. Tanimoto, H., Itoh, S., ten Dijke, P., et al. (2000) Hedgehog creates a gradient of DPP activity in Drosophila wing imaginal discs. *Mol. Cell* **5,** 59–71.
126. Gazzerro, E., Gangji, V., and Canalis, E. (1998) Bone morphogenetic proteins induce the expression of noggin, which limits their activity in cultured rat osteoblasts. *J. Clin. Invest.* **102,** 2106–2114.
127. Kameda, T., Koike, C., Saitoh, K., et al. (1999) Developmental patterning in chondrocytic cultures by morphogenic gradients: BMP induces expression of indian hedgehog and noggin. *Genes Cells* **4,** 175–184.

128. Zhang, J. and Carthew, R. W. (1998) Interactions between Wingless and DFz2 during Drosophila wing development. *Development* **125,** 3075–3085.
129. Cadigan, K. M., Fish, M. P., Rulifson, E. J., et al. (1998) Wingless repression of Drosophila frizzled 2 expression shapes the Wingless morphogen gradient in the wing. *Cell* **93,** 767–77.
130. Chen, Y. and Struhl, G. (1996) Dual roles for patched in sequestering and transducing Hedgehog. *Cell* **87,** 553–563.
131. Briscoe, J., Chen, Y., Jessell, T. M., et al. (2001) A hedgehog-insensitive form of patched provides evidence for direct long-range morphogen activity of sonic hedgehog in the neural tube. *Mol. Cell* **7,** 1279–1291.
132. Chuang, T. and McMahon, A. (1999) Vertebrate Hedgehog signalling modulated by induction of a Hedgehog-binding protein. *Nature* **397,** 617–621.
133. Christian, J. L. (2002) Argosomes: intracellular transport vehicles for intercellular signals? *Sci. STKE* **2002,** E13.
134. Teleman, A. A., Strigini, M., and Cohen, S. M. (2001) Shaping morphogen gradients. *Cell* **105,** 559–562.
135. Seto, E. S., Bellen, H. J., and Lloyd, T. E. (2002) When cell biology meets development: endocytic regulation of signaling pathways. *Genes Devel.* **16,** 1314–1336.
136. Tabata, T. (2001) Genetics of morphogen gradients. *Nat. Rev.* **2,** 620–630.

9
FGF4 and Skeletal Morphogenesis

Valerie Ngo-Muller, Shaoguang Li, Scott A. Schaller, Manjong Han, Jennifer Farrington, Minoru Omi, Rosalie Anderson, and Ken Muneoka

INTRODUCTION

Of vertebrate organ systems, the developing limb has been especially well characterized. Embryological studies combined with molecular manipulations have yielded a wealth of information about the control of pattern formation during limb outgrowth. A number of key signaling pathways have been implicated in the control of numerous aspects of limb development, including the establishment of the early limb field, determination of limb identity, elongation of the limb bud, specification of digit pattern, and sculpting of the digits. Although there is clear evidence that specific signaling pathways that operate in the limb field and early limb bud control the specification of pattern, little is known about how these signals interface with the cell biology of limb development *(1)*. One instance where some progress has been made concerns the role of FGF4 signaling by the apical ectodermal ridge (AER) in the limb bud.

The AER is a developmentally transient ectodermal specialization at the distal tip of the limb bud, where it runs along the distal boundary separating the dorsal and ventral ectodermal surfaces. It is typified by closely grouped, pseudostratified columnar epithelial cells that are linked by gap junctions *(2)* and separated from underlying mesenchymal cells by a basement membrane *(3)*. The AER is indispensable for limb outgrowth *(4,5)* and achieves its function by maintaining underlying mesenchymal cells in an undifferentiated, proliferative state known collectively as the progress zone *(6)*. Pattern specification occurs within the progress zone, and its importance is indicated by the distally localized expression of a number of developmentally important genes, many of which are regulated by the AER. Among these are the 5' members of the *Hoxa* and *Hoxd* gene clusters, which play roles in the regional specification of the limb skeletal pattern (reviewed in Chapter 7). As the limb bud grows, cells leave the progress zone, and differentiation is initiated at proximal levels of the limb bud.

Limb patterning is most frequently related to the pattern of differentiated skeletal elements that can be described along its three primary axes: proximal–distal, anterior–posterior, and dorsal–ventral. The early skeletal pattern is useful for morphological studies because of clear anatomical differences between the various skeletal components that make up the proximal–distal axis. Additionally, the general organization of tissue types is highly conserved among tetrapod vertebrates, even though there is considerable diversity of final morphology *(7)*. The anterior–posterior limb pattern is assessed based on the digit sequence, and there is firm evidence that digit identity is controlled by the production of sonic hedgehog protein (SHH) by the zone of polarizing activity (ZPA) located in the posterior limb bud *(8)*. Digit identity is defined in the early limb bud long before the initiation of differentiation *(9)*,

From: *The Skeleton: Biochemical, Genetic, and Molecular Interactions in Development and Homeostasis*
Edited by: E. J. Massaro and J. M. Rogers © Humana Press Inc., Totowa, NJ

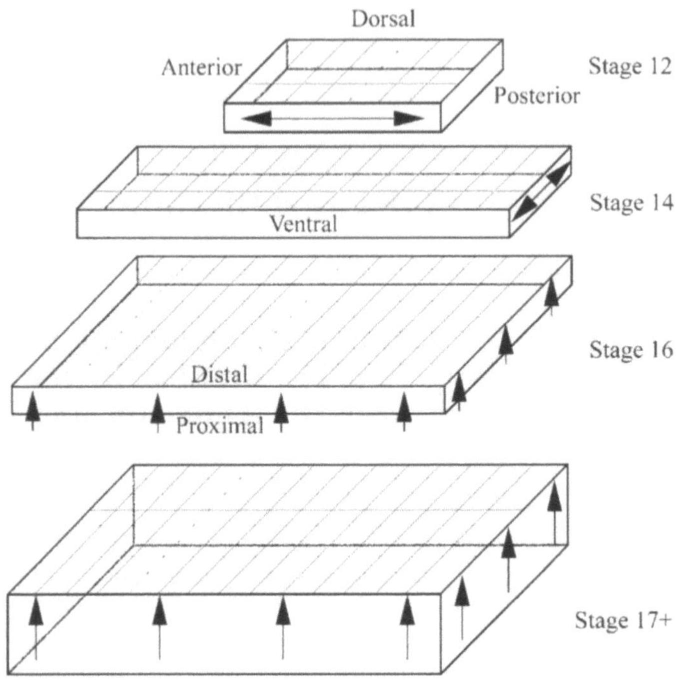

Fig. 1. Schematic illustration depicting changes in limb field size as determined by fate mapping studies. The limb field increases in size in a highly organized manner before the appearance of the limb bud. The size of the limb field changes in only the anterior–posterior dimension between stages 12 and 14; the dorsal–ventral and proximal–distal dimensions remain constant. Between stage 14 and 16, the expansion of the anterior–posterior dimension declines and the dorsal–ventral dimension increases in size. After stage 16, the proximal–distal dimension grows in a disproportionate manner in comparison with the other axes.

but it can be modified even at relatively late stages of limb outgrowth *(10)*. Thus, the developmental window for digit specification is open for a relatively long time. The limb skeleton is first established as a chondrogenic template that is later replaced by bone tissue during endochondrial ossification. In all vertebrates, the pattern of chondrogenesis occurs in a proximal to distal sequence.

The interface between the specification of cell fate in the progress zone and the actual differentiation of limb structures at more proximal levels represents an important area of limb development that is almost completely unexplored. In this review, we provide a model for skeletal morphogenesis that bridges this interface by linking the control of cell movements within the progress zone by the AER to the onset of chondrogenic differentiation at levels proximal to the progress zone.

Fibroblast Growth Factor (FGF) Signaling in the Limb Field

Before the appearance of a limb bud, a field of cells along the embryonic flank acquires the capacity to develop into a limb. In the chick embryo, the limb bud is apparent by stage 17, but explant studies indicate that the wing-forming region has the capacity to form limb structures by stage 12 *(11)*. The stage 12 prebud region has been mapped to an area adjacent to somites 15 to 20 and is approx 480 µm along the anterior–posterior axis, 200 µm along the dorsal–ventral axis, and 120 µm along the prospective proximal–distal axis. Fate mapping studies suggest that this prebud region expands in an organized manner (Fig. 1). During stages 12 to 14, the anterior–posterior dimension more than doubles whereas the dorsal–ventral and proximal–distal dimensions remain constant *(12)*. From stage 14, the anterior–posterior dimension remains relatively constant whereas the dorsal–ventral component increases *(13)*. The proximal–distal dimension expands as the limb bud forms between stages 16 and 17, and this expansion continues with bud elongation *(12)*. Thus, changes in the size of the pre-bud region and the limb bud itself indicates highly coordinated patterns of growth and expansion.

The FGF family of signaling proteins play an important role in setting up the prebud field. FGFs are intercellular signaling molecules that display a strong binding affinity for the extracellular matrix and signal via the FGF receptor (FGFR), a member of the tyrosine kinase superfamily of cell surface receptors *(14)*. The *Fgf* gene family is very large and includes at least seven members expressed during limb development, *Fgf2*, *Fgf4*, *Fgf8*, *Fgf9*, *Fgf10*, *Fgf17*, and *Fgf18 (15,16)*. Of these *Fgf10* and *Fgf18* are expressed only in mesenchymal cells, *Fgf4*, *Fgf8*, *Fgf9*, and *Fgf17* are expressed only in the ectoderm, specifically the AER, and *Fgf2* is expressed in both the ectoderm and the mesenchyme. The *FGFr* gene family includes four members, of which three, *FGFr1*, *FGFr2*, and *FGFr3*, are expressed during limb development. *FGFr1* is expressed predominately in undifferentiated mesenchyme *(17–19)*. There are two isoforms of *FGFr2* expressed in the limb bud; *FGFr2b* is expressed in the limb ectoderm, including the AER, and *FGFr2c* is expressed in the ectoderm and in prechondrogenic condensations *(18–20)*. *FGFr3* is expressed late in skeletogenesis and is associated with differentiating cartilage *(18,19)*.

Fgf10 loss-of-function studies in the mouse result in a limbless phenotype, indicating that FGF10 is required for limb outgrowth *(21,22)*. Similarly, interrupting the action of FGF10 either by overexpressing a soluble, dominant-negative derivative of the *FGFr2B* gene or by the deletion of the FGF binding domain of the *FGFr2* gene results in a limbless or distally truncated phenotype *(23,24)*. In the chick, *Fgf10* is expressed in lateral plate mesoderm at stage 12 when the limb field becomes tissue autonomous *(25)*. At this stage, *Fgf10* is expressed beyond the mapped boundary of the limb; however, it is downregulated in the surrounding tissue so that by stage 15 it is expressed only in the prebud mesoderm.

One downstream target of FGF10 signaling is the AER-specific gene *Fgf8*. *Fgf8* expression in the prebud ectoderm in first observed at stage 16, some 3 h after localization of *Fgf10* expression to the prelimb mesenchymal tissue *(26–30)*. The initial *Fgf8* expression domain encompasses a broad band of ectodermal cells that includes the future AER, and once the bud forms, *Fgf8* expression is exclusively restricted to the AER. Expression of *Fgf8* in the limb ectoderm is FGF10 dependent *(21,22)* and can be induced by ectopic FGF10 application *(25,31)*. FGF8 application in the limb bud induces an expansion of the *Fgf10* expression domain, thus suggesting a reciprocal regulatory loop between mesenchymal FGF10 and ectodermal FGF8 *(14,25)*. The absence of FGF8 during limb outgrowth results in relatively normal limb limbs that display reduced skeletal elements at all levels *(32,33)*. The absence of FGF8 in the limb bud results in the anterior expansion of the Fgf4 expression domain, thus suggesting that *Fgf4* expression in the AER is negatively regulated by FGF8.

Limb defects are not observed in loss of function studies targeting *Fgf2*, *Fgf4*, *Fgf9*, or *Fgf17* genes *(34–37)*; however, gain of function studies in which purified FGF proteins are delivered on slow-release microcarrier beads into the limb-forming region provide evidence that these factors play key roles in the regulation of limb outgrowth. In the chick, nonlimb, embryonic flank tissue (stages 13–17) responds to an ectopic source of FGFs by initially forming an ectopic limb bud that later develops into identifiable limb structures *(38,39)*. The ectopic limb is always of reverse handedness in comparison with the neighboring, endogenous forelimbs and hindlimbs, and the ectopic limb is generally a chimera of both tissues types *(40)*. A number of FGFs have been tested using this assay, including FGF1, FGF2, FGF4, FGF7, FGF8, and FGF10. Of these, only FGF7 failed to induce the formation of ectopic limb structures *(29,30,38,39)*. Ectopic limbs are generally induced by implants of microcarrier beads loaded with purified FGF protein, although implantation of cells expressing different *Fgfs* can induce a similar response *(39)*. Ectopic expression of *Fgf4* or *Fgf8* in flank cells through retroviral infection *(30,41)* or ubiquitous expression of *Fgf2* or *Fgf4* in transgenic models *(42,43)* do not result in ectopic limb formation, thus suggesting that the spatial distribution of FGF is important for this response.

CELL MIGRATION AND A DYNAMIC PROGRESS ZONE

In the chick, the transition between prebud stages to limb bud stages is marked by the lateral bulging of the limb mesenchyme to form the limb bud, a homogeneous population of mesenchymal cells covered by ectoderm. The AER is a prominent ectodermal structure that rims the distal tip of the limb bud in all amniote vertebrates. In the chick, the AER forms soon after the bud is visible, and in the mouse, the AER does not form until limb bud outgrowth is well underway *(44)*. The late appearance of the mouse AER as well as studies of the limbless mutation in the chick shows that initial formation of the limb bud is an AER-independent event *(45)*.

As with limb initiation, the dependency of mesenchymal outgrowth on the AER is known to be a function of FGF activity. Numerous studies have shown that outgrowth can proceed after AER removal in the presence of ectopically applied FGF; thus, FGF signaling is linked to the maintenance of the progress zone. Although this function can be provided for by either FGF2, FGF4, or FGF8 *(30,46–48)*, FGF8 is assumed to be physiologically relevant because it is expressed throughout the AER with no axial bias *(26,27)*. *Fgf2* is present in the dorsal ectoderm and peripheral mesenchyme in addition to the AER *(49,50)*, and Fgf4 transcripts are restricted to the posterior AER in the early limb bud *(51, 52)* but are expressed distally as bud outgrowth proceeds. Both the AER and ectopically applied FGF also induce distal outgrowth of amputated limb buds, thus indicating that FGF signaling is involved in the reformation of the progress zone associated with a regeneration response *(53–55)*.

The outgrowth-promoting properties of FGFs in the limb bud is contrasted by studies showing that ectopic FGF application in the presence of the AER has an inhibitory effect on limb outgrowth *(56,57)*. Studies with ectopic FGF2 bead implantation into the ZPA of an otherwise-normal chick limb bud inhibits limb outgrowth in a dose-dependent manner (Fig. 2A-E). This FGF2 response is position specific in that a similar response is not observed after ectopic application of FGF-2 into the anterior limb bud *(56,58)*. Outgrowth inhibition by FGF2 is associated with dramatic changes in limb bud shape and with the expansion and bifurcation of the *Shh* and *HoxD13* expression domains. Cell marking studies show that ectopic FGF-2 modifies the normal distalward movement of ZPA cells, but not anterior cells, during limb outgrowth. Thus, understanding the role of FGF2 signaling in the limb bud is complicated by the apparent paradoxical result that FGF2 promotes limb outgrowth but also inhibits limb outgrowth *(56)*. A similar set of paradoxical findings are known for both FGF4 and FGF8. Application of FGF4 to the limb bud after AER removal or bud amputation replaces AER function by inducing distal outgrowth *(47,55)*; however, application of FGF4 to a subdistal location of an otherwise-intact limb bud causes localized shortening of the limb bud and reductions in the length of skeletal elements, thus FGF4 inhibits bud outgrowth (Fig. 2F-H). As mentioned above, FGF8 application to the flank of the embryo results in the induction of supernumerary limbs from flank tissues; however, the inhibition of limb bud outgrowth is observed when FGF8 beads are implanted near the endogenous limb field *(30)*.

As a solution to these paradoxical effects of FGFs on limb formation, we have proposed that a major role of FGF signaling by the AER is to control patterns of cell movements important for morphogenesis and pattern formation *(1,57)*. In our in vivo studies, we have found that FGF4 acts as a potent and specific chemoattractive agent for mesenchymal cells of the limb bud (Fig. 3). Thus, an ectopic source of FGF4 can induce posterior limb bud cells to migrate in either an anterior or proximal direction. The in vivo migration response to FGF-4 is dose dependent both in the number of cells stimulated to migrate and the distance migrated. The AER was also found to be a potent chemoattractant, directing the migration of mesenchymal cells within 75 μm of the AER to make contact with the AER within a 24-h period and mesenchymal cells within at least 150 μm to migrate toward the AER. These studies indicate that FGF4 produced by the AER has a long-range chemoattractive function and regulates proximal–distal patterns of cell migration during limb outgrowth. In experiments that result in the inhibition of limb bud outgrowth, we propose that altering the normal migration of these cells results in dramatic and rapid changes in limb bud shape and alters morphogenesis

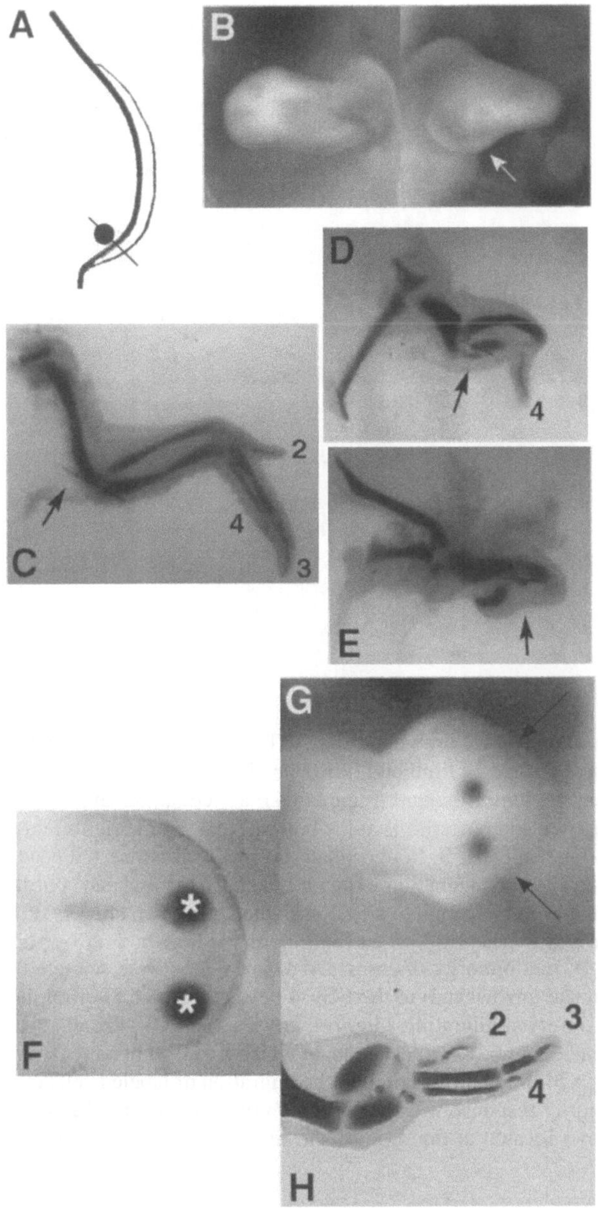

Fig. 2. FGF bead implantation studies demonstrate that FGF2 and FGF4 cause a dramatic alteration of limb bud shape, inhibiting outgrowth and modifying skeletal morphogenesis. Affi-Gel Blue beads containing FGF-2 implanted into the posterior mesenchyme of an otherwise normal wing bud (**A**) induced dramatic alterations of limb bud morphology 18 and 40 h (**B**) after implantation. Distal outgrowth (arrow) of the posterior region of the bud was inhibited as compared with the nonoperated bud on the same embryo (shown on the left). Skeletal morphogenesis is modified from control limbs (untreated bead implantation; **C**), displaying severe loss of digits (**D**) or truncation (**E**) . The arrows in C–E identify implanted beads. Taken from Li et al., 1996 *(56)*. FGF4 bead implantation also inhibits limb outgrowth and skeletal morphogenesis. Two FGF-4 beads (*) implanted into the subapical region of a stage 24 limb bud (**F**) locally inhibits outgrowth (arrows) 24 h later, giving the distal limb bud an "arrowhead" appearance. Skeletal preparation of the resulting limb shows a complete skeletal pattern in which proximal-distal elongation of many skeletal elements is inhibited. Taken from Li and Muneoka, 1999 *(57)*.

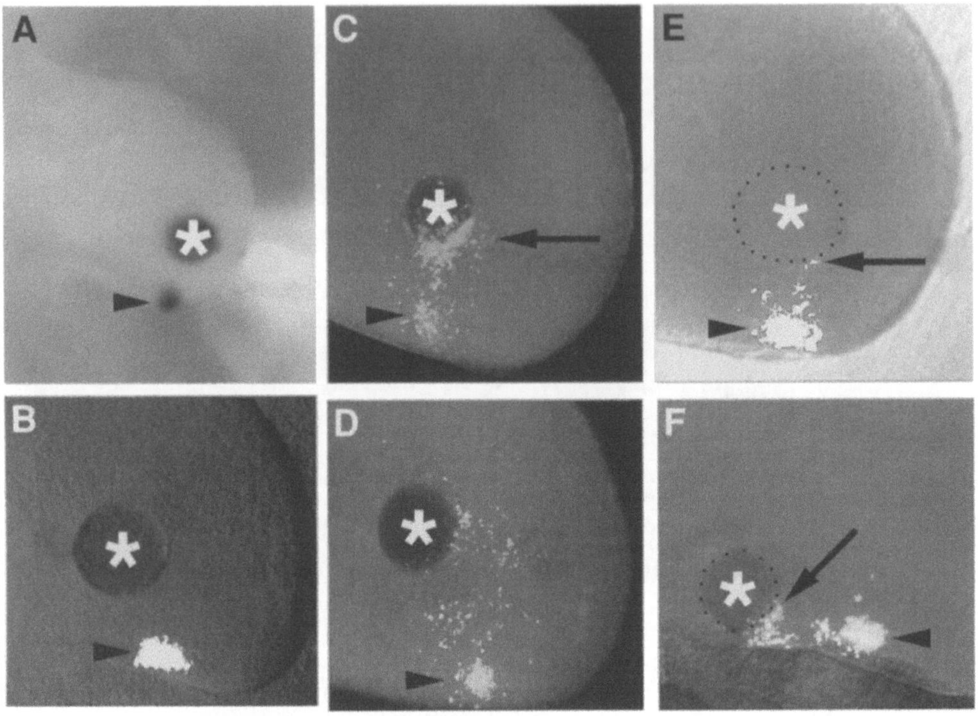

Fig. 3. FGF-4 is a chemoattractant for limb bud cells. **A**, The in vivo assay for migration consisted of DiI labeling of posterior–distal cells of a stage 24 limb bud (arrowhead) and implantation of a carrier bead (*) containing FGF-4 into the central–distal region of the bud. Figures B–F are computer overlays of whole-mount limb buds (dorsal view, distal is to the right and posterior is at the bottom) imaged in bright field and also with fluorescence microscopy to identify DiI-labeled cells. **B**, In phosphate-buffered saline-treated bead implantation control limb buds, DiI-labeled cells after 12 h of incubation expanded distally (arrowhead) but did not migrate toward the implanted bead (*). **C**, 12 h after implantation of a FGF-4-treated bead, two clusters of DiI-labeled cells are apparent: one associated with the FGF-4 bead (*) located centrally in the limb bud (arrow) and a second at the posterior injection site (arrowhead). **D**, In a minority of cases, DiI-labeled cells were scattered along a trail that extended from the posterior injection site (arrowhead) to the FGF-4 bead (*). **E**, 6 h after implantation of a FGF-4 treated bead, DiI-labeled cells are observed migrating anteriorly toward the FGF-4 bead (*) and a few cells can be seen making contact with the bead (arrow). **F**, Experiments in which a FGF-4 bead (*) was implanted proximal to the posterior injection site (stage 24 limb bud) resulted in the migration of labeled cells in a proximal direction. After 12 h of incubation, the majority response was the formation of two clusters of DiI-labeled cells: one associated with the FGF-4 bead (arrow) located at the base of the limb bud and a second at the posterior injection site (arrowhead).

of the skeleton *(57)*. FGF-4 has also been shown to direct the migration of nonlimb cells into the limb bud *(59)*. These findings indicate that the progress zone is a dynamic region of the limb bud where differential cell migration toward the AER results in continuous changes in the type of cell–cell interactions that can occur.

There are a number of implications important for our understanding of limb morphogenesis that result from this dynamic description of the progress zone. Based on direct measurements, we are able to estimate that migrating mesenchymal cells move at a maximum rate of about 50 μm/h (Li and Muneoka, unpublished data). At that rate, migrating cells encounter and move pass about five cells each hour, or one cell every 12 min; thus the nature of cell–cell interactions occurring within the limb bud will be influenced by these cell movements. Because only a subset of cells are migrating to populate the progress zone, it is reasonable to speculate that these cells are uniquely different from their nonmigrating counterparts. The recent demonstration that FGF1-induced migration in NBT-II rat bladder carcinoma cells in vitro is cell cycle dependent *(60)* raises the possibility that a similar cell cycle-specific response occurs in migrating limb bud cells. In the distal limb bud, all cells are proliferating; thus, it is possible that the response to FGF4 signaling could vary in a cell cycle-dependent manner. This possibility can account for our observation that cells that failed to migrate to the FGF4 bead were later found to migrate distally during limb outgrowth *(57)*. One consequence of a cell cycle–dependent migration response in the limb bud is that there will be a tendency for both migrating and nonmigrating cells to become synchronized, and reports of unexplainable regions of synchronized cells in the limb bud have been reported *(61)*. In addition, if G_1 is the migration-responsive phase, as has been shown for cultured cells, then the migration event would also cause an artificial depletion of S-phase cells (low apparent proliferation rate) immediately subjacent to the AER, and an artificial enrichment of S-phase cells (high apparent proliferation rate) at more proximal levels. This unusual and unexplained observation has been noted multiple times in studies characterizing the growth dynamics of the early limb bud *(62–64)*.

It is generally assumed that the AER provides a mitogenic signal that maintains cell proliferation within the progress zone. The AER and FGFs have been shown to be mitogenic for limb bud cells in vitro *(65–68)*; however, the endogenous patterns of cell proliferation in the limb bud do not support the conclusion that the AER produces a unique mitogenic signal. Mesenchymal cell proliferation in the early limb bud is initially uniform, and only after significant elongation and the onset of proximal chondrogenesis are gradients of proliferation evident *(69)*. In the chick limb bud, a distal-to-proximal gradient of cell proliferation is discernible by stage 24, but this gradient is associated with a proximal decline in mitotic rate associated with chondrogenesis in the center of the limb bud. At this same stage, the dorsal–ventral axis also displays a gradient of mesenchymal cell proliferation that is highest at the dorsal and ventral surfaces and lowest at the center of the limb bud where chondrogenesis is commencing. Importantly, growth differences are not apparent when comparing mesenchymal cells at the distal tip to cells at either the ventral or dorsal periphery at proximal levels. Thus, the mitotic gradients in the limb bud are linked to the onset of differentiation and not to specific mitogenic signaling associated with the AER. In support of this conclusion, after AER removal, the rate of ^{3}H-thymidine incorporation in subridge mesoderm is not changed, and the mitotic index is only transiently depressed *(70,71)*. Thus, there is no in vivo evidence for an AER-specific mitogenic signal. Because AER removal inhibits limb outgrowth without modifying cell proliferation rates, the data indicate that cell proliferation and the control of limb elongation by the AER are independent events. However, these data are consistent with a cell migration model in which limb bud outgrowth is driven by distalward cell movements and a relatively uniform rate of cell proliferation. We have proposed that the mitogenic effects of the AER and FGFs in vitro is an indirect consequence of FGF regulated cell migration; limb cell proliferation can be either stimulated or inhibited by FGFs depending on where they are directed to migrate *(57)*.

FGF SIGNALING AND BRANCHING MORPHOGENESIS

The elongating limb bud is characterized by an apical progress zone where pattern specification occurs, a subapical zone of proliferating undifferentiated cells, and a proximal differentiation zone where the onset of differentiation is associated with a decline in cell proliferation. The entire interface between the events important for the specification of patterns that are occurring in the progress zone and the events regulating the differentiation of limb structures is largely a mystery. In the limb, patterning studies have focused almost exclusively on the skeletal pattern, and therefore it is appropriate to target skeletal formation in considering the interact between patterning events and differentiation events. The onset of chondrogenic differentiation is marked by the condensation of mesenchymal cells. These condensations are characterized by an increased packing density, the associated expression of a number of surface proteins (e.g., fibronectin, tenascin, neural cell adhesion molecule, and N-cadherin), and a change in the extracellular matrix composition. Differential adhesion between cells plays a critical role in the initiation of mesenchymal condensations (*see* Chapter 1 by Tuan). Shubin and Alberch *(72)* have proposed that the morphogenesis of the vertebrate limb skeletal pattern occurs through a hierarchical sequence of *de novo* condensation followed by elongation, branching, and segmentation of chondrogenic rudiment. Thus, once initiated, condensations grow by cell recruitment and the skeletal pattern emerges as these condensations elongate, bifurcate, and segment. For example, the proximal long bones of the forelimb, that is, humerus, radius, and ulna, form as a result of elongation with a single bifurcation and segmentation event, and the short bones of the carpal/tarsal region form as a result of multiple bifurcation and segmentation events. Although the actual skeletal pattern is specified early in limb development, the pattern itself is laid down much later by regulating these morphogenetic processes.

The development of the limb skeleton and the evolution of diverse tetrapod limb morphologies can be explained as a result of controlling the spatial–temporal pattern of branching and segmentation events. The axis from which branching events arise is called the metapterygial axis, and it is generally accepted that this axis runs along the proximal–distal axis on the posterior side of the limb and curves from posterior to anterior in congruence with the digital arch *(72,73)*. Skeletal elements proximal to the digits arise from a segmentation/bifurcation mechanism and the digits themselves form by a bifurcation from the digital arch followed by elongation and segmentation without bifurcation. This model of skeletal morphogenesis proposes that alteration in skeletal pattern emerges as a result of physiochemical interactions that regulate whether or not a bifurcation response occurs. During skeletal morphogenesis, the expansion of the prechondrogenic domain reaches a critical mass and induces a mathematical bifurcation as has been proposed in mechanochemical models of skeletal pattern formation *(74)*. In the developing limb bud, these morphogenetic events are occurring at the interface between the undifferentiated subapical zone and the differentiation zone where mesenchyme condensation is initiated.

Ectopic application of FGF4 modifies patterns of cell migration that are associated with changes in limb bud shape and the pattern of chondrogenesis, and we have proposed that these events are causally linked. One obvious way that FGF4-modified cell migration patterns can result in changes in skeletal patterning is by modifying, either directly or indirectly, the processes controlling skeletal morphogenesis. During normal limb outgrowth, we have shown that the AER can influence the migration of cells in the subapical zone; thus, we propose that apical cell migration plays a role in controlling the pattern of skeletal morphogenesis (Fig. 4). One way that this might occur is if the interaction between chondrogenic cells is favored or enhanced by the distal emigration of nonchondrogenic cells toward the AER. Differential cell migration toward the AER in the dynamic progress zone model makes two clear predictions about limb outgrowth. First, undifferentiated cells in the progress zone and the subapical zone migrate distally and remain undifferentiated. Second, nonmigrating cells remain at a proximal location, enter the differentiation zone, and initiate chondrogenesis. One consequence of these differential cell movements is that there will be a reorganization of cells within the subapical zone. Thus, the emigration of distally migrating cells out of this zone results in a concentration of non-migrating cells. We propose that this reorganization of cells in conjunction with the expression of cell adhesion molecules facilitates adhesive interactions between prechondrogenic cells that trigger mesenchymal condensation. In this model, patterns of cell migration that is, in part, under the control of the AER provide the interface between the specification of skeletal pattern and the actual regulation of mesenchymal condensation associated with the establishment of the pattern. This model is supported by the results of fate mapping studies that show anterior or posterior shifts in the migration of mesenchymal cells that are associated with the branching of specific skeletal elements *(75)*.

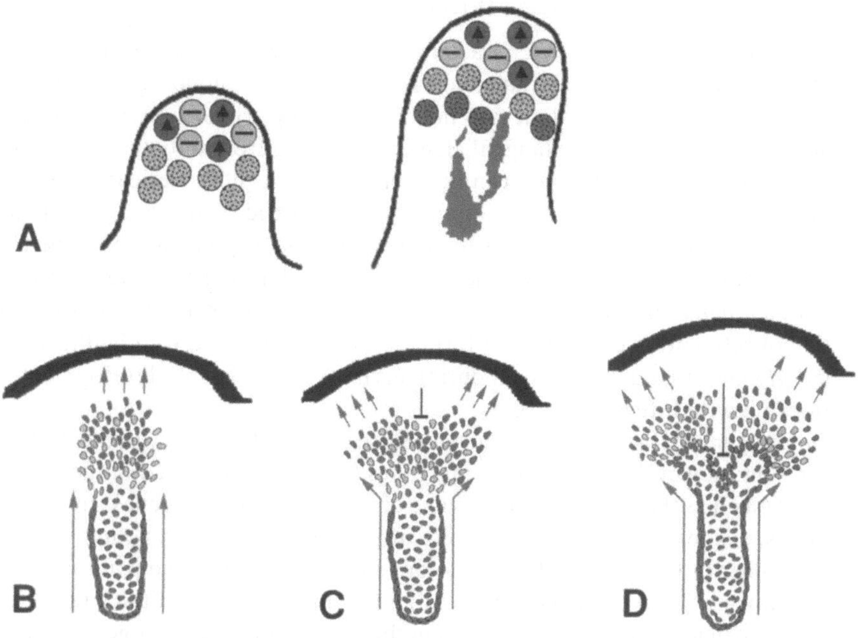

Fig. 4. The dynamic progress zone model for FGF4 directed cell migration and skeletogenesis. **A**, FGF-4 produced by the AER stimulates limb bud outgrowth by selectively directing cell migration distally (arrows), thereby maintaining a progress zone at the tip of the bud and enhancing interactions between nonmigrating (–) chondrogenic cells proximally. Light stippling indicates cells in the undifferentiation zone and dark stippling indicates cells in the differentiation zone. **B–D**, Skeletogenesis is influenced by distal cell migration as a result of emigration, promoting cell–cell interactions between chondrogenic cells. Modifying the direction of cell emigration can influence branching morphogenesis by modulating the size of the mesenchymal condensation.

The hypothesis that FGF signaling is controlling branching morphogenesis of the limb skeletal pattern is supported by studies in other developing organ systems that link the regulation of cell migration by FGF to the control of branching morphogenesis. Organs such as the lung, kidney, and salivary gland in vertebrates develop abnormally or fail to develop at all in mice carrying null mutations for either an FGF family member or an FGF receptor *(21–23,76–78)*. For example, lung development is inhibited in mice carrying a null mutation for *Fgf10 (21,22)* or *FgfR2 (76–78)*, the putative receptor for FGF10. In addition, in vitro experiments indicate that FGF10 functions as a chemotactic signal important for branching during lung formation *(79)*; thus, FGF10 in the developing lung and FGF4 in the developing limb appear to play similar roles. In *Drosophila*, the FGF homolog *branchless* acts via the FGF receptor, *breathless*, in controlling branching of the developing tracheal system, and here the evidence also indicates that *branchless* acts as a chemotactic signal *(80)*.

Beyond the link between FGF signaling and branching morphogenesis, there is considerable evidence that FGF signaling control specific episodes of cell migration in many developing organs. Sex cell migration is controlled in *Caenorhabditis elegans* by the FGF-like protein, EGL-17, which is secreted by the target gonadal cell *(81)*. FGF signaling is required for vertebrate myoblast migration *(82)*, and in vitro experiments indicate that FGF2 and FGF4 act as a chemotactic signals *(83)*. FGF-8 and/or FGF4 have also been shown to be critical for cell migration in gastrulating mouse embryos, and it is required for successful gastrulation *(84)*. Thus, vertebrate FGFs may have evolved from an ancestral gene that functioned in the control of cell movements, and the extensive duplication of *Fgf* genes correlates with the extensive use of cell migration in vertebrate development.

FGF4 AND SKELETAL BIFURCATIONS

Later stages of limb development are characterized by the formation and separation of the digits. The autopodial plate is dorsal-ventrally flattened and fans out with chondrogenic rays that represent the forming digits. Fate maps of these digit rays indicate that they primarily form the metatarsal/metacarpal of the mature digit, with the phalangeal elements forming from only the distal-most region of each ray *(85)*. Individual digit rudiments can develop at ectopic sites, indicating that at this stage each digit rudiment is an autonomously developing morphogenetic field *(86)*. The primary events of digit morphogenesis are distal elongation of the digit blastema, segmentation of the chondrogenic digit ray, and programmed cell death within the interdigital regions that separate the digits. The digits themselves do not normally bifurcate, thus making their formation a potential model system for studying the induction of bifurcation events. Digit formation is also characterized by the downregulation of many of the *Fgf* genes that are expressed during earlier stages of limb development, providing a temporal relationship with bifurcation events.

When prechondrogenic cells of the autopod aggregate to form the digit rays, the AER and the ZPA are no longer present; however, many patterning genes that were expressed in the progress zone of the early limb bud (such as the *Hoxa* and *Hoxd* gene clusters and the *Msx* genes) remain expressed in the digit rudiments, suggesting that the patterning of individual digit rudiments is still incomplete. Furthermore, a number of experimental observations indicating that active patterning of digit rudiments continues into later limb bud stages. First, digit tip amputations result in a rapid level-specific regeneration response that includes re-expression of the AER-dependent *Msx* genes *(86)*. Second, the digit rudiments of mouse limb buds (stage 7/8, E12.5) respond to implantation of a FGF4-releasing microcarrier bead by inducing specific bifurcation of digit IV, indicating that patterning of digit IV is incomplete *(87)*. Third, interdigital cells of the chick autopod are able to form digits in response to wounding or to implantation of transforming growth factor-β-releasing microcarrier beads *(88)*. Fourth, digit identity in the chick hind limb can be modified by interdigital tissues and ectopic BMP application after the formation of the digit ray *(10)*. These studies support the view that patterning of individual digit rudiments continues during later stages of limb development, although endogenous patterning signals that act during digit formation are largely unknown.

Using *exo utero* surgery, we have used ectopic application of FGF4 into the autopod of the mouse hindlimb at a stage shortly after AER regression to study the influence of FGF4 on digit formation *(87)*. Although our studies uncovered a number of FGF4-induced effects on digit formation, two observations are directly relevant for skeletal morphogenesis. First, FGF4 causes a local and transient inhibition of chondrogenesis involving the formed autopodial digit ray. A similar response has been reported in the chick limb *(89,90)*, and FGF signaling has been shown to inhibit chondrogenesis in high density cultures of limb bud cells *(91,92)*. Second, FGF4 induces a bifurcation response by prechondrogenic cells at the tip of digit IV (Fig. 5A). We demonstrate with cell-marking studies that this bifurcation response is associated with an FGF4-induced migration response that results in a reorganization of prechondrogenic cells at the distal tip of the digit ray (Fig. 5B). This response does not involve interdigital cells known to have chondrogenic potential. Consistent with models that predict mathematical bifurcation responses, the FGF4 response is associated with an expansion of the prechondrogenic zone at the digit tip (Fig. 5C). Gene expression studies indicate that this response is associated with the modified expression of number of genes, including *Msx1*, *Igf2*, and the posterior members of the *HoxD* cluster. These findings support our branching morphogenesis model for skeletogenesis by showing that FGF4-induced cell migration is associated with the expansion of the distal prechondrogenic tissue and a skeletal bifurcation response.

SUMMARY

Classical embryological and recent molecular studies have combined to increase our understanding of the complex process of limb development. Although recent years have unarguably broadened

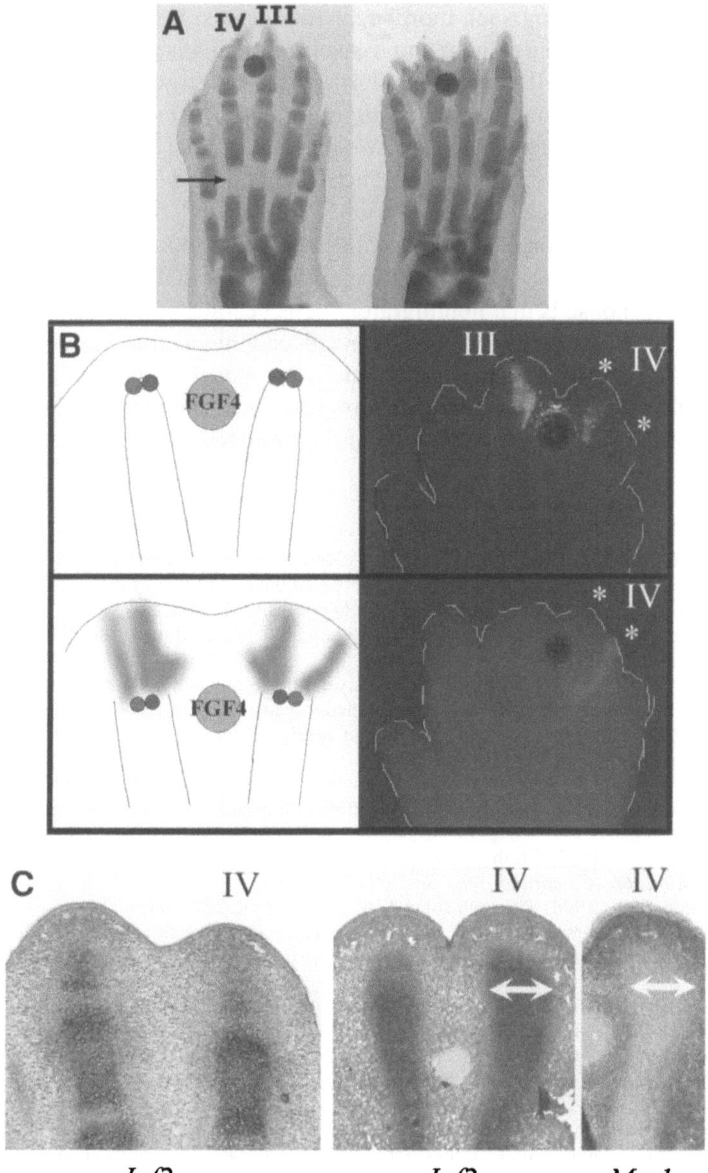

Fig. 5. A, FGF4 bead implantation in E12.5 mouse left hind limb bud causes inhibition of cartilage growth and differentiation (arrow) and the distal bifurcation of digit IV. **B**, FGF4 influences cell migration of digit cells. Cells located at the anterior or posterior digit tip (digit III and IV) were labeled with DiI, and an FGF4 bead was simultaneously implanted in the interdigit III-IV (top left). Anterior is to the left, and distal is toward the top. After 72 h, posterior digit IV cells (away from the bead) were not influenced by the FGF4 bead and migrated distally (lower right), whereas anterior digit IV cells (closest to the bead) migrated toward the bead and established a secondary digit tip (*). A summary map of cell migration in digits III and IV is presented (lower right): red dots represent the location of posterior digit III and anterior digit IV injection sites and green dots represent the location of anterior digit III and posterior digit IV injection sites. **C**, FGF4 influences gene expression and the pattern of condensation in digit tips. *Igf2* gene expression is used as a marker for chondrogenesis and identifies digit tip condensations in control E13.5 day digits (left panel); 48 h after FGF4 bead implantation, *Igf2* expression is distally expanded, indicating a widening of the chondrogenic condensation associated with a bifurcation response (center panel). The widening of *Igf2* expression domain is associated with a *Msx1*-negative domain at the tip of digit IV (right panel).

our information base by identifying such morphogenetic signals, it is less clear how most of these signals influence development at the cellular and tissue level. FGF4 is produced by the AER and functions to regulate mesenchymal cell movements during limb outgrowth. We have shown that FGF4 acts as a chemoattractant and, by regulating cell migration, FGF4 functions to control skeletal bifurcation events important for limb morphogenesis. We present a model for skeletal morphogenesis that integrates both the distalward movement of mesenchymal cells induced by FGF4 and the resulting cell–cell interactions that occur as a result migration. In this model, the view of the progress zone is modified to include distal migration of selective cells that become concentrated under the AER; thus, the progress zone is considered to be dynamically maintained by FGF4 induced migration. One outcome of this migration response is that nonmigratory cells become concentrated proximally, and we propose that this emigration of migrating cells trigger cell–cell interactions between nonmigratory cells necessary for the initiation of chondrogenic condensation. Our model provides a conceptual link between pattern specifying signals that require FGFs in the progress zone, and morphogenetic events important for skeletogenesis that occur in proximal regions of the limb bud.

REFERENCES

1. Schaller, S., Li, S., Ngo-Muller, V., Han, M.-J., Omi, M., Anderson, R., and Muneoka, K. (2001) Cell Biology of Limb Patterning, in *International Review Cytology Volume 203: Cell Lineage Specification and Patterning of the Embryo*, (Etkin, L. D. and Jeon, K. W., eds.), Academic Press, San Diego, CA, pp. 483–517.
2. Allen, F., Tickle, C., and Warner, A. (1990) The role of gap junctions in patterning of the chick limb bud. *Development* **108,** 623–634.
3. Kelley, R. O. and Fallon, J. F. (1976) Ultrastructural analysis of the apical ectodermal ridge during vertebrate limb morphogenesis. 1. the human forelimb with special reference to gap junctions. *Dev. Biol.* **51,** 241–256.
4. Saunders, J. W. Jr. (1948) The proximo-distal sequence of origin of the parts of the chick wing and the role of the ectoderm. *J. Exp. Zool.* **108,** 363–403.
5. Saunders, J. W. Jr. (1998) Apical ectodermal ridge in retrospect. *J. Exp. Zool.* **282,** 669–676.
6. Summerbell, D., Lewis, J. H., and Wolpert, L. (1973) Positional information in chick limb morphogenesis. *Nature* **244,** 492–496.
7. Ettinger, L. and Doljanski, F. (1992) On the generation of form by the continuous interactions between cells and their extracellular matrix. *Biol. Rev. Cambridge Phil. Soc.* **67,** 459–489.
8. Pearse, R. V. and Tabin, C. J. (1998) The molecular ZPA. *J. Exp. Zool.* **282,** 677–690.
9. Hardy, A., Richardson, M. K., Francis-West, P. H., Rodriguez, C., Izpisua-Belmonte, J. C., Duprez, D., et al. (1995) Gene expression, polarising activity and skeletal patterning in reaggregated hind limb mesenchyme. *Development* **121,** 4329–4337.
10. Dahn, R. D. and Fallon, J. F. (2000) Interdigital regulation of digit identity and homeotic transformation by modulated BMP signaling. *Science* **289,** 438–441.
11. Stephens, T. D., Baker, W. C., Cotterell, J. W., Edwards, D. R., Pugmire, D. S., Roberts, S. G., et al. (1993) Evaluation of the chick wing territory as an equipotential self-differentiating system. *Dev. Dyn.* **197,** 157–168.
12. Searls, R. L. and Janner, M. (1971) The initiation of limb bud outgrowth in the embryonic chick. *Dev. Biol.* **24,** 198–213.
13. Chaube, S. (1959) On axiation and symmetry in transplanted wing of the chick. *J. Exp. Zool.* **140,** 29–77.
14. Xu, X., Weinstein, M., Li, C., and Deng, C. (1999) Fibroblast growth factor receptors (FGFRs) and their roles in limb development. *Cell Tissue Res.* **296,** 33–43.
15. Martin, G. R. (1998) The roles of FGFs in the early development of vertebrate limbs. *Genes Dev.* **12,** 1571–1586.
16. Ohuchi, H. and Noji, S. (1999) Fibroblast-growth-factor-induced additional limbs in the study of initiation of limb formation, limb identity, myogenesis, and innervation. *Cell Tissue Res.* **296,** 45–56.
17. Peters, K. G., Werner, S., Chen, G., and Williams, L. T. (1992) Two FGF receptor genes are differentially expressed in epi-thelial and mesenchymal tissues during limb formation and organogenesis in the mouse. *Development* **114,** 233–243.
18. Szebenyi, G., Savage, M. P., Olwin, B. B., and Fallon, J. F. (1995) Changes in the expression of fibroblast growth factor receptors mark distinct stages of chondrogenesis *in vitro* and during chick limb skeletal patterning. *Dev. Dyn.* **204,** 446–456.
19. Delezoide, A. L., Benoist-Lasselin, C., Legeai-Mallet, L., Le Merrer, M., Munnich, A., Vekemans, M., et al. (1998) Spatio-temporal expression of FGFR 1, 2 and 3 genes during human embryo-fetal ossification. *Mech. Dev.* **77,** 19–30.
20. Lizarraga, G., Ferrari, D., Kalinowski, M., Ohuchi, H., Noji, S., Kosher, R. A., et al. (1999) FGFR2 signaling in normal and limbless chick limb buds. *Dev. Genet.* **25,** 331–338.
21. Min, H., Danilenko, D. M., Scully, S. A., Bolon, B., Ring, B. D., Tarpley, J. E., et al. (1998) Fgf-10 is required for both limb and lung development and exhibits striking functional similarity to *Drosophila branchless*. *Genes Dev.* **12,** 3156–3161.

22. Sekine, K., Ohuchi, H., Fujiwara, M., Yamasaki, M., Yoshizawa, T., Sato, T., et al. (1999) *Fgf10* is essential for limb and lung formation. *Nat. Genet.* **21,** 138–141.
23. Celli, G., LaRochelle, W. J., Mackem, S., Sharp, R., and Merlino, G. (1998). Soluble dominant-negative receptor uncovers essential roles for fibroblast growth factors in multi-organ induction and patterning. *EMBO J.* **17,** 1642–1655.
24. Xu, X., Weinstein, M., Li, C., Naski, M., Cohen, R. I., Ornitz, D. M., et al. (1998) Fibroblast growth factor receptor 2 (FGFR2)-mediated reciprocal regulation loop between FGF8 and FGF10 is essential for limb induction. *Development* **125,** 753–765.
25. Ohuchi, H., Nakagawa, T., Yamamoto, A., Araga, A., Ohata, T., Ishimaru, Y., et al. (1997) The mesenchymal factor, FGF10, initiates and maintains the outgrowth of the chick limb bud through interaction with FGF8, an apical ectodermal factor. *Development* **124,** 2235–2244.
26 Heikinheimo, M., Lawshe, A., Shackleford, G. M., Wilson, D. B., and MacArthur, C. A. (1994) Fgf-8 expression in the post-gastrulation mouse suggests roles in the development of the face, limbs and central nervous system. *Mech. Dev.* **48,** 129–138.
27. Ohuchi, H., Yoshioka, H., Tanaka, A., Kawakami, Y., Nohno, T., and Noji, S. (1994) Involvement of androgen-induced growth factor (FGF-8) gene in mouse embryogenesis and morphogenesis. *Biochem. Biophys. Res. Commun.* **204,** 882–888.
28. Crossley, P. H., Minowada, G., Macarthur, C. A., and Martin, G. R. (1996) Roles for FGF8 in the induction, initiation, and maintenance of chick limb development. *Cell* **84,** 127–136.
29. Crossley, P. H. and Martin, G. R. (1995) The mouse *Fgf8* gene encodes a family of polypeptides and is expressed in regions that direct outgrowth and patterning in the developing embryo. *Development* **121,** 439–451.
30. Vogel, A., Rodriguez, C., and Izpisúa-Belmonté, J.C. (1996) Involvement of FGF-8 in initiation, outgrowth and patterning of the vertebrate limb. *Development* **122,** 1737–1750.
31. Yonei-Tamura, S., Endo, T., Yajima, H., Ohuchi, H., Ide, H., and Tamura, K. (1999) FGF7 and FGF10 directly induce the apical ectodermal ridge in chick embryos. *Dev. Biol.* **211,** 133–143.
32. Lewandoski, M., Sun, X., and Martin, G. R. (2000) *Fgf8* signalling from the AER is essential for normal limb development. *Nat. Genet.* **26,** 460–463.
33. Moon, A. M., Boulet, A. M., and Capecchi, M. R. (2000) Normal limb development in conditional mutants of Fgf4. *Development* **127,** 989–996.
34. Zhou, M., Sutliff, R. L., Paul, R. J., Lorenz, J. N., Hoying, J. B., Haudenschild, C. C., et al. (1998) Fibroblast growth factor 2 control of vascular tone. *Nat. Med.* **4,** 201–207.
35. Moon, A. M. and Capecchi, M. R. (2000) *Fgf8* is required for outgrowth and patterning of the limbs. *Nat. Genet.* **26,** 455–459.
36. Sun, X., Lewandoski, M., Meyers, E. N., Liu, Y. H., Maxson, R. E. Jr., and Martin, G .R. (2000) Conditional inactivation of Fgf4 reveals complexity of signalling during limb bud development. *Nat. Genet.* **25,** 83–86.
37. Xu, J., Liu, Z., and Ornitz, D. M. (2000) Temporal and spatial gradients of Fgf8 and Fgf17 regulate proliferation and differentiation of midline cerebellar structures. *Development* **127,** 1833–1843.
38. Cohn, M. J., Izpisúa-Belmonté, J.-C., Abud, H., Heath, J. K., and Tickle, C. (1995) Fibroblast growth factors induce additional limb development from the flank of chick embryos. *Cell* **80,** 739–746.
39. Ohuchi, H., Nakagawa, T., Yamauchi, M., Ohata, T., Yoshioka, H., Kuwana, T., et al. (1995) An additional limb can be induced from the flank of the chick embryo by FGF4. *Biochem. Biophys. Res. Commun.* **209,** 809–816.
40. Ohuchi, H., Takeuchi, J., Yoshioka, H., Ishimaru, Y., Ogura, K., Takahashi, N., et al. (1998) Correlation of wing-leg identity in ectopic FGF-induced chimeric limbs with the differential expression of chick Tbx5 and Tbx4. *Development* **125,** 51–60.
41. Mima, T., Ohuchi, H., Noji, S., and Mikawa, T. (1995) FGF can induce outgrowth of somatic mesoderm both inside and outside of limb-forming regions. *Dev. Biol.* **167,** 617–620.
42. Abud, H. E., Skinner, J. A., McDonald, F. J., Bedford, M. T., Lonai, P., and Heath, J. K. (1996) Ectopic expression of Fgf4 in chimeric mouse embryos induces the expression of early markers of limb development in the lateral ridge. *Dev. Genet.* **19,** 51–65.
43. Lightfoot, P. S., Swisher, R., Coffin, J. D., Doetschman, T. C., and German, R. Z. (1997) Ontogenetic limb bone scaling in basic fibroblast growth factor (FGF-2) transgenic mice. *Growth Dev. Aging* **61,** 127–139.
44. Wanek, N., Muneoka, K., Burton, R., Holler-Dinsmore, G., and Bryant, S.V. (1989) A staging system for mouse limb development. *J. Exp. Zool.* **249,** 41–49.
45. Carrington, J. L. and Fallon, J. F. (1988) Initial limb budding is independent of apical ectodermal ridge activity: evidence from a limbless mutant. *Development* **104,** 361–367.
46. Fallon, J. F., Lopez, A., Ros, M. A., Savage, M. P., Olwin, B. B., and Simandl, B. K. (1994) FGF-2: apical ectodermal ridge growth signal for chick limb development. *Science* **264,** 104–107.
47. Niswander, L., Tickle, C., Vogel, A., Booth, I., and Martin, G. R. (1993) FGF-4 replaces the apical ectodermal ridge and directs outgrowth and patterning of the limb. *Cell* **75,** 579–587.
48. Mahmood, R., Bresnick, J., Hornbruch, A., Mahony, C., Morton, N., Colquhoun, K., et al. (1995) A role for FGF-8 in the initiation and maintenance of vertebrate limb bud outgrowth. *Curr. Biol.* **5,** 797–806.
49. Savage, M. P., Hart, C. E., Riley, B. B., Sasse, J., Olwin, B. B., and Fallon, J. F. (1993) Distribution of FGF-2 suggests it has a role in chick limb bud growth. *Dev. Dyn.* **198,** 159–170.
50. Savage, M. P. and Fallon, J. F. (1995) FGF-2 mRNA and its antisense message are expressed in a developmentally specific manner in the chick limb bud and mesonephros. *Dev. Dyn.* **202,** 343–353.

51. Suzuki, H. R., Sakamoto, H., Yoshida, T., Sugimura, T., Terada, M., and Solursh, M. (1992) Localization of HstI transcripts to the apical ectodermal ridge in the mouse embryo. *Dev. Biol.* **150,** 219–222.
52. Niswander, L. and Martin, G. R. (1992) Fgf-4 expression during gastrulation, myogenesis, limb and tooth development in the mouse. *Development* **114,** 755–768.
53. Hayamizu, T. F., Wanek, N., Taylor, G., Trevino, C., Shi, C., Anderson, R., et al. (1994) Regeneration of HoxD expression domains during pattern regulation in chick wing buds. *Dev. Biol.* **161,** 504–512.
54. Taylor, G., Anderson, R., Reginelli, A. D., and Muneoka, K. (1994) FGF-2 induces regeneration of the chick limb bud. *Dev. Biol.* **163,** 282–284.
55. Kostakopoulou, K., Vogel, A., Brickell, P., and Tickle, C. (1996) 'Regeneration' of wing bud stumps of chick embryos and reactivation of *Msx-1* and *Shh* expression in response to FGF-4 and ridge signals. *Mech. Dev.* **55,** 119–131.
56. Li, S., Anderson, R., Reginelli, A. D., and Muneoka, K. (1996) FGF-2 influences cell movements and gene expression during limb development. *J. Exp. Zool.* **274,** 234–247.
57. Li, S. and Muneoka, K. (1999) Cell migration and chick limb development: chemotactic action of FGF4 and the AER. *Dev. Biol.* **211,** 335–347.
58. Riley, B. B., Savage, M. P., Simandl, B. K., Olwin, B. B., and Fallon, J. F. (1993) Retroviral expression of FGF-2 (bFGF) affects patterning in chick limb bud. *Development* **118,** 95–104.
59. Tanaka, M., Cohn, M. J., Ashby, P., Davey, M., Martin, P., and Tickle, C. (2000) Distribution of polarizing activity and potential for limb formation in mouse and chick embryos and possible relationships to polydactyly. *Development* **127,** 4011–4021.
60. Bonneton, C., Sibarita, J. B., and Thiery, J. P. (1999) Relationship between cell migration and cell cycle during the initiation of epithelial to fibroblastoid transition. *Cell Motil. Cytoskeleton* **43,** 288–295.
61. Hornbruch, A. and Wolpert, L. (1970) Cell division in the early growth and morphogenesis of the chick limb. *Nature* **226,** 764–766.
62. Ede, D. A., Flint, O. P., and Teague, P. (1975) Cell proliferation in the developing wing-bud of normal and talpid3 mutant chick embryos. *J. Embryol. Exp. Morphol.* **34,** 589–607.
63. Smith, A. R. and Crawley, A. M. (1977) The pattern of cell division during growth of the blastema of regenerating newt forelimbs. *J. Embryol. Exp. Morphol.* **37,** 33–48.
64. Cooke, J. and Summerbell, D. (1980) Cell cycle and experimental pattern duplication in the chick wing during embryonic development. *Nature* **287,** 697–701.
65. Globus, M. and Vethamany-Globus, S. (1976) An in vitro analogue of early chick limb bud outgrowth. *Differentiation* **6,** 91–96.
66. Reiter, R. S. and Solursh, M. (1982) Mitogenic property of the apical ectodermal ridge. *Dev. Biol.* **93,** 28–35.
67. Aono, H. and Ide, H. (1988) A gradient of responsiveness to the growth-promoting activity of ZPA (zone of polarizing activity) in the chick limb bud. *Dev. Biol.* **128,** 136–141.
68. Niswander, L. and Martin, G.R. (1993) FGF-4 and BMP-2 have opposite effects on limb growth. *Nature* **361,** 68–71.
69. Summerbell, D. and Wolpert, L. (1972) Cell density and cell division in the early morphogenesis of the chick wing. *Nature* **239,** 24–26.
70. Janner, M. Y. and Searls, R. L. (1971) Effect of removal of the apical ectodermal ridge on the rate of cell division in the subridge mesenchyme of the embryonic chick wing. *Dev. Biol.* **24,** 465–476.
71. Summerbell, D. (1977) Reduction of the rate of outgrowth, cell density, and cell division following removal of the apical ectodermal ridge of the chick limb-bud. *J. Embryol. Exp. Morphol.* **40,** 1–21.
72. Shubin H. and Alberch P. (1986) A morphogenetic approach to the origin and basic organization of the tetrapod limb. *Evol. Biol.* **20,** 319–387.
73. Gerhart, J. and Kirschner, M. (1997) *Cells, Embryos, and Evolution: Toward a Cellular and Developmental Understanding of Phenotypic Variation and Evolutionary Adaptability.* Blackwell Science Inc., London, UK.
74. Oster G. F. and Murray, J. D. (1989) Pattern formation models and developmental constraints. *J. Exp. Zool.* **251,** 186–202.
75. Vargesson, N., Clarke, J. D., Vincent, K., Coles, C., Wolpert, L., and Tickle, C. (1997) Cell fate in the chick limb bud and relationship to gene expression. *Development* **124,** 1909–1918.
76. Arman E., Haffner-Krausz R., Chen, Y., Heath, J. K., and Lonai, P. (1998) Targeted disruption of fibroblast growth factor (FGF) receptor 2 suggests a role for FGF signaling in pregastrulation mammalian development. *Proc. Natl. Acad. Sci. USA* **95,** 5082–5087.
77. De Moerlooze, L., Spencer-Dene, B., Revest, J., Hajihosseini, M., Rosewell, I., and Dickson, C. (2000) An important role for the IIIb isoform of fibroblast growth factor receptor 2 (FGFR2) in mesenchymal-epithelial signalling during mouse organogenesis. *Development* **127,** 483–492.
78. Revest, J. M., Spencer-Dene, B., Kerr, K., De Moerlooze, L., Rosewell, I., and Dickson, C. (2001) Fibroblast growth factor receptor 2-IIIb acts upstream of Shh and Fgf4 and is required for limb bud maintenance but not for the induction of *Fgf8, Fgf10, Msx1,* or *Bmp4. Dev. Biol.* **231,** 47–62.
79. Park, W. Y., Miranda, B., Lebeche, D., Hashimoto, G., and Cardoso W. V. (1998) FGF-10 is a chemotactic factor for distal epithelial buds during lung development. *Dev. Biol.* **201,** 125–134.
80. Zelzer, E. and Shilo, B. Z. (2000) Cell fate choices in Drosophila tracheal morphogenesis. *Bioessays* **22,** 219–226.
81. Branda, C. S. and Stern, M. J. (2000) Mechanisms controlling sex myoblast migration in *Caenorhabditis elegans* hermaphrodites. *Dev. Biol.* **226,** 137–151.
82. Itoh, N., Mima, T., and Mikawa, T. (1996) Loss of fibroblast growth factor receptors is necessary for terminal differentiation of embryonic limb muscle. *Development* **122,** 291–300.

83. Webb, S. E., Lee, K. K., Tang, M. K., and Ede, D. A. (1997) Fibroblast growth factors 2 and 4 stimulate migration of mouse embryonic limb myogenic cells. *Dev. Dyn.* **209,** 206–216.
84. Sun, X., Meyers, E. N., Lewandoski, M., and Martin, G. R. (1999) Targeted disruption of Fgf8 causes failure of cell migration in the gastrulating mouse embryo. *Genes Dev.* **13,** 1834–1846.
85. Muneoka, K., Wanek, N., and Bryant, S. V. (1989) Mammalian limb bud development: In situ fate maps of early hindlimb buds. *J. Exp. Zool.* **249,** 50–54.
86. Reginelli, A. D., Wang, Y., Sassoon, D., and Muneoka, K. (1995) Digit tip regeneration correlates with regions of msx1 (formerly Hox7.1) expression in fetal and newborn mice. *Development* **121,** 1065–1076.
87. Ngo-Muller, V. and Muneoka, K. (2000) Influence of FGF4 on digit morphogenesis during limb development in the mouse. *Develop. Biol.* **219,** 224–236.
88. Macias, D., Ganan, Y., Rodriguez-Leon, J., Merino, R., and Hurle, J. M. (1999) Regulation by members of the transforming growth factor beta superfamily of the digital and interdigital fates of the autopodial limb mesoderm. *Cell Tissue Res.* **296,** 95–102.
89. Buckland, R. A., Collinson, J. M., Graham, E., Davidson, D. R., and Hill, R. E. (1998) Antagonistic effects of FGF4 on BMP induction of apoptosis and chondrogenesis in the chick limb bud. *Mech. Dev.* **71,** 143–150.
90. Merino, R., Gañan, Y., Macias, D., Economides, A. N., Sampath, K. T., et al. (1998) Morphogenesis of digits in the avian limb is controlled by FGFs, TGFbetas, and noggin through BMP signaling. *Dev. Biol.* **200,** 35–45.
91. Anderson, R., Landry, M., and Muneoka, K. (1993) Maintenance of ZPA signaling in cultured mouse limb bud cells. *Development* **117,** 1421–1433.
92. Anderson, R., Landry, M., Reginelli, A., Taylor, G., Achkar, C., Gudas, L., et al. (1994) Conversion of anterior limb bud cells to ZPA signaling cells *in vitro* and *in vivo*. *Dev. Biol.* **164,** 241–257.

10

Retinoid Signaling and Skeletal Development

Andrea D. Weston and T. Michael Underhill

INTRODUCTION: COMPLEXITY OF THE RETINOID SIGNALING SYSTEM

Interest in the role of retinoid signaling during skeletal development was generated as early as the 1930s, when studies revealed the effects of vitamin A on fetal development. Both hyper- and hypovitaminosis A in mothers resulted in offspring with a wide range of severe malformations, with skeletal deformities being particularly dramatic. Since those initial studies, retinoic acid (RA) was found to be a much more potent teratogen than vitamin A *(1)*. An important role for retinoid signaling in many stages of skeletogenesis has been revealed, including the early stages of cartilage formation through to the formation and remodeling of bone. RA inhibits chondrocyte differentiation in vivo and in vitro (for review, *see* ref. *2*), whereas it appears to stimulate chondrocyte hypertrophy. These effects on chondrogenesis correlate with changes in expression of many cartilage-specific genes. RA, therefore, is important at multiple stages during skeletogenesis.

As additional players in the retinoid signaling pathway continue to be identified, the role of the retinoids in skeletogenesis becomes more complex. RA is the natural ligand for a class of nuclear receptors belonging to the steroid hormone family of receptors that are thought to mediate most of the effects of RA on cell behavior *(3)*. These receptors function as ligand-inducible transcription factors and comprise two subfamilies, the RA receptors (RARs) and the retinoid X receptors (RXRs), each consisting of three members, α, β, and γ. The RXRs can form homodimers or can heterodimerize with the RARs to mediate gene transcription through interactions with retinoid X response elements (RXREs) and RA response elements (RAREs), respectively. The importance of the RARs in skeletal development has been studied extensively. Although analysis of mutant embryos lacking the various receptor subtypes suggests a considerable degree of functional redundancy among these receptors, examination of the RAR compound-null fetuses offers strong evidence to suggest that these receptors are the major transducers in the retinoid-signaling pathway. Ligand-induced activity of the receptor dimers involves the displacement of co-repressors followed by the recruitment of co-activators (Fig. 1; ref. *4*). In addition, RAR and RXR activity is modulated through interactions with other signaling pathways, many of which may still be unidentified. Because of the level of complexity of retinoid signaling, the roles of this pathway in skeletal development are only slowly being elucidated.

Nuclear receptors are not the only RA binding proteins present in the cell. Cytoplasmic retinol and RA binding proteins, CRBP and CRABP, respectively, constitute a separate class of intracellular RA binding proteins *(5)*. These proteins are thought to be important in retinoid metabolism, acting to protect cells against excess RA or to sequester RA in those cells in which it is required. The availabil-

From: *The Skeleton: Biochemical, Genetic, and Molecular Interactions in Development and Homeostasis*
Edited by: E. J. Massaro and J. M. Rogers © Humana Press Inc., Totowa, NJ

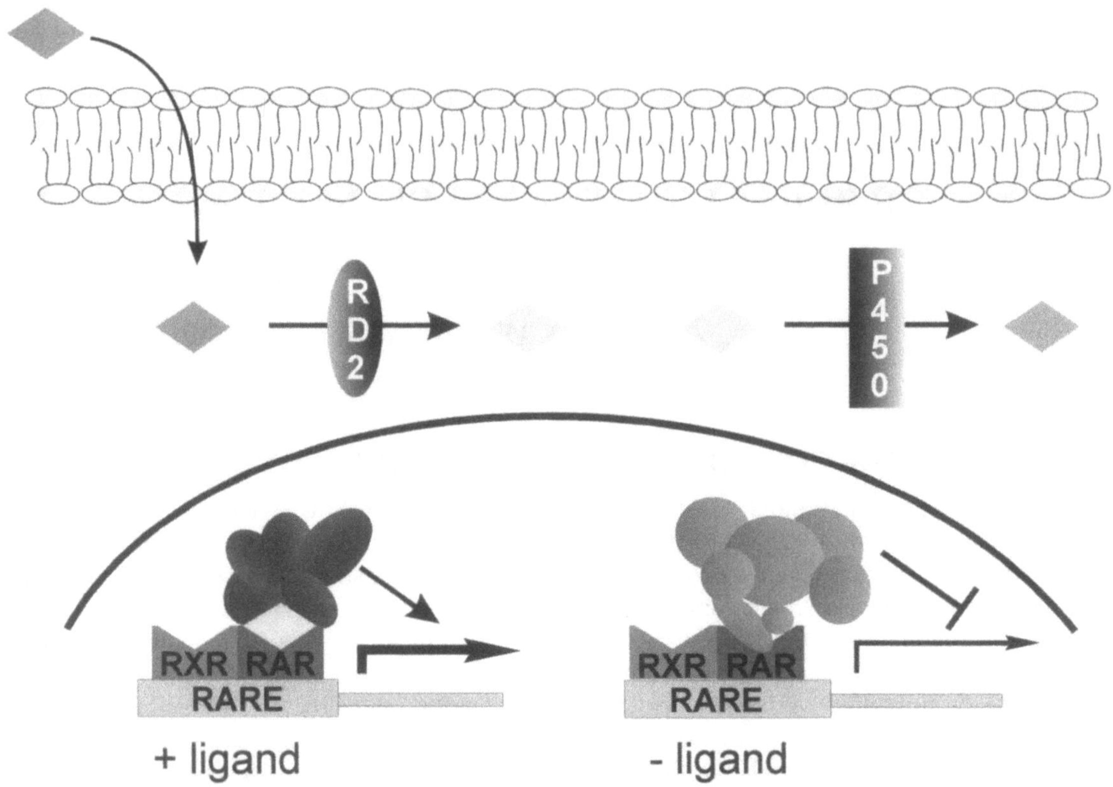

Fig. 1. Overview of retinoid signaling. Retinoids are lipophilic and are thus thought to enter the cell through passive diffusion. Once inside the cell, they interact with a number of cytoplasmic retinoid binding proteins (i.e., CRBPs, CRABPs), some of which may be involved in their metabolism and/or delivery to nuclear receptors. Retinal can be metabolized to its more active form, RA, by RALDH-2 or can degraded to a more polar form(s) by the action of P450RA. All-trans RA binds efficiently to RARs, whereas the 9-cis isomer of RA binds to both RARs and RXRs. In the absence of ligand, an RAR/RXR heterodimer is bound to DNA and is associated with co-repressor complex containing histone deacetylase activity, causing repression of transcription. Ligand binding to the receptors displaces co-repressor and its associated components followed by recruitment of a co-activator complex that in turn acetylates histones, thereby enhancing transcription.

ity of RA is also regulated by enzymes, such as retinaldehyde dehydrogenase (RALDH), which converts retinal to RA, and P450RA, which are cytochrome P450 family members that metabolize RA *(6,7)*. The appropriate expression of these proteins is likely critical in skeletal ontogeny.

A more recent area of retinoid research is becoming popular as specific transcriptional changes in response to activation of retinoid signaling continue to be uncovered. Some of the *Hox* genes are known to contain RAREs and to be under the direct control of RA, and numerous other transcripts are also regulated by RA. With respect to skeletal development, RA induces or represses the expression of many genes that are involved in skeletogenesis. Some of these changes are mediated through the transcriptional regulator AP-1. Cross-coupling with other signaling pathways, such as those regulating AP-1 activity, may underlie many of the effects of RA on skeletogenesis and may represent a common mechanism of RA-induced changes in cell behavior.

The role of retinoid signaling in skeletal development is clearly complex. With numerous stages of skeletal development involving RA and with the multifarious components of the retinoid signaling pathway, it would appear as though we are far from understanding the importance of this pathway in

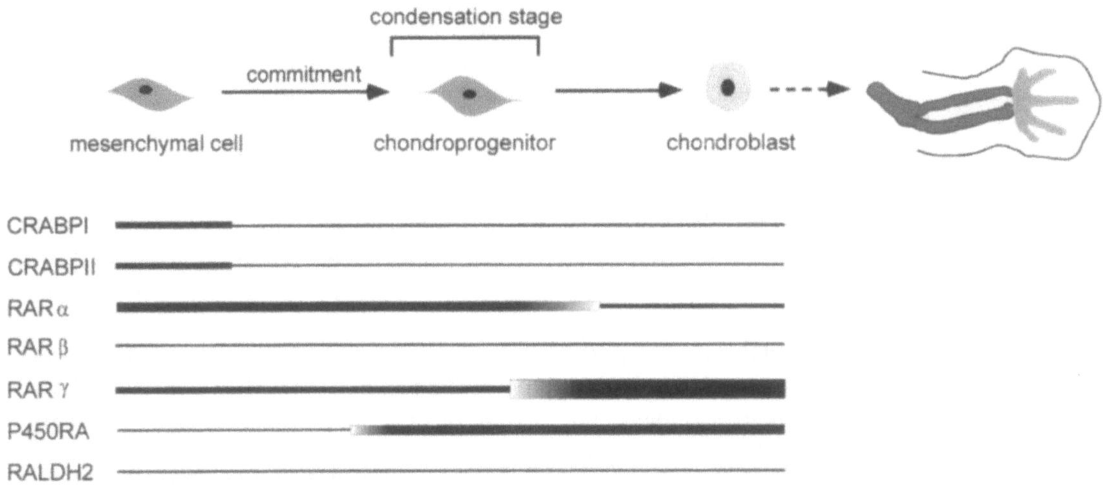

Fig. 2. Expression patterns of the retinoid signaling pathway components during chondrogenesis in the developing mouse limb. CRABPs I and II are expressed early on, in mesenchymal cells, but are undetectable in precartilaginous condensations. RARα and RARγ are expressed in precartilaginous condensations, whereas chondroblast differentiation is accompanied by decreased RARα expression and an increase in the expression of P450RA and RARγ. RARβ and RALDH2 are expressed in proximal mesenchyme early on and at later stages in the IDR. (Intensity of staining corresponds to relative levels of expression.)

skeletogenesis. Nonetheless, substantial progress has been made in this area. As a result of this progress, the retinoid signaling pathway is now recognized as a coordinator at multiple stages of skeletogenesis. This review describes the retinoid signaling pathway's role as a mediator at various levels, but specifically as a regulator of the cell transitions that occur during chondrogenesis.

RETINOID SIGNALING AND CHONDROGENESIS

Chondrogenesis is a critical step in skeletal development in that most of the adult skeleton forms on a cartilage template. Cartilage formation begins when chondroprogenitors aggregate together to form condensations that provide an outline of the future skeleton (reviewed in refs. *8* and *9*). After condensation, cells within the condensate begin differentiating into chondroblasts, which initiate synthesis of a cartilaginous extracellular matrix. As development continues, chondrocytes proliferate then mature into hypertrophic chondrocytes. These hypertrophic chondrocytes eventually die, leaving behind an elaborate matrix to be used by invading osteoblasts as a scaffold for bone formation.

During development, the concentration of RA is spatially and temporally regulated. With respect to skeletal development, activation of RAR-mediated signaling was followed closely in the developing limb using an RAREhspLacZ transgenic mouse model *(10)*. Although detectable RARE activity appears to be only sporadic among chondrocytes within the growth plate, it is highly present in the mesenchyme of the interdigital region (IDR) and in the perichondrium. In addition, Koyama et al. *(11)* used a retinoid bioassay to identify the perichondrium as a rich source of retinoids. RA concentration differences are likely essential in the regulation of skeletogenesis and may be established by the expression of enzymes, such as RALDH-1 and/or -2, and P450RA (Fig. 2). Indeed, RALDH-2 gene expression domains in the developing limb coincide with, but slightly precede, those of RAREhspLacZ activity *(7)*. To date, however, the function of RALDH-2 in skeletogenesis is not entirely clear, and mice with a targeted disruption of the RALDH-2 gene die too early (by E 10.5) to assess a skeletal phenotype *(12)*. P450RAI expression appears to be elevated in chondroprogenitors and chondroblasts and may regulate skeletogenesis indirectly by controlling the amount of RA that remains available to exert its effects *(13)*. Interestingly, the forelimbs of P450RA-null mice do not present with detectable skeletal defects *(14,15)*. This suggests that P450RA may not be important in skeletal development or that as suggested by Abu-Abet et al. *(14)*, P450RAII may be able to substitute for P450RA function in the limb. Furthermore, the P450RA-null mice exhibit a transient increase in RAR activity (as measured by an RAREhspLacZ transgene) in the developing forelimb between E9.5 and E10.5, with this activity returning to levels closer to that of wild-type embryos shortly after this period. Earlier studies have shown that increased levels of RA earlier in limb development have less of an effect on formation of the skeletal elements within the forelimb *(16)*. Thus, a transient increase in RAR activity as observed in P450RA-null embryos may be insufficient to invoke skeletal malformations. In addition to the RALDH and P450RA enzymes, CRABPII has been shown to directly interact with RARs and may be important in delivering ligand to these receptors *(17)*. Mice devoid of CRABPs, however, exhibit only minor skeletal defects, which consist of a single ectopic postaxial bone *(18)*. Moreover, the CRABPs are not expressed in either precartilaginous condensations or in cartilages during appendicular skeletal development. In summary, although there appears to be a tight spatial and temporal regulation of RA concentrations during chondrogenesis, the mechanisms that control these concentrations are only beginning to be understood.

RAR SIGNALING AND THE ESTABLISHMENT OF A CHONDROGENIC TEMPLATE IN THE DEVELOPING LIMB

Several decades ago excess vitamin A was shown to be a skeletal teratogen. More recently, studies performed with RA have revealed skeletal development, particularly chondrogenesis, as a process that is exquisitely sensitive to increased concentrations of RA *(16,19,20)*. Consistent with these observations, numerous studies have shown that RA inhibits cartilage formation both in vivo and in vitro *(21–23)*. In response to RA, chondroprogenitors remain in a mesenchyme-like state instead of differentiating into chondroblasts *(24,25)*. These effects are associated with the continued expression of genes and their products that are abundant during condensation, and with a lack of induction of cartilage-specific genes and proteins *(26,27)*. Contrasting an abundance of data to suggest that RA inhibits cartilage formation, Paulsen et al. *(28,29)* showed, as convincingly, that the addition of physiological concentrations of RA to micromass cultures can stimulate cartilage formation under serum-free conditions and that only higher levels of RA act to inhibit cartilage nodule formation. From these studies, one may presume that the chondrogenic effects of RA are stimulatory under normal physiological conditions; however, other explanations cannot be discounted, including the effects of an absence of growth factors, cytokines, and other components of serum that influence chondrogenesis and may modify the retinoid response.

To better understand the effects of retinoids on skeletal cell behavior, a common approach has been to modulate the activity of specific receptor subtypes. These receptors for RA provide an additional level at which retinoid signaling is regulated. Given that three subfamilies of RARs and RXRs exist, with various isoforms of each, this level of regulation provides much of the diversity of RA responses. This diversity is largely the result of the dynamic spatial and temporal expression of these receptors during development (Fig. 2; ref. *30*). RARα has a relatively ubiquitous distribution in the mouse fetus but is downregulated in newly formed cartilaginous elements of the developing limb and in cartilage nodules in vitro and in vivo *(30,31)*. In contrast, RARγ expression is restricted to cartilaginous elements of the limb bud and the rest of the embryo, whereas RARβ is excluded from many developing tissues that express RARγ, including cartilage. These expression patterns suggest that at least RARα and RARγ are important in early skeletal development. Similar to some of the receptor agonist studies, however, the effects of RAR antagonism on chondrogenesis are unclear because some studies have shown that inhibition of RA signaling stimulates chondrogenesis, whereas others have reported no effect. For instance, addition of RAR-selective antagonists to micromass cultures, such as the pan RAR antagonist AGN 193109 and the RARα-specific antagonist Ro 41-5253, has no observable effect on cartilage formation *(32,33)*. In contrast, treatment of micromass cultures with antisense oligonucleotides to either RARα, β, or γ stimulates chondrogenesis, leading to increased expression of genes encoding matrix proteins *(34)*. Interestingly, this study found that antisense oligonucleotides directed against any of the RARs are equally effective at promoting chondrogenesis. This is somewhat surprising given that RARβ in mice is not normally expressed in precartilaginous condensations or chondroblasts. Expression of a dominant-negative RAR in chondrocytes under the control of a collagen type II promoter results in a decrease in the size of skeletal elements in the limbs of transgenic animals that is speculated to result from decreased chondrocyte proliferation *(35)*. However, transgenic animals that express a weak constitutively active RARα in the developing limbs also exhibit a decrease in the size of limb skeletal elements. In addition to the absent or duplicated bones, many of the malformations seen in transgenic mice phenocopy RA-induced skeletal defects *(31)*. Further examination of the transgenic defect demonstrated that ectopic activation of the RAR-mediated signaling pathway as a result of continued expression of RARα inhibits chondrogenesis, strongly suggesting that downregulation of RARα mRNA is important in cartilage formation. Further analysis of these mice has shown that the transgene-expressing cells have a prechondrogenic phenotype in that they express low levels of type II collagen and exhibit increased expression of type I collagen *(36)*. In addition, this report showed that treatment of wild-type micromass cultures with an RARα-specific antagonist (AGN 194301) stimulates chondroblast differentiation, as indicated by the precocious expression of type II collagen and the cessation of type I collagen expression.

Interestingly, animals devoid of RARα, β, or γ do not exhibit any limb skeletal deficiencies *(37–40)*. Consistent with their expression pattern, however, animals that are deficient in RARα and γ exhibit a number of skeletal deficiencies that result in the loss of skeletal elements or a reduction in their size *(41)*. Surprisingly, these embryos also present with a number of ectopic cartilages that are present in several areas, including the heart, IDR, diaphragm, and meninges *(41,42)*. In addition, RXRα and RXRβ are expressed throughout the developing limb and animals that contain a truncated RXRα and no RXRβ also present with skeletal abnormalities that involve the loss of the radius and some digits *(43)*. Thus, the absence of the RARs appears to inhibit chondrogenesis under certain circumstances while promoting it under others. These results further illustrate the difficulty in interpreting the function of RAR-signaling in skeletal development.

Taken individually, the results from these various studies are not sufficient to formulate a potential function for RAR signaling in chondrogenesis. However, taken together, a coherent theme emerges providing a model that clarifies the function of RA in the developing skeleton. In short, RA signaling appears to regulate the prechondroblast-to-chondroblast transition, with an attenuation of ligand-mediated retinoid signaling, inducing differentiation of chondroprogenitors (Fig. 3). In support of this model, excess RA or overexpression of a weak constitutively active RARα inhibits chondroblast differentiation, favoring the maintenance of the prechondrogenic cell phenotype, whereas an inhibition of RAR signaling promotes expression of the chondroblastic phenotype, limiting the expansion of precartilaginous condensations. Moreover, proteins important in the synthesis or delivery of RA to the receptors, such as the CRABPs and RALDH-2, are not expressed in chondroblastic cells, whereas P450RAI, an enzyme involved in the degradation of RA, is upregulated during formation of embryonic cartilages. This model also reconciles the observations that both decreases and increases in RA signaling yield similar skeletal outcomes, including shortened, fused, or missing elements. With this model, the inappropriate antagonism of RA signaling would be expected to cause premature differentiation of chondroprogenitors, thereby resulting in smaller condensations and smaller cartilages, and in those instances when differentiation occurs too early, there may be insufficient numbers of chondroblasts to support proper formation of an element at all, resulting in the absence of that element. Such premature differentiation may explain why a loss of some skeletal elements is observed in RAR double-null animals. Conversely, enhanced activation of RAR-mediated signaling would

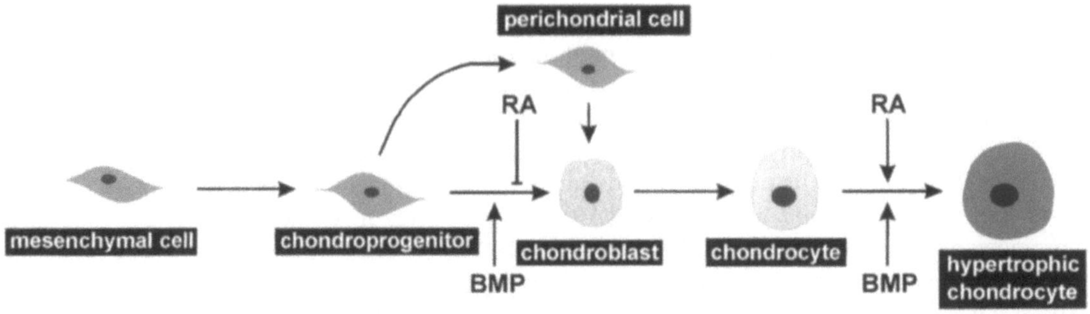

Fig. 3. The importance of RA and other signaling molecules in mediating cell transitions of chondrogenesis in the developing limb. Retinoid signaling appears to be involved in regulating the acquisition of new chondrocytic phenotypes at multiple stages within the developing limb. The expression of the chondroblast phenotype is dependent on a loss of RAR activity, as elevated RAR activity inhibits chondroblast differentiation and an inhibition of RAR signaling promotes expression of chondroblastic markers. At later stages, RA appears to be important in regulating the onset of chondrocyte hypertrophy, as increased concentrations of RA promote hypertrophy, whereas antagonism of RAR signaling suppresses chondrocyte hypertrophy. Localized synthesis of RA in the perichondrium may be important in regulating the transition to hypertrophy and in preventing the premature differentiation of perichondrial cells. In addition, BMPs appear to influence the commitment of mesenchymal cells to the chondrocytic lineage, and evidence suggests that they also regulate chondroblast differentiation.

lead to a decrease in cartilage formation as the result of an inhibition of chondroblast differentiation. Consequently, the skeletal elements would be reduced or absent as observed in RA teratogenicity.

Typically, increased or decreased RA signaling leads to a loss or reduction in skeletal elements; however, both of these conditions can result in the duplication of some elements. For instance, digit duplication observed in response to increased concentrations of RA may be a consequence of effects on early limb patterning cues. In addition, by delaying differentiation of chondroprogenitors, increased RA signaling may act to expand the population of prechondrogenic cells available to form digits. Despite their apoptotic fate, mesenchymal cells of the IDR, in addition to anterior and posterior necrotic zones, have chondrogenic potential *(44)*. Interestingly, RARα/γ double-null mutants and CRABPI/II-null mutant mice present with ectopic cartilages in these regions. In these instances, a loss in RA-mediated signaling may induce cartilage formation before the initiation of the apoptotic program.

Of the two RARs (α and γ) expressed in chondroprogenitors during early murine limb development, it appears that a loss of RARα activity is important in regulating the prechondrogenic-chondroblast transition. Consistent with these observations are the reports that RARα is expressed in condensing mesenchyme but is downregulated during chondroblast differentiation in vivo and in vitro. These observations, however, do not preclude the potential involvement of other RARs in this process because RARα knockout animals do not present with skeletal abnormalities *(39)*. RARα/γ double-null mutants exhibit various appendicular skeletal malformations, suggesting that RARγ can, in part, substitute for RARα in the development of the limb skeletal elements *(41)*; however, a single allele of RARα is sufficient to rescue most of the skeletal defects of the double null mutants further emphasizing a role for RARα in these processes.

RETINOIDS AND BMPS IN CHONDROGENESIS

Aside from the retinoids, numerous molecules have been identified that modulate the expression of the chondrogenic phenotype; however, to date it is unclear as to where, with respect to the network of signals regulating chondrogenesis, the retinoid signaling pathway is placed. Of these molecules, the members of the transforming growth factor-β family, including transforming growth factor-β-1, -2, and -3, and the bone morphogenetic proteins (BMPs) have been shown to regulate many aspects of endochondral bone formation, including the commitment of mesenchymal cells to the chondrocytic lineage and their subsequent differentiation and maturation. During early appendicular skeletal development, *bmp-2* and *-4* are expressed in regions surrounding precartilaginous condensations *(45,46)*. Unfortunately, null mutants die before overt skeletogenesis, making it difficult to ascertain the function of BMPs-2 and -4 in the establishment of limb cartilages *(47,48)*. Subsequent studies using dominant-negative or constitutively active BMP type II receptors in vitro and in vivo have demonstrated that BMP signaling is important at numerous stages of skeletal development *(49)*. Specifically, inhibition of BMP signaling through the expression of dominant-negative BMP type I receptors, noggin, or the generation of BMPR1B-null mutants demonstrates that BMP signaling is required for chondroblast differentiation *(49–51)*. Although both BMP and retinoid signaling have demonstrated regulatory roles in chondroblast differentiation, until recently it was not known whether these two pathways can function independently of one another to coordinate skeletal progenitor differentiation. To this end, a series of experiments was performed in which BMP and/or RA signaling was manipulated to determine the temporal relationship of these two pathways in chondroblast differentiation. Expression of the aforementioned RARα transgene was found to interfere with chondroblast differentiation through a mechanism that could not be rescued by the addition of exogenous BMPs. In contrast, inhibition of endogenous BMP signaling with the addition of Noggin led to decreased chondroblast differentiation that could be restored by the addition of an RAR antagonist *(36)*. Taken together, these results revealed that RA signaling functions either downstream of, or in parallel to, the BMP signaling pathway to regulate the onset of chondroblast differentiation.

MOLECULAR MECHANISMS UNDERLYING RA ACTION IN THE DEVELOPING SKELETON

To date, the mechanisms underlying the demonstrated importance of RA signaling in chondrogenesis are poorly defined. A hallmark of chondroblast differentiation is the dramatic upregulation of col II, a gene encoding the most abundant extracellular protein of cartilage. Within the first intron of col II exists a binding site for the transcription factor Sox9 whose expression is required for induction of col II *(52)*. Prechondrogenic cells devoid of Sox9 do not contribute to cartilage in vivo and haploinsufficiency of Sox9 leads to campomelic dysplasia, a lethal disease associated with severe skeletal defects *(53,54)*. Sox9 is weakly expressed within precartilaginous condensations and becomes more abundantly expressed as condensed cells differentiate into chondroblasts *(55,56)*. In TC6 cells derived from articular cartilage, Sox9 expression increases in response to RA *(57)*. Thus, retinoid signaling appears to influence Sox9 expression, but whether Sox9 represents a direct target of retinoid signaling or is a consequence of RAR-induced chondroblast differentiation remains to be determined.

Aside from the well-characterized induction of col II by Sox9 that accompanies chondroblast differentiation, other factors thought to influence the prechondroblast–chondroblast transition include members of the activating protein-1 (AP-1) transcription factor family. This family of transcription factors is central to many differentiation events, and its members may mediate some of the effects of RA signaling on the differentiation events that occur during skeletogenesis. AP-1 is a dimeric complex composed of either Jun/Jun, Jun/Fos, Jun/ATF, or ATF/ATF components. Each family (Jun, Fos, ATF) contains multiple members, including, c-Jun, Jun B, Jun D in the Jun family; c-Fos, FosB, Fra1, and Fra2 in the Fos family and ATF3 and B-ATF in the ATF family *(58)*. Many studies have shown that prechondrogenic cell differentiation is accompanied by changes in *c-fos* gene expression and AP-1 activity. Prechondrogenic tissues, including condensing mesenchyme, express *c-fos* mRNA, although this protooncogene is undetectable in cartilage. In addition, overexpression of *c-fos* in chick limb buds or in the ATDC5 chondrogenic cell line results in truncation of the long bones and markedly reduced cartilage formation, respectively *(59,60)*. The truncated long bones are caused by severe retardation of differentiation of proliferating chondrocytes into hypertrophic chondrocytes, whereas the cartilage deficiency observed in the ATDC5 cells is the result of markedly reduced differentiation of prechondrogenic cells. Surprisingly, mice lacking functional *c-fos* exhibit no phenotypic changes within the first 10 days after birth. At the growth plates of homozygous animals, however, there is a pronounced reduction in the zone of proliferating chondrocytes with a corresponding increase in the hypertrophic zone.

RA has been shown to be associated with both a negative and positive regulation of AP-1, a discrepancy that is likely the result of cell-specific responses. In addition to binding to RAREs, the RARs affect gene transcription through a mechanism independent of DNA binding but that involves the inhibition of AP-1 assembly *(61,62)*. It has recently been reported that many of the biological functions of another steroid hormone receptor, the glucocorticoid receptor, can also act independently of DNA binding through interactions with AP-1 *(63)*. As mentioned, AP-1 plays an important role in the proliferation and differentiation of skeletal cells; thus, it is reasonable to presume that the actions of retinoids on skeletal cells involve a modulation of AP-1 activity. At this time, however, it is too premature, to speculate on how AP-1 influences chondrogenesis.

In addition to the AP-1 family members, the Hox genes have been shown by various studies to regulate the proliferation and aggregation of precartilaginous condensations. Bona-fide RAREs have been identified in three Hox gene clusters: A, B, and D (reviewed in ref. *64*), and many of these genes, especially those between the A and D clusters, are expressed during early limb development *(65)*. Thus, RAR-mediated signaling may function to control expansion of precartilaginous condensations and/or chondroblast differentiation by regulating the expression of Hox genes.

Several recent reports have described the isolation of genes whose expression is modified in response to manipulation of retinoid signaling *(66)*. Some of these genes represent potential targets for the action of retinoids in the developing skeleton. For instance, a few candidates, namely Stra6 and 13, appear to be expressed in precartilaginous condensations and are subsequently downregulated as cells differentiate into chondroblasts *(67,68)*. At later stages, they are expressed in the perichondrium, but only weakly, if at all, in chondrocytes. In this respect, the expression pattern of Stra6 and 13 is consistent with local sources of retinoids and with ligand activation of the retinoid signaling pathway during skeletogenesis. Thus, retinoid signaling may be functioning, in part, to regulate chondroblast differentiation by controlling the expression of genes, such as Stra6 and 13. Given the varied effects of the retinoid signaling pathway however, these two genes likely represent only a small subset of those mediating retinoid function. Thus, elucidating the function of the retinoids in skeletogenesis will rely largely on the identification of some of these other downstream mediators.

RA SIGNALING AND THE GROWTH PLATE

Retinoid signaling appears to be critical not only in the regulation of chondroblast differentiation but also in regulating chondrocyte hypertrophy. Rats treated systemically with a single dose of RA exhibit a significant reduction in the tibial growth plate height, resulting from a reduced proliferative and hypertrophic zone height *(69)*. This negative regulation of growth plate chondrogenesis was recapitulated in vitro by using a rat metatarsal organ culture system. In this system, a pan RAR-selective antagonist completely reversed the growth-inhibiting effects of RA. Further, Koyoma et al. *(11)* have reported that inhibition of retinoid signaling in the chick growth plate interferes with chondrocyte hypertrophy. Results from these studies also suggest that the perichondrium serves as a source of retinoids that regulates the acquisition of the hypertrophic phenotype. Indian hedgehog (Ihh) has also been shown to be important in controlling chondrocyte hypertrophy and to regulate proliferation of prehypertrophic chondrocytes *(70)*. RA signaling has been recently shown to influence *Ihh* expression within the growth plate *(71)*. Taken together, these results imply that Ihh mediates, at least in part, the actions of RAR signaling during chondrocyte maturation.

The parallels observed between the RA response in prechondroblasts and in growth plate chondrocytes indicate that the retinoid signaling pathway regulates chondrocyte behavior at multiple levels. During the initial stages of cartilage formation, a loss of RAR-mediated signaling appears to regulate the onset of chondroblast differentiation, while at later stages within the growth plate activation of this signaling pathway controls the acquisition of a hypertrophic phenotype. In this respect, both the activation and inhibition of the RA signal transduction cascade controls the onset of new phenotypic characteristics (Fig. 3).

CONCLUSIONS AND PERSPECTIVES

Skeletal development involves a balance between signals regulating proliferation and differentiation. As in many biological systems, retinoid signaling appears to be important in regulating the onset of cellular differentiation. Evidence accumulated from both in vitro and in vivo studies demonstrate that the retinoid signaling cascade functions to regulate many aspects of skeletal development and homeostasis. Unlike other systems, however, during skeletal development, it is an absence of ligand-activated retinoid signaling that appears to trigger the onset of cell differentiation. Thus, RA signaling is critical for maintaining populations of skeletal progenitors in an undifferentiated state, and elevated local concentrations of RA may function to prevent premature differentiation. Too much RA, therefore, negatively affects skeletal development by interfering with skeletal progenitor differentiation. In this manner, RA may regulate the shape of skeletal cartilages by influencing the timing of chondroblast differentiation. To better understand this role, it will be necessary to identify downstream effectors of RAR-mediated signaling and to determine their contribution to the chondrogenic program. In addition, the mechanisms regulating receptor activity in skeletal cells, including ligand availability, levels of expression, post-translational modifications, etc., need to be defined. Resolution of these mechanisms will allow us to determine the placement of the retinoid signaling pathway within the context of the various other molecular networks functioning in skeletogenesis.

ACKNOWLEDGMENTS

We apologize to those colleagues whose work was not cited because of space limitations. A.D.W. was supported by a MRC doctoral fellowship. Some of the research described herein was supported by a grant from the Canadian Institutes of Health and the Canadian Arthritis Network to T.M.U.

REFERENCES

1. Kochhar, D. M. (1967) Teratogenic activity of retinoic acid. *Acta Pathol. Microbiol. Scand.* **70,** 398–404.
2. Underhill, T. M. and Weston, A. D. (1998) Retinoids and their receptors in skeletal development. *Micro. Res. Tech.* **43,** 137–155.
3. Chambon, P. (1996) A decade of molecular biology of retinoic acid receptors. *FASEB J.* **10,** 940–954.
4. Glass, C. K. and Rosenfeld, M. G. (2000) The coregulator exchange in transcriptional functions of nuclear receptors. *Genes Dev.* **14,** 121–141.
5. Giguere, V. (1994) Retinoic acid receptors and cellular retinoid binding proteins: complex interplay in retinoid signaling. *Endo. Rev.* **15,** 61–79.
6. White, J. A., Guo, Y. D., Baetz, K., Beckett-Jones, B., Bonasoro, J., Hsu, K. E., et al. (1996) Identification of the retinoic acid-inducible all-trans-retinoic acid 4-hydroxylase. *J. Biol. Chem.* **271,** 29922–29927.
7. Niederreither, K., McCaffery, P., Drager, U. C., Chambon, P., and Dolle, P. (1997) Restricted expression and retinoic acid-induced downregulation of the retinaldehyde dehydrogenase type 2 (RALDH-2) gene during mouse development. *Mech Dev.* **62,** 67–78.
8. Hall, B. K. and Miyake, T. (1992) The membranous skeleton: The role of cell condensations in vertebrate skeletogenesis. *Anat. Embryol.* **186,** 107–124.
9. Hall, B. K. and Miyake, T. (1995) Divide, accumulate, differentiate: cell condensation in skeletal development revisited. *Int. J. Dev. Biol.* **39,** 881–893.
10. von Schroeder, H. P. and Heersche, J. N. (1998) Retinoic acid responsiveness of cells and tissues in developing fetal limbs evaluated in a RAREhsplacZ transgenic mouse model. *J. Orthop. Res.* **16,** 355–64.
11. Koyama, E., Golden, E. B., Kirsch, T., Adams, S. L., Chandraratna, R. A. S., Michaille, J.-J., et al. (1999) Retinoid signaling is required for chondrocyte maturation and endochondral bone formation during limb skeletogenesis. *Dev. Biol.* **208,** 375–391.
12. Niederreither, K., Subbarayan, V., Dolle, P., and Chambon, P. (1999) Embryonic retinoic acid synthesis is essential for early mouse post-implantation development. *Nat. Genet.* **21,** 444–448.
13. de Roos, K., Sonneveld, E., Compaan, B., ten Berge, D., Durston, A. J., and van der Saag, P. T. (1999) Expression of retinoic acid 4-hydroxylast (CYP26) during mouse and *Xenopus laevis* embryogenesis. *Mech. Dev.* **82,** 205–211.

14. Abu-Abed, S., Dolle, P., Metzger, D., Beckett, B., Chambon, P., and Petkovich, M. (2001) The retinoic acid-metabolizing enzyme, CYP26A1, is essential for normal hindbrain patterning, vertebral identity, and development of posterior structures. *Genes Dev.* **15,** 226–240.
15. Sakai, Y., Meno, C., Fujii, H., Nishino, J., Shiratori, H., Saijoh, Y., et al. (2001) The retinoic acid-inactivating enzyme CYP26 is essential for establishing an uneven distribution of retinoic acid along the anterio-posterior axis within the mouse embryo. *Genes Dev.* **15,** 213–225.
16. Kwasigroch, T. E. and Kochhar, D. M. (1980) Production of congenital limb defects with retinoic acid: phenomenological evidence of progressive differentiation during limb morphogenesis. *Anat. Embryol.* **161,** 105–113.
17. Delva, L., Bastie, J. N., Rochette-Egly, C., Kraiba, R., Balitrand, N., Despouy, G., et al. (1999) Physical and functional interactions between cellular retinoic acid binding protein II and the retinoic acid-dependent nuclear complex. *Mol. Cell. Biol.* **19,** 7158–7167.
18. Lampron, C., Rochette-Egly, C., Gorry, P., Dolle, P., Mark, M., Lufkin, T., et al. (1995) Mice deficient in cellular retinoic acid binding protein II (CRABP II) or in both CRABP I and CRABP II are essentially normal. *Development* **121,** 539–548.
19. Kochhar, D. M. (1973) Limb development in mouse embyros. I. Analysis of teratogenic effects of retinoic acid. *Teratology* **7,** 289–295.
20. Kochhar, D. M. and Aydelotte, M. B. (1974) Susceptible stages and abnormal morphogenesis in the developing mouse limb, analysed in organ culture after transplacental exposure to vitamin A (retinoic acid). *J. Embryol. Exp. Morphol.* **31,** 721–734.
21. Jiang, H., Gyda, M. III, Harnish, D. C., Chandraratna, R. A., Soprano, K. J., Kochhar, D. M., et al. (1994) Teratogenesis by retinoic acid analogs positively correlates with elevation of retinoic acid receptor-β2 mRNA levels in treated embyros. *Teratology* **50,** 38–43.
22. Kwasigroch, T. E., Vannoy, J. F., Church, J. K., and Skalko, R. G. (1986) Retinoic acid enhances and depresses in vitro development of cartilaginous bone anlagen in embryonic mouse limbs. *In Vitro Cell. Dev. Biol.* **22,** 150–156.
23. Kistler, A. (1987) Limb bud cell cultures for estimating the teratogenic potential of compounds. *Arch. Toxicol.* **60,** 403–414.
24. Shapiro, S. S. and Poon, J. P. (1976) Effect of retinoic acid on chondrocyte glycosaminoglycan biosynthesis. *Arch. Biochem. Biophys.* **174,** 74–81.
25. Solursh, M. and Meier, S. (1973) The selective inhibition of mucopolysaccharide synthesis by vitamin A treatment of cultured chick embryo chondrocytes. *Calcif. Tissue Res.* **13,** 131–142.
26. Horton, W. E., Yamada, Y., and Hassell, J. R. (1987) Retinoic acid rapidly reduces cartilage matrix synthesis by altering gene transcription in chondrocytes. *Dev. Biol.* **123,** 508–516.
27. Pennypacker, J. P., Lewis, C. A., and Hassell, J. R. (1978) Altered proteoglycan metabolism in mouse limb mesenchyme cell cultures treated with vitamin A. *Arch. Biochem. Biophys.* **186,** 351–358.
28. Paulsen, D. F., Solursh, M., Langille, R. M., Pang, L., and Chen, W.-D. (1994) Stable, postion-related responses to retinoic acid by chick limb-bud mesenchymal cells in serum-free cultures. *In Vitro Cell. Dev. Biol.* **30A,** 181–186.
29. Paulsen, D. F., Chen, W.-D., Pang, L., Johnson, B., and Okello, D. (1994) Stage- and region-dependent chondrogenesis and growth of chick wing-bud mesenchyme in serum-containing and defined tissue culture media. *Dev. Dyn.* **200,** 39–52.
30. Mollard, R., Viville, S., Ward, S. J., Decimo, D., Chambon, P., and Dolle, P. (2000) Tissue-specific expression of retinoic acid receptor isoform transcripts in the mouse embryo. *Mech Dev.* **94,** 223–232.
31. Cash, D. E., Bock, C., Schughart, K., Linney, E., and Underhill, T. M. (1997) Retinoic acid receptor a function in vertebrate limb skeletogenesis: a modulator of chondrogenesis. *J. Cell Biol.* **136,** 445–457.
32. Eckhardt, K. and Schmitt, G. (1994) A retinoic receptora antagonist counteracts retinoid teratogenicity in vitro and reduced incidence and/or severity of malformations in vivo. *Toxicol. Lett.* **70,** 299–308.
33. Kochhar, D. M., Jiang, H., Penner, J. D., Johnson, A. T., and Chandraratna, R. A. S. (1998) The use of a retinoid receptor antagonist in a new model to study vitamin A-dependent developmental events. *Int. J. Dev. Biol.* **42,** 601–608.
34. Jiang, H., Soprano, D. R., Li, S. W., Soprano, K. J., Penner, J. D., Gyda M, III, and Kochhar, D. M. (1995) Modulation of limb bud chondrogenesis by retinoic acid and retinoic acid receptors. *Int. J. Dev. Biol.* **39,** 617–627.
35. Yamaguchi, M., Nakamoto, M., Honda, H., Nakagawa, T., Fujita, H., Nakamura, T., et al. (1998) Retardation of skeletal development and cervical abnormalities in transgenic mice expressing a dominant-negative retinoic acid receptor in chondrogenic cells. *Proc. Natl. Acad. Sci. USA* **95,** 7491–7496.
36. Weston, A., Rosen, V., Chandraratna, R. A. S., and Underhill, T. M. (2000) Regulation of skeletal progenitor differentiation by the BMP and retinoid signaling pathways. *J. Cell Biol.* **148,** 679–690.
37. Ghyselinck, N. B., Dupe, V., Dierich, A., Messaddeq, N., Garnier, J. M., Rochetteegly, C., et al. (1997) Role of the retinoic acid receptor beta (RAR-β) during mouse development. *Int. J. Dev. Biol.* **41,** 425–447.
38. Lohnes, D., Kastner, P., Dierich, A., Mark, M., LeMeur, M., and Chambon, P. (1993) Function of retinoic acid receptor g in the mouse. *Cell* **73,** 643–658.
39. Lufkin, T., Lohnes, D., Mark, M., Dierich, A., Gorry, P., Gaub, M.-P., et al. (1993) High postnatal lethality and testis degeneration in retinoic acid receptor α mutant mice. *Proc. Natl. Acad. Sci. USA* **90,** 7225–7229.
40. Luo, J., Pasceri, P., Conlon, R. A., Rossant, J., and Giguere, V. (1995) Mice lacking all isoforms of retinoic acid receptor β develop normally and are susceptible to the teratogenic effects of retinoic acid. *Mech. Dev.* **53,** 61–71.
41. Lohnes, D., Mark, M., Mendelsohn, C., Dolle, P., Dierich, A., Gorry, P., et al. (1994) Function of the retinoic acid receptors (RARs) during development (I) Craniofacial and skeletal abnormalities in RAR double mutants. *Development* **120,** 2723–2748.

42. Mendelsohn, C., Lohnes, D., Decimo, D., Lufkin, T., LeMeur, M., Chambon, P., et al. (1994) Function of the retinoic acid receptors (RARs) during development (II) Multiple abnormalities at various stages of organogenesis in RAR double mutants. *Development* **120,** 2749–2771.
43. Mascrez, B., Mark, M., Dierich, A., Ghyselinck, N. B., Kastner, P., and Chambon, P. (1998) The RXR alpha ligand-dependent activation function 2 (AF-2) is important for mouse development. *Development* **125,** 4691–4707.
44. Hurle, J. M., Ganan, Y., and Macias, D. (1989) Experimental analysis of the in vivo chondrogenic potential of the interdigital mesenchyme of the chick leg bud subjected to local ectodermal removal. *Dev. Biol.* **132,** 368–374.
45. Lyons, K. M., Pelton, R. W., and Hogan, B. L. M. (1990) Organogenesis and pattern formation in the mouse: RNA distribution patterns suggest a role for Bone Morphogenetic Protein-2A (BMP-2A). *Development* **109,** 833–844.
46. Jones, C. M., Lyons, K. M., and Hogan, B. L. M. (1991) Involvement of bone morphogenetic protein-4 (BMP-4) and Vgr-1 in morphogenesis and neurogenesis in the mouse. *Development* **111,** 531–542.
47. Zhang, H. and Bradley, A. (1996) Mice deficient for BMP2 are nonviable and have defects in amnion/chorion and cardiac development. *Development* **122,** 2977–2986.
48. Winnier, G., Blessing, M., Labosky, P. A., and Hogan, B. L. M. (1995) Bone morphogenetic protein-4 is required for mesoderm formation and patterning in the mouse. *Genes Dev.* **9,** 2105–2116.
49. Zou, H., Wieser, R., Massague, J., and Niswander, L. (1997) Distinct roles of type I bone morphogenetic protein receptors in the formation and differentiation of cartilage. *Genes Dev.* **11,** 2191–2203.
50. Yi, S. E., Daluiski, A., Pederson, R., Rosen, V., and Lyons, K. M. (2000) The type I BMP receptor BMPRIB is required for chondrogenesis in the mouse limb. *Development* **127,** 621–630.
51. Pizette, S. and Niswander, L. (2000) BMPs are required at two steps of limb chondrogenesis: formation of prechondrogenic condensations and their differentiation into chondrocytes. *Dev. Biol.* **219,** 237–249.
52. Lefebvre, V., Zhou, G., Mukhopadhyay, K., Smith, C. N., Zhang, Z., Eberspaecher, H., et al. (1996) An 18-base-pair sequence in the mouse Pro-alpha-1(II) collagen gene is sufficient for expression in cartilage and binds nuclear proteins that are selectively expressed in chondrocytes. *Mol. Cell. Biol.* **16,** 4512–4523.
53. Bi, W., Deng, J. M., Zhang, Z., Behringer, R. R., and de Crombrugghe, B. (1999) Sox9 is required for cartilage formation. *Nat. Genet.* **22,** 85–89.
54. Wagner, T. (1994) Autosomal sex reversal and campomelic dysplasia are caused by mutations in and around and SRY-related gene. *Cell* **79,** 1111–1120.
55. Wright, E., Hargrave, M. R., Christiansen, J., Cooper, L., Kun, J., Evans, T., et al. (1995) The *Sry*-related gene *Sox9* is expressed during chondrogenesis in mouse embryos. *Nat. Genet.* **9,** 15–20.
56. Zhao, Q., Eberspaecher, H., Lefebvre, V., and De Crombrugghe, B. (1997) Parallel expression of Sox9 and Col2a1 in cells undergoing chondrogenesis. *Dev. Dyn.* **209,** 377–386.
57. Sekiya, I., Tsuji, K., Koopman, P., Watanabe, H., Yamada, Y., Shinomiya, K., et al. (2000) SOX9 enhances aggrecan gene promoter/enhancer activity and is up-regulated by retinoic acid in a cartilage-derived cell line, TC6. *J. Biol. Chem.* **275,** 10738–10744.
58. Karin, M., Liu, Z., and Zandi, E. (1997) AP-1 function and regulation. *Curr. Opin. Cell Biol.* **9,** 240–246.
59. Thomas, D. P., Sunters, A., Gentry, A., and Grigoriadis, A. E. (2000) Inhibition of chondrocyte differentiation in vitro by constitutive and inducible overexpression of the c-fos proto-oncogene. *J. Cell Sci.* **113,** 439–450.
60. Watanabe, H., Saitoh, K., Kameda, T., Murakami, M., Niikura, Y., Okazaki, S., et al. (1997) Chondrocytes as a specific target of ectopic Fos expression in early development. *Proc. Natl. Acad. Sci. USA* **94,** 3994–3999.
61. Zhou, X. F., Shen, X. Q., and Shemshedini, L. (1999) Ligand-activated retinoic acid receptor inhibits AP-1 transactivation by disrupting c-Jun/c-Fos dimerization. *Mol. Endocrinol.* **13,** 276–285.
62. Pfahl, M. (1993) Nuclear receptor/AP-1 interaction. *Endocr. Rev.* **14,** 651–658.
63. Reichardt, H. M., Kaestner, K. H., Tuckermann, J., Kretz, O., Wessely, O., Bock, R., et al. (1998) DNA binding of the glucocorticoid receptor is not essential for survival. *Cell* **93,** 531–541.
64. Underhill, T. M., Kotch, L. E., and Linney, E. (1995) Retinoids and mouse embryonic development. *Vit. Horm.* **51,** 403–457.
65. Nelson, C. E., Morgan, B. A., Burke, A. C., Laufer, E., DiMambro, E., Murtaugh, L. C., et al. (1996) Analysis of Hox gene expression in the chick limb bud. *Development* **122,** 1449–1466.
66. Bouillet, P., Oulad-Abdelghani, M., Vicaire, S., Garnier, J. M., Schuhbaur, B., Dolle, P., et al. (1995) Efficient cloning of cDNAs of retinoic acid-responsive genes in P19 embryonal carcinoma cells and characterization of a novel mouse gene, Stra1 (mouse LERK-2/Eplg2). *Dev. Biol.* **170,** 420–433.
67. Boudjelal, M., Taneja, R., Matsubara, S., Bouillet, P., Dolle, P., and Chambon, P. (1997) Overexpression of Stra13, a novel retinoic acid-inducible gene of the basic helix-loop-helix family, inhibits mesodermal and promotes neuronal differentiation of P19 cells. *Genes Dev.* **11,** 2052–2065.
68. Bouillet, P., Sapin, V., Chazaud, C., Messaddeq, N., Decimo, D., Dolle, P., et al. (1997) Developmental expression pattern of Stra6, a retinoic acid-responsive gene encoding a new type of membrane protein. *Mech Dev.* **63,** 173–186.
69. De Luca, F., Uyeda, J. A., Mericq, V., Mancilla, E. E., Yanovski, J. A., Barnes, K. M., et al. (2000) Retinoic acid is a potent regulator of growth plate chondrogenesis. *Endocrinology* **141,** 346–353.
70. St-Jacques, B., Hammerschmidt, M., and McMahon, A. P. (1999) Indian hedgehog signaling regulates proliferation and differentiation of chondrocytes and is essential for bone formation. *Genes Dev.* **13,** 2072–2086.
71. Koyama, E., Iwamoto, M., Enomoto-Iwamoto, M., Adams, S. L., Chandraratna, R. A., and Pacifici, M. (2000) Regulation of indian hedgehog and CBFA1 expression during chondrocyte maturation by retinoid signaling. *J. Bone Miner. Res.* **15(Suppl 1),** S145.

11

Retinoids and Indian Hedgehog Orchestrate Long Bone Development

Maurizio Pacifici, Chiara Gentili, Eleanor Golden, and Eiki Koyama

INTRODUCTION

Long bone formation is a complex process that has been studied for decades *(1–3)*. It initiates with the emergence, at specific times and sites, of mesenchymal cell condensations that are patterned by the concerted action of the zone of polarizing activity (ZPA), apical ectodermal ridge, and dorsal ectoderm. The condensed cells differentiate into chondrocytes that produce characteristic cartilage matrix components and give rise to readily identifiable cartilaginous elements. The chondrocytes within each element start a process of maturation, which includes a proliferative, prehypertrophic, hypertrophic, and post-hypertrophic phase, and become organized in growth plates. At the same time, diarthrodial synovial joints develop at each epiphyseal end. Once formed, hypertrophic cartilage is invaded by bone, marrow, and vascular progenitor cells from adjacent perichondrial tissues, is eroded, and is finally replaced by endochondral bone and marrow. In addition, perichondrial cells give rise to an intramembranous bone collar surrounding the elements, which is critical to determine diameter and shape of the shaft *(1)*. Maturation, hypertrophy, blood vessel invasion, and ossification first occur in the diaphyseal region and then spread toward the opposing epiphyses with increasing developmental time. Thus, long bone formation requires multiple and topographically restricted events within the cartilaginous elements as well as coordinated events in perichondrial tissues. It is not fully understood how all these processes are set and regulated, what signaling molecules mediate cartilage-perichondrium communication and interactions, and how events in cartilage are coordinated with those in perichondrium.

Studies have indicated that the signaling molecules Indian hedgehog (IHH) and retinoids have critical roles in long bone formation. IHH belongs to the powerful hedgehog family of secreted signaling proteins and is exclusively expressed in prehypertrophic chondrocytes in the growth plate of long bone anlagen *(4–7)*. In contrast, the hedgehog cell surface receptor Patched and the hedgehog nuclear factor GLI are strongly expressed in adjacent proliferative and early hypertrophic zones and in perichondrial tissue surrounding the IHH-expressing prehypertrophic cells *(5,6)*. These and other findings led to the proposal that IHH prominently regulates chondrocyte behavior in the growth plate, inhibits maturation, and determines the overall number of chondrocytes entering and completing the maturation process with the aid of perichondrium-derived parathyroid hormone-related peptide *(5,6)*. Additional work from our group has indicated, however, that IHH may have other important roles in long bone development. We were the first to report that the perichondrial tissue adjacent to the IHH-

From: *The Skeleton: Biochemical, Genetic, and Molecular Interactions in Development and Homeostasis*
Edited by: E. J. Massaro and J. M. Rogers © Humana Press Inc., Totowa, NJ

expressing prehypertrophic chondrocytes is the site of initiation of intramembranous bone collar development *(7,8)*. We then found that treatment of osteoprogenitor cell lines with recombinant IHH induces their differentiation *(9)*. These and other findings led us to propose that IHH is an osteoinductive factor that directs intramembranous ossification along the outer perimeter of developing long bones *(7–9)*. In very good agreement with our proposal, St-Jacques et al. *(10)* have shown that in IHH-null mice there is no ossification in the limbs; interestingly, the IHH-null long bone elements remain cartilaginous and contain disorganized growth plates with much fewer proliferative chondrocytes and more numerous and dispersed hypertrophic chondrocytes. In sum, IHH appears to have multiple key roles in long bone development, and would (1) favor chondrocyte proliferation, (2) limit chondrocyte maturation, and (3) induce intramembranous bone collar formation.

With regard to retinoids, their involvement in skeletogenesis was first suggested by nutrition studies over four decades ago *(11)*. Since then, such connection has been substantiated by work on retinoic nuclear receptors. The receptors comprise two subfamilies, the retinoic acid receptors (RARs) RARα, RARβ, and RARγ, and the retinoid X receptors (RXRs) RXRα, RXRβ and RXRγ *(12,13)*. During limb skeletal development, RARα and RARγ are first expressed broadly; with time, RARγ becomes expressed preferentially in prechondrogenic condensations, RARα remains diffuse and RARβ becomes restricted to perichondrium *(14)*. Gene inactivation studies have shown that loss of a single RAR gene usually causes minor to no skeletal defect, whereas double gene inactivation, such as double-null mutants of RARα and RARγ, produces serious skeletal abnormalities *(15)*. Past and recent work from our group has provided more specific and detailed insights into the roles of retinoid signaling in skeletogenesis. One of our initial findings was that prehypertrophic chondrocytes isolated from developing skeletal elements and maintained in standard culture conditions appeared to be unable to fully mature into hypertrophic mineralizing chondrocytes. The cells, however, promptly did so after treatment with physiologic doses of natural retinoids, such as all-*trans*-retinoic acid or 9-*cis*-retinoic acid *(16)*. We went on to show that retinoids play a similar role in long bone development in the chick limb in vivo *(8)*. We found that the emergence of hypertrophic chondrocytes is invariably accompanied by a marked upregulation of RARγ gene expression and that endogenous retinoids are present in the developing cartilaginous elements. Strikingly, we found that perichondrial tissues adjacent to the elements contain extremely high retinoid levels. This was confirmed by a recent study by others using a transgenic mouse that contains a retinoic acid response element (RARE)/β-galactosidase reporter gene construct to depict endogenous retinoids *(17)*; this study also showed that hypertrophic cartilage contains higher endogenous retinoid amounts than proliferating and prehypertrophic cartilage. When we experimentally blocked retinoid signaling by pharmaceutical means, the chondrocytes were able to reach only the prehypertrophic IHH-expressing stage but could not pass it; thus, no hypertrophic chondrocytes, no expression of hypertrophic gene markers, no vascular invasion of cartilage, and no endochondral bone were present. In sum, our studies have provided clear evidence that retinoid signaling promotes chondrocyte maturation and is required for completion of this process and replacement of hypertrophic mineralized cartilage with endochondral bone.

In the present chapter, we present data form our previous studies to illustrate the roles of IHH and retinoids in long bone development. We also present new data showing that retinoid signaling switches off IHH expression. This could represent a key mechanism by which retinoids promote maturation of prehypertrophic into hypertrophic chondrocytes and bring endochondral ossification to completion.

IHH ROLES IN LONG BONE DEVELOPMENT

Our first clue that IHH may have roles in intramembranous bone collar development came from a study we reported a few years ago *(7)*. That study focused on the question of how the morphogenesis of long bones is regulated and in particular on how the diaphysis comes to acquire its characteristic cylindrical and elongated configuration compared with the three-dimensionally more complex epiphyses. It had been reported at the time that the powerful morphogenetic factor Sonic hedgehog (SHH)

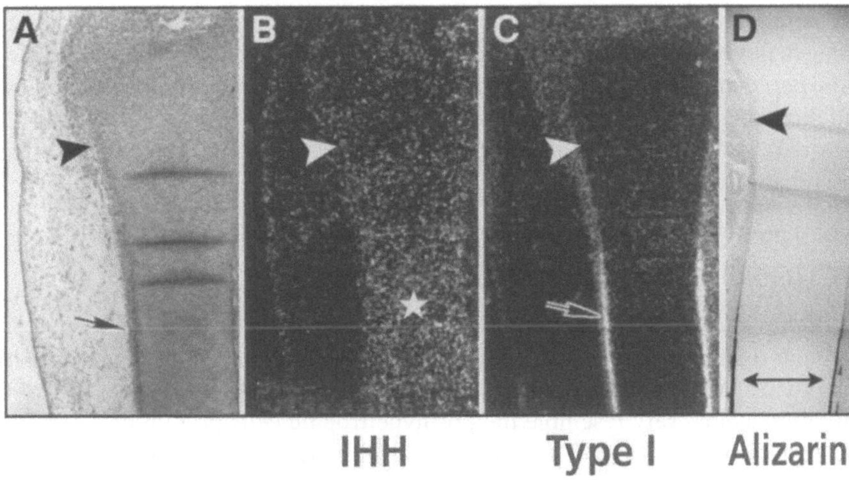

Fig. 1. Analyses of day 8.5 chick embryo skeletal anlage. Longitudinal sections were examined by phase microscopy (**A**); *in situ* hybridization with IHH (**B**); and type I collagen (**C**); cDNA probes and histochemical staining with alizarin red (**D**). Arrows in A, C, and D point to the intramembranous bone collar forming around the IHH-expressing prehypertrophic chondrocytes (star in B).

is expressed in the ZPA located in the posterior part of the limb *(18)*. The ZPA has a critical role in patterning the prechondrogenic mesenchymal condensations during limb development. Thus, we reasoned that SHH itself or another member of its family (i.e., IHH) may be re-expressed in chondrocytes and may have a role in regulating morphogenesis of long bones. To approach this question, we monitored the expression of SHH, IHH, and other relevant genes in developing long bones in chick embryo limbs. We found that IHH gene expression was first turned on in the incipient diaphysis of early long bone cartilaginous anlagen present in day 6–6.5 chick embryo; at this stage, the anlagen were quite primitive and it was hard to precisely establish the maturation stage of the diaphyseal IHH-expressing chondrocytes. Once the anlagen had developed further and displayed recognizable growth plates (Fig. 1A), it became apparent that IHH expression was restricted to prehypertrophic chondrocytes (Fig. 1B, star). Strikingly, the IHH-expressing prehypertrophic chondrocytes were surrounded by a thin intramembranous bone collar that was recognizable histologically (Fig. 1A, arrow) and was characterized by very strong gene expression of type I collagen (Fig. 1C, arrow) and staining by alizarin red (Fig. 1D, arrow). There was no bone collar nor strong type I collagen gene expression in perichondrial tissues adjacent to proliferating or more immature epiphyseal chondrocytes that did not express IHH (Fig. 1A–D, arrowheads). We confirmed our data in a recent study showing selective expression of the bone-characteristic matrix protein osteopontin in the incipient bone collar flanking IHH-expressing prehypertrophic chondrocytes *(8)*. Thus, our data clearly showed that expression of IHH coincides with formation of a bone collar, indicating that the two events may be causally related.

To strengthen that conclusion, we conducted studies *(9)* with two mesenchymal-osteogenic cell lines, C3H10T1/2 and MC3T3-E1. We found that both cell lines express the hedgehog receptor Patched. When the cells were treated with recombinant IHH or SHH, alkaline phosphatase activity and mineralization were induced; these effects were synergistically enhanced by cotreatment with both hedgehog protein and bone morphogenetic protein-2 (BMP-2) compared with hedgehog treatment alone. Reverse transcription polymerase chain reaction analysis revealed that hedgehog protein treatment stimulated expression of Patched, but left expression of BMP-2, -4, -5, -6, and -7 unchanged. Together, the data demonstrated for the first time that hedgehog proteins act directly on osteoprogenitor cells to induce differentiation. They demonstrated also that a positive feedback loop exists in these cells between hedgehog protein and its receptor Patched. This loop may account for the strong and selective expression of Patched in perichondrial cells surrounding IHH-expressing prehypertrophic chondrocytes seen in long bone anlagen in vivo *(5,6,10)*. That is, IHH produced by the prehypertrophic chondrocytes, may diffuse into the perichondrium where it would trigger Patched gene expression as well as osteogenic cell differentiation and bone collar formation (as our model shown in Fig. 6 prescribes). As pointed out above, our data and conclusions are supported by the very recent report that in IHH-null mice there is no ossification in the limb *(10)*.

NEED FOR RETINOID SIGNALING IN ENDOCHONDRAL OSSIFICATION

In a series of previous studies from our laboratory (ref. *16* and refs. therein), we had provided evidence that retinoic signaling promotes the development of immature chondrocytes into hypertrophic chondrocytes in vitro. We found that upon induction by retinoids, the cells progress to the terminal stage of maturation and closely resemble the posthypertrophic cells present at the chondro-osseous border in the growth plate in vivo. The phenotypic traits expressed by the retinoid-induced chondrocytes include a very large cell diameter, production of mineralization-competent matrix vesicles, ability to deposit apatitic crystals and high alkaline phosphatase activity. Because all these traits are actually needed for the transition from mineralized hypertrophic cartilage to endochondral bone, our data suggested that by inducing such traits, retinoid signaling may be required for cartilage-to-bone transition in vivo. Thus, we conducted additional studies to obtain evidence in support of this important conclusion; these studies have been reported *(8)* and only key findings are shown here.

In a first set of experiments, we asked whether expression of retinoid nuclear receptors is upregulated in prehypertrophic and/or hypertrophic chondrocytes. We reasoned that such upregulation may be necessary for retinoids to act on those cells and promote terminal maturation into mineralizing posthypertrophic chondrocytes ready for replacement by bone cells. Thus, we used *in situ* hybridization to monitor expression of RARα, RARβ, and RARγ during long bone development in the embryonic limb. As above, we first examined newly emerged cartilaginous anlagen in young day 5.5 chick embryo limb; these anlagen are composed entirely of immature chondrocytes, display a still primitive morphological organization, and do not contain growth plates. We found that in these anlagen, the expression of RARα and RARγ was quite broad and diffuse throughout the cartilaginous tissue and that RARβ expression was strong in incipient perichondrial cells. We then examined older day 9 through day 18 skeletal elements that display typical elongated morphologies, well-defined diaphysis and epiphyses, and obvious growth plates (Fig. 2A). At these stages, RARα expression remained uniform, broad, and relatively low throughout the cartilaginous tissue (Fig. 2B), whereas RARβ remained confined to perichondrial tissue. Interestingly, expression of RARγ was sharply and selectively upregulated in hypertrophic chondrocytes (Fig. 2C). Identity of the hypertrophic cells was based on their large cell size and location as well as strong expression of a typical marker, type X collagen (Fig. 2D). Equally interesting was the finding that there was a sharp boundary and minimal overlap between RARγ expression in hypertrophic chondrocytes and IHH expression in the preceding prehypertrophic chondrocyte zone (cfr. Fig. 2C,E). Type II collagen was uniformly strong from epiphysis to early hypertropic zone (Fig. 2F).

Having shown that there is a selective upregulation of RARγ in hypertrophic chondrocytes, we conducted a second set of studies to determine whether these and/or other chondrocytes contain endogenous retinoids serving as RAR ligands. To approach this question, we used a bioassay commonly employed to determine endogenous retinoid levels in embryonic tissues; the bioassay is very sensitive, requires small amounts of tissue, and is thus ideal for analyses of scarce specimens such as embryonic tissues *(19)*. It consists of an F9 cell line stably transfected with a retinoid sensitive RARE/β-galactosidase construct; the cell line is exposed to tissue extracts, reporter activity increases in proportion to retinoid content in the extracts, and reporter activity is finally measured biochemically or histochemically. Accordingly, we isolated whole cartilaginous elements from day 5.5, 8.5, and 10 embryos by

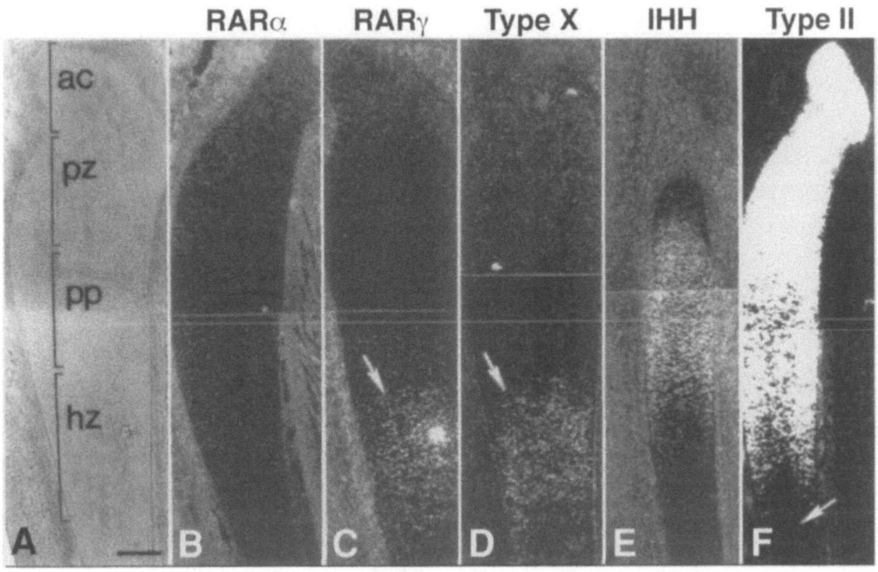

Fig. 2. *In situ* hybridization analysis of expression of indicated genes in day 10 chick embryo ulna. Arrows in **C** and **D** point to hypertrophic chondrocytes expressing RARγ and type X collagen. ac, articular cap; pz, proliferative zone; pp, prehypertrophic zone; and hz, hypertrophic zone. Bar = 185 μm.

microsurgical procedures; for comparison, we isolated other tissues and organs from the same embryos, including the perichondrial tissues immediately adjacent to the cartilages. About 100 mg of each sample were homogenized and extracted, and extracts were added to the reporter cell line; 24 h later, cultures were stained histochemically for β-galactosidase. Standards included cultures receiving known amounts of natural retinoids, such as all-*trans*-retinoic acid or 9-*cis*-retinoic acid. We found that at each stage studied, the cartilaginous elements contained endogenous retinoids (Fig. 3A,C). These levels were higher than those in brain but much lower than those in liver. Surprisingly and unexpectedly, extremely large amounts of retinoids were present in perichondrial tissues (Fig. 3B,D); on a tissue wet weight basis, these amounts were comparable to those in liver. Very similar observations were made in a recent study with a transgenic mouse carrying a RARE/β-galactosidase reporter construct that is activated by endogenous retinoids *(17)*; the authors found that strong β-galactosidase activity (and hence high retinoid content) was present in perichondrial tissues adjacent to the prehypertrophic and hypertrophic zones of long bone growth plate as well as in hypertrophic cartilage itself. The above data, combined with the finding of a specific RARγ upregulation in hypertrophic chondrocytes, set the stage for a third series of experiments in which we asked whether the endogenous retinoids and RARγ are actually required for chondrocyte hypertrophy and ossification in vivo. To approach this question, we made use of powerful pharmacological agents with retinoid antagonistic activity (*see* Fig. 4). Beads containing such agents were placed in the vicinity of newly formed early cartilaginous elements in the chick wing, embryos were reincubated, and effects were determined over developmental time. The major advantage of this pharmacological approach is that the antagonists can be used at specific stages of development and can be placed in contact with specific skeletal elements or portions thereof. Thus, their action and developmental consequences can be studied at the local level, minimizing the possibility that the effects are global and of a systemic nature. The RAR antagonist used was RO 41-5253 from Hoffman-LaRoche *(20)*, which exerts antagonist effects on all RARs. Three to four beads containing the antagonist were placed around the day 4.5–5.5 humeral anlagen, and embryos were examined over time. The results were dramatic. By day 10, humerus in control embryos (implanted with beads containing vehicle) had developed normally and displayed a typical elongated morphology

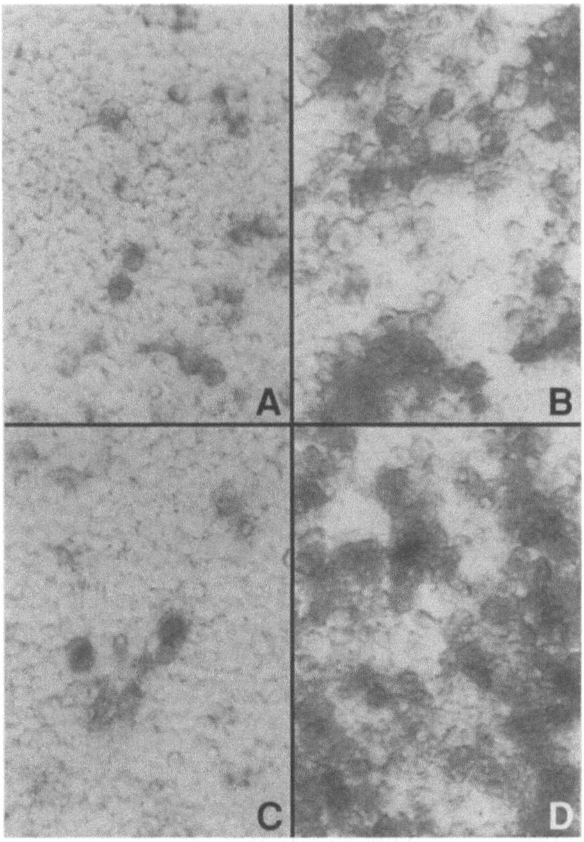

Fig. 3. Bioassay of endogenous retinoid content in cartilage (**A** and **C**) and perichondrial tissues (**B** and **D**) Tissue extracts were used to treat F9 cells stably transfected with a β-galactosidase/RARE reporter construct, and reporter activity was detected histochemically. A and C, day 8.5 and 10 chick embryo cartilage, respectively; B and D, day 8.5 and 10 perichondrial tissues, respectively.

and size; in sharp contrast, the antagonist-treated humerus was about half the length. No effects were seen in radius and ulna, attesting to the fact that the effects were limited to the site of bead implantation and were not systemic.

Histology and *in situ* hybridization provided further insights into the developmental perturbations caused by the block of retinoid signaling (Fig. 4). In control humerus, the growth plate displayed normal zones of proliferating, prehypertrophic, hypertrophic, and mineralizing chondrocytes; the metaphysis was surrounded by an intramembranous bone collar (Fig. 4A, arrowheads), and the diaphysis was undergoing invasion and replacement by endochondral bone and marrow (Fig. 4A, arrow). There was strong and typical gene expression of IHH in prehypertrophic chondrocytes (Fig. 4D, arrow), RARγ in hypertrophic chondrocytes (Fig. 4B, arrow), and osteopontin in endochondral bone (Fig. 4C). As also shown above, osteopontin expression characterized the thin intramembranous bone surrounding the IHH-expressing prehypertrophic chondrocytes (Fig. 4C, arrowhead). In sharp contrast, the antagonist-treated specimens were entirely cartilaginous and displayed no hypertrophic chondrocytes, no endochondral bone and marrow (Fig. 4E) and no expression of RARγ (Fig. 4F). Interestingly, IHH expression was not only present but seemed broader than control (Fig. 4H, arrows), and the metaphyseal–diaphyseal portion was surrounded by a conspicuous intramembranous bone collar (Fig. 4E, arrowhead) strongly expressing osteopontin (Fig. 4G, arrowheads). Thus, interference with retinoid signal-

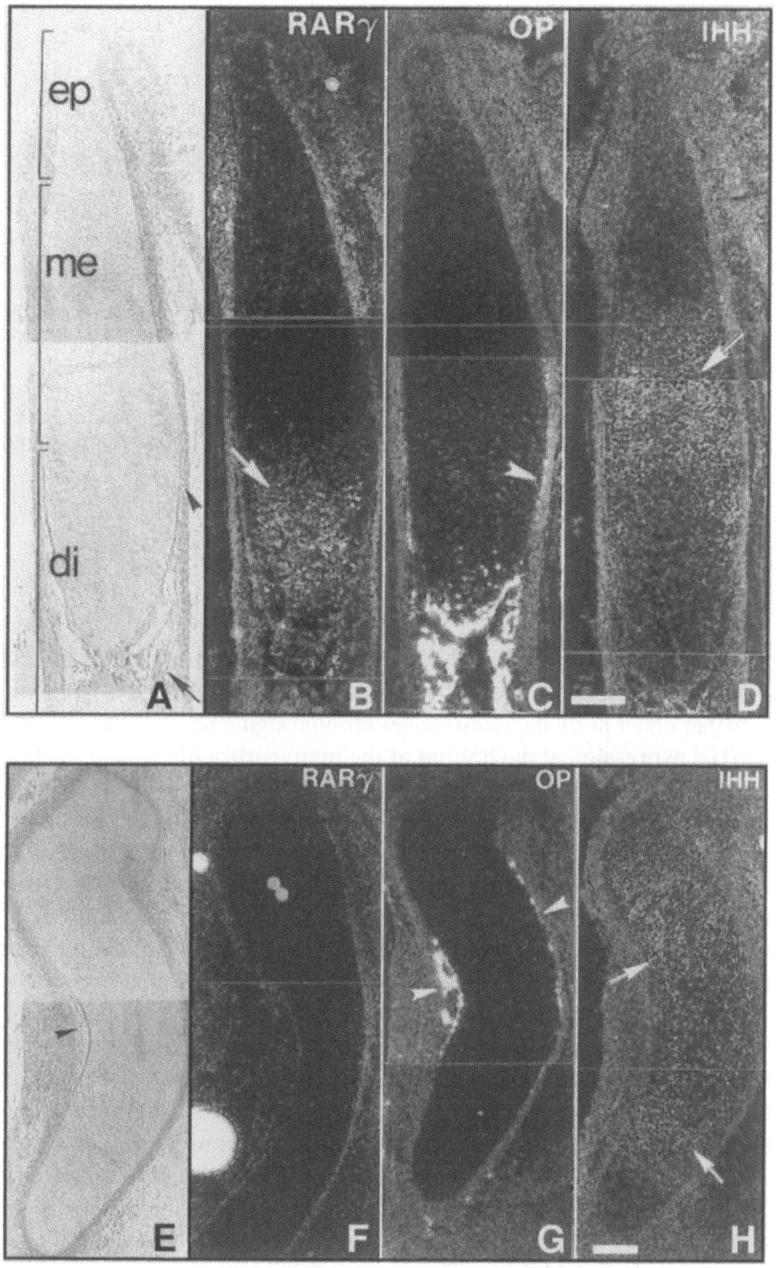

Fig. 4. *In situ* hybridization analysis of expression of indicated genes in control day 10 humerus (**A–D**) and antagonist-treated humerus (**E–H**). *See* text for details. ep, epiphysis; me, metaphysis; and di, diaphysis. Bar = 250 μm.

ing has very specific consequences on long bone development and prevents completion of this process. The chondrocytes can reach the prehypertrophic IHH-expressing stage but cannot pass it; likewise, the intramembranous bone collar forms but there is no formation of endochondral bone and marrow invasion. Retinoid signaling thus appears to be required for normal progression through the terminal phases of long bone development (*see* our model in Fig. 6).

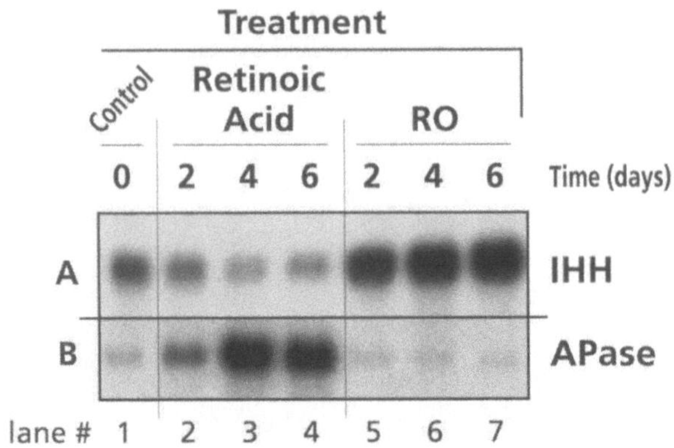

Fig. 5. Northern blot analysis of IHH and APase gene expression in cultured chondrocytes. Cells were left untreated (lane 1) or were treated with all-*trans*-retinoic acid (lanes 2–4) or antagonist (lanes 5–7) for 2, 4, and 6 d.

RETINOID SIGNALING AND IHH EXPRESSION

The *in situ* in the previous section indicate that IHH gene expression is not only maintained in antagonist-treated skeletal anlagen but appears to be broader and more extensive than in control specimens. This led us to ask whether under normal circumstances retinoid signaling may actually represent a mechanism to switch off IHH expression at the bottom of the prehypertrophic zone, thus favoring progression to the hypertrophic phase. It is worth reiterating here that turning off IHH expression may be a very important step in chondrocyte maturation because constitutive IHH expression prevents chondrocyte hypertrophy *(6)* and IHH gene ablation results in excessive and disorganized hypertrophy *(10)*. To test our hypothesis, we conducted studies with cultured chondrocytes (these preliminary experiments have not been reported and will be described in full here). As a source of chondrocytes, we used the chick embryo sternum, which allows efficient and effective isolation of chondrocyte populations at specific stages of maturation, compared with the more cumbersome long bone growth plate *(21)*. Accordingly, chondrocytes were isolated from the cephalic core portion of day 16 chick embryo sterna, which contains prehypertrophic-early hypertrophic chondrocytes at this stage *(21)*. Cells were seeded in monolayer culture and allowed to grow for a few days in complete serum-containing medium to recover from the enzymatic isolation procedure. The cells were then treated with 30 n*M* all-*trans*-retinoic acid for 2, 4, and 6 d; RNA was isolated from each culture and processed for northern blot analysis, using a cDNA probe encoding IHH. This retinoid was chosen because it is a natural retinoid and is present in the developing limb *(22)*; the dose used is precisely within the range seen in the developing limb as well *(22)*. For comparison, we determined the effects of the retinoid antagonist used above, namely RO 41-5253. The results of these experiments were clear-cut. Control untreated chondrocytes displayed obvious expression of IHH (Fig. 5A, lane 1). Upon treatment with all-*trans*-retinoic acid, IHH RNA levels were decreased markedly (Fig. 5A, lanes 2–4); on the contrary, treatment with 50 n*M* retinoid antagonist boosted IHH gene expression by several fold (Fig. 5A, lanes 5–7), in good correlation with the *in situ* data (*see* Fig. 4H). Clearly, retinoid signaling appears to represent a powerful and effective switch by which IHH gene expression is inhibited in maturing chondrocytes.

Retinoids should not only turn off gene expression of IHH but also should promote maturation and expression of hypertrophic chondrocyte-characteristic traits. Thus, we examined in the above cultures whether treatment with all-*trans*-retinoic acid or RO 41-5253 affected expression of alkaline phosphatase (APase), a typical hypertrophic cell trait. Northern hybridization showed that treatment with all-*trans*-retinoic acid led to a powerful increase in APase gene expression (Fig. 5B, lanes 2–4) compared with control values (Fig. 5B, lane 1), whereas antagonist treatment decreased it (Fig. 5B, lanes 5–7). Thus, retinoid signaling downregulates traits characteristic of prehypertrophic chondrocytes (i.e., IHH) and induces expression of hypertrophic traits (i.e., APase).

PERICHONDRIAL TISSUES AS POSITIVE REGULATORS OF CHONDROCYTE MATURATION

Perichondrial tissues adjacent to the prehypertrophic to hypertrophic zones of growth plate contain large amounts of endogenous retinoids (*see* Fig. 3), which in turn could exert a positive effect on neighboring chondrocytes and favor their maturation. To gain support for our hypothesis, we conducted the following studies.

We reasoned that if perichondrial tissues were to provide positive signals for chondrocyte maturation, hypertrophic chondrocytes should first emerge along the chondroperichondrial border in an early developing long bone anlage because chondrocytes in that location would be closer to the source of positive perichondrially derived signals. To test this possibility, we systematically examined the development of long bone anlagen between day 7.5 and day 9.0 of chick embryogenesis. We knew from previous observations that a day 7.5 anlage contains chondrocytes up to the prehypertrophic stage but does not contain hypertrophic cells yet; conversely, a day 9 anlage displays a clear hypertrophic zone in the diaphysis. Thus, we prepared longitudinal sections of limbs from day 7.5 through day 9 chick embryos and processed them for histology and *in situ* hybridization by using type X collagen as a molecular marker of chondrocyte hypertrophy. We found that the first hypertrophic type X collagen-expressing hypertrophic chondrocytes emerged on day 8.5 of development and were indeed located along the chondroperichondrial border; no such cells were present in the center where the distance from the border is greater (not shown; *see* Fig. 8 in ref. *8*). By day 9, hypertrophic chondrocytes had formed a "zone," that is, they were uniformly present from border to border.

To corroborate this finding, we performed another experiment. We implanted a single bead containing the retinoid antagonist RO 41-5253 next to the incipient diaphysis of a day 5.5 humerus anlage and reincubated the embryos until day 8.5. Because the antagonist emanates from a single bead, it creates a concentration gradient in its surroundings *(23)*, including one from the near side (closest to the bead) to the far site of anlage's diaphysis. If so, the antagonist should block the emergence of type X collagen-expressing chondrocytes in the near side but may not do so in the far side. *In situ* hybridization on longitudinal sections of day 8.5 control and antagonist-treated humerus showed that this prediction was correct. Type X collagen-containing chondrocytes were present only on the far side and were absent in the near side (not shown; manuscript in preparation). Together, the data clearly indicate that the chondroperichondrial border serves as the initial site for emergence of hypertrophic chondrocytes. This site may thus have special promaturation properties, including presence of promaturation retinoids.

CONCLUSIONS AND A MODEL

The lines of evidence presented here and in previous reports provide strong evidence that the hedgehog and retinoid signaling pathways participate in, and regulate, long bone development. These pathways act within zones of the growth plate to regulate behavior and function of resident cells as well as amongst different growth plate zones. The latter is exemplified by the ability of IHH produced in the prehypertrophic zone to influence mitotic activity in the preceding proliferative zone. In addition, these pathways appear to be able to mediate interactions between chondrocytes and surrounding perichondrial tissues. This is suggested by the involvement of chondrocyte-derived IHH in bone collar formation and of perichondrium-derived retinoids in chondrocyte function. Thus, these pathways represent critical signaling mechanisms that are interrelated and interdependent, counteract and counterbalance each other's actions, and ultimately orchestrate long bone development. Their respective roles are depicted in the model shown in Fig. 6, which can be summarized as follows: (1) In the growth

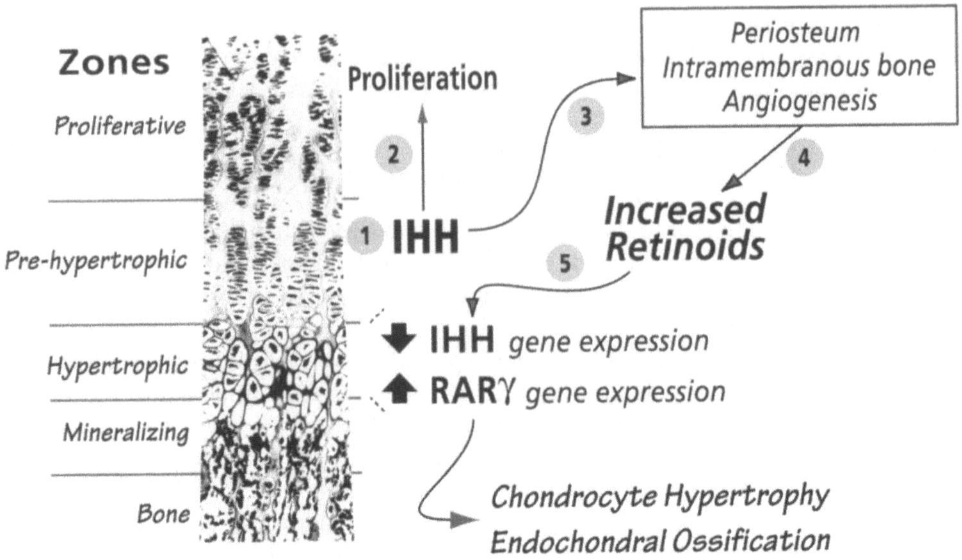

Fig. 6. Model depicting the distinct but interrelated roles of IHH and retinoid signaling in long bone development. *See* text for details.

plate of developing long bone anlagen, IHH expression is turned on in prehypertrophic chondrocytes (step 1); (2) IHH diffuses, reaches chondrocytes in the preceding proliferative zone, and regulates their mitotic activity and maturation rates (step 2); (3) IHH also reaches perichondrial cells and induces intramembranous ossification. This would require a transition from perichondrium to periosteum, angiogenesis and/or vessel recruitment, and osteogenesis (step 3); (4) The intramembranous process causes or is accompanied by a marked upregulation of retinoid synthesis or delivery of retinoids from perichondrium/periosteum-associated blood vessels (step 4); and (5) The retinoids diffuse into the adjacent cartilage, switch off IHH expression and turn on RARγ expression, and promote terminal maturation of chondrocytes and endochondral ossification (step 5).

The model correlates well with recent data on the roles of IHH in chondrocyte proliferation and osteogenesis in developing long bones *(24–27)*. For example, we and others have shown that IHH is a direct stimulator of chondrocyte proliferation *(25–27)* and that IHH is located in both prehypertrophic and proliferative zones of the growth plate *(28,29)*. In addition, the importance of retinoid signaling in cartilage maturation, matrix mineralization and osteogenesis has been reiterated by elegant recent studies *(30–32)*. One particularly interesting insight is that retinoid signaling regulates expression of Cbfa1/Runx2 *(31–33)*, a master regulator of chondrocyte hypertrophy and osteoblast differentiation *(34)*. The model prescribes also that angiogenesis is an important aspect of long bone development and may actually have previously unsuspected roles *(8)*. Blood vessels have long been known to be required for osteogenesis and marrow formation. In step 4 of the above model, however, we speculate that blood vessels may also be required at an earlier step during long bone development that is at the level of prehypertrophic/hypertrophic chondrocytes where the vessels would deliver retinoids or stimulate local production of them. The resulting increase in retinoid signaling would promote further cartilage maturation, hypertrophy and endochondral ossification. Indeed, we and others have shown recently that pharmacological or genetic interference with angiogenesis has severe repercussions on not only osteogenesis but also chondrocyte maturation in developing long bones *(28,35)*. When blood vessels did not form normally, chondrocyte maturation was delayed and the cells failed to display traits of their terminally mature phenotype.

It is important to point out here work by others indicating that perichondrium is a negative regulator of cartilage maturation *(36,37)* rather than a positive regulator as we propose. Before addressing this important issue, it should be remembered that perichondrium is not a homogeneous and static structure. It is composed of cell layers with different organization, phenotype and function *(38,39)*, and its phenotype and gene expression patterns change dramatically depending on its location along the epiphyseal–diaphyseal axis *(40,41)*. Thus, it is actually possible that perichondrium has both negative and positive roles in long bone development and such differing functions depend on its topographical location/phenotype. In the epiphyses and proximal metaphyses where immature chondrocytes reside, perichondrium could have a negative role on maturation, would help the cells to remain proliferative and immature, and would clearly demarcate the cartilage boundary. In distal metaphyseal and diaphyseal regions instead, perichondrium would undergo a phenotypic change and favor/permit maturation as well as invasion of hypertrophic cartilage by progenitor bone and marrow cells and vessels. Although speculative at the moment, this possibility offers an explanation for the fact that cartilage does become hypertrophic and thus, mechanisms must exist to allow it to do so. Should perichondrium be such a powerful negative regulator of maturation as suggested by others, cartilage would never mature. These considerations and speculations underline the fact that much remains to be learned about long bone development and that exciting insights are to be expected by current unabating interest in limb skeletogenesis.

ACKNOWLEDGMENTS

We thank Dr. W. Abrams for help with preparation of figures and our colleagues Drs. S. L. Adams, T. Kirsch, and M. Iwamoto, who participated in the original studies upon which this chapter is based. Original work was supported by NIH grants AR46000 and AR47543 to M.P.

REFERENCES

1. Fell, H. B. (1925) The histogenesis of cartilage and bone in the long bones of the embryonic fowl. *J. Morphol. Physiol.* **40,** 417–459.
2. Thorogood, P. (1983) Morphogenesis of cartilage, in *Cartilage* (Hall, B. K., ed.), vol. 2. Academic Press, New York, pp. 223–254.
3. Hinchcliffe, J. R. and Johnson, D. R. (1990) *The Development of the Vertebrate Limb*, Clarendon Press, Oxford.
4. Bitgood, M. J. and McMahon, A. P. (1995) Hedgehog and Bmp genes are coexpressed at many diverse sites of cell-cell interaction in the mouse embryo. *Dev. Biol.* **172,** 126–138.
5. Vortkamp, A., Lee, K., Lanske, B., Segre, G. V., Kronenberg, H. M., and Tabin, C. J. (1996) Regulation of the rate of cartilage differentiation by Indian hedgehog and PTH-related protein. *Science* **273,** 613–622.
6. Vortkampt, A., Pathi, S., Peretti, G. M., Caruso, E. M., Zaleske, D. J., and Tabin, C. J. (1998) Recapitulation of signals regulating embryonic bone formation during postnatal growth and in fracture repair. *Mech. Dev.* **71,** 65–76.
7. Koyama, E., Leatherman, J. L., Noji, S., and Pacifici, M. (1996) Early chick limb cartilaginous elements possess polarizing activity and express hedgehog-related morphogenetic factors. *Dev. Dyn.* **207,** 344–354.
8. Koyama, E., Golden, E. B., Vaias, L., Kirsch, T., Adams, S. L., Chandraratna, R. A. S., et al. (1999) Retinoid signaling is required for chondrocyte maturation and endochondral bone formation during limb skeletogenesis. *Dev. Biol.* **208,** 375–391.
9. Nakamura, T., Aikawa, T., Enomoto-Iwamoto, M., Iwamoto, M., Higuchi, Y., Pacifici, M., et al. (1997) Induction of osteogenic differentiation by hedgehog proteins. *Biochem. Biophys. Res. Commun.* **237,** 465–469.
10. St-Jacques, B., Hammerschidt, M., and McMahon, A. P. (1999) Indian hedgehog signaling regulates proliferation and differentiation of chondrocytes and is essential for bone formation. *Genes Dev.* **13,** 2076–2086.
11. Walbach, S. B. and Hegsted, D. M. (1952) Vitamin A deficiency in the duck. Skeletal growth and the central nervous system. *Arch. Pathol.* **54,** 548–563.
12. Chambon, P. (1994) The retinoid signaling pathway: molecular and genetic analyses. *Semin. Cell Biol.* **5,** 115–125.
13. Mangelsdorf, D. J., Umesono, K., and Evans, R. M. (1994) The retinoid receptors, in *The Retinoids: Biology, Chemistry, and Medicine.* (Sporn, M. B., et al., eds.), Raven Press, New York, pp. 319–349.
14. Dolle, P., Ruberte, E., Kastner, P., Petkovich, M., Stoner, C. M., Gudas, L. J., et al. (1989) Differential expression of genes encoding α, β and γ retinoic acid receptors and CRABP in the developing limbs of the mouse. *Nature* **342,** 702–705.
15. Mendelsohn, C., Lohnes, D., Decimo, D., Lufkin, T., LeLeur, M., Chambon, P., et al. (1994) Function of the retinoic acid receptors (RARs) during development. II. Multiple abnormalities at various stages of organogenesis in RAR double mutants. *Development* **120,** 2749–2771.

16. Iwamoto, M., Shapiro, I. M., Yagami, K., Boskey, A. L., Leboy, P. S., Adams, S. L., et al. (1993) Retinoic acid induces rapid mineralization and expression of mineralization-related genes in chondrocytes. *Exp. Cell Res.* **207,** 413–420.
17. von Schroder, H. P. and Heersche, J. N. M. (1998) Retinoic acid responsiveness of cells and tissues in developing fetal limbs evaluated in a RAREhsplacZ transgenic mouse model. *J. Orthop. Res.* **16,** 355–364.
18. Riddle, R. D., Johnson, R. L., Laufer, E., and Tabin, C. (1993) Sonic hedgehog mediates the polarizing activity of the ZPA. *Cell* **75,** 1401–1416.
19. Wagner, M., Han, B., and Jessell, T. M. (1992) Regional differences in retinoid release from embryonic neural tissue detected by an in vitro reporter assay. *Development* **116,** 55–66.
20. Keidel, S., LeMotte, P., and Apfel, C. (1994) Different agonist- and antagonist-induced conformational changes in retinoic acid receptors analyzed by protease mapping. *Mol. Cell Biol.* **14,** 287–298.
21. Gibson, G. J. and Flint, M. H. (1985) Type X collagen syntheiss by chick sternal cartilage and its relationship to endochondral development. *J. Cell Biol.* **101,** 277–284.
22. Eichele, G. and Thaller, C. (1987) Characterization of concentration gradients of a morphogenetically active retinoid in the chick limb bud. *J. Cell Biol.* **105,** 1917–1923.
23. Eichele, G., Tickle, C., and Alberts, B. (1984) Micro-controlled release of biologically active compounds in chick embryos: beads of 200-μm diameter for the local release of retinoids. *Anal. Biochem.* **142,** 542–555.
24. Chung, U.-I., Schipani, E., McMahon, A. P., and Kronenberg, H. M. (2001) Indian hedgehog couples chondrogenesis to osteogenesis in endochondral bone development. *J. Clin. Invest.* **107,** 295–304.
25. Long, F., Zhang, X. M., Karp, S., Yang, Y., and McMahon, A. P. (2001) Genetic manipulation of hedgehog signaling in the endochondral skeleton reveals a direct role in the regulation of chondrocyte proliferation. *Development* **128,** 5099–5108.
26. Wu, Q., Zhang, Y., and Chen, Q. (2001) Indian hedgehog is an essential component of mechanotransduction complex to stimulate chondrocyte proliferation. *J. Biol. Chem.* **276,** 35290–35296.
27. Gentili, C., Koyama, E., Iwamoto, M., and Pacifici, M. (2002) Indian hedgehog mediates multiple chondrocyte functions in the growth plate. *Trans. Orth. Res. Soc.* **48,** 122.
28. Yin, M., Gentili, C., Koyama, E., Zasloff, M., and Pacifici, M. (2002) Antiangiogenic treatment delays chondrocyte maturation and bone formation during limb skeletogenesis. *J. Bone Miner. Res.* **17,** 56–65.
29. Gritli-Linde, A., Lewis, P., McMahon, A. P., and Linde, A. (2001) The whereabouts of a morphogen: direct evidence for short- and graded long-range activity of hedgehog signaling peptides. *Dev. Biol.* **236,** 364–386.
30. Wang, W. and Kirsch, T. (2002) Retinoic acid stimulates annexin-mediated growth plate chondrocyte mineralization. *J. Cell Biol.* **157,** 1061–1070.
31. Jimenez, M. J., Balbin, M., Alvarez, J., Komori, T., Bianco, P., Holmbeck, K., et al. (2001) A regulatory cascade involving retinoic acid, Cbfa1, and matrix metalloproteinases is coupled to the development of a process of perichondrial invasion and osteogenic differentiation during bone formation. *J. Cell Biol.* **155,** 1333–1344.
32. Iwamoto, M., Koyama, E., Enomoto-Iwamoto, M., Golden, E. B., Adams, S. L., and Pacifici, M. (2001) Indian hedgehog and Cbfa1 expression in growth plate chondrocytes is regulated by retinoid signaling. *Proc. Orthop. Res. Soc.* **47,** 352.
33. Iwamoto, M., Kitagaki, J., Tamamura, Y., Gentili, C., Koyama, E., Enomoto, H., et al. (2003) Runx2 expression and action in chondrocytes are regulated by retinoid signaling and parathyroid hormone-related peptide. *Osteoarthr. Cart.* **11,** 6–15.
34. Komori, T., Yagi, H., Nomura, S., Yamaguchi, A., Sasaki, K., Deguchi, K., et al. (1997) Targeted disruption of Cbfa1 results in a complete lack of bone formation owing to maturation arrest of osteoblasts. *Cell* **89,** 755–764.
35. Zelser, E., McLean, W., Ng, Y., Fukai, N., Reginato, A. M., Lovejoy, S., et al. (2002) Skeletal defects in $VEGF^{120/120}$ mice reveal multiple roles for VEGF in skeletogenesis. *Development* **129,** 1893–1904.
36. Long, F. and Linsenmayer, T. F. (1998) Regulation of growth region cartilage proliferation and differentiation by perichondrium. *Development* **125,** 1067–1073.
37. Alvarez, J., Sohn, P., Zeng, X., Doetschman, T., Robbins, D. J., and Serra, R. (2002) TGFβ2 mediates the effects of hedgehog on hypertrophic differentiation and PTHrP expression. *Development* **129,** 1913–1924.
38. Pechak, D. G., Kujawa, M. J., and Caplan, A. I. (1986) Morphological and histochemical events during first bone formation in embryonic chick limbs. *Bone* **7,** 441–458.
39. Gigante, A., Specchia, N., Nori, S., and Greco, F. (1996) Distribution of elastic fiber types in the epiphyseal region. *J. Orthop. Res.* **14,** 810–817.
40. Koyama, E., Shimazu, A., Leatherman, J. L., Golden, E. B., Nah, H.-D., and Pacifici, M. (1996) Expression of syndecan-3 and tenascin-C: possible involvement in periosteum development. *J. Orthop. Res.* **14,** 403–412.
41. Koyama, E., Leatherman, J. L., Shimazu, A., Nah, H.-D., and Pacifici, M. (1995) Syndecan-3, tenascin-C, and the development of cartilaginous skeletal elements and joints in chick limbs. *Dev. Dyn.* **203,** 152–162.

III
Osteoblastic Cell Differentiation

12

Synergy Between Osteogenic Protein-1 and Osteotropic Factors in the Stimulation of Rat Osteoblastic Cell Differentiation

John C. Lee and Lee-Chuan C. Yeh

INTRODUCTION

Osteoblastic cell differentiation and proliferation are multistep processes involving numerous growth factors and signaling molecules in a regulated manner that is highly complex and not yet fully understood. Osteogenic Protein-1 (OP-1), a member of the bone morphogenetic protein (BMP) subfamily of the transforming growth factor-β (TGF-β) superfamily *(1–5)*, induces new bone formation in vivo *(6,7)*. In different osteoblastic cell cultures, including fetal rat calvaria (FRC) cells and human osteosarcoma cell lines, the recombinant human OP-1 stimulates synthesis of various biochemical markers characteristic of osteoblastic cell differentiation in a defined spatial and temporal manner *(6,8–12)*. OP-1 also stimulates synthesis of other growth factors, such as insulin-like growth factor (IGF)-I *(13–15)*. Knowledge of the functional relationship between OP-1 and these growth factors will not only further our understanding of the mechanism of the inductive action of OP-1 but also the osteoblastic cell differentiation.

The fact that OP-1 stimulates osteoblastic cell differentiation and IGF-I gene expression led to the hypothesis that the action of OP-1 on osteoblastic cell differentiation is, at least in part, through the IGF-I system. Several recent findings lend credence to this hypothesis. First, OP-1 and IGF-I synergistically stimulate FRC cell differentiation and proliferation in a dose- and time-dependent manner *(16)*. Maximal enhancement between OP-1 and IGF-I was observed when both proteins were added simultaneously. Synergy was not observed in FRC cells pretreated with IGF-I. These observations suggest that IGF-I acts on OP-1-sensitized cells. Second, coincubation of OP-1 and an antisense oligonucleotide corresponding to the IGF-I mRNA sequence reduced the OP-1-induced elevation in alkaline phosphatase (AP) activity by approx 40% *(15)*. Third, we recently reported that OP-1 and interleukin (IL)-6 in the presence of its soluble receptor (IL-6sR) synergistically stimulated FRC cell differentiation without having a significant effect on cell proliferation *(17)*. Maximal synergy was observed in cells treated with OP-1, IL-6, and IL-6sR simultaneously. IL-6 and IL-6sR are known to enhance IGF-I gene expression in FRC cells *(18)*. However, the possibility that other signaling pathways, in addition to the IGF-I pathway, might also be involved in the synergy between OP-1 and IL-6 plus IL-6sR should not be overlooked.

The objective of the present work was to examine the effects of osteotropic factors on OP-1 action. Three factors that are known to affect IGF-I expression were selected for the present study: human growth

From: *The Skeleton: Biochemical, Genetic, and Molecular Interactions in Development and Homeostasis*
Edited by: E. J. Massaro and J. M. Rogers © Humana Press Inc., Totowa, NJ

hormone (hGH), prostaglandin E2 (PGE2), and parathyroid hormone (PTH). Several excellent reviews have been published recently on these factors (e.g., refs. *19–22*), the following provides only a brief review of these factors, focusing on their actions on gene expression at the cellular level and on those that are closely related to the current topic.

Human Growth Hormone

Numerous studies show that hGH is required for normal bone remodeling (*see* reviews in refs. *19* and *20*). At the cellular level, the high-affinity GH receptors are present in osteoblasts and the binding capacity is higher in differentiated cells. The binding of GH stimulates osteoblastic cell proliferation *(23)*, IGF-I synthesis *(24)*, and IL-6 synthesis *(25)*. Conversely, the IGF binding protein-5 stimulates GH synthesis in the osteosarcoma UMR cells *(26)*. A feedback regulatory pathway between GH and IGF-I has been proposed *(27)*. Additionally, GH induces BMP-2 and -4 expression and BMPR-IA in developing rat periodontium *(28)*.

Prostaglandins

Ample data show that prostaglandins have important physiological roles in skeletal metabolism *(21)*. PGE2 stimulates IGF-I synthesis, upregulates the IGF-I receptor, and increases both the synthesis and the degradation of IGFBP-5 *(29–34)*. PGE2 also stimulates OP-1 expression *(35)* and bone nodule formation in adult rat calvaria cells *(36)*.

PTH

The effects of PTH, a protein consisting of 82 amino acids, on bone formation have been widely studied both in vivo and in vitro, although the mechanisms of action remain to be fully established *(22)*. Most intriguing is the fact that PTH exhibits both anabolic and catabolic effects, presumably dependent on the mode of administration. An anabolic effect usually results when PTH is administrated intermittently, and a catabolic effect results when it is continuously administrated. At the cellular level, PTH affects gene expression in osteoblasts. For example, PTH stimulates *c-fos* expression *(37)* and several nuclear matrix proteins *(38)* but inhibits expression of type I collagen *(39)*. PTH also stimulates matrix metalloproteinases and cytokines that regulate matrix metabolism, for example, IL-6 and IL-11 *(40–42)*. PTH stimulates IGF-I mRNA and protein in cultured newborn rat calvaria cells *(43)* as well as in vivo *(44)*.

RESULTS

Effects of OP-1 and hGH on FRC Cell Differentiation

To examine whether hGH affects OP-1 action in primary cultures of FRC cells, confluent cultures were treated with OP-1 in the presence of varying concentrations of hGH. Two markers were used to monitor the effects: AP activity, as a short-term biochemical marker, and nodule formation, as a long-term marker of bone formation in cell cultures. Figure 1 shows that hGH alone in the concentration range tested did not alter the basal AP activity. OP-1 stimulated AP activity by approximately twofold above the control. Treatment of FRC cells with a combination of a fixed concentration of OP-1 with varying concentrations of hGH resulted in a dose-dependent enhancement of the OP-1-induced AP activity. A maximum of approx 7- and 3.5-fold stimulation beyond the control and the OP-1 alone-treated cultures, respectively, was observed at 1000 ng/mL of hGH.

Continuous treatment of long-term cultures (15 d) of FRC cells with hGH significantly enhanced the number of mineralized bone nodule formed (Fig. 2). In agreement with the AP results, low concentrations of hGH did not affect the OP-1-induced bone nodule formation. Higher concentrations of hGH (>10 ng/mL) potentiated the OP-1-induced formation of nodules. The enhancement of OP-1-induced nodule formation was most evident in cultures treated with 200 ng/mL of OP-1 and 100 ng/mL of hGH.

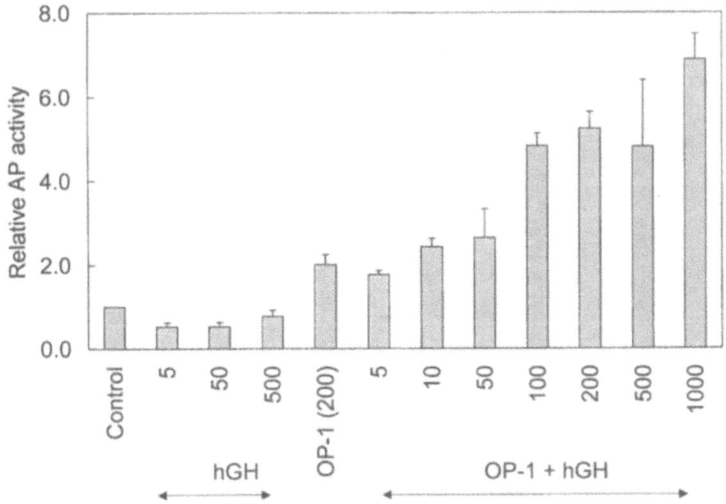

Fig. 1. Effects of recombinant hGH on the OP-1-induced AP activity in FRC cells. Confluent cells were treated with solvent, OP-1 (200 ng/mL) alone, recombinant hGH (5, 50, or 500 ng/mL) alone, or OP-1 (200 ng/mL) in the presence of varying concentrations of hGH (5 to 1000 ng/mL) for 48 h with one change of media after the first 24 h. Total AP activity in these cultures was determined. Results are normalized to the AP activity in the vehicle-treated control. Values are the means ± SEM of 12 replicates of each condition with two different FRC cell preparations.

OP-1	0	0	200	200	200	200	(ng/ml)
hGH	0	10	0	1	10	100	(ng/ml)

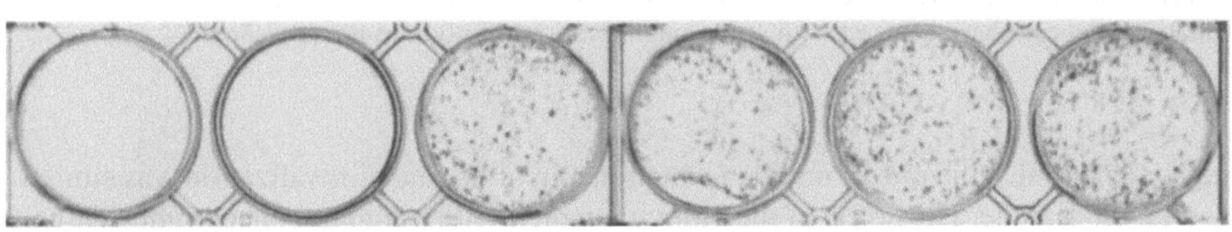

1 2 3 4 5 6

Fig. 2. Effects of recombinant hGH on the OP-1-induced bone nodule formation in FRC cells. Confluent cells grown in 12-well plates were treated with either solvent vehicle, 200 ng/mL OP-1, or OP-1 + varying concentrations of GH in αMEM+5% fetal bovine serum (supplemented with 30 μg/mL gentamicin, 100 μg/mL ascorbic acid, and 5 mM β-glycerolphosphate). Media were refreshed with the same treatments every 3 d. Progress of nodule formation was monitored every 3 d. After 15 d, the cells were fixed with formalin and photographed. Bone nodules are visible as white areas and mineralized bone nodules as dark areas.

A 23 ± 3% increase in the number of nodules was observed, in comparison with the OP-1 alone-treated cultures. hGH alone did not stimulate mineralized bone nodule formation in cultures treated continuously for as long as 15 d.

The rate of nodule formation in FRC cells treated with a fixed concentration of OP-1 and varying concentrations of hGH was also studied by following and capturing the images of individual bone nodules at regular time intervals (Fig. 3). In the OP-1-treated cultures, bone nodules (visible as white areas) were visible after 3 d of treatment and mineralized bone nodules (visible as dark nodules) were observed after 9 d of treatment. In the cultures treated with the combination of OP-1 and a low concentration of

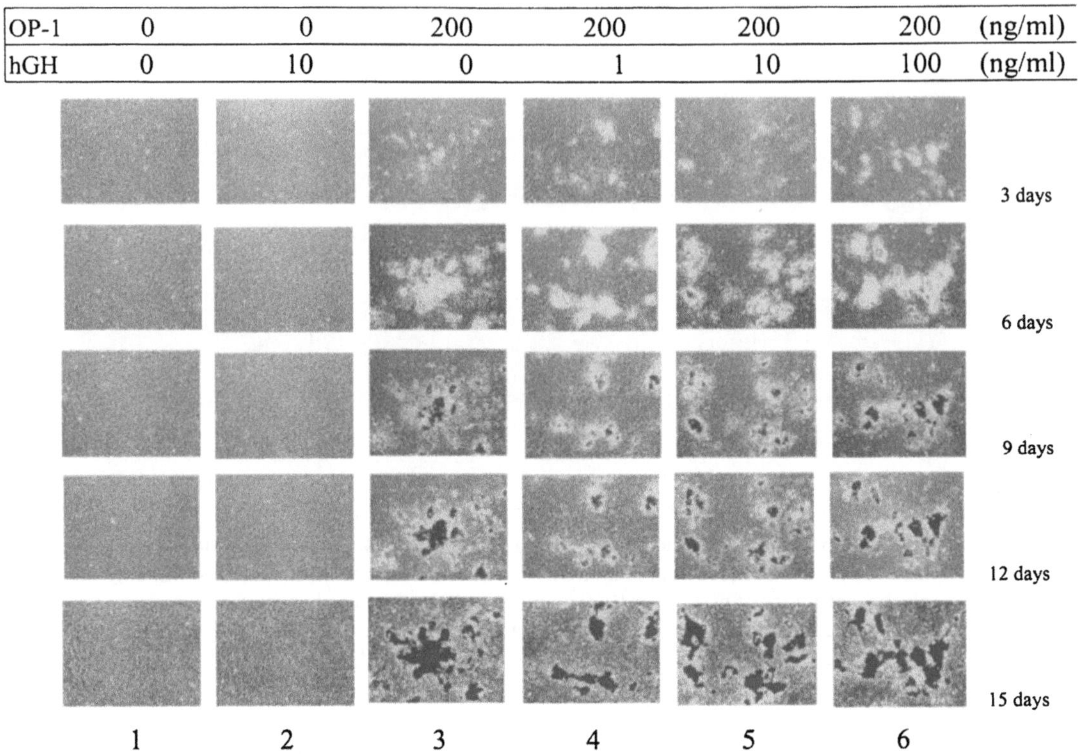

Fig. 3. Effects of recombinant hGH on the rate of bone nodule formation. Confluent FRC cells, grown in 12-well plates, were treated as described in the legend of Fig. 2. Progression of nodule formation was monitored and captured using an Olympus CK2 inverted microscope (Olympus America, Inc.) equipped with a CCD camera. Representative images (phase contrast with 100× magnification) of nodules are presented.

hGH (e.g., <10 ng/mL), the rate of nodule formation and of nodule mineralization was similar to that treated with OP-1 alone. However, in the cultures treated with a higher concentration of hGH (100 ng/mL) in the presence of OP-1, there were more mineralized nodules as early as 9 d compared with those treated with OP-1 alone. The size and number of mineralized nodules continued to increase as a function of time in culture.

Effects of OP-1 and PGE2 on FRC Cell Differentiation

To examine effects of exogenous PGE2 on the action of OP-1 in FRC cells, confluent FRC cells were treated with OP-1 in the presence of different concentrations of PGE2. The total cellular AP activity in these cultures was measured. Figure 4 shows that PGE2 alone in the concentration range tested did not alter the basal AP activity. OP-1 alone stimulated AP activity by approx twofold, and the OP-1-induced AP activity was further elevated by exogenous PGE2 in a dose-dependent manner. At 0.5 n*M* PGE2, an approx 3- and 1.5-fold stimulation was observed, compared with the control and the OP-1-induced activity, respectively. The enhancement of the OP-1-induced AP activity by PGE2 approached saturation at 0.5 n*M*.

The effect of a long-term exposure of PGE2 on OP-1-treated FRC cells was also examined. Figure 5 shows that the number of OP-1-induced bone nodules was enhanced by the presence of PGE2 in a dose-dependent manner, reaching a maximum of 46 ± 9% increase at 5 n*M* of PGE2 compared with the OP-1 alone-treated cultures. PGE2 alone did not stimulate mineralized bone nodule formation after 15 d of continuous treatment.

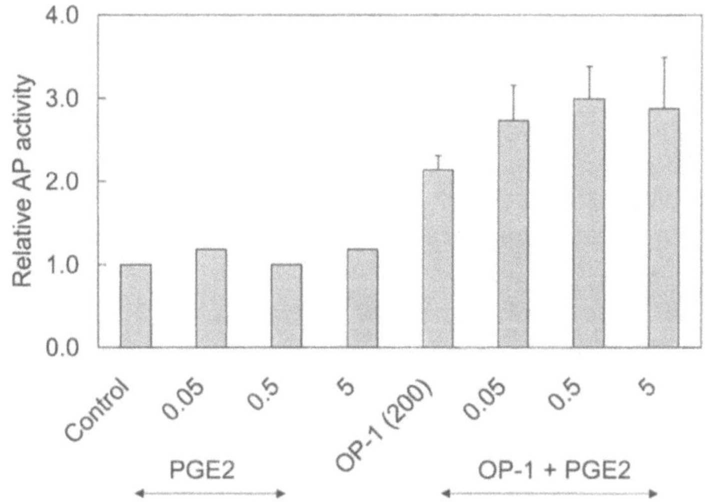

Fig. 4. Effect of PGE2 on the OP-1-induced AP activity in FRC cells. Confluent cell cultures were treated with solvent, OP-1 (200 ng/mL) alone, PGE2 (0.05, 0.5, or 5 nM) alone, or OP-1 (200 ng/mL) in the presence of varying concentrations of PGE2. *See* Fig. 1 legend for additional experimental detail. Values are the mean ± SEM of five replicates of each condition with two different FRC cell preparations.

OP-1	0	0	200	200	200	200	(ng/ml)
PGE2	0	0.5	0	0.05	0.5	5	(nM)

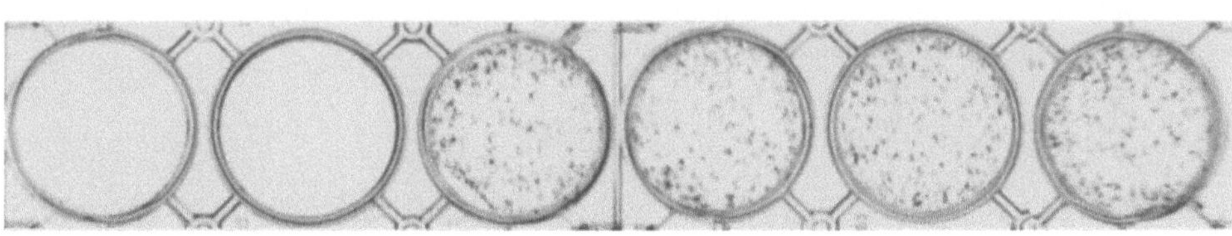

1 2 3 4 5 6

Fig. 5. Effect of PGE2 on the OP-1-induced bone nodule formation in FRC cells. Confluent cells were treated with solvent, PGE2 (0.5 nM) alone, OP-1 (200 ng/mL) alone, or OP-1 (200 ng/mL) in the presence of 0.05, 0.5, or 5 nM PGE2. *See* Fig. 2 legend for additional experimental details.

The rate of nodule formation in FRC cells treated with a fixed concentration of OP-1 and varying concentrations of PGE2 was also studied (Fig. 6). In the OP-1-treated culture, bone nodules were visible after 3 d of treatment. Mineralized bone nodules began to be detectable after 9 d of OP-1 treatment. The size and number of nodules continued to increase as a function of time in culture. In the cultures treated with the combination of OP-1 and PGE2, the rates of nodule formation and of mineralization were increased compared with those treated with OP-1 alone, in a PGE2 concentration-dependent manner. The size and number of mineralized bone nodules were significantly enhanced by PGE2.

Effects of OP-1 and PTH on FRC Cell Differentiation

The effect of exogenous PTH on OP-1 action in FRC cells was examined by treating confluent cultures with a fixed OP-1 concentration and different concentrations of PTH (1-34) for 48 h. Total cellular AP

OP-1	0	0	200	200	200	200	(ng/ml)
PGE2	0	0.5	0	0.05	0.5	5	(nM)

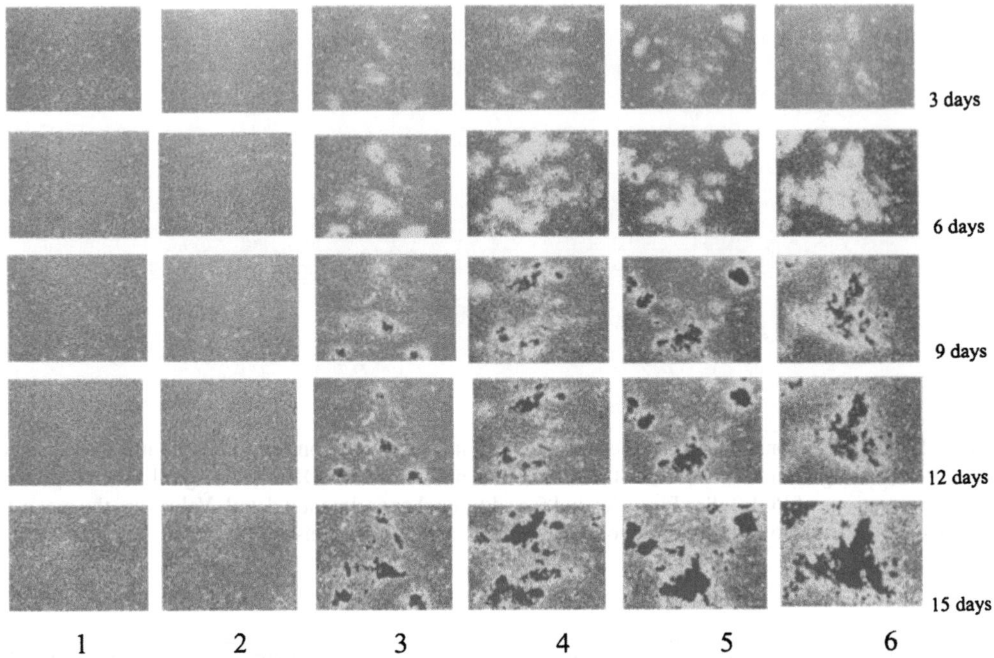

Fig. 6. Effect of PGE2 on the rate of OP-1-induced bone nodule formation in FRC cells. Confluent cells were treated with solvent, PGE2 (0.5 nM) alone, OP-1 (200 ng/mL) alone, or OP-1 (200 ng/mL) in the presence of 0.05, 0.5, or 5 nM PGE2. *See* Fig. 3 legend for additional experimental details. Representative images (phase contrast with 100× magnification) of nodules are presented.

activity was measured. As shown in Fig. 7, OP-1 by itself stimulated AP activity by approx 2.5-fold. Exogenous synthetic PTH (1-34) stimulated the OP-1-induced AP activity in FRC cells. At 0.1 n*M* PTH, a maximum stimulation of 4- and 1.7-fold above the control and the OP-1 alone-treated cultures, respectively, was observed. However, higher concentrations of PTH were less effective in increasing the OP-1-induced AP activity. PTH alone, in the concentration range tested, did not change the basal AP activity.

The effect of long-term, continuous treatment of FRC cells with PTH was also studied. Figure 8 shows that PTH alone did not stimulate bone nodule formation in FRC cells under these experimental conditions. OP-1 potentiated the formation of mineralized bone nodules. PTH inhibited the OP-1-induced formation of mineralized bone nodule (visible as dark areas) in a dose-dependent manner. However, a closer examination of the cultures treated with OP-1 and PTH (>0.1 n*M*) revealed the presence of nonmineralized nodules (visible as white areas), which increased in both size and number with increasing PTH concentration. It became more evident, as shown in Fig. 9, that PTH enhanced the OP-1-induced formation of bone nodules (visible as white areas), but inhibited the mineralization process in a dose-dependent manner.

DISCUSSION

The results presented in this report confirm that OP-1 is capable of inducing the differentiation and proliferation of FRC cells and further reveal that the induction could be significantly and syner-

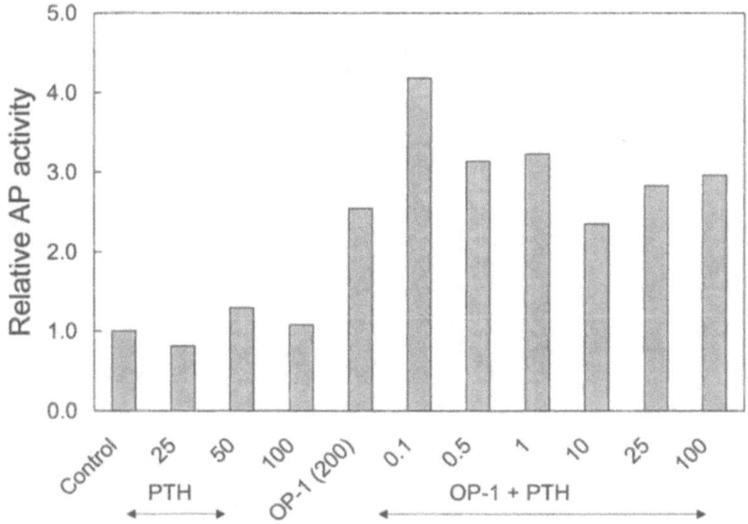

Fig. 7. Effect of PTH on the OP-1-induced AP activity in FRC cells. Confluent cell cultures were treated with solvent, OP-1 (200 ng/mL) alone, PTH (25, 50, or 100 nM) alone, or OP-1 (200 ng/mL) in the presence of varying concentrations of PTH. *See* Fig. 1 legend for additional experimental details. Values are the mean ± SEM of five replicates of each condition with two different FRC cell preparations.

OP-1	0	0	200	200	200	200	200 (ng/ml)
PTH	0	0.5	0	0.1	0.5	1	10 (nM)

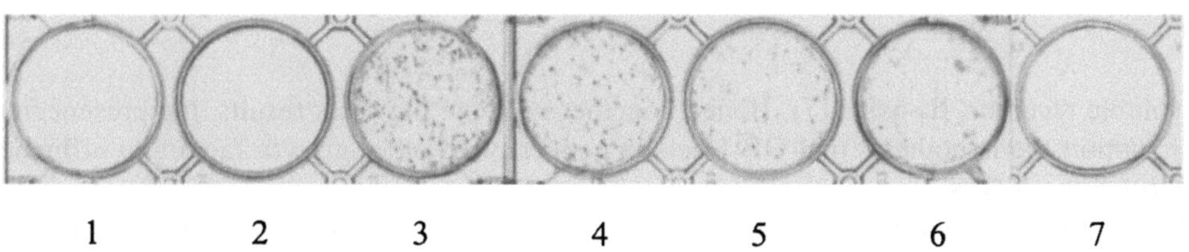

Fig. 8. Effect of exogenous PTH on the OP-1-induced bone nodule formation in FRC cells. Confluent cell cultures were treated solvent, PTH (0.5 nM) alone, OP-1 (200 ng/mL) alone, or OP-1 (200 ng/mL) in the presence of 0.1, 0.5, 1.0, or 10 nM PTH. *See* Fig. 2 legend for additional experimental details.

gistically stimulated by hGH, PGE2, and PTH. The current study shows that exogenous hGH, PGE2, and PTH did not affect the AP activity, a biochemical marker of osteoblast differentiation. A combination of OP-1 and any one of these osteotropic factors resulted in a greater stimulation of AP activity compared to OP-1 alone. Furthermore, hGH and PGE2 enhanced the OP-1 action in stimulating mineralized bone nodule formation, a hallmark of bone formation in cell cultures. PTH also enhanced the OP-1 action in stimulating nodule formation but inhibited the mineralization of these nodules. Taken together, the present studies provide biochemical and morphological evidence supporting the idea that these osteotropic agents synergistically enhance the differentiation activity of OP-1 in primary cultures of osteoblastic cells.

Previously, our laboratory showed that OP-1 and IGF-I synergistically enhance FRC cell differentiation and proliferation *(16)*. We subsequently showed synergism between OP-1 and IL-6 in the presence

OP-1	0	0	200	200	200	200	200 (ng/ml)
PTH	0	0.5	0	0.1	0.5	1	10 (nM)

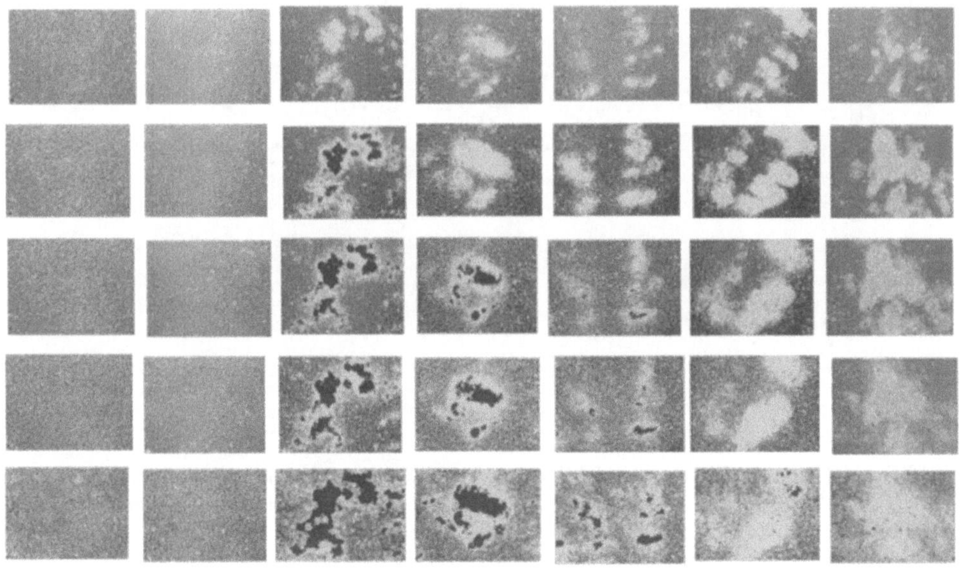

Fig. 9. Effect of PTH on the rate of OP-1-induced mineralized bone nodule formation in FRC cells. Confluent cells were treated solvent, PTH (0.5 nM) alone, OP-1 (200 ng/mL) alone, or OP-1 (200 ng/mL) in the presence of 0.1, 0.5, 1.0, or 10 nM PTH. *See* Fig. 3 legend for additional experimental details.

of its soluble receptor, IL-6sR (17). Hence, together with the previous results, the present findings further support the hypothesis that OP-1 acts in concert with other growth factors to influence the bone formation process.

Although the molecular mechanism of synergy between OP-1 and these osteotropic factors is not known at present, a common outcome of the tested osteotropic factors on a variety of osteoblastic cells is that the IGF-I expression is elevated. hGH stimulates IGF-I synthesis in human osteoblastic cells derived from trabecular explants *(24)*. PGE2 stimulates synthesis of IGF-I and several components of the IGF-I system in FRC cells *(29–34)*. PTH stimulates IGF-I mRNA and protein in cultured newborn rat calvaria cells *(43)* and in vivo *(44)*. In addition, experiments with IGF-I knockout mice showed that PTH treatment did not increase AP activity or bone mineral density, in contrast to the results obtained with the wild-type animal. The data suggest that the anabolic effects of PTH on bone formation require the presence of IGF-I *(45)*. Moreover, IL-6 with IL-6sR also enhances the levels of IGF-I mRNA and protein in a time- and dose-dependent manner in FRC cells *(18)*. Thus, we are tempted to speculate that the observed synergy between OP-1 and these different osteotropic factors may be mediated, at least partly, by the stimulation of IGF-I expression.

That additional mechanism(s) and different signal transduction systems may also be involved in the observed synergy cannot be overlooked. For example, PGE2 also stimulates OP-1 expression *(35)*. The increased OP-1 expression thus could elevate the OP-1 concentration in the cell culture media, resulting in an autocrine effect that further stimulates FRC cell differentiation. GH has also been shown to stimulate BMPR-IA expression in rat periodontium *(28)*. It is conceivable that the increase in BMPR-IA expression could also lead to enhancement of the OP-1 action.

Our observation that PTH enhanced the OP-1-induced AP activity as well as nodule formation but inhibited the mineralization process is intriguing. One possible explanation may lie on the observed differences in the in vivo effect of PTH when given continuously versus intermittently *(22)*. An earlier in vitro study revealed that PTH exerts incongruent effects on osteoblast differentiation depending on the mode of administration *(46)*.

It is noteworthy that, in several clonal cell lines, vitamin D and retinoic acid increased the actions of BMP-2 and -3, which share 60% and 42% amino acid sequence homology with OP-1 *(47–49)*. The BMP-2 stimulated AP activity was enhanced by β-estradiol, dexamethasone, and vitamin D3 in MC3T3 cells *(50)*, and, in rat bone marrow stromal cell cultures, by dexamethasone *(51)* as well as basic fibroblast growth factor *(52)*. On the contrary, higher doses of bFGF inhibited BMP-2 effect in vivo *(53)*. The combination of PGE1 and BMP-2 led to a significant increase in the mechanical strength of the cranial bone of rabbits *(54)*. Also of interest is the observation that the inductive effects of BMP-2, -4, and -6 on a fetal rat secondary calvaria cell culture system were potentiated by co- or pretreatment with the glucocorticoid triamcinolone *(55)*. Another report revealed that vitamin D3 affected osteoblastic cells in an opposite manner to OP-1 and TGF-β *(56)*. TGF-β1 has been reported to stimulate the action of OP-1 in adult baboons *(57)*. Hence, most data support the notion that a combination of BMPs with other factors may improve osteoblastic cell differentiation.

In summary, we have demonstrated a synergy between OP-1 and hGH, PGE2, and PTH in the stimulation of biochemical and morphological markers characteristic of bone cell differentiation in the primary culture of fetal rat calvaria cells. These data further suggest that a combination of OP-1 and other osteotropic factors may enhance bone formation and repair, and that the availability of growth factors locally may contribute significantly in influencing the induction of bone formation by OP-1 in vivo.

ACKNOWLEDGMENTS

This research was supported by Stryker Biotech.

REFERENCES

1. Kingsley, D. M. (1994) The TGF-beta superfamily: new members, new receptors, and new genetic tests of function in different organisms. *Genes Dev.* **8,** 133–146.
2. Ozkaynak, E., Rueger, D. C., Drier, E. A., Corbett, C., Ridge, R. J., Sampath, T. K., et al. (1990) OP-1 cDNA encodes an osteogenic protein in the TGF-beta family. *EMBO J.* **9,** 2085–2093.
3. Reddi, A. H. (2000) Bone morphogenetic proteins and skeletal development: the kidney-bone connection (review). *Pediatr. Nephrol.* **14,** 598–601.
4. Sampath, T. K., Coughlin, J. E., Whetstone, R. M., Banach, D., Corbett, C., Ridge, R. J., et al. (1990) Bovine osteogenic protein is composed of dimers of OP-1 and BMP-2A, two members of the transforming growth factor-beta superfamily. *J. Biol. Chem.* **265,** 13198–13205.
5. Wozney, J. M. and Rosen, V. (1998) Bone morphogenetic protein and bone morphogenetic protein gene family in bone formation and repair. *Clin. Orthop.* **346,** 26–37.
6. Sampath, T. K., Maliakal, J. C., Hauschka, P. V., Jones, W. K., Sasak, H., Tucker, R. F., et al. (1992) Recombinant human osteogenic protein-1 (hOP-1) induces new bone formation in vivo with a specific activity comparable with natural bovine osteogenic protein and stimulates osteoblast proliferation and differentiation in vitro. *J. Biol. Chem.* **267,** 20352–20362.
7. Cook, S. D. (1999) Preclinical and clinical evaluation of osteogenic protein-1 (BMP-7) in bony sites (see comments). *Orthopedics* **22,** 669–671.
8. Andrews, P. W., Damjanov, I., Berends, J., Kumpf, S., Zappavigna, V., Mavilio, F., et al. (1994) Inhibition of proliferation and induction of differentiation of pluripotent human embryonal carcinoma cells by osteogenic protein-1 (or bone morphogenetic protein-7). *Lab. Invest.* **71,** 243–251.
9. Maliakal, J. C., Asahina, I., Hauschka, P. V., and Sampath, T. K. (1994) Osteogenic protein-1 (BMP-7) inhibits cell proliferation and stimulates the expression of markers characteristic of osteoblast phenotype in rat osteosarcoma (17/2.8) cells. *Growth Factors* **11,** 227–234.
10. Knutsen, R., Wergedal, J. E., Sampath, T. K., Baylink, D. J., and Mohan, S. (1993) Osteogenic protein-1 stimulates proliferation and differentiation of human bone cells in vitro. *Biochem. Biophys. Res. Commun.* **194,** 1352–1358.
11. Kitten, A. M., Lee, J. C., and Olson, M. S. (1995) Osteogenic protein-1 enhances phenotypic expression in ROS 17/2.8 cells. *Am. J. Physiol.* **269,** E918–E926.

12. Asahina, I., Sampath, T. K., Nishimura, I., and Hauschka, P. V. (1993) Human osteogenic protein-1 induces both chondroblastic and osteoblastic differentiation of osteoprogenitor cells derived from newborn rat calvaria. *J. Cell Biol.* **123,** 921–933.
13. Dudley, A. T., Lyons, K. M., and Robertson, E. J. (1995) A requirement for bone morphogenetic protein-7 during development of the mammalian kidney and eye. *Genes Dev.* **9,** 2795–2807.
14. Knutsen, R., Honda, Y., Strong, D. D., Sampath, T. K., Baylink, D. J., and Mohan, S. (1995) Regulation of insulin-like growth factor system components by osteogenic protein-1 in human bone cells. *Endocrinology* **136,** 857–865.
15. Yeh, L. C., Adamo, M. L., Kitten, A. M., Olson, M. S., and Lee, J. C. (1996) Osteogenic protein-1-mediated insulin-like growth factor gene expression in primary cultures of rat osteoblastic cells. *Endocrinology* **137,** 1921–1931.
16. Yeh, L. C., Adamo, M. L., Olson, M. S., and Lee, J. C. (1997) Osteogenic protein-1 and insulin-like growth factor I synergistically stimulate rat osteoblastic cell differentiation and proliferation. *Endocrinology* **138,** 4181–4190.
17. Yeh, L. C., Zavala, M. C., and Lee, J. C. (2002) Osteogenic protein-1 and interleukin-6 with its soluble receptor synergistically stimulate rat osteoblastic cell differentiation. *J. Cell. Physiol.* **190,** 322–331.
18. Franchimont, N., Gangji, V., Durant, D., and Canalis, E. (1997) Interleukin-6 with its soluble receptor enhances the expression of insulin-like growth factor-I in osteoblasts. *Endocrinology* **138,** 5248–5255.
19. Ohlsson, C., Bergtsson, B.-A., Isoksson, O. G. P., Andreassen, T. T., and Slootweg, M. C. (1998) Growth hormone and bone. *Endocr. Rev.* **19,** 55–79.
20. Rosen, C. J. (2002) Growth hormone and insulin-like growth factor-I treatment for metabolic bone diseases, in *Principles of Bone Biology*, Vol 2 (Bilezikian, J. P., Raisz, L. G., and Rodan, G. A., eds.), Academic Press, New York, pp. 1441–1453.
21. Pilbeam, C. C., Harrison, J. R., and Raisz, L. G. (2002) Prostaglandins and bone metabolism, in *Principles of Bone Biology*, Vol. 1 (Bilezikian, J. P., Raisz, L. G., and Rodan, G. A., eds.), Academic Press, New York, pp. 979–994.
22. Hock, J. M., Fitzpatrick, L. A., and Bilezikian, J. P. (2002) Actions of parathyroid hormone, in *Principles of Bone Biology,* Vol 1 (Bilezikian, J. P., Raisz, L. G. and Rodan, G. A., eds.), Academic Press, New York, pp. 463–481.
23. Barnard, R., Ng, K. W., Martin, T. J., and Waters, M. J. (1991) GH receptors on clonal osteoblasts-like cells mediate a mitogenic response to GH. *Endocrinology* **128,** 1459–1464.
24. Langdahl, B. L., Kassem, M., Moller, M. K., and Eriksen, E. F. (1998) The effects of IGF-I and IGF-II on proliferation and differentiation of human osteoblasts and interactions with growth hormone. *Eur. J. Clin. Invest.* **28,** 176–183.
25. Wang, D. S., Sato, K., Demura, H., Kato, Y., Maruo, N., and Miyachi, Y. (1999) Osteo-anabolic effects of human growth hormone with 22K- and 20K Daltons on human osteoblast-like cells. *Endocr. J.* **46,** 125–132.
26. Slootweg, M. C., Ohlsson, C., van Elk, E. J., Netelenbos, J. C., and Andress, D. L. (1996) Growth hormone receptor activity is stimulated by insulin-like growth factor binding protein 5 in rat osteosarcoma cells. *Growth Regul.* **6,** 238–246.
27. Leung, K., Rajkovic, I. A., Peters, E., Markus, I., Van Wyk, J. J., and Ho, K. K. (1996) Insulin-like growth factor I and insulin down-regulate growth hormone (GH) receptors in rat osteoblasts: evidence for a peripheral feedback loop regulating GH action. *Endocrinology* **137,** 2694–2702.
28. Li, H., Bartold, P. M., Young, W. G., Xiao, Y., and Waters, M. J. (2001) Growth hormone induces bone morphogenetic proteins and bone-related proteins in the developing rat periodontium. *J. Bone Miner. Res.* **16,** 1068–1076.
29. McCarthy, T. L., Centrella, M., Raisz, L. G., and Canalis, E. (1991) Prostaglandin E2 stimulates insulin-like growth factor I synthesis in osteoblast-enriched cultures from fetal rat bone. *Endocrinology* **128,** 2895–2900.
30. McCarthy, T. L., Casinghino, S., Centrella, M., and Canalis, E. (1994) Complex pattern of insulin-like growth factor binding protein expression in primary rat osteoblast enriched cultures: regulation by prostaglandin E2, growth hormone, and the insulin-like growth factors. *J. Cell. Physiol.* **160,** 163–175.
31. Pash, J. M., Delany, A. M., Adamo, M. L., Roberts, C. T. Jr., LeRoith, D., and Canalis, E. (1995) Regulation of insulin-like growth factor I transcription by prostaglandin E2 in osteoblast cells. *Endocrinology* **136,** 33–38.
32. Pash, J. M. and Canalis, E. (1996) Transcriptional regulation of insulin-like growth factor-binding protein-5 by prostaglandin E2 in osteoblast cells. *Endocrinology* **137,** 2375–2382.
33. Raisz, L. G., Fall, P. M., Gabbitas, B. Y., McCarthy, T. L., Kream, B. E., and Canalis, E. (1993) Effects of prostaglandin E2 on bone formation in cultured fetal rat calvariae: role of insulin-like growth factor-I. *Endocrinology* **133,** 1504–1510.
34. Schmid, C., Schlapfer, I., Waldvogel, M., Zapf, J., and Froesch, E. R. (1992) Prostaglandin E2 stimulates synthesis of insulin-like growth factor binding protein-3 in rat bone cells in vitro. *J. Bone Miner. Res.* **7,** 1157–1163.
35. Paralkar, V. M., Grasser, W. A., Mansolf, A. L., Baumann, A. P., Owen, T. A., Smock, S. L., et al. (2002) Regulation of BMP-7 expression by retinoic acid and prostaglandin E(2). *J. Cell. Physiol.* **190,** 207–217.
36. Kaneki, H., Takasugi, I., Fujieda, M., Kiriu, M., Mizuochi, S., and Ide, H. (1999) Prostaglandin E2 stimulates the formation of mineralized bone nodules by a cAMP-independent mechanism in the culture of adult rat calvarial osteoblasts. *J. Cell. Biochem.* **73,** 36–48.
37. Clohisy, J. C., Scott, D. K., Brakenhoff, K. D., Quinn, C. O., and Partridge, N. C. (1992) Parathyroid hormone induces c-fos and c-jun messenger RNA in rat osteoblastic cells. *Mol. Endocrinol.* **6,** 1834–1842.
38. Bidwell, J. P., Alvarez, M., Feister, H., Onyia, J., and Hock, J. (1998) Nuclear matrix proteins and osteoblast gene expression. *J. Bone Miner. Res.* **13,** 155–167.
39. Bogdanovic, Z., Huang, Y. F., Dodig, M., Clark, S. H., Lichtler, A. C., and Kream, B. E. (2000) Parathyroid hormone inhibits collagen synthesis and the activity of rat col1a1 transgenes mainly by a cAMP-mediated pathway in mouse calvariae. *J. Cell. Biochem.* **77,** 149–158.
40. McClelland, P., Onyia, J. E., Miles, R. R., Tu, Y., Liang, J., Harvey, A. K., et al. (1998) Intermittent administration of parathyroid hormone (1-34) stimulates matrix metalloproteinase-9 (MMP-9) expression in rat long bone. *J. Cell. Biochem.* **70,** 391–401.

41. Greenfield, E. M., Horowitz, M. C., and Lavish, S. A. (1996) Stimulation by parathyroid hormone of interleukin-6 and leukemia inhibitory factor expression in osteoblasts is an immediate-early gene response induced by cAMP signal transduction. *J. Biol. Chem.* **271,** 10984–10989.
42. Huang, Y. F., Harrison, J. R., Lorenzo, J. A., and Kream, B. E. (1998) Parathyroid hormone induces interleukin-6 heterogeneous nuclear and messenger RNA expression in murine calvarial organ cultures. *Bone* **23,** 327–332.
43. Schmid, C., Schlapfer, I., Futo, E., Waldvogel, M., Schwander, J., Zapf, J., et al. (1992) Triiodothyronine (T3) stimulates insulin-like growth factor (IGF)-1 and IGF binding protein (IGFBP)-2 production by rat osteoblasts in vitro. *Acta Endocrinol. (Copenh.)* **126,** 467–473.
44. Pfeilschifter, J., Laukhuf, F., Muller-Beckmann, B., Blum, W. F., Pfister, T., and Ziegler, R. (1995) Parathyroid hormone increases the concentration of insulin-like growth factor-I and transforming growth factor beta 1 in rat bone. *J. Clin. Invest.* **96,** 767–774.
45. Miyakoshi, N., Kasukawa, Y., Linkhart, T. A., Baylink, D. J., and Mohan, S. (2001) Evidence that anabolic effects of PTH on bone require IGF-I in growing mice. *Endocrinology* **142,** 4349–4356.
46. Ishizuya, T., Yokose, S., Hori, M., Noda, T., Suda, T., Yoshiki, S., and Yamaguchi, A. (1997) Parathyroid hormone exerts disparate effects on osteoblast differentiation depending on exposure time in rat osteoblastic cells. *J. Clin. Invest.* **99,** 2961–2970.
47. Benayahu, D., Fried, A., and Wientroub, S. (1995) PTH and 1,25(OH)2 vitamin D priming to growth factors differentially regulates the osteoblastic markers in MBA-15 clonal subpopulations. *Biochem. Biophys. Res. Commun.* **210(1),** 197–204.
48. Benayahu, D., Fried, A., Shamay, A., Cunningham, N., Blumberg, S., and Wientroub, S. (1994) Differential effects of retinoic acid and growth factors on osteoblastic markers and CD10/NEP activity in stromal-derived osteoblasts. *J. Cell. Biochem.* **56,** 62–73.
49. Kawamura, M. and Urist, M. R. (1988) Growth factors, mitogens, cytokines, and bone morphogenetic protein in induced chondrogenesis in tissue culture. *Dev. Biol.* **130,** 435–442.
50. Takuwa, Y., Ohse, C., Wang, E. A., Wozney, J. M., and Yamashita, K. (1991) Bone morphogenetic protein-2 stimulates alkaline phosphatase activity and collagen synthesis in cultured osteoblastic cells, MC3T3-E1. *Biochem. Biophys. Res. Commun.* **174,** 96–101.
51. Rickard, D. J., Sullivan, T. A., Shenker, B. J., Leboy, P. S., and Kazhdan, I. (1994) Induction of rapid osteoblast differentiation in rat bone marrow stromal cell cultures by dexamethasone and BMP-2. *Dev. Biol.* **161,** 218–228.
52. Hanada, K., Dennis, J. E., and Caplan, A. I. (1997) Stimulatory effects of basic fibroblast growth factor and bone morphogenetic protein-2 on osteogenic differentiation of rat bone marrow-derived mesenchymal stem cells. *J. Bone Miner. Res.* **12,** 1606–1614.
53. Wang, J. S. and Aspenberg, P. (1993) Basic fibroblast growth factor and bone induction in rats. *Acta Orthop. Scand.* **64,** 557–561.
54. Ono, I., Tateshita, T., and Kuboki, Y. (1999) Prostaglandin E1 and recombinant bone morphogenetic protein effect on strength of hydroxyapatite implants. *J. Biomed. Mater. Res.* **45,** 337–344.
55. Boden, S. D., McCuaig, K., Hair, G., Racine, M., Titus, L., Wozney, J. M., et al. (1996) Differential effects and glucocorticoid potentiation of bone morphogenetic protein action during rat osteoblast differentiation in vitro. *Endocrinology* **137,** 3401–3407.
56. Eichner, A., Brock, J., Heldin, C. H., and Souchelnytskyi, S. (2002) Bone morphogenetic protein-7 (OP1) and transforming growth factor-beta1 modulate 1,25(OH)2-vitamin D3-induced differentiation of human osteoblasts. *Exp. Cell Res.* **275,** 132–142.
57. Ripamonti, U., Duneas, N., Van Den Heever, B., Bosch, C., and Crooks, J. (1997) Recombinant transforming growth factor-beta1 induces endochondral bone in the baboon and synergizes with recombinant osteogenic protein-1 (bone morphogenetic protein-7) to initiate rapid bone formation. *J. Bone Miner. Res.* **12,** 1584–1595.

13

Bone Morphogenic Proteins, Osteoblast Differentiation, and Cell Survival During Osteogenesis

Cun-Yu Wang

INTRODUCTION

Osteogenesis or bone formation is a well-coordinated process mediated by osteoblasts. Understanding the molecular regulation of osteogenesis has important clinical implications for bone regeneration and the treatment of bone disorders. Osteoblasts are believed to differentiate from pluripotent mesenchymal stem cells in a tightly regulated sequence of events mediated by a variety of growth factors and cytokines *(1–4)*. Among these factors and cytokines, bone morphogenetic proteins (BMPs) appear to be the most potent inducers of osteoblast differentiation *(5,6)*. BMPs are members of the transforming growth factor-β (TGF-β) superfamily and were originally identified by their unique ability to induce osteoblast differentiation in nonosseous cell lineages in vitro and bone formation in vivo *(5–10)*. BMPs are dimeric molecules with two polypeptide chains linked by a single disulfide bond. Recent discoveries and the elucidation of signal transduction pathways mediated by BMPs in the last decade have provided an important insight into the molecular mechanisms governing osteogenesis and skeletal development. Given their unique capacity as osteoinducers, multiple approaches have been developed and applied in human clinical trials to deliver BMPs to stimulate bone regeneration and repair *(5)*.

BASIC SIGNALING MECHANISMS OF BMP

BMP Signaling Is Mediated Through Smads

Like other growth factors, BMPs activate intracellular signaling cascades after binding to their cognate receptors. There are two known transmembrane serine–threonine kinase receptors for BMP ligands, designated type I (BMPR1) and type II (BMPR2). Upon BMP stimulation, the constitutively active type II receptors phosphorylate and activate type I receptors. Type I receptors, in turn, phosphorylate a specific group of Smad proteins that are then responsible to transduce the signal to the nucleus *(1,4,7)*. To date, eight Smad proteins, Smad1 through Smad8, have been identified and characterized. Smads are divided into three classes according to their signaling functions: receptor-regulated Smads (R-Smad), common-Smads (Co-Smad), and inhibitory Smads (I-Smad; refs. *1,4,7)*. R-Smads are ligand specific and include Smad1, Smad2, Smad3, Smad5, and Smad8. Among these R-Smads, Smad1, 5, and 8 are involved in the BMPs-activated signaling pathway *(9,11–16)*. Active BMPR1 phosphorylates Smads 1, 5, and 8 at a specific SSXS motif in the carboxy terminus, which leads to their dissociation from the receptor. These dissociated Smads then form a heterotrimeric complex with

From: *The Skeleton: Biochemical, Genetic, and Molecular Interactions in Development and Homeostasis*
Edited by: E. J. Massaro and J. M. Rogers © Humana Press Inc., Totowa, NJ

Co-Smad, Smad 4, in the cytoplasm, which then translocates to the nucleus to activate gene transcription *(4,11)*. R-Smads Smad2 and 3 are activated by TGF and activin *(7)*. I-Smads Smad6 and 7 inhibit BMP signaling by competitively interfering with R-Smad phosphorylation by BMPR1. Additionally, Smad6 inhibits BMP signaling by impeding the formation of the cytosolic heterotrimeric Smad complex *(4,11,17,18)*.

In addition to serving as transcriptional activators through the Smads, BMPs also stimulate several important kinase-signaling pathways, including the extracellular signal-related kinase (ERK) and p38 *(4,11,19)*. A cascade of phosphorylation events mediates the activation of these pathways, and they play important roles in stimulating cell proliferation, differentiation, survival, and growth. Although it is not clear how BMPs activate these signaling pathways, TAK1, a mitogen-activated protein kinase kinase kinase (MAPKKK), and its activator, TAB1 (TGF-β-activated kinase-binding protein), have been identified as components of BMP-mediated kinase-signaling pathways. Additionally, X-linked inhibitor of apoptosis protein (XIAP), a broad inhibitor of the caspases, has been found to interact with the BMP type I receptor. It appears that XIAP functions to connect BMP-mediated signaling to downstream signaling molecules TAB1 and TAK1 *(4,11)*.

Regulation of BMP Signaling

Given the importance of BMPs in development, BMP signaling is tightly regulated. Like other important cytokines, BMPs induce genes that feed back to regulate their own function. The I-Smad Smad7 is induced by BMPs in a feedback loop that inhibits Smad1 and Smad5 phosphorylation by BMPR1 *(4,11)*. Recently, Tob, a member of a novel antiproliferative family of proteins, was shown to be regulated by BMPs *(20)*. Tob potently suppressed BMP-induced Smad-dependent transcription through an interaction with Smads1, 5, and 8. Interestingly, Tob also was associated with Smad4. Cofocal microscope image analysis found that Tob specifically regulated the subcellular localization of R-Smads. Upon BMP-2 stimulation, Tob colocalized with R-Smad in nuclear bodies. Therefore, Tob together with the Smad proteins may form a transcription regulatory complex and control the expression of genes relevant to BMP2-induced cell growth and development *(20)*.

An additional level of regulation of BMPs signal transduction that involves the degradation of Smads by Smurf1 and Smurf2 has recently been identified *(21)*. These Smurfs are ubiquitin-protein ligases found in human and *Xenopus* cells. Ubiquitin–protein ligases, known as E3 proteins, mediate the final steps in the process of protein ubiquitination, which begins with an ATP-dependent activation of ubiquitin and culminates with its conjugation to the specific substrates. E3s have high substrate specificity and often act in a regulated fashion to control signaling pathways and cellular function. Smurf1 was identified by a two-hybrid screen for proteins that interact with Smad1. Smurf1 selectively interacts with R-Smads specific to BMP ligand-mediated signaling pathways to trigger their ubiquitination and degradation. In *Xenopus*, Smurf1 messenger RNA is localized to the animal pole of the egg. Ectopic expression of Smurf1 inhibits the transmission of BMP signals, thereby affecting pattern formation in *Xenopus* embryos *(4,11,22)*. Currently, the role of Smurf1 and Smurf2 in osteoblast differentiation and bone formation is unknown. The gene inactivation of Smurf1 and/or Smurf2 should greatly advance our understanding in this regard.

MOLECULAR REGULATION OF OSTEOBLAST DIFFERENTIATION BY BMP

BMP Induction of Osteoblast Differentiation Is Dependent on Smad Signaling

Gene knockout experiments have demonstrated that BMPs are involved at multiple stages of development and embryogenesis. Although a single BMP gene deletion has not demonstrated effects on skeleton development, great evidence supports that BMPs play a pivotal role in osteoblast differentiation and bone formation *(3,11)*. Histological studies have found that BMPs are localized to the region around bone growth. Importantly, several key transcription factors induced by BMPs, which is dependent on Smad signaling, have been found to play an essential role in osteoblast differentiation and bone formation in vivo and in vitro *(1,3,4,11)*. Inhibition of the Smad signaling pathway with dominant-negative mutants has demonstrated that Smads play an essential role in BMP-induced osteoblast differentiation *(13)*.

BMP-Inducible Runt-Related Gene 2 (RUNX2), Also Known as Cbfa1 (Core-Binding Factor A1), Is Essential for Osteoblast Differentiation and Bone Formation

Because the small gla protein osteocalcin is a specific bone matrix protein that is predominantly expressed by osteoblasts, studies have focused extensively on the elucidation of regulatory mechanisms that transcriptionally control osteocalcin gene expression. These studies have lead to the identification of Runx-2 as an important regulator of osteoblast differentiation *(23–26)*. There are three Runx-2 transcription factors, Runx-2 (Osf2), Runx-1 (also called Pepb2aB and AML1), and Runx-3 (Pepb2aC and AML2). Among these factors, Runx-2 is a key player in osteoblast differentiation and skeleton development *(1,3,23)*. Runx-2 expression is initiated during the mesenchymal condensation of the developing skeleton and is strictly restricted to hypertrophic chondrocytes and cells of the osteoblast lineage *(23)*. Many studies have demonstrated that Runx-2 binds to and regulates the expression of multiple genes expressed in osteoblasts, including osteocalcin, type I collagen, osteopontin, bone sialoprotein, and fibronectin *(12,23)*. Ectopic expression of Runx-2 in cells of nonosteoblastic lineages induces the expression of osteoblast-specific proteins. Several studies have demonstrated that BMPs induce Smad-dependent Runx-2 expression *(3,11)*. Importantly, the role of Runx-2 in osteoblast differentiation has been confirmed through in vivo gene deletion studies. Histological examination of Runx-2-deficiant embryos revealed a complete lack of ossification, whereas chondrocyte differentiation was largely unaffected. The expression of the genes encoding bone matrix proteins, such as osteocalcin, osteopontin, and type I collagen, are either not detected or weakly expressed in Runx-2-deficient embryos. These studies establish an essential role of Runx-2 in osteoblast differentiation and osteogenesis *(24,25)*.

To further study the role of Runx-2 in bone formation after birth, Ducy et al. *(27)* generated transgenic mice that overexpressed a dominant-negative mutant of Runx-2 (DN-Runx-2) under the control of the osteocalcin promoter in differentiated osteoblasts. Mice expressing the DN-Cbfa1 presented a normal skeleton at birth but develop an osteopenic phenotype thereafter. Dynamic histomorphometric studies found that the osteopenia was caused by a major decrease in the bone formation rate, whereas the number of osteoblasts was normal. Molecular analyses revealed that the expression of the genes encoding bone extracellular matrix proteins was nearly abolished in these mice *(27)*. These results indicate that Runx-2 also transcriptionally controls the function of mature osteoblasts. Conversely, Liu et al. *(28)* generated transgenic mice that overexpressed wild-type Runx-2 under the control of the type I collagen promoter in osteoblasts. Paradoxically, they found that Runx-2 transgenic mice also had severe osteopenia and suffered from bone fractures within a few weeks after birth. Although the number of neonatal osteoblasts was increased, their function was impaired in matrix production and mineralization. The number of mature osteoblast and osteocytes were significantly decreased *(28)*. In contrast to the works by Ducy et al. *(27)* that suggested Runx-2 plays an important role in maturation of osteoblasts, studies by Liu et al. *(28)* indicated that Runx-2 inhibits osteoblast differentiation at a late stage. However, it should be pointed out that superphysiological overexpression of Runx-2 in osteoblasts may have a myriad of side effects and perhaps cannot reflect the true function of Runx-2.

Regulation of Runx-2 Transactivation by Smad Signaling

Given the fact that Runx-2 plays an essential role in osteoblast differentiation in vivo and in vitro, it is conceivable that the transcription potential of Runx-2 is regulated by multiple factors and signaling pathways. The expression of Runx-2 induced by BMP is dependent on the Smad signaling pathway.

Interestingly, several recent studies have shown that BMP-activated R-Smads are also important for Runx-2 transactivation by interacting with Runx-2. Cleidocranial dysplasia (CCD), an autosomal-dominant human bone disease, is caused by heterozygous mutations to Runx-2 *(24,29)*. To understand the mechanism underlying the pathogenesis of CCD, Zhang et al. *(29)* studied crosstalk between Runx-2 and the BMPs/Smad signaling pathway. They found that Smad1 interacted with wild-type Runx-2 in vivo and in vitro to enhance the transactivation of Runx-2 as a coactivator. Moreover, they found the interaction between Runx-2 and Smad1 to be dependent on BMP stimulation. In contrast, a mutant of Runx-2, CCDA376, failed to interact with or respond to Smads, and was unable to induce an osteoblast-like phenotype in C2C12 mesenchymal cells upon stimulation with BMPs *(29)*. CCDA376 was isolated from a patient with CCD, and it was a nonsense mutation in the Runx-2 gene that yielded a truncated Runx-2 protein *(24)*. These results suggest the pathogenesis of CCD may be related to an impaired BMP/Smad signaling pathway, which targets the transcription activity of Runx-2 during bone formation.

Interestingly, studies by Alliston et al. *(30)* found that TGF-β-activated R-Smads play an opposite role in Runx-2 transactivation. It is known that TGF-β is present in high levels in bone extracellular matrix and inhibits osteoblast differentiation by unknown mechanisms. As osteoclasts resorb mature bone during the process of bone remodeling, TGF-β is released from the matrix and becomes available to osteoblasts in the bone marrow microenvironment. To understand the molecular mechanism by which TGF-β negatively regulates osteoblast differentiation, Alliston et al. *(30)* studied the effects of TGF-β and its effectors, the Smads, on the expression and function of Runx-2. They found that TGF-β inhibited the expression of Runx-2-induced genes in osteoblast-like cell lines. This inhibition was mediated by Smad3, which interacted physically with Runx-2 and repressed its transcriptional activity. The repression of Runx-2 function by Smad3 contrasted with previous observations that Smad1 functions as a transcription activator. They also found that Smad3-mediated Runx-2 transcription repression specifically occurred in mesenchymal but not epithelial cells and depended on the promoter sequence. The demonstration that Smad3-mediated repression of Runx-2 has provided a regulatory mechanism for the inhibition of osteoblast differentiation by TGF-β *(30)*.

Regulation of Smad Signaling by a Tumor Suppressor Retinoblastoma Protein (pRb)

pRb belongs to the pocket protein family, which includes p107 and p130. pRb acts as a generic corepressor of the E2F family of transcription factors and is inactivated in many human cancers *(31)*. Specifically, pRb mutation has been associated with osteosarcoma, and viral oncoproteins that block pRb function potently inhibit osteoblast differentiation. To understand how pRb regulates osteoblast differentiation, Thomas et al. *(31)* examined the interaction between pRb and Runx-2. They found that pRb played a key role in facilitating expression of late markers of osteoblast differentiation through a physical association with Runx-2. Loss of pRb, but not p107 or p130, severely impaired late osteoblast differentiation. Chromatin immunoprecipitation analysis found that pRb was associated with Runx-2 and bound to osteoblast-specific promoters in vivo in a Runx-2-dependent manner. pRb stimulated Runx-2-mediated transactivation of an osteoblast-specific reporter by the direct interaction with Runx-2 and the transcriptional machinery. Moreover, tumor-derived pRb mutants were unable to interact with Runx-2 and failed to potentiate Runx-2-mediated transactivation. These results suggest that pRb functions as a direct transcriptional coactivator of Runx-2 to promote osteoblast differentiation.

Regulation of Runx-2 Function by MAPK (Mitogen-Activated Protein Kinase) Signaling

Like other general transcription factors, the transactivation potential of Runx-2 is regulated by phosphorylation. Xiao et al. *(32)* have found that the MAPK signal cascade phosphorylates Runx-2 in vitro and in vivo during the induction of osteoblast differentiation. The transcriptional activity of Runx-2 was significantly potentiated by the overexpression of active MEK. Stimulation of MAPK through the transfection of a constitutively active form of MEK1 into MC3T3-E1 preosteoblast cells increased the expression of endogenous osteocalcin mRNA. In contrast, overexpression of a dominant-negative mutant of MEK1 inhibited the expression of osteocalcin. The active MEK1 also stimulated activity of the osteocalcin promoter, and this stimulation required the DNA binding site for Runx-2. The specific MAPK inhibitor, PD98059, blocked extracellular matrix-dependent upregulation of the osteocalcin promoter. These results indicate that the MAPK pathway and, presumably, Runx-2 phosphorylation are also required for the responsiveness of osteoblasts to extracellular matrix signals. The findings may also provide an explanation for the observation in several studies that BMP-induced osteoblast differentiation is required for the MAPK signaling *(32,33)*.

BMP-Inducible Transcription Factor Osterix Is Essential for Osteoblast Differentiation

Very recently, another BMP-inducible transcription factor dubbed Osterix (Osx) was found to play an essential role in osteoblast differentiation. Osx was identified and cloned through a differential display analysis that sought to identify BMP-induced genes. Osx is a novel zinc finger-containing transcription factor that is specifically expressed in developing bones. Osx contains a proline- and serine-rich transcription activation domain. The DNA binding domain of Osx consists of three zinc fingers at its C-terminus that share a high degree of homology with motifs in transcription factors Sp1, Sp3, and Sp4. Although to a lesser degree, Osx also has homology to motifs in the Krüppel-like factor family. Biochemical characterization of Osx demonstrated that Osx bound to Sp1 consensus sequences and to other specific G/C-rich sequences. Such G/C-rich sequences are present in the promoters of bone matrix genes, including collagen I. Ectopic expression of Osx in nonosteoblastic lineages induced expression of osteocalcin and collagen I *(34)*.

Gene deletion studies in mice have demonstrated that Osx functions downstream from Cbfa1 and is essential for osteoblast differentiation. In the absence of Osx, neither cortical nor trabecular bone was generated through intramembranous or endochondral ossification. During the normal endochondral bone formation, the degradation of the mineralized cartilage matrix by osteoclasts/chondroclasts and the deposition of new bone matrix by osteoblasts are tightly coordinated. Histological studies found that both osteoclast differentiation and active cartilage matrix degradation were not affected in Osx null mutants. However, mesenchymal cells that comigrated with osteoclasts could not deposit bone matrix, and no ossification was found in the mesenchyme. Similarly, no ossification was found in the condensed mesenchyme of membranous skeletal elements in Osx-null mutants *(34)*.

Because Runx-2 is essential for osteoblast differentiation as described above, Nakashima et al. *(34)* further examined whether bone formation defects in Osx-null mutant mice may be caused by disregulation of Runx-2 expression. Interestingly, they discovered that osteogenic cells from Osx-null mutants express Runx-2 at levels comparable to wild-type osteoblasts, indicating that Osx was not required for Runx-2 expression. In contrast, they found that Osx was not expressed in Runx-2-deficient embryos, indicating that Runx-2 was required for the expression of Osx. However, currently, it is unknown how Cbfa1 controls Osx expression. Taken together, elegant studies by Nakashima suggest that Osx is an essential transcription factor for skeleton development and acts downstream from Runx-2 to induce osteoblast differentiation *(34)*.

REGULATION OF OSTEOBLAST APOPTOSIS BY BMP

Bone Development and Apoptosis

Apoptosis or programmed cell death is an important biological process that orchestrates cell removal required to maintain cell turnover and integrity in multicellular organisms. Apoptosis is characterized by caspase activation, DNA fragmentation, and condensation of the nucleus *(35,36)*. Although Ker et al. formally proposed the concept of apoptosis in 1972, biologists have been aware that cell death occurs in bone since the early 1960s. Frost et al. described empty osteocyte lacunae in human bone specimens and suggested they were derived as a consequence of cell death *(36–38)*. Emerging evidence indicates that apoptosis is an important component in skeletal development and remodeling. Well-coordinated homeostatic apoptosis of hypertropic chondrocytes in their terminal differentiation stage is essential for the progression of endochondral bone formation. Abnormal apoptosis of osteoblasts may be associated with bone disorders such as osteoporosis and Paget's disease of bone. It is widely accepted that once they have completed their bone-forming function, osteoblasts are either entrapped in bone matrix and become osteocytes or remain on the surfaces as lining cells. Studies since Frost's have shown that the terminal stages of the osteocyte life cycle are structurally and functionally consistent with the morphological modifications associated with apoptosis. Specifically, electron micrographs have shown osteocytes with irregularly shaped nuclei containing condensed heterochromatin and interrupted nuclear envelopes consistent with morphological characteristics of apoptotic cells. Apoptotic osteoblasts or osteocytes have also been detected in vivo with the terminal UTP nick end labeling (TUNEL) assay, which specifically labels fragmented nucleosome-sized DNA strands *(36,38)*.

In an elegant experiment using mouse fetal calvaria-derived osteoblasts, Lynch et al. *(37)* presented evidence of cell death by apoptosis in the development of bone-like tissue in vitro. In this model system, osteoblast differentiation can be divided into three well-characterized stages: a proliferation period; a matrix maturation period where cell growth is arrested, abundant amounts of Type I collagen are deposited and genes marking a bone cell phenotype are induced; and finally a mineralization stage characterized by the expression of bone-specific genes. With the use of TUNEL and DNA laddering assays, Lynch et al. *(37)* found cells that terminally differentiated to the mature bone cell phenotype underwent apoptosis. During the proliferative period, only a small percentage of isolated apoptotic cells were observed. As nodules form, more apoptotic cells were identified in the premineralized multilayered cell nodule. With progressive development of mineral nodules in the extracellular matrix, a marked increase in the proportion of apoptotic cells dispersed throughout the nodule was observed. Additionally, they found that apoptosis of differentiated osteoblasts was associated with several pro-apoptotic genes including p53 and Bax. Bax and p53, which can accelerate apoptosis, are expressed in heavily mineralized bone tissue nodules. These findings provide important evidence that indicates apoptosis in osteogenesis is essential to bone homeostasis and mineralized nodule formation *(37)*.

Apoptosis and Bone Disorder

Recently, several studies have found that abnormal osteoblastic apoptosis may be associated with osteoporosis *(22,36,38,39)*. Bone mass can be increased by intermittent parathyroid hormone (PTH) administration, but the mechanism of this phenomenon remains unknown. Jilka et al. *(40)* reported that daily PTH injections in mice with osteopenia caused by defective osteoblastogenesis increased bone formation without affecting the generation of new osteoblasts. Instead, PTH prolonged the life span of mature osteoblasts by inhibiting apoptosis and thereby extended their matrix-producing function. Using primary rodent and human osteoblasts in an in vitro study, they demonstrated that the anti-apoptotic effect of PTH required the hormone to bind to the PTH/PTHrP receptor of osteoblasts and was mediated by the c-AMP signaling pathway. The evidence from these studies provides proof of the basic principle that the promotion of bone formation may be obtained through suppression of osteoblast apoptosis.

On the contrary, several studies suggested that osteoporosis mediated by glucocorticoid is caused, in part, by increased apoptosis of osteocytes and osteoblasts *(36,38,41)*. Experimental and clinical studies have demonstrated that bisphosphonates (BPs) are effective agents in the prevention of glucocorticoid-mediated osteoporosis. To understand BP-mediated therapeutic effects, Plotkin et al. *(41)*

examined whether BPs modulated apoptosis of bone cells. They found that BPs blocked apoptosis of primary murine osteoblastic cells in vitro induced by multiple stimuli, including etoposide, tumor necrosis factor (TNF) and the synthetic glucocorticoid dexamethasone. BP-mediated antiapoptotic effect was correlated with a rapid increase in the phosphorylated fraction of ERKs. Inhibition of ERK activation abolished BP-mediated survival function. Moreover, BPs significantly suppressed apoptosis in vertebral cancellous bone osteocytes and osteoblasts that followed glucocorticoid administration in mice. These results suggest that the therapeutic efficacy of BPs, which is currently used to treat Paget's disease of bone and glucocorticoid-induced osteoporosis, may be caused by their ability to prevent osteocyte and osteoblast apoptosis *(41)*. Therefore, the regulation of osteoblast lifespan may provide an important therapeutic strategy to treat osteoporosis.

Regulation of Osteoblast Apoptosis by BMPs

Induction of apoptosis by BMP was originally reported in studies focused on interdigital cell death that leads to the regression of soft tissue between embryonic digits in many vertebrates. Results from these experiments indicate that BMP signaling actively mediates cell death in the embryonic limb *(11, 35)*. Consistent with BMP pro-apoptotic activity in development, Hay et al. *(42)* observed that BMP-2 promoted apoptosis in primary human calvaria osteoblasts and in immortalized human neonatal calvaria osteoblasts, as shown by TUNEL analysis. Moreover, BMP-2 induced the release of mitochondrial cytochrome c into the cytosol. Subsequently, BMP-2 increased caspase-9 and caspase-3, -6, and -7 activity. Inhibition of caspase-9 activity suppressed BMP-2-induced apoptosis. However, overexpression of dominant-negative Smad1 effectively blocks BMP-2-induced Runx-2 expression but not the activation of caspases or apoptosis induced by BMP-2, indicating that the BMP-2-induced apoptosis was independent of the Smad1 signaling pathway. They found that the proapoptotic effect of BMP-2 was dependent on activation of protein kinase C (PKC). The inhibition of PKC by the selective PKC inhibitor calphostin C blocked the BMP-2-induced increase in the Bax/Bcl-2 ratio, caspase activity, and apoptosis. In contrast, the cAMP-dependent protein kinase A (PKA) inhibitor H89, the p38 MAPK inhibitor SB203580, and the MEK inhibitor PD-98059 did not affect BMP-2-induced apoptosis. Therefore, Hay et al. *(42)* proposed that BMP-2 modulated apoptosis through a Smad-independent, PKC-dependent pathway that uses Bax/Bcl-2, cytochrome c, and a caspase cascade that involves caspases-9, 3, 6, and 7 in human osteoblasts.

To address the general concern that apoptosis induction in Hay et al.'s studies *(42)* was very weak, we explored whether BMP played a role in the regulation of apoptosis during the induction of osteoblast differentiation using mesenchymal cells *(35)* . Using the death receptor inducer TNF, we found that BMP-2 and BMP-4 inhibited TNF-mediated apoptosis by blocking caspase-8 activation in C2C12 cells, which are pluripotent mesenchymal cells that differentiate into osteoblasts when stimulated with BMPs. Moreover, the antiapoptotic activity of BMPs functioned through the Smad signaling pathway and inhibition of Smad signaling rendered cells sensitive to TNF-induced apoptosis. Our results suggest that BMPs not only stimulate osteoblast differentiation but can also promote cell survival during the induction of osteoblast differentiation. Currently, we cannot explain the conflicting pro- and antiapoptotic properties of BMPs reported by us and by others. This disparity may underline the importance of cell context and stimuli. Interestingly, studies from Smad5-deficient mice suggest BMP-mediated Smad signaling may play a role in survival of mesenchymal cells, the cells from which osteoblasts are differentiated *(43)*. Mice homozygous for the Smad5 mutation die between days 10.5 and 11.5 of gestation because of defects in angiogenesis and apoptosis. Histological analysis showed that embryos lacked mesenchyme and that massive apoptosis was present in head mesenchyme. The apoptosis was most concentrated in the mesenchyme of the head and somites, where Smad5 was highly expressed. Because Smad5 is a BMPs-specific signaling molecule and osteoblasts are differentiated from mesenchymal cells, these results strongly support the notion that signaling by BMPs has antiapoptotic functions, at least, during the early stage of osteoblast differentiation *(43)*.

SUMMARY

The induction of osteoblast differentiation and osteogenesis by BMPs are well coordinated dynamic processes. BMP-mediated osteoblast differentiation is dependent on the Smad signaling pathway. BMP-inducible transcription factors, Cbfa1 and Osx, play an essential role in osteoblast differentiation and osteogenesis. Additionally, BMP may regulate osteoblast cell survival during the induction of differentiation from mesenchymal stem cells. It will be interesting to know whether Cbfal or Osx regulates osteoblast survival in the future. The regulatory functions of BMPs on osteoblast differentiation and survival are currently the focus of many laboratories around the world. A more clear understanding of these regulatory mechanisms is critical to the elucidation of the origin of bone diseases and to the development of exciting new therapies.

REFERENCES

1. Ducy, P., Schinke, T., and Karsenty, G. (2000) The osteoblast: a sophisticated fibroblast under central surveillance. *Science* **289,** 1501–1504.
2. Karsenty, G. (1999) The genetic transformation of bone biology. *Genes Dev.* **13,** 3037–3051.
3. Wagner, E. F. and Karsenty, G. (2001) Genetic control of skeletal development. *Curr. Opin. Genet. Dev.* **11,** 527–532.
4. Yamaguchi, A., Komori, T., and Suda, T. (2000) Regulation of osteoblast differentiation mediated by bone morphogenetic proteins, hedgehogs, and Cbfa1. *Endocr. Rev.* **21,** 393–411.
5. Reddi, A. H. (1997) Bone morphogenetic proteins: an unconventional approach to isolation of first mammalian morphogens. *Cytokine Growth Factor Rev.* **8,** 11–20.
6. Wang, E. A., Rosen, V., D'Alessandro, J. S., Bauduy, M., Cordes, P., Harada, T., et al. (1990) Recombinant human bone morphogenetic protein induces bone formation. *Proc. Natl. Acad. Sci. USA* **87,** 2220–2224.
7. Derynck, R., Akhurst, R. J., and Balmain, A. (2001) TGF-β signaling in tumor suppression and cancer progression. *Nat. Genet.* **29,** 117–129.
8. Ebisawa, T., Tada, K., Kitajima, I., Tojo, K., Sampath, T. K., Kawabata, M., et al. (1999) Characterization of bone morphogenetic protein-6 signaling pathways in osteoblast differentiation. *J. Cell Sci.* **112,** 3519–3527.
9. Nohe, A., Hassel, S., Ehrlich, M., Neubauer, F., Sebald, W., Henis, Y. I., et al. (2002) The mode of bone morphogenetic protein (BMP) receptor oligomerization determines different BMP-2 signaling pathways. *J. Biol. Chem.* **277,** 5330–5338.
10. Yang, X., Ji, X., Shi, X., and Cao, X. (2000) Smad1 domains interacting with Hoxc-8 induce osteoblast differentiation. *J. Biol. Chem.* **275,** 1065–1072.
11. Kawabata, M., Imamura, T., and Miyazono, K. (1998) Signal transduction by bone morphogenetic proteins. *Cytokine Growth Factors Rev.* **9,** 49–61.
12. Lee, K. S., Kim, H. J., Li, Q. L., Chi, X. Z., Ueta, C., Komori, T., et al. (2000) Runx2 is a common target of transforming growth factor beta1 and bone morphogenetic protein 2, and cooperation between Runx2 and Smad5 induces osteoblast-specific gene expression in the pluripotent mesenchymal precursor cell line C2C12. *Mol. Cell. Biol.* **20,** 8783–8792.
13. Nishimura, R., Kato, Y., Chen, D., Harris, S. E., Mundy, G. R., and Yoneda, T. (1998) Smad5 and DPC4 are key molecules in mediating BMP-2-induced osteoblastic differentiation of the pluripotent mesenchymal precursor cell line C2C12. *J. Biol. Chem.* **273,** 1872–1879.
14. Tamura, Y., Takeuchi, Y., Suzawa, M., Fukumoto, S., Kato, M., Miyazono, K., and Fujita, T. (2001) Focal adhesion kinase activity is required for bone morphogenetic protein–Smad1 signaling and osteoblastic differentiation in murine MC3T3-E1 cells. *J. Bone Miner. Res.* **16,** 1772–1779.
15. Tamaki, K., Souchelnytskyi, S., Itoh, S., Nakao, A., Sampath, K., Heldin, C. H., and ten Dijke, P. (1998) Intracellular signaling of osteogenic protein-1 through Smad5 activation. *J. Cell. Physiol.* **177,** 355–363.
16. Yamamoto, N., Akiyama, S., Katagiri, T., Namiki, M., Kurokawa, T., and Suda, T. (1997) Smad1 and smad5 act downstream of intracellular signalings of BMP-2 that inhibits myogenic differentiation and induces osteoblast differentiation in C2C12 myoblasts. *Biochem. Biophys. Res. Commun.* **238,** 574–580.
17. Imamura, T., Takase, M., Nishihara, A., Oeda, E., Hanai, J., Kawabata, M., and Miyazono, K. (1997) Smad6 inhibits signaling by the TGF-beta superfamily. *Nature* **389,** 622–626.
18. Ishida, W., Hamamoto, T., Kusanagi, K., Yagi, K., Kawabata, M., Takehara, K., et al. (2000) Smad6 is a Smad1/5-induced smad inhibitor. Characterization of bone morphogenetic protein-responsive element in the mouse Smad6 promoter. *J. Biol. Chem.* **275,** 6075–6079.
19. Lou, J., Tu, Y., Li, S., and Manske, P. R. (2000) Involvement of ERK in BMP-2 induced osteoblastic differentiation of mesenchymal progenitor cell line C3H10T1/2. *Biochem. Biophys. Res. Commun.* **268,** 757–762.
20. Yoshida, Y., Tanaka, S., Umemori, H., Minowa, O., Usui, M., Ikematsu, N., et al. (2000) Negative regulation of BMP/Smad signaling by Tob in osteoblasts. *Cell* **103,** 1085–1097.
21. Zhu, H., Kavsak, P., Abdollah, S., Wrana, J. L., and Thomsen, G. H. (1999) A Smad ubiquitin ligase targets the BMP pathway and affects embryonic pattern formation. *Nature* **400,** 687–693.

22. Zhao, W., Byrne, M. H., Wang, Y., and Krane, S. M. (2000) Osteocyte and osteoblast apoptosis and excessive bone deposition accompany failure of collagenase cleavage of collagen. *J. Clin. Invest.* **106,** 941–949.
23. Ducy, P., Zhang, R., Geoffroy, V., Ridall, A. L., and Karsenty, G. (1997) Osf2/Cbfa1: a transcriptional activator of osteoblast differentiation. *Cell* **89,** 747–754.
24. Mundlos, S., Otto, F., Mundlos, C., Mulliken, J. B., Aylsworth, A. S., Albright, S., et al. (1997) Mutations involving the transcription factor CBFA1 cause cleidocranial dysplasia. *Cell* **89,** 773–779.
25. Komori, T., Yagi, H., Nomura, S., Yamaguchi, A., Sasaki, K., Deguchi, K., et al. (1997) Targeted disruption of Cbfa1 results in a complete lack of bone formation owing to maturational arrest of osteoblasts. *Cell* **89,** 755–764.
26. Otto, F., Thornell, A. P., Crompton, T., Denzel, A., Gilmour, K. C., Rosewell, I. R., et al. (1997) Cbfa1, a candidate gene for cleidocranial dysplasia syndrome, is essential for osteoblast differentiation and bone development. *Cell* **89,** 765–771.
27. Ducy, P., Starbuck, M., Priemel, M., Shen, J., Pinero, G., Geoffroy, V., et al. (1999) A Cbfa1-dependent genetic pathway controls bone formation beyond embryonic development. *Genes Dev.* **13,** 1025–1036.
28. Liu, W., Toyosawa, S., Furuichi, T., Kanatani, N., Yoshida, C., Liu, Y., et al. (2001) Overexpression of Cbfa1 in osteoblasts inhibits osteoblast maturation and causes osteopenia with multiple fractures. *J. Cell Biol.* **155,** 157–166.
29. Zhang, Y. W., Yasui, N., Ito, K., Huang, G., Fujii, M., Hanai, J., et al. (2000) A RUNX2/PEBP2alpha A/CBFA1 mutation displaying impaired transactivation and Smad interaction in cleidocranial dysplasia. *Proc. Nat. Acad. Sci. USA* **97,** 10549–10554.
30. Alliston, T., Choy, L., Ducy, P., Karsenty, G., and Derynck, R. (2001) TGF-β-induced repression of CBFA1 by Smad3 decreases cbfa1 and osteocalcin expression and inhibits osteoblast differentiation. *EMBO J.* **20,** 2254–2272.
31. Thomas, D. M., Carty, S. A., Piscopo, D. M., Lee, J., Wang, W., Forrester, W. C., et al. (2001) The retinoblastoma protein acts as a transcriptional coactivator required for osteogenic differentiation. *Mol. Cell* **8,** 303–316.
32. Xiao, G., Jiang, D., Thomas, P., Benson, M. D., Guan, K., Karsenty, G., et al. (2000) MAPK pathways activate and phosphorylate the osteoblast-specific transcription factor, Cbfa1. *J. Biol. Chem.* **275,** 4453–4459.
33. Gallea, S., Lallemand, F., Atfi, A., Rawadi, G., Ramez, V., Spinella-Jaegle, S., et al. (2001) Activation of mitogen-activated protein kinase cascades is involved in regulation of bone morphogenetic protein-2-induced osteoblast differentiation in pluripotent C2C12 cells. *Bone* **28,** 491–498.
34. Nakashima, K., Zhou, X., Kunkel, G., Zhang, Z., Deng, J. M., Behringer, R. R., and de Crombrugghe, B. (2002) The novel zinc finger-containing transcription factor osterix is required for osteoblast differentiation and bone formation. *Cell* **108,** 17–29.
35. Chen, S., Guttridge, D. C., Tang, E., Shi, S., Guan, K., and Wang, C. Y. (2001) Suppression of tumor necrosis factor-mediated apoptosis by nuclear factor kappaB-independent bone morphogenetic protein/Smad signaling. *J. Biol. Chem.* **276,** 39259–39263.
36. Hock, J. M., Krishnan, V., Onyia, J. E., Bidwell, J. P., Milas, J., and Stanislaus, D. (2001) Osteoblast apoptosis and bone turnover. *J. Bone Miner. Res.* **16,** 975–984.
37. Lynch, M. P., Capparelli, C., Stein, J. L., Stein, G. S., and Lian, J. B. (1998) Apoptosis during bone-like tissue development in vitro. *J. Cell. Biochem.* **68,** 31–49.
38. Weinstein, R. S. and Manolagas, S. C. (2000) Apoptosis and osteoporosis. *Am. J. Med.* **108,** 153–164.
39. Hill, P.A., Tumber, A., and Meikle, M. C. (1997) Multiple extracellular signals promote osteoblast survival and apoptosis. *Endocrinology* **138,** 3849–3858.
40. Jilka, R. L., Weinstein, R. S., Bellido, T., Roberson, P., Parfitt, A. M., and Manolagas, S. C. (1999) Increased bone formation by prevention of osteoblast apoptosis with parathyroid hormone. *J. Clin. Invest.* **104,** 439–446.
41. Plotkin, L. I., Weinstein, R. S., Parfitt, A. M., Roberson, P. K., Manolagas, S. C., and Bellido, T. (1999) Prevention of osteocyte and osteoblast apoptosis by bisphosphonates and calcitonin. *J. Clin. Invest.* **104,** 1363–1374.
42. Hay, E., Lemonnier, J., Fromigue, O., and Marie, P. J. (2001) Bone morphogenetic protein-2 promotes osteoblast apoptosis through a Smad-independent, protein kinase C-dependent signaling pathway. *J. Biol. Chem.* **276,** 29028–29036.
43. Yang, X., Castilla, L. H., Xu, X., Li, C., Gotay, J., Weinstein, M., et al. (1999) Angiogenesis defects and mesenchymal apoptosis in mice lacking SMAD5. *Development* **126,** 1571–1580.

14
Osteoclast Differentiation

Sakamuri V. Reddy and G. David Roodman

INTRODUCTION

The osteoclast is the primary bone-resorbing cell and the majority of evidence favors that it is derived from the monocyte–macrophage lineage, although recently there have been reports that early B lymphocytes, B220+ cells can also form osteoclasts (1). The earliest identifiable osteoclast precursor is the granulocyte-macrophage colony-forming unit (CFU-GM), the granulocyte-macrophage progenitor cells that proliferate and differentiate into committed precursors for the osteoclast *(2)*. These committed precursors are postmitotic and fuse to form multinucleated osteoclasts. These multinucleated cells (MNCs) are then activated to form bone-resorbing osteoclasts. After a prescribed period of time, the cells undergo apoptosis. The life cycle of the osteoclast is depicted in Fig. 1. The molecular and cellular events involved in osteoclast differentiation and the large array of factors regulating osteoclast formation and activity are just beginning to be defined. In this review, the factors that are known to be critical to osteoclast differentiation and the genes involved in this process will be discussed.

PHENOTYPIC AND INTRACELLULAR CHANGES ASSOCIATED WITH OSTEOCLAST DIFFERENTIATION

As noted above, during osteoclast differentiation, multipotent osteoclast precursors, which can form both osteoclasts and monocyte–macrophages, proliferate and differentiate to become unipotent committed postmitotic osteoclast precursors. The early precursor differentiates and begins to express CD11b, CD45, and the Kn22 antigen *(3)*. The Kn22 antigen is expressed on cells that are still bipotent and can form monocyte–macrophages or osteoclasts. As these cells differentiate further, they begin to express vitronectin receptors, which can be identified by the 23c6 monoclonal antibody *(4)*, and calcitonin receptors (CTRs). The mature human osteoclast expresses the interleukin-6 receptor, c-fms, the receptor for macrophage colony-stimulating factor (M-CSF), vitronectin receptor, and CTR.

Suda and coworkers *(5)* have reported that 1,25-$(OH)_2D_3$ specifically stimulated the expression of the third component of complement (C3) on osteoclasts in bone in vitro and in vivo. They also reported that an anti-C3 antibody inhibits osteoclast formation when added between days 2–4 of the total 6-d culture period needed for osteoclast development in marrow cultures. This time period corresponds to the late proliferative phase and the early differentiation phase of osteoclast development. This study also demonstrated that C3 protein, produced by the stromal cells in response to

From: *The Skeleton: Biochemical, Genetic, and Molecular Interactions in Development and Homeostasis*
Edited by: E. J. Massaro and J. M. Rogers © Humana Press Inc., Totowa, NJ

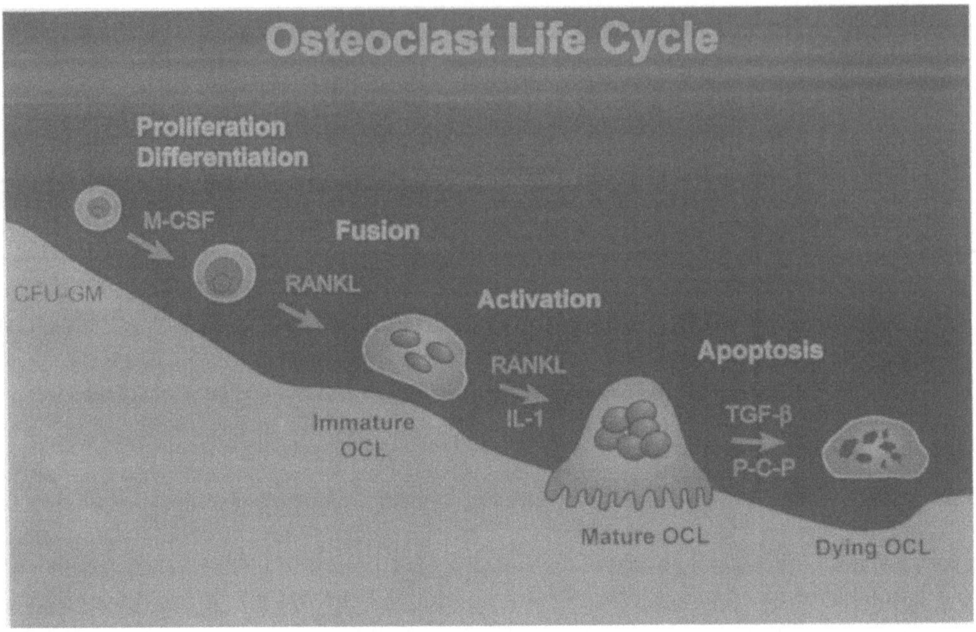

Fig. 1. Life cycle of the osteoclast.

1,25-$(OH)_2D_3$, is involved in osteoclast development by potentiating M-CSF-dependent proliferation of bone marrow cells and induction of osteoclast differentiation.

Kania et al. *(6)* determined that CD44, a cell surface glycoprotein that is known to function as an adhesion receptor, is also involved in osteoclast differentiation. They demonstrated that CD44 is expressed on mouse osteoclasts that develop in primary bone marrow cultures treated with 1,25-$(OH)_2D_3$. Monoclonal antibodies against CD44 inhibited osteoclast formation in these cultures in a dose-dependent manner. Similarly, coculture experiments with mouse spleen cells and ST2 bone marrow stromal cells to form osteoclasts indicated that the inhibitory effects of the CD44 antibody were directed against hematopoietic cells rather than stromal cells. However, CD44 antibodies did not inhibit the bone-resorptive activity of mature osteoclasts, suggesting that this surface antigen plays a role predominantly in osteoclast formation.

In addition to changes in the surface phenotype that occur during osteoclast differentiation, early osteoclast precursors but not macrophages express tartrate-resistant acid phosphatase (TRAP) in vivo, which is a marker enzyme for the osteoclast. Expression of TRAP has been detected in early proliferating osteoclast precursors and is expressed at high levels in committed osteoclast precursors that fuse to form mature osteoclasts *(7)*. However, this in itself is not a reliable marker for osteoclast differentiation because human macrophages will express TRAP in vitro. The functional role of TRAP in the osteoclast is unknown. Studies using homologous recombination to inactivate the TRAP gene have demonstrated that these animals appear to have relatively normal bone resorption and in fact have problems with endochondral bone formation and mild osteopetrosis *(8)*. A substrate for this phosphatase activity has not been clearly identified in the osteoclast, but Halleen et al *(9)* have reported that TRAP can generate reactive oxygen species in osteoclasts that facilitate fragmentation of collagen degradation products that are transcytosed through the osteoclasts. In addition to TRAP, studies using chick osteoclast culture systems have also suggested that tensin and cortactin expression may be useful as osteoclast differentiation markers *(10)*.

AUTOCRINE/PARACRINE REGULATION OF OSTEOCLASTOGENESIS

Osteoclast itself is an abundant source of cytokines. Ousler et al. *(11)* have shown that osteoclasts produce transforming growth factor (TGF)-β, which can inhibit or enhance osteoclast formation and bone resorption, depending on its concentration. We have used an expression cloning approach with a human osteoclast cDNA library and identified Annexin II, which stimulates osteoclast formation *(12)*. We further demonstrated that Annexin II enhanced GM-CSF production by bone marrow T-lymphocytes and stromal cells, increasing the proliferation of osteoclast precursors, and resulting in increased osteoclastogenesis *(13)*. We have also identified a novel intracellular signaling molecule, termed osteoclast stimulatory factor, that interact with the spinal muscular atrophy-determining gene product and results in release of soluble factors that enhance osteoclast differentiation *(14)*. Using a similar approach, we also identified inhibitory factors, such as osteoclast inhibitory peptide-1 (OIP-1/hSca) and OIP-II (legumain), which inhibit osteoclast development and bone resorption *(15,16)*. OIP-1/hSca is expressed by osteoclast precursor cells and activated T-lymphocytes *(17)*. We have recently shown that interferon-γ enhances OIP-1/hSca expression in osteoclast precursors and that cytokines, such as interleukin (IL)-1, enhance OIP-II expression *(18)*. Similarly, using cDNA subtractive hybridization methods, ADAM8 (a disintegrin and metalloproteinase) has been shown to be highly expressed in mature osteoclasts. ADAM8 affects the later stages of osteoclast differentiation increasing bone resorption capacity of these cells *(19)*.

Takahashi and coworkers *(20)* developed a coculture system with mouse spleen cells and osteoblastic cells to examine the role of osteoblasts in osteoclast formation. They demonstrated that when mouse spleen cells and osteoblastic cells, isolated from fetal mouse calvariae, were cocultured in the presence of 1,25-$(OH)_2D_3$, numerous multinucleated cells that expressed an osteoclast phenotype were formed. However, no osteoclast-like cells were formed when the spleen cells and osteoblastic cells were separated by a membrane filter in the coculture, suggesting that cell-to-cell contact with osteoblastic cells is required for the differentiation of osteoclast progenitors from splenic tissue into mature osteoclasts. The membrane factor expressed by osteoblasts and stromal cells that induces osteoclastogenesis has subsequently been identified as receptor activator of NF-κB (RANK) ligand.

The importance of stromal cell involvement in osteoclast differentiation has also been reported by Kukita et al. *(21)*. They showed that rat hematopoietic progenitor cells could differentiate into mononuclear osteoclast-like precursor cells in the absence of stromal cells. The fusion of these preosteoclasts to form multinucleated cells occurred only in the presence of 1,25-$(OH)_2D_3$ and stromal cells. The preosteoclasts also did not resorb dentine but could differentiate into functional bone resorbing multinucleated osteoclast-like cells in the presence of primary rat osteoblasts. Similarly, the bone marrow-derived stromal cell lines MC3T3-G2/PA6 and ST2 also support osteoclast-like cell differentiation in cocultures with mouse spleen cells *(22)*. Chambers et al. *(23)* have developed clonal bone marrow stromal cell lines that have the capacity to support osteoclast differentiation in cocultures with bone marrow cells. Hill et al. *(24)* have shown that insulin-like growth factors (IGF) I and II indirectly stimulate osteoclast activity through their action on osteoblastic cells, and that the type I but not the type II IGF receptor is involved in their response. Similarly, Shevde et al. *(25)* reported that stimulation of osteoclastogenesis by PTH or 1,251,25-$(OH)_2D_3$ is mediated indirectly by inducing production of factors by normal marrow stromal cells that enhance osteoclast formation. We have previously established and characterized a human marrow-derived stromal cell line (Saka) that enhances osteoclast-like cell formation in human marrow cultures *(26)*. Cultures of human bone marrow and Saka cells separated by a Millipore membrane did not enhance MNC formation. Addition of a neutralizing antibody to IL-6 or IL-1β blocked the effects of Saka cells on MNC formation. These results suggest that marrow stromal cells and osteoblasts enhance osteoclast formation through direct cell-to-cell contact and through production of IL-6 and/or IL-1β and other osteotropic factors, such as M-CSF and RANK ligand. Recently fibroblastic stromal cells have been reported to express RANKL and support osteoclast differentiation *(27)*.

TRANSCRIPTION FACTORS

Several transcription factors and/or protein kinases appear to be critical to osteoclast differentiation.

Nuclear Factor-κB (NF-κB)

NF-κB is an important transcription factor involved in osteoclast differentiation. Mice deficient in both the p50 and p52 subunits of NF-κB develop severe osteopetrosis *(28)*. Deletion of only the p50 or p52 subunit does not result in a bone phenotype. NF-κB plays a critical role in expression of a variety of cytokines involved in osteoclast differentiation, including IL-1, tumor necrosis factor (TNF)-α, IL-6, GM-CSF, and RANK ligand, and deletion of both p50 and p52 may affect the production of growth factors critical for osteoclast differentiation as well as RANK ligand signaling. Recently, Xing et al *(29)* showed that NF-κB p50 and p52 expression is not required for formation of RANK-expressing osteoclast progenitors but is essential for RANK-expressing osteoclast precursors to differentiate into osteoclasts in response to RANKL and other osteoclastogenic cytokines.

PU.1

Tondravi and coworkers *(30)* reported that the myeloid and B-cell specific transcription factor, PU.1, was critical for osteoclast differentiation. They showed that PU.1 expression progressively increased as marrow macrophages expressed the osteoclast phenotype in vitro. Furthermore, PU.1 expression increased with the induction of osteoclastogenesis by $1,25\text{-}(OH)_2D_3$ and dexamethasone. These workers also developed PU.1-deficient mice and found that these mice were osteopetrotic. Transplantation of normal marrow into these mice resulted in complete restoration of osteoclast and macrophage differentiation. The absence of both osteoclasts and macrophages in PU.1-deficient mice suggests that this transcription factor regulates the initial stages of macrophage differentiation. PU.1 has been shown to interact with the microphthalmia transcription factor to regulate TRAP gene expression and osteoclast differentiation *(31)*.

c-fos

c-fos, a proto-oncogene normally associated with osteosarcomas, also appears to be a key regulator of osteoclast differentiation. Grigoriadis and coworkers *(32)* have shown by using the techniques of homologous recombination, that mice lacking the *c-fos* proto-oncogene develop osteopetrosis and have normal macrophage differentiation. The *fos*-deficient mice have a block in differentiation at the branch point between monocyte–macrophages and osteoclasts and only form macrophages. Furthermore, transfection of *c-fos* cDNA into avian osteoclast precursors induced a twofold increase in TRAP activity and osteoclastic bone resorption activity as compared with controls. These data suggest that prolonged expression of *c-fos* can enhance osteoclast differentiation. Hoyland and Sharpe *(33)* have also shown that *c-fos* proto-oncogene expression is upregulated in osteoclasts from patients with Paget's disease. Owens and coworkers *(34)* transduced osteoclast precursors with *c-fos* or Fra-1 using retroviral constructs. Overexpression of Fra-1 but not *c-fos* in an immortalized bipotential osteoclast/macrophage precursor cell line caused a significant increase in the proportion of these precursors that developed calcitonin receptors and subsequent bone resorption. These data suggest that Fra-1 may play a role in osteoclast differentiation distinct from that of *c-fos*. Recently, Fleischmann et al. *(35)* reported that Fra-1, but none of the Jun proteins *(c-Jun, Jun-B, and Jun-D)* rescued the block in osteoclast differentiation when the Fra-1 gene is knocked-in to *c-fos*-deficient mice and this effect was gene dose dependent. Matsuo et al. *(36)* also found that the N-terminal portion and the core region of Fos proteins were sufficient for osteoclast differentiation. Recently, these investigators have also shown that RANKL induces transcription of Fosl1 in a *c-fos*-dependent manner, thereby establishing a link between RANK signaling and the expression of AP-1 proteins in osteoclast differentiation *(37)*.

Udagawa and coworkers *(38)* reported that *c-fos* plays an important role in the proliferative phase of osteoclast progenitors but not in the terminal differentiation phase or in the bone-resorbing activity of mature osteoclasts. This study demonstrated that treatment of cocultures of mouse bone marrow with primary osteoblastic cells with *c-fos* antisense oligomers for the first 4 d of culture inhibited osteoclast formation. However, when *c-fos* antisense oligomers were added during the second phase of coculture *(days 4 through 6)*, osteoclast formation was unaffected, suggesting a role for *c-fos* in osteoclast progenitor proliferation. Taken together, these data suggest that *c-fos* plays a critical role in the differentiation of osteoclast precursors at the branch point where the osteoclast lineage diverges from the macrophage and has a primary effect on the proliferative phase of osteoclast development.

c-src

c-src, a proto-oncogene, plays a critical role in the activation of quiescent osteoclasts to become bone-resorbing osteoclasts. Osteoclast formation is normal in animals lacking the c-src gene. However, they develop osteopetrosis because the osteoclasts are unable to resorb bone *(39)* because the osteoclasts cannot form ruffled borders *(40)*. These animals can be rescued by transplantation of normal hematopoietic precursors from animals expressing c-src *(41)*. The substrate for src appears to be cortactin, which plays a critical role in attachment of osteoclasts to bone surfaces. However, it is unclear if the enzyme activity of c-src, which is a nonreceptor tyrosine kinase, is required for osteoclast activity. Schwartzberg and coworkers *(42)* generated transgenic mice that had the wild-type or mutated versions of c-src proto-oncogene targeted to the osteoclast using the TRAP gene promoter. They demonstrated that expression of the wild-type transgene in only a limited number of tissues can fully rescue the c-src–deficient phenotype. Interestingly, they reported that expression of kinase defective mutants of c-src in c-src–deficient mice also reduces osteopetrosis. These data suggest that there are essential kinase-independent functions for c-src in vivo. Abu-Amer et al. *(43)*, using double antibody immunoconfocal microscopy, demonstrated that c-src associated with tubulin only when avian osteoclasts were adherent to bone. This would suggest that matrix recognition by osteoclasts induces c-src to associate with microtubules that traffic proteins to the cell surface. Tanaka et al. *(44)* have suggested that the lack of phosphorylation of c-cbl is the important step in osteoclast activation in c-src–deficient animals, that c-cbl forms molecular complexes with src and Pyk2 and regulates src kinase to regulate osteoclast adhesion and motility *(45)*.

Tax

Inoue and coworkers *(46)* developed transgenic mice expressing the human T cell leukemia virus type I-tax under the control of human T cell leukemia virus type I-long terminal repeat promoter and found that these transgenic mice had skeletal abnormalities characterized by high bone turnover. Tax gene expression in bone was restricted to osteoclasts, was dependent on treatment of osteoclast precursors with 1,25-$(OH)_2D_3$, and coincided with TRAP expression in mononuclear osteoclast precursors and mature osteoclasts. These investigators have also identified an osteoclast-specific nuclear transcription factor, NFOC-1, whose expression is enhanced by Tax. NFOC-1 is absent in macrophages and conserved in osteoclasts from different species, including humans. These data suggest that this nuclear factor may have a role in commitment of cells to the osteoclast lineage and/or osteoclast differentiation.

Microphthalmic Transcription Factor (MITF)

MITF is required for terminal osteoclast differentiation. Mice lacking the MITF gene developed osteopetrosis. Mansky et al. *(47)* have shown that MITF is involved in the RANK ligand signaling pathway and that phosphorylation of MITF results in activation of target genes in osteoclasts. Weilbaecher and coworkers *(48)* showed that M-CSF induces phosphorylation of MITF and that MITF and the TFE3 transcription factor are required for osteoclast gene activation. MITF and TFE3 are closely related helix–loop–helix transcription factors that have been implicated in osteoclast development and function. The data demonstrate the link between cytokine signaling with gene expression vital to osteoclast differentiation and function. Mansky et al *(49)* have also shown that the microphthalmia transcription factor and the related helix–loop–helix factor TFE-3 and TFE-C collaborate to activate the TRAP gene promoter during osteoclast differentiation.

c-Myc

Recently, RANKL has been reported to strongly induce c-myc proto-oncogene expression during osteoclast differentiation of RAW 264.7 cells *(50)*. However, c-myc expression is absent in undifferentiated cells. Furthermore, expression of a dominant-negative myc in these cells results in blockade of RANKL-induced osteoclast formation. These results suggest that c-myc is a downstream target of RANKL and its expression is required for RANKL-induced osteoclastogenesis.

REGULATION OF OSTEOCLAST DIFFERENTIATION BY CYTOKINES, GROWTH FACTORS AND HORMONES

Cytokines and Growth Factors

RANKL

RANKL is a recently described member of the TNF family that is induced upon T cell receptor binding *(51)* and activates c-Jun N-terminal kinase after binding with its putative receptor, RANK. RANKL inhibits apoptosis of mouse bone marrow-derived dendritic cells and human monocyte-derived dendritic cells in vitro *(52)*. RANKL also upregulates Bcl-X_L expression, suggesting a potential mechanism for the enhanced dendritic cell survival. RANKL is critical for osteoclast formation and is produced by osteoblasts and stromal cells. RANKL in combination with M-CSF is all that is needed to induce osteoclast formation by spleen cells in the absence of osteoblasts *(53)*. Yasuda et al. *(54)* have reported that RANKL also binds to osteoprotegerin, a novel member of the TNF receptor family that inhibits osteoclast formation and bone resorption. Lacey et al. *(55)* have shown that RANKL is essential but not sufficient for osteoclast survival and that endogenous CSF-1 levels are insufficient to maintain osteoclast viability in the absence of RANKL. Kojima et al. *(56)* further demonstrated that RANKL inhibits rDrak1, a kinase that is highly expressed in active osteoclasts and induces apoptosis.

M-CSF

M-CSF, also called CSF-1, is produced by murine osteoblast/stromal cells and is the critical factor in combination with RANKL that is responsible for the effects of marrow stromal cells on osteoclast development in coculture systems. The role of M-CSF in osteoclast differentiation has been clearly demonstrated in the op/op mouse *(57)*. A frame-shift mutation in the coding region of the M-CSF gene in these mice results in an osteopetrotic phenotype as a result of lack of functionally active M-CSF *(58)*. However, the administration of recombinant M-CSF to these mice reversed the osteopetrotic phenotype. The addition of M-CSF together with 1,25-$(OH)_2D_3$ to the cocultures of op/op osteoblastic cells and normal spleen cells restored osteoclast formation in vitro *(59)*. In these studies, when M-CSF was added throughout the 6-d culture period, osteoclasts were formed in response to 1,25-$(OH)_2D_3$. However, absence of M-CSF either for the first 4 d (proliferative phase) or for the final 2 d (differentiation phase) blocked osteoclast formation. Furthermore, osteoclasts were formed in cocultures of spleen cells obtained from op/op mice and osteoblastic cells from normal mice. However, osteoclasts never formed in cocultures of normal spleen cells and op/op osteoblastic cells. These results clearly indicate that osteoclast deficiency in op/op mice is caused by a defect in M-CSF production by osteoblastic cells but not in spleen cells *(60)*. Halasy and Hofstetter *(61)* have recently examined the expression of the secreted and membrane bound M-CSF in bone during development of osteoclasts by quantitative polymerase chain reaction in the fetal metatarsal model of osteoclast formation. This study demonstrated that in vivo the highest levels of M-CSF are expressed during the late differentiation stage of osteoclast formation and are required for activation of osteoclasts. It also supports the hypothesis that locally produced M-CSF may act in a paracrine manner during osteoclastogenesis and that both forms, secreted and membrane bound, are required for the full biological action of the cytokine. Yamane et al. *(62)* have reported that expansion of osteoclast precursors and terminal differentiation of mature osteoclasts was affected by treatment of embryonic stem cells with an antibody to the M-CSF receptor, c-fms. This resulted in <75% reduction in the number of osteoclasts produced. Transition of embryonic stem cells to other hematopoietic lineages was not blocked by an antibody to c-fms. Fan et al. *(63)* have also recently reported that M-CSF downregulates c-fms expression and that the entry of osteoclast progenitors into the osteoclast lineage in murine bone marrow cultures. Nilsson and coworkers *(64)* have reported that the osteopetrosis in op/op mice improves with age, suggesting that M-CSF is required for osteoclast development in younger animals. Therefore, M-CSF produced by osteoblasts appears to be indispensable for proliferation and differentiation of osteoclast progenitors, but can be substituted by other factors. Lean et al. *(65)* have shown that FLT3 ligand can partly substitute for M-CSF in support of osteoclast differentiation and function in osteopetrotic (op/op) mice.

Osteoprotegerin (OPG)

OPG is a novel secreted glycoprotein that regulates bone resorption. Osteoprotegerin, also called osteoclastogenesis inhibitory factor, is a member of TNF receptor superfamily that has been identified recently *(53,66)*. In vitro and in vivo osteoclast differentiation from precursor cells is blocked in a dose-dependent manner by recombinant OPG. OPG is produced by most cell types and appears to block the fusion/differentiation stage of osteoclast differentiation rather than the proliferative phase. It binds to a single class of high-affinity binding sites on the ST2 mouse marrow stromal cell line treated with 1,25-$(OH)_2D_3$ *(53)*. Yasuda and coworkers *(54)* have recently demonstrated that RANKL, produced by osteoblasts, binds to OPG and blocks the inhibitory actions of OPG on osteoclastogenesis. OPG blocks osteoclast precursor formation and osteoclast differentiation supported by osteoblasts *(67)*. The expression of OPG and RANKL has been shown to be developmentally regulated in the stromal–osteoblast lineage. Osteoblast differentiation resulted in decreased RANKL and increased OPG mRNA levels *(68)*. Furthermore, a number of local factors as well as systemic hormones induce RANKL expression through diverse cellular signal transduction mechanisms. These include 1,25-$(OH)_2D_3$ signaling through vitamin D receptor; parathyroid hormone (PTH), parathyroid hormone-related peptide (PTHrP), prostaglandin E_2 (PGE_2), and IL-1 signaling through protein kinase A; and IL-6, IL-11, oncostatin M, leukemia inhibitory factor signaling through gp 130 *(5)*. However, IL-1β and TNF-α but not IL-6 stimulated RANKL expression in human osteoblastic cells *(69)*. Furthermore, Horwood et al. *(70)* have shown that osteotropic agents such as 1,25 dihydroxy vitamin D3, PTH, or IL-11 promoted an increase in the ratio of RANKL:OPG in osteoblastic stromal cells. TGF-β has also been shown to induce OPG expression in murine stroma/osteoblast cells *(71)*.

TNF

TNF-α and TNF-β stimulate both osteoclast formation and osteoclastic bone resorption both in murine and human marrow cultures *(72)*. TNF appears to induce both the proliferation and differentiation of osteoclast precursors, as well as activating preformed osteoclasts to resorb bone. Uy and coworkers *(73)* have demonstrated that TNF acts on the more differentiated osteoclast precursor rather than CFU-GM and does not have a CSF-like activity. Similarly, TNF-β, also called lymphotoxin, can stimulate osteoclast formation and osteoclastic bone resorption *(72)*. TNF-α has also been implicated as a potential mediator of the increased bone loss in patients with postmenopausal osteoporosis and may work in concert with IL-1 to increase bone resorption in mice that have undergone ovariectomy *(74)*. TNF-α has been reported to stimulate osteoclast differentiation by a mechanism independent of RANK-RANKL interaction *(75)*, but Lam et al *(76)* showed that trace amounts of RANKL are required with TNF-α to promote osteoclastogenesis.

IL-1

IL-1 is a cytokine produced by a variety of cell types, including monocyte–macrophages and marrow stromal cells. It is also produced by osteoclasts. IL-1 can stimulate bone resorption in vitro and in vivo *(72,77)*.

Uy et al. *(78)* have used an in vivo model of osteoclast formation to examine the systemic effects of IL-1 on different stages of osteoclast development. IL-1 induced hypercalcemia and enhanced the growth and differentiation of CFU-GM, the earliest identifiable osteoclast precursor. It also increased the number of more committed mononuclear osteoclast precursors and stimulated mature osteoclasts to resorb bone. These data demonstrate that IL-1 affects all stages of osteoclast development and may explain its potent effects on bone turnover in vivo. It has also been shown that indomethacin did not block the effects of IL-1 in vivo, suggesting that the effects of IL-1 on osteoclasts are not mediated by prostaglandins *(77)*.

We have previously established a human bone marrow stromal cell line (Saka) that supports osteoclast formation in human marrow culture system. Addition of neutralizing antibodies to IL-1β or IL-6 blocked the stimulatory effect of Saka cells on osteoclast formation *(26)*, suggesting that IL-1 can mediate in part the effects of marrow stromal cells on osteoclast formation. Pacifici *(74)* has also implicated IL-1 as a mediator for the increased bone resorption seen after estrogen withdrawal in mice and in postmenopausal women. IL-1 induces the expression of nitric oxide synthase *(iNOS)* and studies in vitro and in vivo studies showed that iNOS-deficient mice exhibited profound defects of IL-1–induced osteoclastic bone resorption but responded normally to 1,25 dihydroxy vitamin D3. Furthermore, iNOS-deficient mice showed abnormalities in IL-1 induced nuclear translocation of the p65 component of NF-κB and in NF-κB DNA binding *(79)*. IL-1 directly stimulates actin ring formation and survival of osteoclasts ex vivo *(80)*.

IL-4

IL-4 is a lymphocyte growth factor that exerts a potent inhibitory effect on osteoclast activity. Although IL-4 can stimulate M-CSF expression, its inhibitory effect on osteoclast recruitment was not prevented by anti-M-CSF antibodies *(81)*. Furthermore, recombinant murine IL-4 blocks PTHrP-stimulated osteoclast formation and bone resorption in vivo *(82)*. However, transgenic mice overexpressing IL-4 develop an osteopenic syndrome that is similar to osteoporosis *(83)*. These data suggest that high levels of IL-4 may also inhibit bone formation as well as bone resorption in vivo. Recently, Abu-Amer *(84)* has shown that IL-4 abrogates osteoclastogenesis through STAT6-dependent inhibition of NF-κB activation.

IL-6

High levels of interleukin-6 (IL-6) have been associated with several bone diseases, including Paget's disease, multiple myeloma, osteoporosis, and Gorham-Stout disease *(85)*. Furthermore, IL-6 can act as an autocrine/paracrine factor that stimulates osteoclast formation in human marrow cultures in the absence of added IL-6 receptors *(86)*. We have also demonstrated that addition of a neutralizing antibody to IL-6 or antisense deoxyoligonucleotides to IL-6 mRNA can block bone resorption by human osteoclasts isolated from giant cell tumors of bone *(87,88)*. Devlin et al. *(89)* demonstrated that IL-6 mediates the effects of IL-1 and TNF-α on osteoclast formation in human marrow cultures. However, Udagawa et al. *(90)*, using osteoblastic cells from transgenic mice constitutively overexpressing human IL-6 receptors, showed that the ability of IL-6 to induce osteoclast differentiation depended on signal transduction mediated by IL-6 receptors expressed on osteoblastic cells but not on osteoclast progenitors. Suda and coworkers *(5)* have also reported the essential role of membrane-bound IL-6 receptors on osteoblastic cells in IL-6-mediated osteoclast formation. They have also shown that when osteoblastic cells and bone marrow cells were cocultured without direct contact, no osteoclasts were formed even in the presence of IL-6.

In contrast with studies with human osteoclasts, Holt et al. *(91)* reported that although IL-6 levels are elevated in response to PGE_2 and PTH in the neonatal mouse bone resorption assay, IL-6 did not mediate osteoclast differentiation or bone resorption in these organ cultures. Addition of a neutralizing antibody to IL-6 in quantities sufficient to block the increased IL-6 activity in these organ cultures did not inhibit osteoclast formation.

Passeri et al. *(92)* have demonstrated that estrogen loss causes an upregulation of IL-6 production in murine bone marrow cell cultures in response to either 1,25-$(OH)_2D_3$ or PTH and that a similar phenomenon can be elicited by withdrawal of 17β-estradiol from primary cell cultures of mouse calvarial cells. These authors suggested that IL-6 may mediate the increased bone resorption after estrogen withdrawal. IL-6 in murine systems can induce RANKL expression on osteoblasts but does not induce RANKL expression in human systems *(93)*.

IL-11

IL-11 is produced by mesenchymal-derived stromal cells of the bone marrow *(94)*. Girasole et al. *(95)* reported that IL-11 induced the formation of osteoclasts in cocultures of murine bone marrow and calvarial cells. Osteoclasts formed in the presence of IL-11 showed a high degree of ploidy and formed resorption lacunae on calcified matrices. This study also demonstrated that a neutralizing antibody against IL-11 suppressed osteoclast development induced by either 1,25-$(OH)_2D_3$, PTH, IL-1, or TNF. These data also suggest that a variety of osteotropic factors can induce osteoblasts to produce IL-11. The effects of IL-11 on osteoclast differentiation appear to be mediated by inducing prostaglandin synthesis, since indomethacin blocked the effects of IL-11 on osteoclast development.

Osteoclast differentiation was also reported to be stimulated by rhIL-11 and PGE_2 in porcine bone marrow cultures *(96)*. Similar to IL-6, IL-11 acts synergistically with IL-3 and IL-4 to stimulate CFU-GM formation in vitro, and they both use the gp130 signal transduction pathway *(97)*. Suda and coworkers *(5)* have suggested that in addition to IL-6, IL-11 and other bone-resorbing factors, such as oncostatin M and leukemia inhibitory factor, which transduce signals through gp130, may induce a critical common membrane-bound factor(s) on osteoblastic stromal cells, which interacts with osteoclast progenitors to trigger differentiation. This factor has been identified as RANK ligand.

TGF-β

TGF-β is secreted by osteoblasts and osteoclasts and may act as an autocrine/paracrine factor to inhibit osteoclast formation and stimulate osteoblastic bone formation. Oursler *(11)* showed that osteoclasts express TGF-β messenger RNA and that latent TGF-β produced by osteoclasts was activated when it was secreted by the osteoclasts. TGF-β is a potent inhibitor of osteoclastic bone resorption, and Chenu and coworkers *(98)* showed that TGF-β inhibits both the proliferation and fusion of human osteoclast precursors. In addition, TGF-β appears to preferentially induce granulocytic rather than monocyte–macrophage differentiation of early monocyte precursors. These data demonstrate that TGF-β, in addition to inhibiting all stages of osteoclast differentiation, also appears to deplete the precursor pool for osteoclasts by shifting the differentiation of immature precursor cells toward the granulocytic lineage. Recent studies have shown that very low concentrations of TGF-β_1 can enhance osteoclast formation and bone resorption *(99)*. These data suggest that the effects of TGF-β on osteoclast activity differ depending on the amount of TGF-β that is present.

Interferons

Interferon (IFN)-γ inhibits osteoclastic bone resorption in organ cultures stimulated either by IL-1 or TNF *(100)*. In addition to inhibiting the bone-resorbing capacity of preformed osteoclasts, interferons also inhibit osteoclast formation in human marrow culture systems. Takahashi and coworkers *(101)* showed that IFN-γ inhibited the formation of osteoclast-like cells in human marrow cultures, and Kurihara and Roodman *(102)* have also shown that IFN-γ can inhibit osteoclast formation in these cultures. These data suggest that interferons represent a class of inhibitors of both osteoclast formation and bone resorption.

Immune cell products, such as IFNs, that are released in response to inflammatory stimuli or viral infections have been reported as important local negative regulators for bone remodeling *(100)*. IFN-γ inhibited 1,25 dihydroxy vitamin D3-induced osteoclast formation in long-term human bone marrow cultures. In addition, IFNs inhibit CFU-GM growth and recruitment of osteoclast precursors to fuse and form multinucleated osteoclasts *(101)*. T-cell production of IFN-γ also strongly suppresses osteoclastogenesis by interfering with the RANKL–RANK signaling pathway *(103)*. IFN-γ induces rapid degradation of the RANK adaptor protein, TRAF6, which results in strong inhibition of the RANKL-induced NF-κB activation and c-jun kinase activity. These studies suggested there is cross-talk between TNF and IFN families of cytokines, through which IFN provides a negative link between T-cell activation and bone resorption. IFN-γ exerts a direct effect on osteoclast progenitors and TGF-β antagonizes the effect of IFN-γ *(104)*. IFN-γ has been shown to inhibit IL-1 and TNF-α-stimulated bone resorption by strongly stimulating nitric oxide synthesis *(105)*. Recently, it has been shown that RANKL induces the interferon-β gene in osteoclast precursor cells and that IFN-β inhibits osteoclast differentiation by interfering with the RANKL induced expression of *c-fos* to maintain bone homeostasis *(106)*.

Hormones

Calcitriol

Metabolites of vitamin D_3 are potent stimulators of osteoclastic bone resorption and osteoclast formation. The most active metabolite, 1,25-$(OH)_2D_3$, acts as a fusigen for committed osteoclast precursors *(107)*. It is unknown whether 1,25-$(OH)_2D_3$ acts on mature osteoclasts directly or indirectly through osteoblasts, although mature osteoclasts express vitamin D receptors *(108)*, because 1,25 $(OH)_2$ is a potent stimulator of RANKL expression by stromal cells *(53)*. Feyen et al. *(109)* have reported that1,25-$(OH)_2D_3$ can induce IL-1 production and IL-6 production by osteoblasts, factors that stimulate osteoclastic bone resorption. Furthermore, 1,25-$(OH)_2D_3$ also enhances osteoclastic bone resorption stimulated by PTH. Mice treated with 1,25-$(OH)_2D_3$ develop hypercalcemia, and analogs of 1,25-$(OH)_2D_3$ have variable effects on osteoclast activity *(110)*. In contrast, Woods et al. *(111)* demonstrated an antagonistic role for vitamin D_3 and retinoic acid on the induction of chicken macrophages to become osteoclast progenitors. Importantly, osteoclast formation in vitamin D_3 receptor knockout mice is normal, suggesting that in murine system, 1,25-$(OH)_2D_3$ is not absolutely required for osteoclast formation.

PTH/PTHrP

PTH is a peptide produced by the parathyroid glands that is important in the maintenance of normal calcium homeostasis because of its stimulatory effects on osteoclastic bone resorptive activity and renal reabsorption of calcium. PTHrP is the mediator of the humoral hypercalcemia of malignancy and is produced by a variety of cells *(112)*. PTHrP has 70% homology with the first 13 amino acids of PTH. PTHrP binds the PTH receptor and activates cAMP. Uy et al. *(78)* have studied the effects of PTH and PTHrP on osteoclasts and osteoclast precursors in vivo. This study demonstrated that neither PTH nor PTHrP had an effect on early osteoclast precursors, but increased the number of more committed mononuclear osteoclast progenitors as well as mature osteoclasts.

The primary target cell for PTH appears to be the osteoblast *(113)*. Isolated osteoclasts do not resorb bone in response to PTH and only do so when osteoblasts or osteoblastic cell lines are added to the cultures *(114)*. Greenfield et al. *(115)* have suggested that stimulation of osteoclast activity by PTH is dependent on activation of the cAMP signal transduction pathway and secretion of IL-6 by osteoblasts. However, Kurihara et al. *(116)* have reported that PTH is a mitogen for highly purified human osteoclast precursors.

Until recently, it was thought that osteoclasts did not express PTH receptors. However, Agarwala and Gay *(117)* and Teti et al. *(118)* have reported that murine or avian osteoclasts express PTH receptors. Hakeda et al. *(119)* previously reported, by using immunocytochemical techniques, that osteoclast precursors derived from murine hematopoietic blast cells expressed PTH receptors and suggested that PTH may act directly on osteoclast precursors to induce their differentiation. Orlandini et al. *(120)* also reported that addition of PTH to the coculture of human clonal cell lines of osteoclast precursors (FLG 29.1) and osteoblastic cells (Saos-2) further potentiated the differentiation of the preosteoclasts. Radiolabeled PTH binds to osteoclasts in vitro *(118)* and data obtained by reverse transcription polymerase chain reaction demonstrated that microisolated rat and mouse osteoclasts express the mRNA for the PTH/PTHrP receptor *(121)*. More recently, Kartsogiannis et al. *(122)*, by using immunocytochemical staining and *in situ* hybridization methods, also provided evidence for the expression of PTHrP mRNA and protein by mouse, rabbit, and human osteoclasts derived from in vitro and in vivo sources. The presence of a nucleolar localization signal sequence within PTHrP and evidence for cell cycle-linked expression of PTHrP strongly support a possible intracrine role for PTHrP related to growth, differentiation, and other functions in cells that express PTHrP. However, PTHrP and PTH exert their effects on osteoclast formation through increasing expression of RANKL on marrow stromal cells.

Calcitonin

Calcitonin is a peptide hormone secreted by the parafollicular cells of the thyroid gland and is a potent inhibitor of osteoclastic bone resorption. CTRs are expressed on committed osteoclast precursors and mature osteoclasts *(123)*. Calcitonin downregulates expression of calcitonin receptors in osteoclast precursors and mature osteoclasts and inhibits CTR mRNA expression *(7)*. Calcitonin acts on osteoclasts by stimulating adenylcyclase activity and cAMP accumulation, which results in immobilization of the osteoclast and contraction of the osteoclast away from the bone surface *(124)*. Osteoclasts continuously exposed to calcitonin can escape the effects of calcitonin. The mechanism responsible for this escape phenomenon is unclear but may be caused by the effects of calcitonin on transcriptional regulation of CTR gene expression and downregulation of CTR on the surface of the osteoclast.

Estradiol

Estrogen negatively regulates osteoclastogenic cytokines produced by stromal cells, such as IL-1, TNF, and IL-6. Recent studies *(125)* demonstrate that estrogen modulate osteoclast formation by direct suppression of RANKL-induced osteoclast differentiation. Estadiol can stimulate OPG mRNA levels and protein secretion in human osteoblast cells through activation of the estrogen receptor. This was caused by the enhancement of OPG gene transcription rather than stabilizing the message *(126)*. Szulc et al. *(127)* showed that serum osteoprotegrin levels in elderly men correlated with free estradiol levels.

Prostaglandins

The effect of prostaglandins on osteoclast formation and osteoclastic bone resorption may be dependent on the dose administered and the assay system used. Prostaglandins are stimulators of osteoclastic bone resorption in bone organ culture systems and osteoclast formation in murine marrow cultures *(128)*. However, PGE_2 inhibits osteoclastic bone resorption and formation in human marrow systems *(129)*. Quinn and coworkers *(130)* have also examined the inhibitory effect of PGE_2 on osteoclast differentiation. To identify the cellular mechanisms responsible for this inhibitory effect of PGE_2 and to determine whether PGE_2 inhibition was dependent on the stromal cells supporting osteoclast differentiation, PGE_2 was added to murine monocyte/rat UMR 106 osteoblastic cells and murine monocyte/ST2 stromal cell cocultures before and during specific phases of differentiation. PGE_2 exerts an inhibitory effect on osteoclast differentiation in the monocyte/UMR 106 coculture system and in contrast stimulates osteoclast formation and bone resorption in monocyte/ST2 cocultures. These data suggest that prostaglandins strongly influence the differentiation of osteoclast precursors, and this effect is also dependent not only on the type and dose of prostaglandin administered but the nature of bone-derived stromal cells that support osteoclast formation. Roux et al. *(131)* have reported that PGE_2 has an inhibitory effect on human osteoclast differentiation from cord blood monocytes, possibly by reducing precursor proliferation in these cultures. They have also proposed that PGE_2 may reduce osteoclast differentiation by increasing the proportion of precursor cells that differentiate into macrophages.

Tashjian and coworkers *(132)* have reported that a variety of factors that stimulate osteoclastic bone resorption in the mouse calvarial organ culture system do so by generating prostaglandins. These data suggest that PGE_2 may be an important second message for cytokines that enhance bone resorption. Wani and coworkers *(133)* have shown that in addition to stimulating RANKL expression, PGE_2 can enhance the effects of RANKL on osteoclast formation.

Gallwitz et al. *(134)* showed that other arachidonic acid metabolites, such as the peptidoleukotrienes, as well as 5-hydroxyeiocatetraenoic acid, stimulate isolated osteoclasts to resorb bone. These 5-lipoxygenase metabolites are produced by stromal cells isolated from giant cell tumors of bone, suggesting that they may serve as a means for stromal cell enhancement of osteoclast activity. These arachidonic metabolites may also play an important role in bone resorption in areas of chronic inflammation, in addition to the effects of tumor necrosis factor alpha and IL-1. Franchi-Miller and Saffar *(135)* also examined the role of leukotrienes on bone resorption by inhibiting their biosynthesis with BWA4C, a specific inhibitor of 5-lipoxygenase. Rats treated with this compound demonstrated a dramatic decrease in the number of TRAP-positive mononucleated preosteoclasts compared with the sham-treated group. This decrease in osteoclast precursors also correlated with a significant decrease in the number of osteoclasts, further supporting a role for leukotrienes in the recruitment of osteoclast progenitors and/or their differentiation into preosteoclasts. Garcia and coworkers *(136)* have also studied the effects of 5-lipoxygenase metabolites on osteoclastic bone resorption both in vitro and in vivo. They have shown that LTC4, LTD4 or LTE4, and 5-HETE induce osteoclastic bone resorption and that receptors for LTD4 are present on isolated avian osteoclast-like cells. Another metabolite, LTB4, increased osteoclastic bone resorption in vivo and in vitro in organ cultures of neonatal mice.

OTHER FACTORS/AGENTS AFFECTING OSTEOCLAST DIFFERENTIATION

Calcium (Ca^{2+})

Ca^{2+}-ATPase inhibitors and Ca^{2+} ionophores can stimulate osteoclast formation in cocultures of mouse calvaria-derived stromal cells and bone marrow/spleen cells *(137)*. However, the differentiation of hematopoietic cells into osteoclasts induced by these compounds required the presence of calvarial cells, further suggesting that intracellular Ca^{2+} levels may be a part of the signaling pathways that induce osteoclast differentiation. Takami et al. *(138)* have shown that increases in intracellular calcium levels in osteoblasts upregulates RANKL mRNA expression.

Zinc

Zinc is an abundant element in the bone and may act as a local regulator of bone cells, although its actions are controversial. Zinc is a prosthetic group in carbonic anhydrase *(139)*, a critical enzyme required for bone resorption. Zinc also inhibits the activity of TRAP. Both enzymes are highly expressed in OCL. Zinc is a potent and selective inhibitor of OCL bone resorption in vitro *(140)*, and decreases production of prostaglandin E_2, a potent stimulator of OCL activity in organ cultures *(141)*. Kishi and Yamaguchi *(142,143)* also reported that zinc compounds block OCL formation by having an inhibitory effect on preosteoclastic cells in mouse bone marrow cultures. In contrast, Holloway and coworkers

(144) reported that zinc increased the number of OCL but inhibited bone resorption in neonatal rats and OCL culture systems.

Cadmium

Chronic exposure to cadmium has been linked to bone loss *(145)*. Addition of cadmium to normal canine bone marrow cell cultures accelerated osteoclast differentiation from their progenitors and also activated the mature osteoclasts.

Ipriflavone

Notoya et al. *(146)* showed that ipriflavone inhibits both the activation of mature osteoclasts and the formation of new osteoclasts. When ipriflavone was added to unfractionated bone cell cultures containing mature osteoclasts from femur and tibia of newborn mice, there was a decrease in the number of osteoclast-like TRAP-positive multinucleated cells and bone resorption. In contrast, no increase in the number of TRAP-positive multinucleated osteoclasts was observed in the presence of vitamin D_3. Furthermore, Miyauchi et al. *(147)* recently demonstrated the presence of novel specific ipriflavone receptors that are coupled to Ca^{2+} influx in OCL and their precursor cells that may regulate OCL differentiation/function.

pH

Shibutani and Heersche *(148)* studied the effect of pH on osteoclast formation in neonatal rabbit osteoclast cultures. Osteoclast differentiation and proliferation were optimal at pH 7.0–7.5 but decreased at pH 6.5. Arnett and coworkers *(149)* have extensively studied the effects of pH on osteoclast formation and osteoclastic bone resorption. Acidosis stimulates bone resorption by activating mature osteoclasts present in calvaria and inducing formation of new osteoclasts. Furthermore at low pH, osteoclast formation is markedly enhanced in vitro compared to neutral pH levels. These data suggest a critical role for acid base balance in controlling osteoclast function *(150)*. These results imply that the pH of the bone microenvironment can affect osteoclast formation/differentiation.

Bone Matrix Factors

Osteopontin (OPN)

Osteopontin is an acidic phosphoprotein synthesized by osteoblasts and osteoclasts that is localized to the mineralized phase of bone matrix. Tani-Ishii et al. *(151)* demonstrated that addition of OPN antisense oligomers to cocultures of mouse bone marrow cells with MC3T3-G2/PA6 cells decreased the number of osteoclasts formed, suggesting that OPN may play a role in osteoclast differentiation and bone resorption. Recently, Asou et al. *(152)* showed that OPN facilitated accumulation of osteoclasts in ectopic bone.

Bone Morphogenetic Proteins (BMPs)

Kaneko et al. *(153)* have examined the direct effects of BMPs on osteoclastic bone resorbing activity in cultures of highly purified rabbit mature osteoclasts. BMP-2 and BMP-4 appeared to stimulate osteoclastic bone resorption. BMP-2 also increased cathepsin K and carbonic anhydrase mRNA expression, enzymes that participate in degradation of organic and inorganic matrices respectively.

Ascorbic Acid

Recently it has been shown that treatment of ST2 cells with ascorbic acid resulted in fivefold induction of RANKL and that inhibitors of collagen formation blocked ascorbic acid induced expression of RANKL. These data suggest that extracellular matrix play important role in ascorbic-induced osteoclast formation *(154)*.

SUMMARY

Osteoclast differentiation is a complex process that is regulated by both soluble and membrane-bound factors. Cells in the marrow microenvironment, including osteoblasts and marrow stromal cells, play critical roles in controlling this process by producing M-CSF and RANKL and blocking the effects of OPG. Loss of transcription factors that induce monocyte/macrophage differentiation, such as PU.1 and *c-fos*, result in the absence of osteoclast formation. Furthermore, cytokines, such as M-CSF, IL-1, IL-6, IL-11, RANKL, and TNF-α are important regulators of osteoclast differentiation in normal and pathologic conditions that result in increased bone resorption. Further studies should provide important insights into the molecular events associated with commitment of multipotent precursor cells to the osteoclast lineage and identify potential molecular targets for modulating osteoclast formation and activity in pathologic conditions associated with bone destruction.

REFERENCES

1. Sato, T., Shibata, T., Ikeda, K., and Watanabe, K. (2001) Generation of bone resorbing osteoclasts from B220+ cells: its role in accelerated osteoclastogenesis due to estrogen deficiency. *J. Bone Miner Res.* **16,** 2215–2221.
2. Menaa, C., Kurihara, N., and Roodman, G. D. (2000) CFU-GM-derived cells form osteoclasts at a very high efficiency. *Biochem. Biophys. Res. Commun.* **267,** 943–946.
3. Kukita, T. and Roodman, G. D. (1989) Development of a monoclonal antibody to osteoclasts formed in vitro which recognizes mononuclear osteoclast precursors in the marrow. *Endocrinology* **125,** 630–637.
4. Horton, M. A., Lewis, D., McNulty, K., Pringle, J. A. S., and Chambers, T. J. (1985) Monoclonal antibodies to osteoclastomas (giant cell bone tumors): definition of osteoclast-specific cellular antigens. *Cancer Res.* **45,** 5663–5669.
5. Suda, T., Udagawa, N., Nakamura, I., Miyaura, C., and Takahashi, N. (1995) Modulation of osteoclast differentiation by local factors. *Bone* **17,** 87S–91S.
6. Kania, J. R., Kehat-Stadler, T., and Kupfer, S. R. (1997) CD44 antibodies inhibit osteoclast formation. *J. Bone Miner. Res.* **12,** 1155–1164.
7. Takahashi, S., Goldring, S., Katz, M., Hilsenbeck, S., Williams, R., and Roodman, G. D. (1995) Downregulation of calcitonin receptor mRNA expression by calcitonin during human osteoclast-like cell differentiation. *J. Clin. Invest.* **95,** 167–171.
8. Hayman, A. R., Jones, S. J., Boyde, A., Foster, D., Colledge, W. H., Carlton, M. B., et al. (1996) Mice lacking tartrate-resistant acid phosphatase (Acp 5) have disrupted endochondral ossification and mild osteopetrosis. *Development* **122,** 3151–3162.
9. Halleen, J. M., Raisanen, S., Salo, J. J., Reddy, S. V., Roodman, G. D., Hentunen, T. A., et al. (1999) Intracellular fragmentation of bone resorption products by reactive oxygen species generated by osteoclastic tartrate resistant acid phosphatase. *J. Biol. Chem.* **274,** 22907–22910.
10. Sato, T., Abe, E., Jin, C. H., Hong, M. H., Katagiri, T., Kinoshita, T., et al. (1993) The biological roles of the third component of complement in osteoclast formation. *Endocrinology* **133,** 397–404.
11. Oursler, M. J. (1994) Osteoclast synthesis, secretion and activation of latent transforming growth factor beta. *J. Bone Miner. Res.* **9,** 443–452
12. Takahashi, S., Reddy, S. V., Chirgwin, J. M., Devlin, R. D., Haipek, C., Anderson, J., et al. (1994) Cloning and characterization of Annexin II as an autocrine/paracrine factor that increases osteoclast formation and bone resorption. *J. Biol. Chem.* **269,** 28696–28701.
13. Menaa, C., Devlin, R. D., Reddy, S. V., Gazitt, Y., Choi, S., and Roodman, G. D. (1999) Annexin II increases osteoclast formation by stimulating the proliferation of osteoclast precursors in human marrow cultures. *J. Clin. Invest.* **103,** 1605–1613.
14. Kurihara, N., Menaa, C., Haile, D. J., and Reddy, S. V. (2001) Osteoclast stimulatory factor (OSF) interacts with the spinal muscular atrophy (SMA) gene product to stimulate osteoclast formation. *J. Biol. Chem.* **276,** 41035–41039.
15. Choi, S., Devlin, R. D., Menaa, C., Chung, H., and Roodman, G. D., and Reddy S. V. (1988) Cloning and identification of human Sca as a novel inhibitor of osteoclast formation and bone resorption. *J. Clin. Invest.* **102,** 1360–1368.
16. Choi, S., Reddy, S. V., Devlin, R. D., Menaa, C., Chung, H., Boyce, B. F., et al. 1999) Identification of human Asparaginyl endopeptidase (Legumain) as an inhibitor of osteoclast formation and bone resorption. *J. Biol. Chem.* **274,** 27747–27753.
17. Koide, M., Kurihara, N., Maeda, H., and Reddy, S. V. (2002) Identification of the functional domain of osteoclast inhibitory peptide-1/hSca. *J. Bone Miner. Res.* **17,** 111–118.
18. Koide, M., Maeda, H., Roccisana, J. L., and Reddy, S. V. (2003) Cytokine regulation and the signaling mechanism of osteoclast inhibitory peptide-1 (OIP-1/hSca) to inhibit osteoclast formation. *J. Bone Miner. Res.* **18,** 458–465.
19. Choi, S. J., Han, J. H., and Roodman, G. D. (2001) ADAM8: a novel osteoclast stimulating factor. *J. Bone Miner. Res.* **16,** 814–822.
20. Takahashi, N., Akatsu, T., Udagawa, N., Sasaki, T., Yamaguchi, A., Moseley, J. M., et al. (1988) Osteoblastic cells are involved in osteoclast formation. *Endocrinology* **123,** 2600–2602.

21. Kukita, A., Kukita, T., Shin, J. H., and Kohashi, O. (1993) Induction of mononuclear precursor cells with osteoclastic phenotypes in a rat bone marrow culture system depleted of stromal cells. *Biochem. Biophys. Res. Commun.* **196,** 1389–1389.
22. Udagawa, N., Takahashi, N., Akatsu, T., Sasaki, T., Yamaguchi, A., Kodama, H., et al. (1989) The bone marrow-derived stromal cell lines MC3T3-G2/PA6 and ST2 support osteoclast-like cell differentiation in cocultures with mouse spleen cells. *Endocrinology* **125,** 1805–1813.
23. Chambers, T. J., Owens, J. M., Hattersley, G., Jat, P. S., and Noble, M. D. (1993) Generation of osteoclast-inductive and osteoclastogenic cell lines from the H-2KbtsA58 transgenic mouse. *Proc. Natl. Acad. Sci. USA* **90,** 5578–5582.
24. Hill, P. A., Reynolds, J. J., and Meikle, M. C. (1995) Osteoblasts mediate insulin-like growth factor-I and -II stimulated osteoclast formation and function. *Endocrinology* **136,** 124–131.
25. Shevde, N., Anklesaria, P., Greenberger, J. S., Bleiberg, I., and Glowacki, J. (1994) Stromal cell-mediated stimulation of osteoclastogenesis. *Proc. Soc. Exp. Biol. Med.* **205,** 306–315.
26. Takahashi, S., Reddy, S. V., Dallas, M., Devlin, R., Chou, J. Y., and Roodman, G. D. (1995) Development and characterization of a human marrow stromal cell line that enhances osteoclast-like cell formation. *Endocrinology* **136,** 1441–1449.
27. Quinn, J. M., Horwood, N. J., Elliott, J., Gillespie, M. T., and Martin, T. J. (2000) Fibroblastic stromal cells express receptor activator of NF kappa B ligand and support osteoclast differentiation. *J. Bone Miner. Res.* **15,** 1459–1466.
28. Franzoso, G., Carlson, L., Xing, L., Poljak, L., Shores, E. W., Brown, K. D., et al. (1997) Requirement for NF-kappaB in osteoclast and B-cell development. *Genes Dev.* **11,** 3482–3496.
29. Xing, L., Bushnell, T. P., Carlson, L., Tai, Z., Tondravi, M., Siebenlist, U., et al. (2002) NF-kappaB p50 and p52 expression is not required for RANK expressing osteoclast progenitor formation but is essential for RANK and cytokine mediated osteoclastogenesis. *J. Bone Miner. Res.* **17,** 1200–1210.
30. Tondravi, M. M., McKercher, S. R., Anderson, K., Erdmann, J. M., Quiroz, M., Maki, R., et al. (1997) Osteopetrosis in mice lacking hematopoietic transcription factor PU.1. *Nature* **386,** 81–84.
31. Luchin, A., Suchting, S., Merson, T., Rosol, T. J., Hume, D. A., Cassady, A. I., et al. (2001) Genetic and physical interactions between micropththalmia transcription factor and PU.1 are necessary for osteoclast gene expression and differentiation. *J. Biol. Chem.* **276,** 36703–36710.
32. Grigoriadis, A. E., Wang, Z. Q., Cecchini, M. G., Hofstetter, W., Felix, R., Fleisch, H. A., et al. (1994) *c-fos*: a key regulator of osteoclast-macrophage lineage determination and bone remodeling. *Science* **266,** 443–448.
33. Hoyland, J. and Sharpe, P. T. (1994): Upregulation of *c-fos* proto-oncogene expression in pagetic osteoclasts. *J. Bone Miner. Res.* **9,** 1191–1194.
34. Owens, J. M., Matsuo, K., Nicholson, G. C., Wagner, E. F., and Chambers, T. J. (1999) Fra-I stimulates osteoclastic differentiation in osteoclast macrophage precursor cell lines. *J. Cell Physiol.* **179,** 170–178.
35. Fleischmann, A., Hafezi, F., Elliott, C., Reme, C. E., Ruther, U., and Wagner, E. F. (2000) Fra-1 replaces *c-fos* dependent functions in mice. *Genes Dev.* **14,** 2695–2700.
36. Matsuo, K., Jochum, W., Owens, J. M., Chambers, T. J., and Wagner, E. F. (1999) Function of Fos proteins in bone cell differentiation. *Bone* **25,** 141.
37. Matsuo, K., Owens, J. M., Tonko, M., Elliott, C., Chambers, T. J., and Wagner, E. F. (2000) Fosl1 is a transcriptional target of *c-fos* during osteoclast differentiation. *Nat. Genet.* **24,** 184–187.
38. Udagawa, N., Chan, J., Wada, S., Findlay, D. M., Hamilton, J. A., and Martin, T. J. (1996) *c-fos* antisense DNA inhibits proliferation of osteoclast progenitors in osteoclast development but not macrophage differentiation in vitro. *Bone* **18,** 511–516.
39. Soriano, P., Montgomery, C., Geske, R., and Bradley, A. (1991) Targeted disruption of the c-src proto-oncogene leads to osteopetrosis in mice. *Cell* **64,** 693–702.
40. Boyce, B. F., Yoneda, T., Lowe, C., Soriano, P., and Mundy, G. R. (1992) Requirement of pp60c-src expression for osteoclasts to form ruffled borders and resorb bone in mice. *J. Clin. Invest.* **90,** 1622–1627.
41. Lowe, C., Yoneda, T., Boyce, B. F., Chen, H., Mundy, G. R., and Soriano, P. (1993) Osteopetrosis in src-deficient mice is due to an autonomous defect of osteoclasts. *Proc. Natl. Acad. Sci. USA* **90,** 4485–4489.
42. Schwartzberg, P. L., Xing, L., Hoffmann, O., Lowell, C. A., Garrett, L., Boyce, B. F., et al. (1997) Rescue of osteoclast function by transgenic expression of kinase-deficient src in src-1- mutant mice. *Genes Dev.* **11,** 2835–2844.
43. Abu-Amer, Y., Ross, F. P., Schlesinger, P., Tondravi, M. M., and Teitelbaum, S. L. (1997) Substrate recognition by osteoclast precursors induces c-src/microtubule association. *J. Cell Biol.* **137,** 247–258.
44. Tanaka, S., Amling, M., Neff, L., Peyman, A., Uhlmann, E., Levy, J. B., and Baron, R. (1996) C-cbl is downstream of -src in a signaling pathway necessary for bone resorption. *Nature* **383,** 528–531.
45. Sanjay, A., Houghton, A., Neff, L., DiDomenico, E., Bardelay, C., Antoine, E., et al. (2001) Cbl associates with Pyk2 and Src to regulate Src kinase activity, alpha(v) beta(3) integrin mediated signaling, cell adhesion and osteoclast motility. *J. Cell Biol.* **152,** 181–195.
46. Inoue, D., Santiago, P., Horne, W. C., and Baron, R. (1997) Identification of an osteoclast transcription factor that binds to the human T cell leukemia virus type I-long terminal repeat enhancer element. *J. Biol. Chem.* **272,** 25386–25393.
47. Mansky, K. C., Sankar, U., Han, J., and Ostrowski, M. C. (2002) Micropththalmia transcription factor (MITF) is a target of the p38 MAPK pathway in response to receptor activator of NF-kB ligand signaling. *J. Biol. Chem.* **277,** 11077–11083.
48. Weilbaecher, K. N., Motyckova, G., Huber, W. E., Takemoto, C. M., Hemesath, T. J., Xu, Y., et al. (2001) Linkage of M-CSF signaling to Mitf, TFE3, and the osteoclast defect in Mitf(mi/mi) mice. *Mol. Cell.* **8,** 749–758.

49. Mansky, K. C., Sulzbacher, S., Purdom, G., Nelsen, L., Hume, D. A., Rehli, M., et al. (2002) The micropthalmia transcription factor and the related helix-loop-helix zipper factors TFE3 and TFE-C collaborate to activate the tartrate resistant acid phosphatase promoter. *J. Leukoc. Biol.* **71,** 304–310.
50. Battaglino, R., Kim, D., Fu, J., Vaage, B., Fu, X. Y., and Stashenko, P. (2002) c-myc is required for osteoclast differentiation. *J. Bone Miner. Res.* **17,** 763–773.
51. Anderson, B. M., Maraskovsky, E., Billingsley, W. L., Dougall, W. C., Tometsko, M. E., Roux, E. R., et al. (1997) A homologue of the TNF receptor and its ligand enhance T-cell growth and dendritic-cell function. *Nature* **390,** 175–179.
52. Wong, B. R., Josien, R., Lee, S. Y., Sauter, B., Li, H. L., Steinman, R. M., et al. (1997) TRANCE (tumor necrosis factor [TNF]-related activation-induced cytokine), a new TNF family member predominantly expressed in T cells, is a dendritic cell-specific survival factor. *J. Exp. Med.* **186,** 2075–2080.
53. Yasuda, H., Shima, N., Nakagawa, N., Mochizuki, S., Yano, K., Fujise, N., et al. (1998) Identity of osteoclastogenesis inhibitory factor (OCIF) and osteoprotegerin (OPG): A mechanism by which OPG/OCIF inhibits osteoclastogenesis in vitro. *Endrocrinology* **139,** 1329–1337.
54. Yasuda, H., Shima, N., Nakagawa, N., Yamaguchi, K., Kinosaki, M., Mochizuki, S., et al. (1998) Osteoclast differentiation factor is a ligand for osteoprotegerin/osteoclastogenesis-inhibitory factor and is identical to TRANCE/RANKL. *Proc. Natl. Acad. Sci. USA* **95,** 3597–3602.
55. Lacey, D. L., Tan, H. L., Lu, J., Kaugman, S., Van, G., Qiu, W., et al. (2000) Osteoprotegerin ligand modulates murine osteoclast survival in vitro and in vivo. *Am. J. Pathol.* **157,** 35–48.
56. Kojima, H., Nemoto, A., Uemura, T., Honma, R., Ogura, M., and Liu, Y. (2001) rDrak1, a novel kinase related to apoptosis, is strongly expressed in active osteoclasts and induces apoptosis. *J. Biol. Chem.* **276,** 19238–19243.
57. Felix, R., Cecchini, M. C., and Fleisch, H. (1990) Macrophage colony-stimulating factor restores in vivo bone resorption in the op/op osteopetrotic mouse. *Endocrinology* **127,** 2592–2594.
58. Yoshida, H., Hayashi, S., Kunisada, T., Ogawa, M., Nishikawa, S., Okumura, H., et al. (1990) The murine mutation osteopetrosis is in the coding region of the macrophage colony-stimulating factor gene. *Nature* **345,** 442–444.
59. Tanaka, S., Takahashi, N., Udagawa, N., Tamura, T., Akatsu, T., Stanley, E. R., et al. (1993) Macrophage colony-stimulating factor is indispensable for both proliferation and differentiation of osteoclast progenitors. *J. Clin. Invest.* **91,** 257–263.
60. Takahashi, N., Udagawa, N., Akatsu, T., Tanaka, H., Isogai, Y., and Suda, T. (1991) Deficiency of osteoclasts in osteopetrotic mice is due to a defect in the local microenvironment provided by osteoblastic cells. *Endocrinology* **128,** 1792–1796.
61. Halasy, J. and Hofstetter, W. (1998) Expression of colony-stimulating factor-1 (CSF-1) during the formation of osteoclasts in vivo. *J. Bone Miner. Res.* **13,** 1267–1274.
62. Yamane, T., Kunisada, T., Yamazaki, H., Era, T., Nakano, T., and Hayashi, S. I. (1997) Development of osteoclasts from embryonic stem cells through a pathway that is c-fms but not c-kit dependent. *Blood* **90,** 3516–3523.
63. Fan, X., Biskobing, D. M., Fan, D., Hofstetter, W., and Rubin, J. (1997) Macrophage colony stimulating factor down-regulates M-CSF receptor expression and entity of progenitors into the osteoclast lineage. *J. Bone Miner. Res.* **12,** 1387–1395.
64. Nilsson, S. K., Lieschke, G. J., Garcia-Wijnen, C. C., Williams, B., Tzelepis, D., Hodgson, G., et al. (1995) Granulocyte-macrophage colony-stimulating factor is not responsible for the correction of hematopoietic deficiencies in the maturing op/op mouse. *Blood* **86,** 66–72.
65. Lean, J. M., Fuller, K., and Chambers, T. J. (2001) FLT3 ligand can substitute for macrophage colony stimulating factor in support of osteoclast differentiation and function. *Blood* **98,** 2707–2713.
66. Simonet, W. S., Lacey, D. L., Dunstan, C. R., Kelley, M., et al. (1997) Osteoprotegerin: a novel secreted protein involved in the regulation of bone density. *Cell* **89,** 309–319.
67. Tsurukai, T., Udagawa, N., Masuzaki, K., Takahashi, N., and Suda, T. (2000) Roles of macrophage-colony stimulating factor and osteoclast differentiation factor in osteoclastogenesis. *J. Bone Miner. Res.* **18,** 177–184.
68. Gori, F., Hofbauer, L. C., Dunstan, C. R., Spelsberg, T. C., Khosla, S., and Riggs, B. L. (2000) The expression of osteoprotegerin and RANK ligand and the support of osteoclast formation by stromal-osteoblast lineage cells is developmentally regulated. *Endocrinology* **141,** 4768–4776.
69. Hofbauer, L. C., Gori, F., Riggs, B. L., Lacey, D. L., Dunstan, C. R., Spelsberg, T. C., et al. (1999) Stimulation of osteoprotegerin ligand and inhibition of osteoprotegerin production by glucocorticoids in human osteoblastic lineage cells: potential paracrine mechanisms of glucocorticoid induced osteoporosis. *Endocrinology* **140,** 4382–4389.
70. Horwood, N. J., Elliott, J., Martin, T. J., and Gillespie, M. T. (1998) Osteotropic agents regulate the expression of osteoclast differentiation factor and osteoprotegerin in osteoblastic stromal cells. *Endocrinology* **139,** 4743–4746.
71. Thirunavukkarasu, K., Miles, R. R., Halladay, D. L., Yang, X., Galvin, R. J., Chandrasekhar, S., et al. (2001) Stimulation of osteoprotegerin (OPG) gene expression by transforming growth factor-beta (TGF-beta). Mapping of the OPG promoter region that mediates TGF beta effects. *J. Biol. Chem.* **276,** 3641–3650.
72. Pfeilschifter, J., Chenu, C., Bird, A., Mundy, G. R., and Roodman, G. D. (1989) Interleukin-1 and tumor necrosis factor stimulate the formation of human osteoclast-like cells in vitro. *J. Bone Miner. Res.* **4,** 113–118.
73. Uy, H. L., Mundy, G. R., Boyce, B. F., Story, B. M., Dunstan, C. R., Yin, J. J., et al. (1997) Tumor necrosis factor enhances parathyroid hormone-related protein-induced hypercalcemia and bone resorption without inhibiting bone formation in vivo. *Cancer Res.* **573,** 3194–3199.
74. Pacifici, R. (1996) Estrogen, cytokines and pathogenesis of postmenopausal osteoporosis. *J. Bone Miner. Res.* **11,** 1043–1051.

75. Kobayashi, K., Takahashi, N., Jimi, E., Udagawa, N., Takami, M., Kotake, S., et al. (2000) Tumor necrosis factor alpha stimulates osteoclast differentiation by a mechanism independent of the ODF/RANKL-RANK interaction. *J. Exp. Med.* **191,** 275–286.
76. Lam, J., Takeshita, S., Barker, J. E., Kanagawa, O., Ross, F. P., and Teitelbaum, S. L. (2000) TNF alpha induces osteoclastogenesis by direct stimulation of macrophages exposed to permissive levels of RANK ligand. *J. Clin. Invest.* **106,** 1481–1488.
77. Boyce, B. F., Aufdemorte, T. B., Garrett, I. R., Yates, A. J., and Mundy, G. R. (1989) Effects of interleukin-1 on bone turnover in normal mice. *Endocrinology* **125,** 1142–1150.
78. Uy, H. L., Guise, T. A., De La Mata, J., Taylor, S. D., Story, B. M., Dallas, M. R., et al. (1995) Effects of parathyroid hormone-related protein and PTH on osteoclasts and osteoclast precursors in vivo. *Endocrinology* **136,** 3207–3212.
79. Van't Hof, R. J., Armour, K. J., Smith, L. M., Armour, K. E., Wei, X. Q., Liew, F. Y., et al. (2000) Requirement of the inducible nitric oxide synthase pathway for IL-1 induced osteoclastic bone resorption. *Proc. Natl. Acad. Sci. USA* **97,** 7993–7998.
80. Fox, S. W., Fuller, K., and Chambers, T. J. (2000) Activation of osteoclasts by interleukin-1: divergent responsiveness in osteoclasts formed in vivo and in vitro. *J. Cell Physiol.* **184,** 334–340.
81. Riancho, J. A., Zarrabeitia, M. T., and Gonzalez-Macias, J. (1993) Interleukin-4 modulates osteoclast differentiation and inhibits the formation of resorption pits in mouse osteoclast cultures. *Biochem. Biophys. Res. Commun.* **196,** 678–685.
82. Nakano, Y., Watanabe, K., Morimoto, I., Okada, Y., Ura, K., Sato, K., et al. (1994) Interleukin-4 inhibits spontaneous and parathyroid hormone-related protein-stimulated osteoclast formation in mice. *J. Bone Miner. Res.* **9,** 1533–1539.
83. Lewis, D. B., Liggitt, H. D., Effmann, E. L., Motley, S. T., Teitelbaum, S. L., Jepsen, K. J., et al. (1993) Osteoporosis induced in mice by overproduction of interleukin 4. *Proc. Natl. Acad. Sci. USA* **90,** 11618–11622.
84. Abu-Amer, Y. (2001) IL-4 abrogates osteoclastogenesis through STAT6 dependent inhibition of NF-κB. *J. Clin Invest.* **107,** 1375–1385.
85. Roodman, G. D. (1996) Advances in bone biology: the osteoclast. *Endocr. Rev.* **17,** 308–332.
86. Kurihara, N., Bertolini, D., Suda, T., Akiyama, Y., and Roodman, G. D. (1990) IL-6 stimulates osteoclast-like multinucleated cell formation in long-term human marrow cultures by inducing IL-1 release. *J. Immunol.* **144,** 4226–4230.
87. Ohsaki, Y., Takahashi, S., Scarcez, T., Demulder, A., Nishihara, T., Williams, R., et al. (1992) Evidence for an autocrine/paracrine role for IL-6 in bone resorption by giant cell tumors of bone. *Endocrinology* **131,** 2229–2234.
88. Reddy, S. V., Takahashi, S., Dallas, M., Williams, R. E., Neckers, L., and Roodman, G. D. (1994) IL-6 antisense deoxyoligonucleotides inhibit bone resorption by giant cells from human giant cell tumors of bone. *J. Bone Miner. Res.* **9,** 753–757.
89. Devlin, R. D., Reddy, S. V., Savino, R., Ciliberto, G., and Roodman, G. D. (1998) IL-6 mediates the effects of IL-1 or TNF, but not PTHrP or 1,25$(OH)_2D_3$ on osteoclast-like cell formation in normal human bone marrow culture. *J. Bone Miner. Res.* **13,** 393–399.
90. Udagawa, N., Takahashi, N., Katagiri, T., Tamura, T., Wada, S., Findlay, D. M., et al. (1995) Interleukin-6 induction of osteoclast differentiation depends on IL-6 receptors expressed on osteoblastic cells but not on osteoclast progenitors. *J. Exp. Med.* **182,** 1461–1468.
91. Holt, I., Davie, M. W., Braidman, I. P., and Marshall, M. J. (1994) Interleukin-6 does not mediate the stimulation by prostaglandin E2, parathyroid hormone, or 1,25 dihydroxyvitamin D3 of osteoclast differentiation and bone resorption in neonatal mouse parietal bones. *Calcif. Tissue Int.* **52,** 114–119.
92. Passeri, G., Girasole, G., Jilka, R. L., and Manolagas, S. C. (1993) Increased interleukin-6 production by murine bone marrow and bone cells after estrogen withdrawal. *Endocrinology* **133,** 822–828.
93. Han. J. H., Choi, S. J., Kurihara, N., Koide, M., Oba, Y., and Roodman, G. D. (2001) Macrophage inflammatory protein-1 alpha is an osteoclastogenic factor in myeloma that is independent of receptor activator of nuclear factor kappaB ligand. *Blood* **97,** 3349–3353.
94. Paul, S. R., Bennett, F., Calvetti, J. A., Kelleher, K., Wood, C. R., O'Hara, R. M., et al. (1990) Molecular cloning of a cDNA encoding interleukin-ll, a stromal cell-derived lymphopoietic and hematopoietic cytokine. *Proc. Natl. Acad. Sci. USA* **87,** 7512–7516.
95. Girasole, G., Passeri, G., Jilka, R. L., and Manolagas, S. C. (1994) Interleukin 11: a new cytokine critical for osteoclast development. *J. Clin. Invest.* **93,** 1516–1524.
96. Galvin, R. J., Bryan, P., Horn, J. W., Rippy, M. K., and Thomas, J. E. (1996) Development and characterization of a porcine model to study osteoclast differentiation and activity. *Bone* **19,** 271–279.
97. Musashi, M., Yang, Y. C., Paul, S. R., Clark, S. C., Sudo, T., and Ogawa, M. (1991) Direct and synergistic effects of interleukin-11 on murine hemopoiesis in culture. *Proc. Natl. Acad. Sci. USA* **88,** 765–769.
98. Chenu, C., Pfeilschifter, J., Mundy, G. R., and Roodman, G. D. (1988) Transforming growth factor beta inhibits formation of osteoclast-like cells in long-term human marrow cultures. *Proc. Natl. Acad. Sci. USA* **85,** 5683–5687.
99. Yan, T., Riggs, B. L., Boyle, W. J., and Khosla, S. (2001) Regulation of osteoclastogenesis and RANK expression by TGE-beta1. *J. Cell Biochem.* **4,** 1041–1049.
100. Gowen, M. and Mundy, G. R. (1986) Actions of recombinant interleukin-1, interleukin-2, and interferon gamma on bone resorption in vitro. *J. Immunol.* **136,** 2478–2482.
101. Takahashi, N., Mundy, G. R., and Roodman, G. D. (1986) Recombinant human interferon-γ inhibits formation of human osteoclast-like cells. *J. Immunol.* **137,** 3544–3549.
102. Kurihara, N. and Roodman, G. D. (1990) Interferons-α and -γ inhibit interleukin-1β-stimulated osteoclast-like cell formation in long-term human marrow cultures. *J. Interferon Res.* **10,** 541–547.

103. Takayanagi, H., Ogasawara, K., Hida, S., Chiba, T., Murata, S., Sato, K., et al. (2000) T-cell-mediated regulation of osteoclastogenesis by signaling cross-talk between RANKL and IFN-γ. *Nature* **408,** 600–605.
104. Fox, S. W. and Chambers, T. J. (2000) Interferon-γ directly inhibits TRANCE induced osteoclastogenesis. *Biochem. Biophys. Res. Commun.* **276,** 868–872.
105. van't Hof, R. J. and Ralston, S. H. (2001) Nitric oxide and bone. *Immunology* **103,** 255–261.
106. Takayanagi, H., Kim, S., Matsuo, K., Suzuki, H., Suzuki, T., Sato, K., et al. (2002) RANKL maintains bone homeostasis through c-Fos dependent induction of interferon-β. *Nature* **416,** 744–749.
107. Kurihara, N., Chenu, C., Civin, C. I., and Roodman, G. D. (1990) Identification of committed mononuclear precursors for osteoclast-like cells formed in long-term marrow cultures. *Endocrinology* **126,** 2733–2741.
108. Menaa, C., Barsony, J., Reddy, S. V., Cornish, J., Cundy, T., and Roodman, G. D. (2000) 1,25 dihydroxyvitamin D3 hypersensitivity of osteoclast precursors from patients with Paget's disease, *J. Bone Miner. Res.* **15,** 228–236.
109. Feyen, J. H., Elford, P., Di Padova, F. E., and Trechsel, U. (1989) Interleukin-6 is produced by bone and modulated by parathyroid hormone. *J. Bone Miner. Res.* **4,** 633–638.
110. Abe, J., Takita, Y., Nakano, T., Miyaura, C., Suda, T., and Nishii, Y. (1989) A synthetic analogue of vitamin D3, 22-oxa-1 alpha, 25-dihydroxyvitamin D3, is a potent modulator of in vivo immunoregulating activity without inducing hypercalcemia in mice. *Endocrinology* **124,** 2645–2647.
111. Woods, C., Domenget, C., Solari, F., Gandrillon, O., Lazarides, E., and Judic, P. (1995) Antagonistic role of vitamin D3 and retinoic acid on the differentiation of chicken hematopoietic macrophages into osteoclast precursor cells. *Endocrinology* **136,** 85–95.
112. Chirgwin, J. M. and Guise, T. (2000) Molecular mechanisms of tumor-bone interactions in osteolytic metastasis. *Crit. Rev. Eukaryot. Gene Exp.* **10,** 159–78.
113. Rodan, G. A. and Martin, T. J. (1981) Role of osteoblasts in hormonal control of bone resorption: a hypothesis. *Calcif. Tissue Int.* **33,** 349–351.
114. McSheehy, P. M. J. and Chambers, T. J. (1986) Osteoblastic cells mediate osteoclastic responsiveness to parathyroid hormone. *Endocrinology* **118,** 824–828.
115. Greenfield, E. M., Horowitz, M. C., and Lavish, S. A. (1996) Stimulation by parathyroid hormone of interleukin-6 and leukemia inhibitory factor expression in osteoblasts is an immediate-early gene response induced by cAMP signal transduction. *J. Biol. Chem.* **271,** 10984–10989.
116. Kurihara, N., Civin, C., and Roodman, G. D. (1991) Osteotropic factor responsiveness of highly purified populations of early and late precursors for human multinucleated cells expressing the osteoclast phenotype. *J. Bone Miner. Res.* **6,** 257–261.
117. Agarwala, N. and Gay, C. V. (1992) Specific binding of parathyroid hormone to living osteoclasts. *J. Bone Miner. Res.* **7,** 531–539.
118. Teti, A., Rizzoli, R., and Zambonin-Zallone, A. (1991) A parathyroid hormone binding to cultured avian osteoclasts. *Biochem. Biophys. Res. Commun.* **174,** 1217–1222.
119. Hakeda, Y., Hiura, K., Sato, T., Olazaki, R., Matsumoto, T., Ogata, E., et al. (1989) Existence of parathyroid hormone binding sites on murine hemopoietic blast cells. *Biochem. Biophys. Res. Commun.* **163,** 1481–1486.
120. Orlandini, S. Z., Formigli, L., Benvenuti, S., Lasagni, L., Franchi, A., Masi, L., et al. (1995) Functional and structural interactions between osteoblastic and preosteoclastic cells in vitro. *Cell Tissue Res.* **281,** 33–42.
121. Tong, H., Lin, H., Wang, H., Sakai, D., and Minkin, C. (1995) Osteoclasts respond to parathyroid hormone and express mRNA for its receptor. *J. Bone Miner. Res.* **10,** S322.
122. Kartsogiannis, V., Udagawa, N., Martin, T. J., Moseley, J. M., and Zhou, H. (1998) Localization of parathyroid hormone-related protein in osteoclasts by in situ hybridization and immunohistochemistry. *Bone* **22,** 189–194.
123. Lee, S. K., Goldring, S. R., and Lorenzo, J. A. (1995) Expression of the calcitonin receptor in bone marrow cell cultures and in bone: a specific marker of the differentiated osteoclast that is regulated by calcitonin. *Endocrinology* **136,** 4572–4581.
124. Gorn, A. H., Rudolph, S. M., Flannery, M. R., Morton, C. C., Weremowicz, S., Wang, T. Z., et al. (1995) Expression of two human skeletal calcitonin receptor isoforms cloned from a giant cell tumor of bone. The first intracellular domain modulates ligand binding and signal transduction. *J. Clin. Invest.* **95,** 2680–2691.
125. Shevde, N. K., Bendixen, A. C., Dienger, K. M., and Pike, J. M. (2000) Estrogens suppress RANK ligand-induced osteoclast differentiation via a stromal cell independent mechanism involving c-Jun repression. *Proc. Natl. Acad. Sci. USA* **97,** 7829–7834.
126. Viereck, V., Grundker, C., Blaschke, S., Siggelkow, H., Emons, G., and Hofbauer, L. C. (2002) Phytoestrogen genistein stimulates the production of osteoprotegerin by human trabecular osteoblasts. *J. Cell Biochem.* **84,** 725–735.
127. Szulc, P., Hofbauer, L. C., Heufelder, A. E., Roth, S., and Delmas, P. D. (2001) Osteoprotegerin serum levels in men: correlation with age, estrogen and testosterone status. *J. Clin. Endocrinol. Metab.* **86,** 3162–3165.
128. Takahashi, N., Yamana, H., Yoshiki, S., Roodman, G. D., Mundy, G. R., Jones, S. J., et al. (1988) Osteoclast-like cell formation and its regulation by osteotropic hormones in mouse bone marrow cultures. *Endocrinology* **122,** 1373–1382.
129. Chenu, C., Kurihara, N., Mundy, G. R., and Roodman, G. D. (1990) Prostaglandin E_2 inhibits formation of osteoclast-like cells in long-term human marrow cultures but is not a mediator of the inhibitory effects of transforming growth factor-β. *J. Bone Miner. Res.* 5, 677–681.
130. Quinn, J. M. W., Sabokbar, A., Denne, M., de Vernejoul, M. C., McGee, J. O. D., and Athanasou, N. A. (1997) Inhibitory and stimulatory effects of prostaglandins on osteoclast differentiation. *Calcif. Tissue Int.* **60,** 63–70.

131. Roux, S., Pichaud, F., Quinn, J., Lalande, A., Morieux, C., Jullienne, A., et al. (1997) Effects of prostaglandins on human hematopoietic osteoclast precursors. *Endocrinology* **138,** 1476–1482.
132. Tashjian, A. H., Voelkel, E. F., Lazzaro, M., Goad, D., Bosma, T., and Levine, L. (1985) Alpha and beta transforming growth factors stimulate prostaglandin production and bone resorption in cultured mouse calvaria. *Proc. Natl. Acad. Sci. USA* **82,** 4535–4538.
133. Wani, M. R., Fuller, K., Kim, N. S., Choi, Y., and Chambers, T. (1999) Prostaglandin E2 cooperates with TRANCE in osteoclast induction from hemopoietic precursors: synergistic activation of differentiation, cell spreading, and fusion. *Endocrinology* **140,** 1927–1935.
134. Gallwitz, W. E., Mundy, G. R., Lee, C. H., Qiao, M., Roodman, G. D., Raftery, M., et al. (1993) 5-Lipoxygenase metabolites of arachidonic acid stimulate isolated osteoclasts to resorb calcified matrices. *J. Biol. Chem.* **268,** 10087–10094.
135. Franchi-Miller, C. and Saffar, J. L. (1995) The 5-lipoxygenase inhibitor BWA4C impairs osteoclastic resorption in a synchronized model of bone remodeling. *Bone* **17,** 185–191.
136. Garcia, C., Boyce, B. F., Gilles, J., Dallas, M., Qiao, M., Mundy, G. R., et al. (1996) Leukotriene B4 stimulates osteoclastic bone resorption both in vitro and in vivo. *J. Bone Miner. Res.* **11,** 1619–1627.
137. Takami, M., Woo, J. T., Takahashi, N., Suda, T., and Nagai, K. (1997) Ca2+-ATPase inhibitors and Ca2+ ionophore induce osteoclast-like cell formation in the cocultures of mouse bone marrow cells and calvarial cells. *Biochem. Biophys. Res. Commun.* **237,** 111–115.
138. Takami, A., Takahashi, N., Udagawa, N., Miyaura, C., Suda, K., Woo, J. T., et al. (2000) Intracellular calcium and protein kinase C mediate expression of receptor activator of nuclear factor-kappa B ligand and osteoprotegerin in osteoblasts. *Endocrinology* **141,** 4711–4719.
139. Biskobing, D. M., Fan, D., and Rubin, J. (1997) Induction of carbonic anhydrase II expression in osteoclast progenitors requires physical contact with stromal cells. *Endocrinology* **138,** 4852–4857.
140. Moonga, B. S. and Dempster, D. W. (1995) Zinc is a potent inhibitor of osteoclastic bone resorption in vitro. *J. Bone Miner. Res.* **10,** 453–457.
141. Suzuki, Y., Morita, I., Yamane, Y., and Murota, S. (1990) Preventive effect of zinc against cadmium-induced bone resorption. *Toxicology* **62,** 27–34.
142. Kishi, S. and Yamaguchi, M. (1994) The inhibitory effects of zinc compounds on osteoclast-like cell formation in mouse marrow cultures. *Biochem. Pharmacol.* **48,** 1225–1230.
143. Kishi, S. and Yamaguchi, M. (1997) Characterization of zinc effect to inhibit osteoclast-like cell formation in mouse bone marrow cultures: Interactions with dexamethasone. *Mol. Cell. Biochem.* **166,** 145–151.
144. Holloway, W. R., Collier, F. M., Herbst, R. E., Hodge, J. M., and Nicholson, G. C. (1996) Osteoblast-mediated effects of zinc on isolated rat osteoclasts: inhibition of bone resorption and enhancement of osteoclast number. *Bone* **19,** 137–142.
145. Wilson, A. K., Cerny, E. A., Smith, B. D., Wagh, A., and Bhattacharyya, M. H. (1996) Effect of cadmium on osteoclast formation and activity in vitro. *Toxicol. Appl. Pharm.* **140,** 451–460.
146. Notoya, K., Yoshida, K., Taketomi, S., Yamazaki, I., and Kumegawa, M. (1993) Inhibitory effect of ipriflavone on osteoclast mediated bone resorption and new osteoclast formation in long-term cultures of mouse unfractionated bone cells. *Calc. Tissue Int.* **53,** 206–209.
147. Miyauchi, A., Notoya, K., Taketomi, S., Takagi, Y., Fujii, Y., Jinnai, K., et al. (1996) Novel ipriflavone receptors coupled to calcium influx regulate osteoclast differentiation and function. *Endocrinology* **137,** 3544–3550.
148. Shibutani, T. and Heersche, J. N. (1993) Effect of medium pH on osteoclast activity and osteoclast formation in cultures of dispersed rabbit osteoclasts. *J. Bone Miner. Res.* **8,** 331–336.
149. Arnett, T. R. and Dempster, D. W. (1990) Protons and osteoclasts. *J. Bone Miner. Res.* **5,** 1099–1103
150. Meghji, S., Morrison, M. S., Henderson, B., and Arnett, T. R. (2001) pH dependence of bone resorption: mouse calvarial osteoclasts are activated by acidosis. *Am. J. Physiol. Endocrinol. Metab.* **280,** E112–E119.
151. Tani-Ishii, N., Tsunoda, A., and Umemoto, T. (1997) Osteopontin antisense deoxyoligonucleotides inhibit bone resorption by mouse osteoclasts in vitro. *J. Periodont. Res.* **32,** 480–486.
152. Asou, Y., Rittling, S. R., Yoshitake, H., Tsuji, K., Shinomiya, K., Nifuji, A., et al. (2001) Osteopontin facilitates angiogenesis, accumulation of osteoclasts and resorption in ectopic bone. *Endocrinology* **142,** 1325–1332.
153. Kaneko, H., Arakawa, T., Mano, H., Kaneda, T., Ogasawara, A., Nakagawa, M., et al. (2000) Direct stimulation of osteoclastic bone resorption by bone morphogenetic protein (BMP-2) and expression of BMP receptors in mature osteoclasts. *Bone* **27,** 479–486.
154. Otsuka, E., Kato, Y., Hirose, S., and Hagiwara, H. (2000) Role of ascorbic acid in the osteoclast formation: induction of osteoclast differentiation factor with formation of the extracellular collagen matrix. *Endocrinology* **141,** 3006–3011.

[illegible]

IV
Bone Induction, Growth, and Remodeling

15

Soluble Signals and Insoluble Substrata

Novel Molecular Cues Instructing the Induction of Bone

Ugo Ripamonti, Nathaniel L. Ramoshebi, Janet Patton, Thato Matsaba, June Teare, and Louise Renton

MOLECULAR SIGNALS OF THE TRANSFORMING GROWTH FACTOR-β (TGF-β) SUPERFAMILY

The repair and regeneration of bone is a complex process that is temporally and spatially regulated by soluble and insoluble signals *(1)*. The initiation of bone formation during embryonic development and postnatal osteogenesis involves a complex cascade of molecular and morphogenetic processes that ultimately lead to the architectural sculpturing of precisely organized multicellular structures.

Which are the molecular signals that initiate *de novo* bone differentiation? Identification of bone morphogenetic proteins capable of initiating *de novo* bone formation has been a difficult task because of the relative inaccessibility of rather small quantities of soluble signals tightly bound to both organic and inorganic components of the extracellular matrix of bone.

The discovery that demineralized bone matrix implanted in intramuscular or subcutaneous sites of rodents induced bone formation by induction *(2–4)* was of paramount importance to understanding that the devitalized matrix contained morphogenetic factors capable of inducing the differentiation of resident extraskeletal mesenchymal cells first into chondroblasts and then osteoblasts, culminating in the differentiation of hemopoietic marrow within the newly formed ossicles *de novo* generated in extraskeletal sites *(1–4)*. The discovery of bone formation by induction was later followed by the demonstration that the intact demineralized matrix could be dissociatively extracted and inactivated with chaotropic agents and that the osteoinductive activity could be restored by reconstituting the inactive residue (mainly insoluble collagenous matrix) with solubilized protein fractions obtained after the extraction of the bone matrix *(5)*. This major biological advance provided the starting point for the isolation and purification of osteoinductive/osteogenic proteins from bovine and baboon bone matrices *(1)*. This has led to the identification of an entirely new family of protein initiators that induce cartilage and bone differentiation in vivo, collectively called the bone morphogenetic proteins/osteogenic proteins (BMPs/OPs) *(1,6)*. Expression cloning and continuous research has helped to identify at least twenty BMP isoforms of the BMP/OP family of proteins. These gene products show marked sequence homologies with members of the TGF-β family of proteins, and together with other morphogens comprise the TGF-β superfamily, gene products that have major activities in the mechanisms of morphogenesis, axial growth, soft- and hard-tissue development, maintenance, and repair, including but not limited to organs and tissues as diverse as bone, cartilage, kidney, lung, the periodontal ligament, the root cementum, and the central and peripheral nervous systems *(1,6–14)*.

From: *The Skeleton: Biochemical, Genetic, and Molecular Interactions in Development and Homeostasis*
Edited by: E. J. Massaro and J. M. Rogers © Humana Press Inc., Totowa, NJ

Elucidating the nature and interaction of the signaling molecules that direct the generation of tissue-specific patterns during the initiation of endochondral bone formation by induction is a major challenge for contemporary molecular, cellular, developmental, and tissue-engineering biology. Common molecular mechanisms are selectively regulated to provide the emergence of specialized tissues and organs. The induction of bone in postnatal life recapitulates events that occur in the normal course of embryonic development and morphogenesis *(1,9,11,14)*. Both embryonic development and postnatal tissue regeneration are equally regulated by a selected few and highly conserved families of morphogens.

BONE INDUCTION BY BMPs/OPs AND OTHER MEMBERS OF THE TGF-β SUPERFAMILY

BMPs/OPs, members of the TGF-β supergene family, are morphogens endowed with the striking prerogative of initiating *de novo* bone formation by induction in heterotopic extra skeletal sites of animal models *(1,7,8,11–14)*. The three most important requirements for successful tissue engineering of bone are a suitable extracellular matrix substratum, capable-responding cells, and soluble osteoinductive signals, members of the TGF-β supergene family *(1,11,12,14)*. The reconstitution of BMPs/OPs (the soluble signals) with biomimetic matrices (the insoluble signal or substratum) provides a bioassay for bona fide initiators of bone differentiation as well as the operational concept of delivery systems for therapeutic local osteogenesis in preclinical and clinical contexts *(1,11–16)*. Naturally-derived BMPs/OPs and recombinant human osteogenic protein-1 (hOP-1), also known as BMP-7, induce osteogenesis in nonhuman and human primates (Fig. 1; refs. *13–16*). Long-term experiments in the adult primate *Papio ursinus* have shown that γ-irradiated osteogenic devices composed of hOP-1 delivered by a xenogeneic bovine collagenous matrix completely regenerated and maintained the architecture of the induced bone up to 1 yr after treatment of nonhealing calvarial defects with single applications of doses of 0.5 and 2.5 mg hOP-1 per gram of xenogeneic matrix (Fig. 1B; refs. *12,14*).

In the quest to continuously investigate biomimetic carrier matrices, we have recently reported a novel delivery system for BMPs/OPs for the induction of endochondral bone formation in the heterotopic rodent bioassay using the basement membrane Matrigel *(17)*. We have shown that Matrigel biomatrix is a very effective carrier of osteogenic soluble signals so much so that naturally-derived BMPs/OPs were delivered by injecting aliquots of Matrigel in lumbar vertebrae affected by systemic bone loss *(17)*. The use of Matrigel biomatrix delivering human recombinant morphogens is an innovative approach to induce with local injections bone formation by induction in systemic bone loss such as osteoporosis *(17)*.

Mechanistically and importantly for further understanding of novel molecular strategies in clinical contexts, is to gain insights into the distinct spatial and temporal patterns of expression of other TGF-β superfamily members during bone regeneration *(14)*. We have studied gene products elicited by single applications of doses of hOP-1 implanted both in heterotopic and orthotopic sites of *Papio ursinus*. Ultimately, it will be necessary to elucidate the expression of potential distinct spatial and temporal expression of TGF-β family members during morphogenesis and regeneration elicited by single applications of doses of hOP-1 *(12,14)*. In vivo studies should now design therapeutic approaches based on gene regulation by hOP-1.

Fig. 1. *(opposite page)* Induction of bone formation by naturally derived and recombinant hBMPs/OPs in human and nonhuman primates. **A**, Newly formed and mineralized bone (blue) surfaced by continuous osteoid seams (orange–red, arrows) 90 d after implantation of naturally derived BMPs/OPs extracted and purified from bovine bone matrix in a human mandibular defect. **B**, Complete regeneration of a nonhealing calvarial defect of the primate *P. ursinus* 90 d after implantation of 100 μg hOP-1 delivered by 1 g of xenogeneic bovine collagenous matrix as carrier. **C**, Tissue engineering and "*restitutio ad integrum*" of a periodontally induced furcation defect in the primate *P. ursinus* 365 d after implantation of 2.5 mg hOP-1 per 1 g of xenogeneic bovine collagenous matrix as carrier. Original magnification: A, ×9; B, ×3; C, ×9.

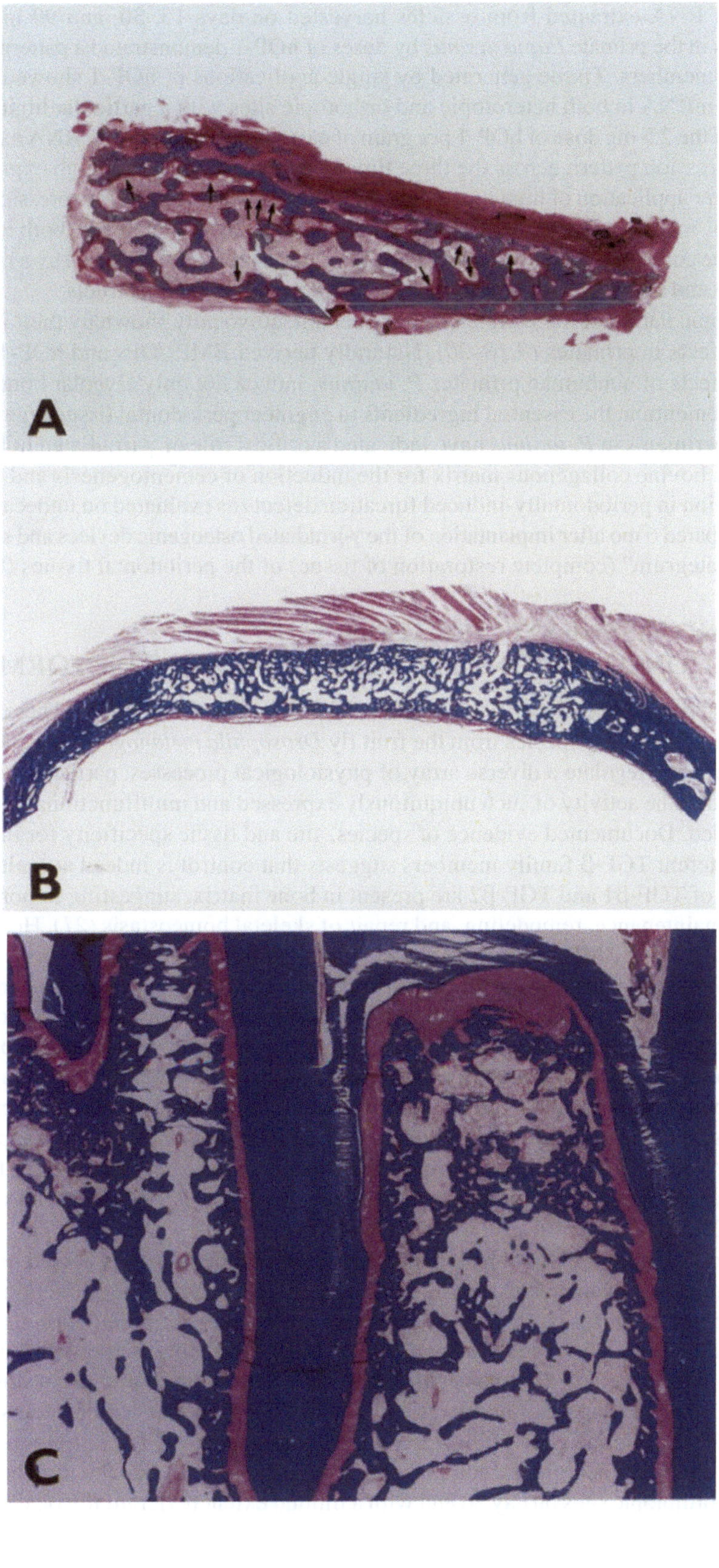
A
B
C

Analyses of RNA extracted from ossicles harvested on days 15, 30, and 90 in heterotopic and orthotopic sites in the primate *Papio ursinus* by doses of hOP-1 demonstrated a pattern of expression of TGF-β family members. Tissue generated by single applications of hOP-1 showed high expression levels of OP-1 mRNA in both heterotopic and orthotopic sites with a particular high expression after implantation of the 2.5 mg dose of hOP-1 per gram of carrier matrix. BMP-3 mRNA expression showed a common expression pattern across the three time periods with relatively high expression in heterotopic tissues after application of high doses of hOP-1 but a rather low mRNA expression as evaluated in orthotopic sites. mRNA expression of TGF-β1 was found to be low on day 15 both in heterotopic and orthotopic tissue constructs with a relatively high expression on day 30 followed by a rather low expression on day 90 and again in both heterotopic and orthotopic tissue constructs.

The pleiotropic nature of the BMPs/OPs has been unequivocally shown by their implantation into periodontal defects in primates *(9,18–20)*. Naturally derived BMPs/OPs and hOP-1, when tested in periodontal defects of nonhuman primates *P. ursinus*, induce not only alveolar bone but periodontal ligament and cementum, the essential ingredients to engineer periodontal tissue regeneration *(18,19)*. Long-term experiments in *P. ursinus* have indicated a critical role of γ-irradiated hOP-1 delivered by the xenogeneic bovine collagenous matrix for the induction of cementogenesis and periodontal ligament regeneration in periodontally-induced furcation defects as evaluated on undecalcified histological sections prepared 6 mo after implantation of the γ-irradiated osteogenic devices and showing complete "restitutio ad integrum" (complete restoration of tissue) of the periodontal tissues (Fig. 1C; ref. *20*).

SPECIES AND TISSUE SPECIFICITY OF ENDOCHONDRAL BONE INDUCTION BY TGF-β ISOFORMS

The TGF-β superfamily includes five distinct TGF-β isoforms *(1,6–8,11,14)*. These proteins are evolutionarily conserved across species from the fruit fly *Drosophila melanogaster* to mammalian species *(1,6–8)*. The proteins regulate a diverse array of physiological processes, particularly in morphogenesis, indicating that the activity of such ubiquitously expressed and multifunctional molecules must be tightly controlled. Documented evidence of species, site and tissue specificity for the osteoinductive capacity of different TGF-β family members suggests that control is indeed at multiple levels.

High levels of TGF-β1 and TGF-β2 are present in bone matrix, suggesting important roles during the initiation, maintenance, remodeling, and repair of skeletal homeostasis *(21)*. However, in marked contrast to results using BMPs/OPs, extra skeletal implantation of TGF-β proteins consistently failed to initiate endochondral bone by induction in rodents *(22,23)*. From a human perspective, results obtained using nonhuman primates as the in vivo model for tissue engineering of bone must be considered more relevant because *P. ursinus* share 98% DNA homology with human primates *(24)*.

Contrary to all the results obtained in the rodent bioassay, heterotopic implantation of naturally derived or recombinant human (h) TGF-β isoforms induces endochondral bone induction in the *rectus abdominis* muscle of the adult primate *P. ursinus (25–27)*. In addition, the binary applications of relatively low doses of hTGF-β1 with recombinant hBMPs/OPs interact synergistically to rapidly induce massive heterotopic and orthotopic ossicles in the *rectus abdominis* muscle and calvarial defects, respectively *(25,26)*.

The pleiotropy of the signaling molecules of the TGF-β superfamily is indeed highlighted by the apparent redundancy of molecular signals initiating endochondral bone induction, yet only in the primate. In the rodent bioassay, the TGF-β isoforms are inducers of granulation tissue with marked fibrosis only *(22,23)*. In marked contrast, strikingly, TGF-β proteins are powerful inducers of endochondral bone when implanted in the *rectus abdominis* muscle of *P. ursinus* at doses of 5, 25, and 125 μg per 100 mg of collagenous matrix as carrier *(25–27)*. A further striking and significant observation is that the osteoinductivity of the TGF-β isoforms so far tested in our laboratories is site and tissue specific. TGF-β proteins in the adult primate *P. ursinus* induce endochondral bone in heterotopic sites but not in orthotopic sites on day 30 and with a limited extent pericranially on day 90 (Fig. 2; refs.

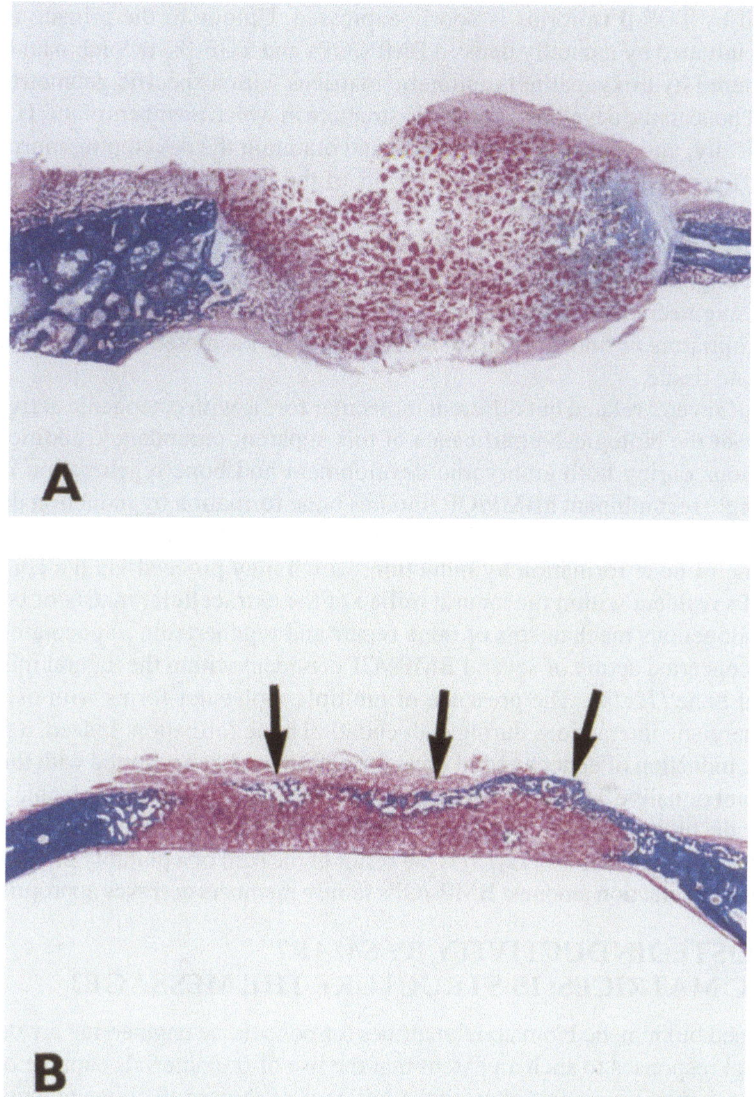

Fig. 2. Morphology of calvarial regeneration by recombinant hTGF-β2 in conjunction with allogeneic baboon collagenous matrix as carrier. **A**, Lack of bone formation upon implantation of 100 μg of hTGF-β2 on day 30 with prominent mesenchymal tissue influx and displacement of the collagenous matrix. **B**, Limited osteogenesis and only pericranially (arrows) upon implantation of 100 μg hTGF-β2 in a calvarial specimen harvested 90 d after implantation. Original magnification: **A** and **B**, ×3.

26–28). Ossicles generated in heterotropic sites by TGF-βs express mRNAs of OP-1, BMP-3, TGF-β1, and GDF-10.

At the cellular level, there is strict regulation of TGF-β-induced activity. Every step of TGF-β synthesis and signal transduction is tightly controlled *(28)*. Regulation may occur at the level of receptor expression and availability or distal to receptor activation. For instance, one mechanism of intracellular negative regulation of TGF-β-mediated signaling is by upregulation of the inhibitory Smad proteins, Smad-6 and Smad-7 *(29)*.

Experiments in our laboratories indicate the influence of downstream antagonists of TGF-β signaling, Smad-6 and -7, at least in heterotopic sites, because mRNA expression of Smad-6 and -7 in heterotopic ossicles generated by TGF-β isoforms is poorly expressed. Unique to the primate only, heterotopic bone induction is initiated by naturally derived BMPs/OPs and TGF-βs, recombinant hBMPs/OPs and hTGFβs, and sintered hydroxyapatite biomimetic matrices with a specific geometric configuration. This indicates that bone tissue develops as a mosaic structure in which members of the TGF-β superfamily singly, synergistically, and synchronously initiate and maintain the developing morphological structures and play different roles at different time points of the morphogenetic cascade *(12–14,25–27)*.

The discovery of endochondral osteoinductivity albeit only heterotopically and only in primates by TGF-β isoforms will have an important and substantial impact on the biological and clinical understanding of tissue engineering of bone that is changing the modus operandi of molecular and cellular biologists, tissue engineers, and surgeons alike. Fundamentally thus, the TGF-β isoforms need now to be considered initiators of bone formation rather than only promoters during the maintenance and remodeling of bone tissue.

The presence of several related but different molecular forms with osteogenic activity poses important questions about the biological significance of this apparent redundancy, additionally indicating multiple interactions during both embryonic development and bone regeneration in postnatal life. The fact that a single recombinant hBMP/OP initiates bone formation by induction does not preclude the requirement and interactions of other morphogens deployed synchronously and synergistically during the cascade of bone formation by induction, which may proceed via the combined action of several BMPs/OPs resident within the natural milieu of the extracellular matrix of bone *(12,14)*. It is likely that the endogenous mechanisms of bone repair and regeneration in postnatal life require the deployment and concerted action of several BMPs/OPs resident within the natural milieu of the extracellular matrix of bone *(12,14)*. The presence of multiple molecular forms with osteogenic activity also points to synergistic interactions during endochondral bone formation. Indeed, a potent and accelerated synergistic induction of endochondral bone formation has been reported with the binary application of recombinant or native TGF-β1 with hOP-1 both in heterotopic and orthotopic sites of primates *(25,26)*. Whether the biological activity of partially purified BMPs/OPs as shown in long-term experiments in the adult primate *P. ursinus (12,13)* is the result of the sum of a plurality of BMPs/OPs activities or a truly synergistic interaction amongst BMPs/OPs family members deserves appropriate investigation.

INTRINSIC OSTEOINDUCTIVITY BY *SMART* BIOMIMETIC MATRICES: IS STRUCTURE THE MESSAGE?

Newly developed biomimetic biomaterial matrices for bone tissue engineering are designed to obtain specific biological responses to such an extent that the use of biomaterials capable of initiating bone formation via osteoinductivity is fast altering the horizons of therapeutic bone regeneration (Fig. 3A). A critical issue in bone tissue engineering is the development of osteoinductive biomaterials capable of optimizing not only the delivery and biological activity of BMPs/OPs but also the osteogenic activity of low doses of recombinant hBMPs/OPs in clinical contexts (Fig. 3B,C; refs. *30–32*).

The insoluble signal, the carrier substratum, when combined with osteogenic proteins of the TGF-β superfamily, triggers the bone induction cascade, additionally providing an exciting and novel concept of tissue engineering of bone. Biomimetic matrices have been developed that can *per se* induce specific and selective responses from the host tissues without the addition of exogenously applied BMPs/OPs (Fig. 3A; refs. *30–33*). Morphological, biochemical, and molecular evidence has been harnessed in our laboratories to guide the incorporation of specific angiogenic and osteogenic activities into

Fig. 3. (*opposite page*) Bone induction in sintered biomimetic matrices of highly crystalline hydroxyapatite and effect of geometry of the substratum on tissue induction and morphogenesis. **A**, Induction of bone formation in a sintered porous hydroxyapatite harvested from the *rectus abdominis* of an adult primate on day 90. Note intrinsic and spontaneous induction of bone formation within the porous spaces of the hydroxyapatite essentially initiating in concavities of the substratum (arrows). **B**, Low-power photomicrograph of a sintered porous hydroxy-

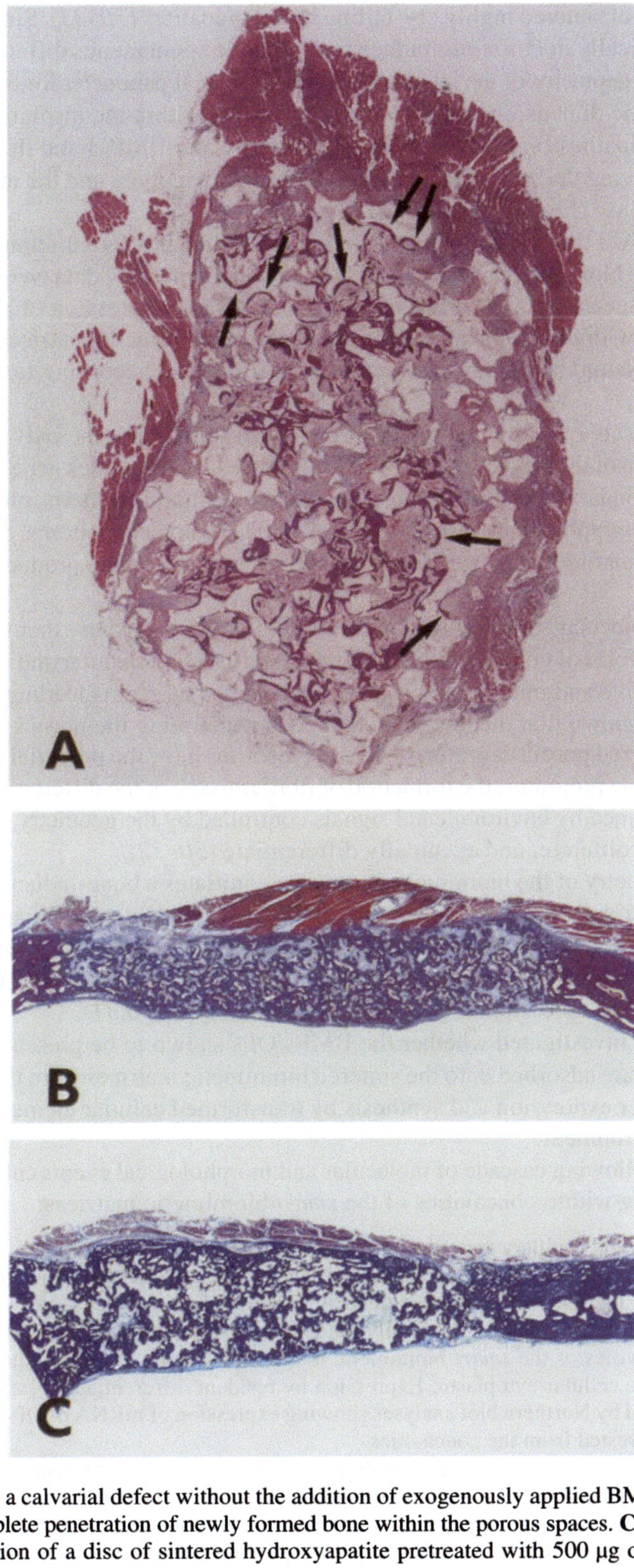

apatite disc implanted in a calvarial defect without the addition of exogenously applied BMPs/OPs and harvested on day 90; note the complete penetration of newly formed bone within the porous spaces. **C**, Bone induction 365 d after calvarial implantation of a disc of sintered hydroxyapatite pretreated with 500 μg of recombinant hOP-1. Original magnification: **A**, ×10; **B** and **C**, ×3.

biomimetic matrices of sintered highly crystalline hydroxyapatites *(30–33)*. Sintered hydroxyapatites implanted heterotopically in *P. ursinus* induce reproducible spontaneous differentiation of bone (Fig. 3A; refs. *30,31*). The geometry of the insoluble signal is a critical parameter for bone induction to occur: concavities of specific dimensions prepared and assembled within the insoluble signal of the highly crystalline hydroxyapatites bind BMPs/OPs, that is, OP-1 and BMP-3 and then initiate a sequential cascade of events driving the emergence of the osteogenic phenotype and the morphogenesis of bone as a secondary response (Fig. 3A; refs. *30,31*).

We have now shown that the spontaneous induction of bone differentiation initiates even in concavities of resorbable biomimetic matrices. Additional complementary data were deduced by Northern blot analyses using specific cDNA probes to study the mRNA expression of gene products induced by responding cells within the concavities of the sintered biomimetic matrices and showing critical differences in expression of mRNA markers of bone formation according to the type of implanted biomatrices.

Results have indicated that the geometry of the substratum is not the only driving force because the structure of the insoluble signal dramatically influences and regulates gene expression and induction of bone as a secondary response. Soluble signals induce morphogenesis, physical forces imparted by the geometric topography of the insoluble signal dictate biological patterns, constructing the induction of bone and regulating the expression of selective mRNA of gene products as a function of the structure.

However, our molecular, biochemical, and morphological data show that the specific geometric configuration in the form of concavities is the foremost driving molecular and morphogenetic microenvironment conducive and inductive to a specific sequence of events leading to bone formation by induction. We have shown that the mesenchymal cells penetrating the porous spaces of the concave geometry of the sintered porous biomimetic hydroxyapatites have the potential to express at least two distinct morphogenetic programs, the formation of fibrous tissue or the differentiation of bone, and that this choice is determined by environmental signals controlled by the geometry of the substratum onto which they attach, proliferate, and eventually differentiate *(30–32)*.

The specific geometry of the biomimetic biomaterial initiates a bone-inductive microenvironment by providing geometrical structures biologically and architecturally conducive and inducible to optimal sequestration and synthesis of BMPs/OPs but particularly capable of stimulating angiogenesis, a prerequisite for osteogenesis. Angiogenesis may indeed provide a temporally regulated flow of cell populations capable of expression of the osteogenic phenotype *(30,31)*.

We have recently investigated whether the BMPs/OPs shown to be present in the concavities by immunolocalization are adsorbed onto the sintered biomimetic matrices from the circulation or rather produced locally after expression and synthesis by transformed cellular elements resident within the concavity microenvironment.

We propose the following cascade of molecular and morphological events culminating in the induction of bone initiating within concavities of the *smart* biomimetic matrices:

1. Vascular invasion and capillary sprouting within the invading tissue with capillary elongation in close contact with the hydroxyapatite biomatrix. Attachment and differentiation of mesenchymal cells at the hydroxyapatite/soft tissue interface of the concavities.
2. Expression of TGF-β and BMPs/OPs family members in osteoblast-like cells resident and differentiated within the concavities of the *smart* biomimetic matrices as shown by immunolocalization of OP-1 and BMP-3 within the cellular cytoplasm. Expression by resident differentiated osteoblast-like cells is additionally confirmed by Northern blot analyses showing expression of mRNA of OP-1 and BMP-3 in homogenized tissue harvested from the concavities.
3. Expression and synthesis of specific BMP/OP from transformed resident osteoblast-like cells onto the sintered crystalline hydroxypatite as shown by immunolocalization of OP-1 and BMP-3.
4. Intrinsic osteoinduction with further differentiation into osteoblastic cells and intrinsic osteoinduction depending on a critical threshold of endogenously produced BMPs/OPs initiating bone formation as a secondary response.

The concavities per se are geometric regulators of growth endowed with shape memory, recapitulating events which occur in the normal course of embryonic development and appearing to act as gates, giving or withholding permission to growth and differentiation *(31)*. The concavities as prepared in the biomimetic matrices act as powerful geometric attractants for capillary invasion and bone-forming cells, differentiating within the concavities and initiating bone formation by induction.

ANGIOGENIC SIGNALS DURING BONE FORMATION

Adequate vascularization is an essential element for comprehensive bone formation by induction because an adequate development of a new blood vessel system is necessary for transporting and delivering oxygen, nutrients, supplementary bone-forming mesenchymal cells, and additional bone-inducing molecules (i.e., BMPs/OPs and TGF-βs) to the site of new bone formation *(1,34,35)*. Previous data have shown that BMPs/OPs and TGF-β1 bind to extracellular matrix components of the basement membrane of invading capillaries further highlighting the role of capillaries delivering both angiogenic and osteogenic molecules *(1,14,36,37)*. Great benefits can thus be attained from manipulating and enhancing the vascular supply during the formation of bone.

Angiogenic molecules induced and expressed at sites of osteogenesis and bone formation by induction include fibroblast growth factor, vascular endothelial growth factor, type IV collagen, and angiopoietins *(38–41)*. In addition, other molecules delivered in the blood supply include proteases that are required for the degradation of the extracellular matrix *(42)* and facilitating the deposition of an anatomically contiguous bone with bone marrow in the spaces created within the matrix.

For the promotion of increased vascularization during bone formation by induction, is highly desirable to use a delivery system that is conducive and inducible to blood vessel invasion. The geometric topography of the insoluble signal via the design of novel biomimetic matrices is a deciding factor for the extent of vascularization. The importance of the geometric configuration of biomimetic matrices has been openly highlighted by the expansive condensation of newly formed blood vessels and capillary juxtaposed to the newly induced bone within the concavities of the *smart* biomimetic matrices of highly crystalline hydroxyapatite *(30,31)*.

The specific geometric and surface characteristics of the substratum induce rapid vessel ingrowth and capillary sprouting within the early mesenchyme that penetrates the porous spaces. In previous experiments *(43)*, histological, immunohistochemical, and molecular data have suggested that osteogenetic vessels, as defined by Trueta in 1963 *(44)*, might have provided a temporally regulated flow of cell populations capable of the expression of the osteogenic phenotype *(30,43)*. Angiogenesis may indeed provide a temporally regulated flow of cell populations capable of expression of the osteogenic phenotype. The affinity of BMPs/OPs for type IV collagen, a major component of the vascular basement membrane *(36)*, provides a further mechanistic insight, particularly in the light of morphological evidence of substantial angiogenesis localized in the mesenchymal tissue invading the concavities of the biomimetic matrices *(30,31)*. The discovery of the affinity of osteogenin (BMP-3) for type IV collagen may link angiogenesis to osteogenesis *(36)*, additionally providing a conceptual framework for the supramolecular assembly of the extracellular matrix of bone. Type IV collagen and other basement membrane components around the endothelial cells of the invading capillaries may function as a delivery system by sequestering both angiogenic and bone morphogenetic proteins and present them locally in an immobilized form to responding mesenchymal and osteoprogenitor cells to initiate osteogenesis and function as delivery systems by sequestering both initiators and promoters involved in angiogenesis and endochondral bone differentiation by induction.

ACKNOWLEDGMENTS

This work is supported by grants of the South African Medical Research Council, the University of the Witwatersrand, Johannesburg, the National Research Foundation, and by ad hoc grants of the Bone Research Unit. We thank Barbara van den Heever, Laura Yeates, Manolis Heliotis, and Jean Crooks for critical help in experiments. We thank Michael Thomas and Wim Richter (Council for Scientific and Industrial Research, Manufacturing and Materials Technology Group, Pretoria) for the preparation of the biomimetic matrices of sintered hydroxyapatite.

REFERENCES

1. Reddi, A. H. (2000) Morphogenesis and tissue engineering of bone and cartilage: inductive signals, stem cells, and biomimetic biomaterials. *Tissue Eng.* **6,** 351–359.
2. Urist, M. R. (1965) Bone: formation by autoinduction. *Science* **159,** 893–899.
3. Reddi, A. H. and Huggins, C. B. (1972) Biochemical sequences in the transformation of normal fibroblasts in adolescent rats. *Proc. Natl. Acad. Sci. USA* **69,** 1601–1605.
4. Reddi, A. H. (1981) Cell biology and biochemistry of endochondral bone development. *Collagen Rel. Res.* **1,** 209–226.
5. Sampath, T. K. and Reddi, A. H. (1981) Dissociative extraction and reconstitution of extracellular matrix components involved in local bone differentiation. *Proc. Natl. Acad. Sci. USA* **78,** 7599–7603.
6. Wozney, J. M., Rosen, V., Celeste, A. J., Mitsock, L. M., Whitters, M. J., Kriz, R. W., et al. (1988) Novel regulators of bone formation: molecular clones and activities. *Science* **242,** 1528–1534.
7. Wozney, J. M. (1992) The bone morphogenetic protein family and osteogenesis. *Mol. Reprod. Dev.* **32,** 160–167.
8. Reddi, A. H. (1992) Regulation of cartilage and bone differentiation by bone morphogenetic proteins. *Curr. Opin. Cell. Biol.* **4,** 850–855.
9. Ripamonti, U. and Reddi, A. H. (1997) Tissue engineering, morphogenesis and regeneration of the periodontal tissues by bone morphogenetic proteins. *Crit. Rev. Oral Biol. Med.* **8,** 154–163.
10. Thomadakis, G., Ramoshebi, L. N., Crooks, J., Rueger, D. C., and Ripamonti, U. (1999) Immunolocalization of bone morphogenetic protein-2 and -3 and osteogenic protein-1 during murine tooth root morphogenesis and in other craniofacial structures. *Eur. J. Oral Sci.* **107,** 368–377.
11. Ripamonti, U. and Duneas, N. (1998) Tissue morphogenesis and regeneration by bone morphogenetic proteins. *Plast. Reconstr. Surg.* **101,** 227–239.
12. Ripamonti, U., van den Heever, B., Crooks, J., Tucker, M. M.., Sampath, T. K., Rueger, D. C., et al. (2000) Long term evaluation of bone formation by osteogenic protein-1 in the baboon and relative efficacy of bone-derived bone morphogenetic proteins delivered by irradiated xenogeneic collagenous matrices. *J. Bone Miner. Res.* **15,** 1798–1809.
13. Ripamonti, U., Ma, S., Cunningham, N., Yeates, L., and Reddi, A. H. (1992) Initiation of bone regeneration in adult baboons by osteogenin, a bone morphogenetic protein. *Matrix* **12,** 369–380.
14. Ripamonti, U., Ramoshebi, L. N., Matsaba, T., Tasker, J., Crooks, J., and Teare, J. (2001) Bone induction by BMPs/OPs and related family members in primates. The critical role of delivery systems. *J. Bone Joint Surg. Am.* **83-A,** S1116–S1127.
15. Groeneveld, E. H. J. and Burger, E. H. (2002) Bone morphogenetic proteins in human bone regeneration. *Eur. J. Endocrinol.* **142,** 9–21.
16. Ferretti, C. and Ripamonti, U. (2002) Human segmental mandibular defect treated with naturally derived bone morphogenetic proteins. *J. Craniofacial Surg.* **3,** 434–444.
17. Ripamonti, U., van den Heever, B., Heliotis, M., Dal Mas, I., Hähnle, U. R., and Biscardi, A. (2002) Local delivery of bone morphogenetic proteins in primates using a reconstituted basement membrane gel: tissue engineering with Matrigel. *S. Afr. J. Sci.* **98,** 429–433.
18. Ripamonti, U., Heliotis, M., van den Heever B., and Reddi, A. H. (1994) Bone morphogenetic proteins induce periodontal regeneration in the baboon (*Papio ursinus*). *J. Periodont. Res.* **29,** 439–445.
19. Ripamonti, U., Heliotis, M., Rueger, D. C., and Sampath, T. K. (1996) Induction of cementogenesis by recombinant human osteogenic protein-1 (hOP-1/BMP-7) in the baboon. *Arch. Oral Biol.* **41,** 121–126.
20. Ripamonti, U., Crooks, J., Teare, J., Petit. J.-C., and Rueger, D. C. (2002) Periodontal tissue regeneration by recombinant human osteogenic protein-1 in periodontally-induced furcation defects of the primate *Papio ursinus. S. Afr. J. Sci.* **98,** 361–368.
21. Centrella, M., Horowitz, M., Wozney, J. M., and McCarthy, T. L. (1994) Transforming growth factor β (TGF-β) family members and bone. *Endocr. Rev.* **15,** 27–39.
22. Roberts, A. B., Sporn, M. B., Assoian, R. K., Smith, J. M., Roche, N. S., Wakefield, L. M., et al. (1986) Transforming growth factor type β: rapid induction of fibrosis and angiogenesis in vivo and stimulation of collagen formation in vitro. *Proc. Natl. Acad. Sci. USA* **83,** 4167–4171.
23. Shinozaki, M., Kawara, S., Hayashi, N., Kakinuba, T., Igarashi, A., and Takehara, K. (1997) Induction of subcutaneous tissue fibrosis in newborn mice by transforming growth factor-β: simultaneous application with basic fibroblast growth factor causes persistent fibrosis. *Biochem. Biophys. Res. Commun.* **237,** 292–296.
24. Raven, P. H. and Johnson, G. B. (1989) Evolutionary History of the Earth, in *Biology* 2nd ed. (Brake, D. K., ed), Times Mirror/Mosby College, St. Louis, pp. 419–441.
25. Ripamonti, U., Duneas, N., van den Heever, B., Bosch, C., and Crooks, J. (1997) Recombinant transforming growth factor-β1 induces endochondral bone in the baboon and synergizes with recombinant osteogenic protein-1 (bone morphogenetic protein-7) to initiate rapid bone formation. *J. Bone Miner. Res.* **12,** 1584–1595.
26. Duneas, N., Crooks, J., and Ripamonti, U. (1998) Transforming growth factors β1: Induction of bone morphogenetic protein genes expression during endochondral bone formation in the baboon, and synergistic interaction with osteogenic protein-1 (BMP-7) *Growth Factors* **15,** 259–277.

27. Ripamonti, U., Crooks, J., Matsaba, T., and Tasker, J. (2000) Induction of endochondral bone formation by recombinant human transforming growth factor-β2 in the baboon (*Papio ursinus*). *Growth Factors* **17,** 269–285.
28. Ripamonti U., Teare, J., Matsaba, T., and Renton, L. (2001) Site, tissue and organ specificity of endochondral bone induction and morphogenesis by TGF-β isoforms in the primate *Papio ursinus*. Proceedings FASEB Summer Conference: The TGF-β superfamily: signaling and development, Tucson Arizona, USA, July 7–12.
29. Miyazono, K., Ten Dijke, P., and Heldin, C.-H. (2002) TGF-β signaling by Smad proteins. *Adv. Immunol.* **75,** 115–157.
30. Ripamonti, U., Crooks, J., and Kirkbride, A. N. (1999) Sintered porous hydroxyapatites with intrinsic osteoinductive activity: geometric induction of bone formation. *S. Afr. J. Sci.* **95,** 335–343.
31. Ripamonti, U. (2000) Smart biomaterials with intrinsic osteoinductivity: geometric control of bone differentiation, in *Bone Engineering* (Davies, J. E., ed.), EM2 Corporation, Toronto, Canada, pp. 215–222.
32. Ripamonti, U., Crooks, J., and Rueger D. C. (2001) Induction of bone formation by recombinant human osteogenic protein-1 and sintered porous hydroxyapatite in adult primates. *Plast. Reconstr. Surg.* **107,** 977–988.
33. Ripamonti, U. and Duneas, N. (1996) Tissue engineering of bone by osteoinductive biomaterials. *MRS Bull.* **21,** 36–39.
34. Gerber, H. P. and Ferrare, N. (2000) Angiogenesis and bone growth. *Trends Cardiovasc. Med.* **10,** 223–228.
35. Colnot, C. I. and Helms, J. A. (2001) A molecular analysis of matrix remodeling and angiogenesis during long bone development. *Mech. Dynamics* **100,** 245–250.
36. Paralkar, V. M., Nandedkar, A. K. N., Pointer, R. H., Kleinman, H. K., and Reddi, A. H. (1990) Interaction of osteogenin, a heparin binding bone morphogenetic protein, with type IV collagen. *J. Biol. Chem.* **265,** 17281–17284.
37. Heliotis, M. and Ripamonti, U. (1994) Phenotypic modulation of endothelial cells by bone morphogenetic protein fractions in vitro. *In Vitro Cell. Dev. Biol.* **30A,** 353–355.
38. Wang, J. S. and Aspenberg, P. (1993) Basic fibroblast growth factor and bone induction in rats. *Acta. Orthop. Scand.* **64,** 557–561.
39. Takita, H., Tsuruga, E., Ono, I., and Kuboki, Y. (1997) Enhancement by bFGF of osteogenesis induced by rhBMP-2 in rats. *Eur. J. Oral. Sci.* **105,** 588–592.
40. Gerber, H. P., Vu, T. H., Ryan, A. M., Kowalski, J., Werb, Z., and Ferrara, N. (1999) VEGF couples hypertrophic cartilage remodeling, ossification and angiogenesis during endochondral bone formation. *Nat. Med.* **5,** 623–628.
41. Horner A., Bord S., Kelsall, A. W., Coleman, N., and Compston, J. E. (2001) Tie2 ligands angiopoietin-1 and angiopoietin-2 are coexpressed with vascular endothelial cell growth factor in growing human bone. *Bone* **28,** 65–71.
42. Delaissé, J. M., Ensig, M. T., Everts, V., del Carmen Ovejero, M., Ferreras, M., Lund, L., et al. (2000) Proteinases in bone resorption: obvious and less obvious roles. *Clin. Chim. Acta* **291,** 223–234.
43. Ripamonti, U., van den Heever, B., and Van Wyk, J. (1993) Expression of the osteogenic phenotype in porous hydroxyapatite implanted extraskeletally in baboons. *Matrix.* **13,** 491–502.
44. Trueta, J. (1963) The role of the vessels in osteogeneis. *J. Bone Joint Surg.* **45B,** 402–418.

16

Perichondrial and Periosteal Regulation of Endochondral Growth

Dana L. Di Nino and Thomas F. Linsenmayer

INTRODUCTION

Limb development requires the precise spatial and temporal regulation of the growth of skeletal elements *(1)*. All long bones originate as cartilage rudiments that are surrounded by a fibrous connective tissue, the perichondrium. Longitudinal growth of these cartilaginous templates occurs by endochondral ossification. During this process, chondrocytes undergo rapid proliferation and then enter a maturation phase, where they cease proliferation and increase their synthesis and deposition of extracellular matrix. Subsequently they undergo hypertrophy and then synthesize and secrete a specialized extracellular matrix component, type X collagen *(2–4)*. After progressing through the hypertrophic zone, the cells either undergo cell death or further differentiate into osteoblast-like cells *(5,6)*. This removal of chondrocytes, concomitant with the invasion of blood vessels, leads to the formation of the marrow cavity. Where the bony shaft has formed, the perichondrium (PC) differentiates into the periosteum (PO), whose cells provide the osteoblasts for appositional bone growth *(7)*.

To ensure the correct rate of cartilage elongation and its subsequent removal and replacement by bone and marrow, regulation must occur at all stages of endochondral development. The mechanisms of regulation must therefore involve chondrocyte proliferation, differentiation, and removal *(2,5)* and the subsequent progression of the bone collar.

This precise regulation of cartilage growth and development is necessary to ensure the proper formation of long bones. Disturbances in the regulation of chondrocyte proliferation and/or hypertrophy can result in either delayed or accelerated ossification. Both types of abnormalities can result in the same phenotype: eventual shortening of bones, or dwarfism. Studies, including our own *(2,8,9)*, suggest that negative regulation is the major type of regulation controlling the growth of skeletal elements, and that both chondrocyte proliferation and hypertrophy are affected. However, positive regulation must also exist to promote growth.

FACTORS INVOLVED IN CARTILAGE GROWTH REGULATION

Regulatory interactions between the cartilage and perichondrium were first suggested from studies on the Indian hedgehog/parathyroid hormone-related peptide signaling pathway *(8,10)*. The model for this pathway is a negative feedback loop, which is initiated in the prehypertrophic zone of the cartilage template by the expression of Indian hedgehog (Ihh; ref. *8*). The Ihh protein secreted by chondrocytes

From: *The Skeleton: Biochemical, Genetic, and Molecular Interactions in Development and Homeostasis*
Edited by: E. J. Massaro and J. M. Rogers © Humana Press Inc., Totowa, NJ

signals through its receptor, Patched (Ptc; ref. *11*). Ptc and Gli, another downstream target of Ihh, are expressed in high levels in the perichondrium, suggesting that this tissue is a primary target of Ihh. In response to Ihh, the perichondrium signals back to the cartilage to delay its growth and to decrease the expression of Ihh itself. The Ihh signal is propagated by the articular perichondrium through its production of parathyroid hormone-related peptide (PTHrP). A connection between Ihh and PTHrP was suggested from PTHrP –/– mice, in which Ihh is no longer capable of negatively regulating cartilage growth. This observation suggested that the Ihh signal is mediated through PTHrP *(8)*.

In addition to the negative regulatory role of Ihh in this pathway, this factor is also capable of effecting positive regulation of chondrocyte proliferation *(12,13)*. Somewhat surprisingly, an increase in proliferation results in dwarfism—as does a decrease in proliferation. That the same phenotype results from opposite effects on proliferation is caused most likely by subsequent disturbances that occur in the hypertrophic zone, as hypertrophy has been shown to be a major factor in overall growth *(14)*. An increase in the number of proliferating chondrocytes is accompanied by a decrease in the rate of hypertrophy. Likewise, a decrease in the number of proliferating chondrocytes leaves fewer cells available to undergo hypertrophy. Therefore, in both situations, the result is an overall decrease in longitudinal growth as a result of fewer hypertrophic chondrocytes.

The bone morphogenic proteins (BMPs) are another family of signaling molecules that have been implicated in the regulation of cartilage development *(15)*. The BMPs, which constitute a subgroup of the transforming growth factor-β (TGF-β) superfamily, were first identified by their ability to produce ectopic bone when injected subcutaneously into developing embryos *(16)*. Subsequently, the BMPs have been shown to be involved in many events in the developing embryo, such as heart development and interdigital apoptosis *(17,18)*. In developing long bones, a number of BMPs are expressed in the perichondrium, whereas in hypertrophic cartilage only BMP6 has been detected *(7)*. In the perichondrium, BMP7 is expressed in the region adjacent to the expression of Ihh; BMPs 2 and 4 are expressed in this same region, but their expression also extends towards the epiphysis, and BMP5 is expressed more towards the epiphysis. The perichondrial expression patterns of these BMPs suggest a role in their mediating the Ihh signal received by Ptc to the articular perichondrium, which in turn leads to the expression of PTHrP. Consistent with this, retroviral overexpression of BMPs 2 and 4 results in an increase in proliferation of chondrocytes and a delay in their hypertrophy. In addition, overexpression of BMP receptor 1A results in an increase of PTHrP expression and a phenotype similar to Ihh ectopic overexpression, without directly affecting the levels of Ihh *(19)*. This further supports that BMP signaling acts either downstream of Ihh, or in parallel with the Ihh pathway.

Additional factors, although less well studied, have also been shown to be involved in chondrocyte proliferation and differentiation. These include the fibroblast growth factors (FGFs), TGFs, and retinoic acid (RA). All of these have been further examined by us, as presented in detail later.

Signaling through the fibroblast growth factor receptor 3 (FGFR3) inhibits chondrocyte proliferation, as determined by upregulation in transgenic and knockout mice *(9,20)*, and a form of human dwarfism, achondrodysplasia, is caused by an activating point mutation in FGFR3 *(21)*. FGFR3 is expressed by chondrocytes in the proliferative zone. It mediates intracellular signaling in response to FGFs but is also capable of responding to other ligands, including extracellular matrix molecules *(22)*. Thus, it is a promiscuous receptor. Although in cartilage it is not known what ligands signal through FGFR3, three different FGFs (FGF 1–3) have been identified and localized in the growth plate. And, functionally, studies of rat metatarsal organ cultures have suggested that FGF-2 acts to negatively regulate both chondrocyte proliferation and hypertrophy *(23)*.

TGF-β family members have also been implicated in regulating cartilage growth. *In situ* hybridization has shown that TGF-βs 1–3 are all expressed in the mouse perichondrium and periosteum *(24)*. Functionally, disruption of TGF-β signaling (by the expression of a dominant negative type II receptor) in the perichondrium and periosteum and in the lower hypertrophic zone results in increased hypertrophy and Ihh expression *(25)*. This suggests that TGF-β signaling, as mediated by this receptor, normally functions to inhibit the progression of chondrocytes to hypertrophy. However, it is likely that TGF-β1 does not affect chondrocyte hypertrophy directly, instead acting through the perichondrium. In support of this, TGF-β1 overexpression leads to ectopic expression of PTHrP in the perichondrium *(26)*. This observation raises the question of whether TGF-β1 is capable of directly affecting cartilage growth or whether it acts partially or even entirely, through the perichondrium by eliciting secondary signals from this tissue.

Cartilage growth can also be affected by RA, which is capable of interfering with cartilage maturation at hyper- or hypodietary levels *(27)*. RA has been shown to be synthesized in cartilage, but much higher levels are made in the perichondrium *(28)*. In addition, three nuclear receptors for RA are expressed in developing cartilage anlagen, with RA receptor (RAR)β being expressed in the perichondrium and RARs α and γ in the cartilage itself *(29)*. Also, the addition of RA to organ cultures of fetal rat metatarsals caused an inhibition of longitudinal growth, similar to that observed with the systemic administration of RA *(30)*. This inhibition of cartilage growth could be reversed by the addition of RAR antagonists, thus restoring normal growth *(30)*. These studies suggest that RA produced by the perichondrium is capable of negatively regulating cartilage growth. However, the significance of the expression of RA receptors in these different locations (cartilage and perichondrium) is not known.

REGULATION OF CARTILAGE GROWTH BY THE PERICHONDRIUM AND PERIOSTEUM: ANALYSES BY ORGAN CULTURE

The aforementioned studies indicate that the PC acts to regulate cartilage growth. Most of these studies examined the patterns of expression of potential regulatory factors, and the phenotypes resulting from their overexpression or elimination, frequently producing abnormal shortening or elongation, which we refer to as "overcompensation," described in the Additional Factors That Act Through the Perichondrium to Effect Negative Regulation of Cartilage Growth section.

We have taken a different approach to examine regulation by the PC and also by the PO *(2,31,32)*. The model system we devised compares organ cultures of contralateral pairs of tibiotarsal long bone anlagen from 12-d chicken embryos. Generally, in these pairs one tibiotarsus has had its PC and PO removed (PC/PO-free cultures), whereas in the contralateral tibiotarsus these tissues are left intact (intact cultures). The use of such organ cultures, depending on the experimental design, can (1) maintain the integrity of the anlagen and the inherent cell and tissue interactions involved in its normal development, (2) allow for analysis of interactions between the component tissues through their differential removal, and (3) allow testing the effects of putative regulatory factors through their addition to the culture medium. These factors can be unknown factors, in the form of conditioned medium collected from cell cultures of the tissues to be examined, or known factors (either purified or recombinant). In our studies (presented next) we have used most of these approaches.

In our initial studies using this system *(2)*, we observed that removal of the PC and PO from the tibiotarsi before culture resulted in a greater growth in length of these PC/PO-free tibiotarsi as compared to intact cultures of contralateral tibiotarsi (*see* Fig. 1A). Both the intact and the PC/PO-free cultures undergo growth in length, and virtually all of this is in the intact cartilaginous portion of the long bone anlagen, with the bony portion remaining essentially unchanged *(2)*. Thus, removal of the PC and PO resulted in "extended growth" in length of the limb cartilage (defined in more detail later, Fig. 1B). This result, in itself, suggested that one, or both, of the removed tissues normally function in the negative regulation of the growth of endochondral cartilage.

Further analysis performed in this initial study showed that the extended growth of the cartilage that resulted from removal of the PC and PO involved enlargement of both the zones of proliferation (demonstrated by BrdU incorporation) and hypertrophy (identified by immunofluorescence for the hypertrophic cartilage specific collagen, type X; ref. *1*). Also, the regulation of these parameters by the PC/PO was observed to be a local effect because removal of the PC/PO from one side of the

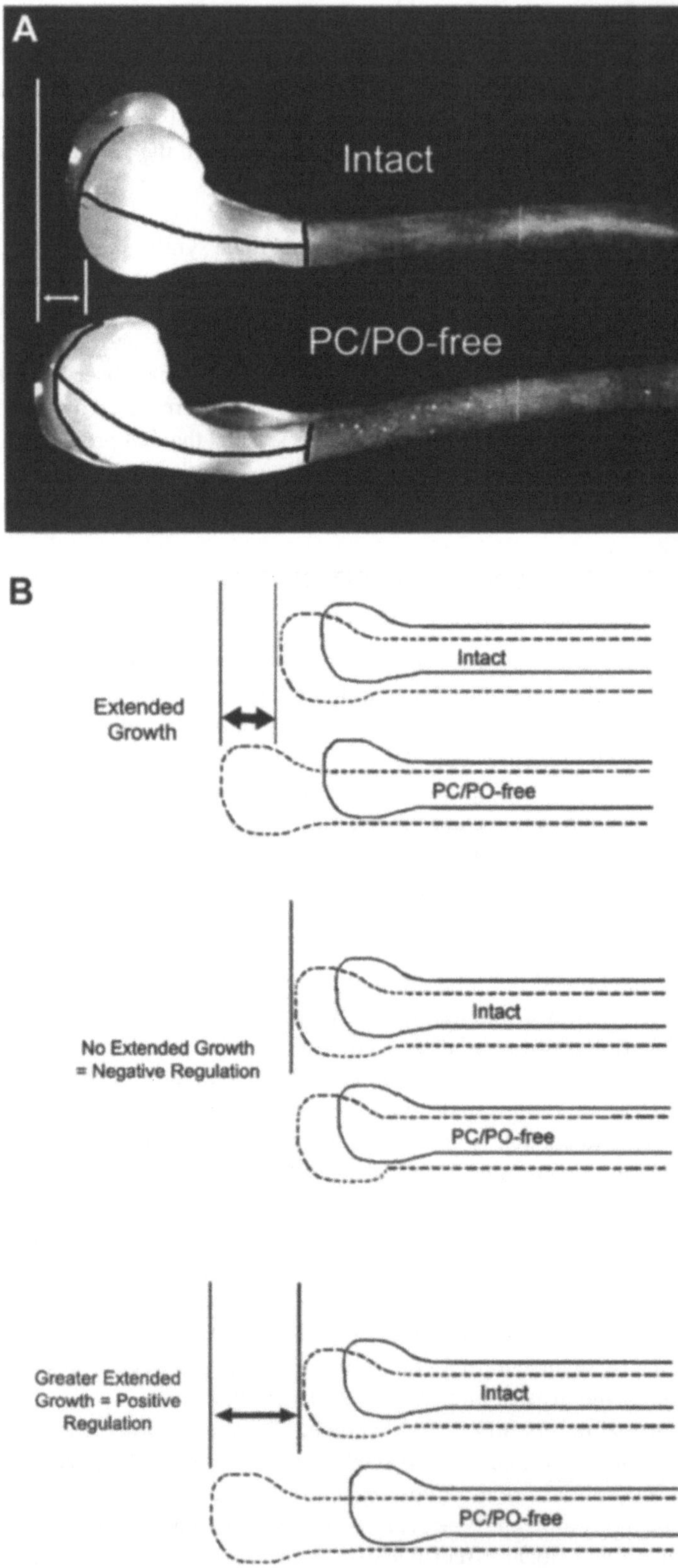
A
Intact
PC/PO-free
B
Extended Growth
Intact
PC/PO-free
No Extended Growth = Negative Regulation
Intact
PC/PO-free
Greater Extended Growth = Positive Regulation
Intact
PC/PO-free

anlagen led to expansion of both the type X-positive domain and the BrdU-positive zones at the site of removal but not where the PC/PO remained intact. Furthermore, we observed that the PC/PO-free cultures responded to the addition of PTH, consistent with the involvement of PTHrP and the perichondrium in the Vortkamp model of growth regulation *(8)*. This addition of PTH to the PC/PO-free cultures reversed the expansion of the collagen type X-positive domain but not that of the proliferative zone. This suggests that the regulation of chondrocyte differentiation (hypertrophy) is dependent on the PTH/PTHrP receptor, but proliferation is likely to be independent of it. However, precisely where PTH/PTHrP fits into the PC/PO-mediated regulation we have observed here and examined further (as described next) is still not known.

Cooperative Negative Regulation by Factors from the Perichondrium and Periosteum

One possibility for the observed effect of PC and PO in the negative regulation of cartilage growth in the developing long bone was that this regulation was mediated through the production of diffusible factors secreted by these tissues. To examine this possibility, we *(31)* examined the ability of various conditioned media (serum-free) from cell cultures of PC and PO cells to regulate cartilage growth when added to PC/PO-free organ cultures vs the PC/PO-intact ones. To compare and evaluate the results, we further characterized and quantified the parameter "extended growth" with extended growth being defined, for each tibiotarsal pair, as the difference in length of the tarsal-end cartilage of the PC/PO-free culture vs that of the intact culture (*see* Fig. 1 A,B, top panel). This method of evaluating the data uses the intact tibiotarsus of each pair as the internal control for "normal" longitudinal growth. It therefore reduces any differences that exist between individual embryos within the population *(33)*, such as the initial sizes of the tibiotarsi when removed for culture or inherent differences in growth rates.

Using this definition, an "extended growth" of zero would represent complete compensation for removal of the PC and PO (i.e., the factor(s) present in the conditioned medium effected net negative regulation of cartilage growth, precisely to the same extent as the endogenous PC and PO of the intact limb; Fig. 1B, middle panel). The other result that might be expected was that the conditioned medium produced an extended growth greater than that of cultures grown in control medium, which would suggest that the factors present were involved in positive regulation of cartilage growth (Fig. 1B, bottom panel).

In these experiments, as well as all of the subsequent ones, each member of the tibiotarsal pair was cultured for 3 d, the time period during which linear growth occurred *(2)*. Consistent with these results *(2)*, in control medium (serum-free), the cartilages of both the intact and PC/PO-free cultures underwent longitudinal growth and removal of PC and PO resulted in "extended growth" of the cartilaginous

---

Fig. 1. (*opposite page*) **A**, A tibiotarsal pair cultured in serum-free (control) medium showing the extended growth of cartilage in the PC/PO-free tibiotarsus vs the intact contralateral tibiotarsus. In all experiments, the measurements of cartilage growth are made along the midline from the articular surface to the boney collar (as shown by the solid lines). **B**, Top diagram depicts extended growth (arrows) of cartilage as defined by the increased length of the PC/PO-free tibiotarsus compared with its intact counterpart after culture in serum-free control medium. The diagrams with the solid lines depict original size of the tibiotarsus and the corresponding diagrams with the dotted lines depict the results after culture. Extended growth is depicted by the two-headed arrow. Middle diagram depicts the result predicted for a negative regulatory factor(s) that produces precise negative regulation. When such a factor is added to the medium, it precisely compensates for the removal of the endogenous perichondrium and periosteum (i.e., the growth of the PC/PO-free culture is the same as that of the intact culture). Lower diagram depicts the result predicted for a factor(s) effecting positive regulation (stimulation) of growth. Here, the extended growth of the PC/PO-free culture to which the factor is added is greater than the extended growth observed in cultures in control (serum-free) medium (compare this diagram to the top diagram). Modified from Di Nino et al. *(31)*.

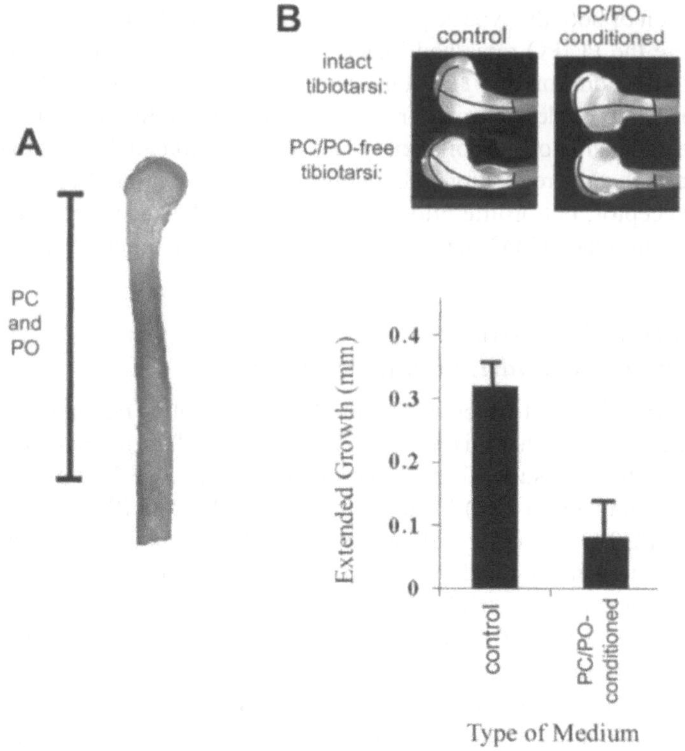

Fig. 2. A, Depiction of the region along the length of a tibiotarsus used to initiate cell cultures for PC/PO conditioned medium. **B**, Photographic examples and a bar graph showing extended cartilage growth of organ culture pairs grown in control medium vs PC/PO-conditioned medium. Note that the extended growth for the PC/PO-free tibiotarsus in control medium is 0.3 mm and that this is essentially eliminated by growth in PC/PO-conditioned medium. Thus, the factor(s) in the PC/PO-conditioned medium effect precise negative regulation, compensating for removal of the endogenous PC and PO. Modified from Di Nino et al. *(31)*.

region (Fig. 2B, "control"). Quantification showed that in most experiments the average extended growth was 0.3 mm (Fig. 2B, lower panel, "control"). Conversely, the bony shaft showed little extended growth, if any at all (not shown; *see* ref. *2*).

Using this control value (0.3 mm) for "extended growth" (of the cartilage) as the baseline difference between the intact cultures and PC/PO-free cultures, we were able to test whether the negative regulation effected by the PC and/or the PO resulted from the secretion of diffusible factors secreted by these tissues, or possibly by physical constraints exerted by them when present. For this, we performed a variety of experiments in which cells from the PC and PO were grown as cell cultures, and the conditioned media from these cultures (containing the putative regulatory factors) were added to organ cultures to determine their effect on "extended growth." The results, as described next, suggested that the PC and PO do secrete negative regulatory factors that compensate for removal of the endogenous PC and PO, and in addition they secrete positive stimulators effecting increased growth.

Using this approach, our initial experiments *(31)* examined whether the conditioned medium from mixed cultures of PC and PO cells, when added to PC/PO-free organ cultures, would effect negative regulation and, if so, whether this would compensate exactly for removal of the endogenous PC and PO (i.e., the regulation would be precise). One way to initiate mixed cultures of PC and PO cells was to use, as the source of cells, the entire length of the PC and PO (*see* diagram in Fig. 2A); another way was to use the narrow "border" region where the PC and PO overlap (*see* diagram in Fig. 3A). In both

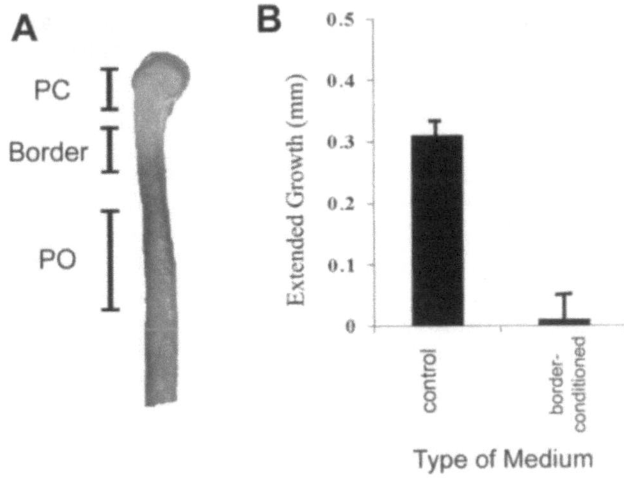

Fig. 3. A, Depiction of the regions along the length of a tibiotarsus used to generate cell cultures for PC-conditioned medium, PO-conditioned medium, and border region-conditioned medium. **B**, Bar graph showing the extended cartilage growth of the organ culture pairs in control medium and conditioned medium from cultures of cells taken from the border region border conditioned. Note that the extended growth in the border-conditioned medium is zero, showing again that the factor(s) effect precise negative regulation (i.e., they compensate precisely for removal of the endogenous PC and PO). Modified from Di Nino et al. *(31)*.

cases, the cultures of cells from these regions produced a conditioned medium which, when added to the PC/PO-free cultures, produced an "extended growth" of zero (i.e., the growth was the same as that of the intact culture; Fig. 2B, PC/PO conditioned; and 3B, border conditioned). Thus, the factors in these conditioned media effected negative regulation that precisely compensated for removal of the endogenous PC and PO. This result is consistent with the negative regulation on cartilage growth effected by the PC and/or the PO, resulting largely, if not entirely, through the secretion of diffusible regulatory factors. This also largely eliminates an involvement of physical constraints by these tissues, at least within the limits of this assay.

During the period that the PC/PO cells are in culture, some of PC cells differentiate into chondrocytes (Fig. 4), which is not unexpected as one of the functions of the PC in vivo is the production of chondrocytes for appositional growth of the cartilage. However, further experiments suggest that it is unlikely that these chondrocytes themselves are responsible for the negative regulation, as conditioned medium from pure cultures of nonhypertrophic or hypertrophic chondrocytes showed no negative regulatory properties. In fact, the conditioned medium from the hypertrophic chondrocytes produced increased growth, raising the possibility that chondrocytes have an inherent tendency to stimulate their own growth, possibly through an autocrine mechanism(s).

To test further for the cell-type specificity of the conditioned medium, and to eliminate the possibility that the observed negative regulation was caused by a trivial reason, such as a general depletion of nutrients in the conditioned medium, we examined the effect of conditioned medium from scleral (ocular) fibroblasts, a cell type that produces dense multilayer cultures that should provide an adequate test for depletion of nutrients. When this conditioned medium was tested on the PC/PO-free cultures, there was no detectible effect.

Requirement for Both PC and PO in Negative Regulation of Cartilage Growth

These experiments (and others not described; *see* ref. *31*) are consistent with the PC and PO negatively regulating cartilage growth through the secretion of diffusible factors. However, they do not distinguish whether these negative regulatory properties of the PC/PO-conditioned medium could result

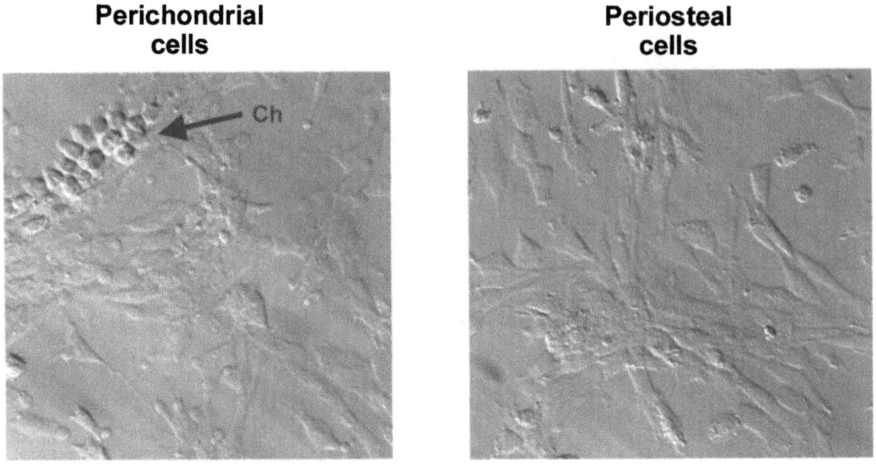

Fig. 4. Photomicrographs of cultures of the perichondrial cells and periosteal cells from which the conditioned media are harvested. In the perichondral cultures, small nests of chondrocytes occasionally form (Ch).

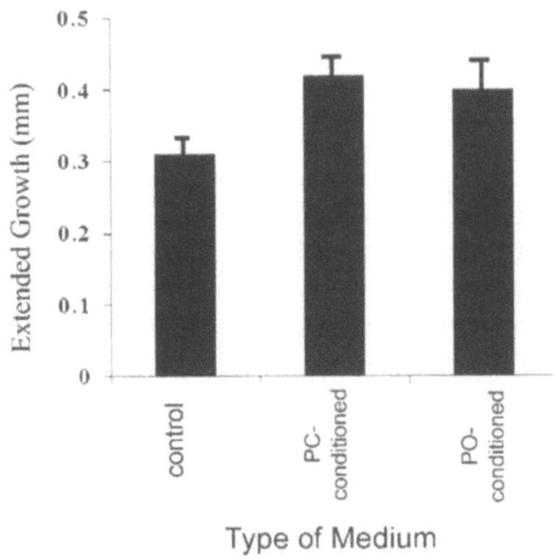

Fig. 5. Extended growth of PC/PO-free cultures observed with conditioned medium from either PC or PO cell cultures vs control medium. Note that the extended growth in medium from either the PC or PO cells is greater than that in the control medium suggesting that either cell type, by itself, produces a factor(s) that stimulates growth (i.e., a positive regulator). Modified from Di Nino et al. *(31)*.

from the same factors being produced by both cell types, or from different factors produced by each tissue. Furthermore, these could work in concert or independently to produce the inhibitory effect.

To test these possibilities, the cell cultures used to produce conditioned medium were initiated from separate regions of the PC and the PO (*see* diagram in Fig. 3A). When the conditioned media from these regions were tested separately on the PC/PO-free cultures, neither showed negative regulation. In fact, the "extended growth" observed with either of these media was greater than in the control medium (Fig. 5).

These results suggested that the negative regulation either might involve an interaction between the PC and PO cells but could not distinguish whether this required direct cell–cell interactions or, alternatively, could be mediated by diffusible factors produced by each cell type.

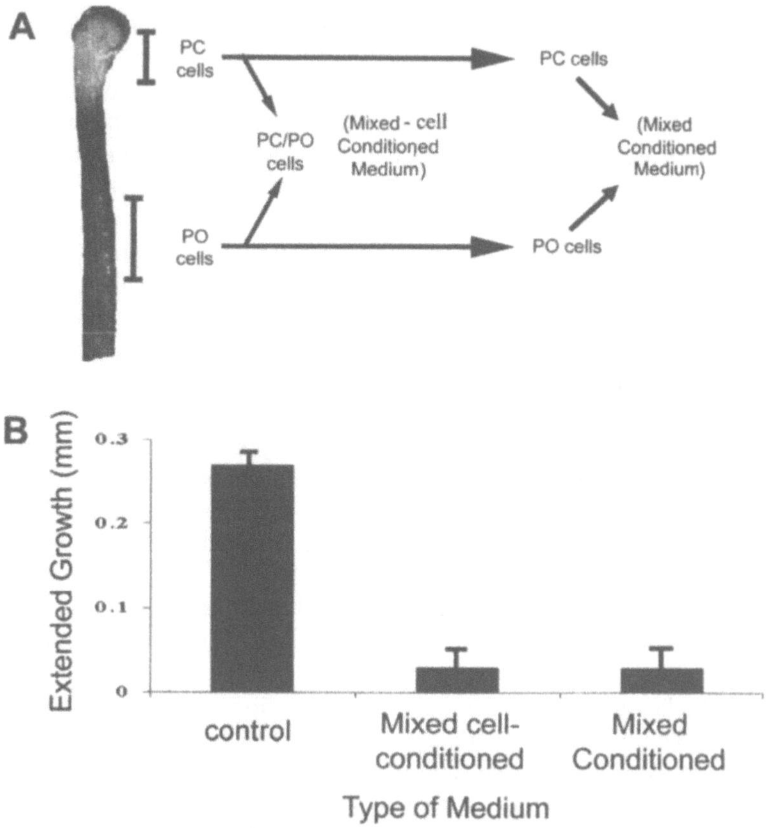

Fig. 6. A, Depiction of the regions of the PC and PO used to generate "mixed cell-conditioned medium" (when the PC and PO cells themselves were mixed together and cocultured) and "mixed-conditioned medium" (when the conditioned media from separate cultures of PC cells and PO cells were collected and subsequently mixed together). **B**, Bar graph showing the extended growth of organ culture pairs in each of these mixed media, as compared to those in control medium. Note that either type of mixed medium results in an extended growth of zero (i.e., they effect precise negative regulation). Modified from Di Nino et al. *(31)*.

To test these possibilities, the conditioned media produced in two different types of "mixing" experiments were examined for their ability to effect negative regulation in the PC/PO-free cultures (diagramed in Fig. 6A). In the first type of experiment, the conditioned medium was harvested from co-cultures of PC and PO cells that were mixed before culture ("mixed-cell" conditioned medium); in the second type of experiment, conditioned media were harvested from separate cultures of PC and PO cells and then were subsequently combined to yield "mixed conditioned medium". Both types of conditioned medium, when added to the PC/PO-free cultures, produced negative regulation resulting in an "extended growth" of zero (i.e., they effected precise regulation; Fig. 6B). The mixed PC- and PO-conditioned media reduced the overall length of the tarsal cartilage to that of the intact cartilage. However, the above experiments do not address the possibility that the putative factors in the "mixed media" may have an effect over and above that of the PC and PO in the intact cartilages. To test this, organ culture pairs were examined in which both tibiotarsi were intact (their PC /PO were not removed). One tibiotarsus in each pair was grown in control serum-free medium, whereas the other was grown in conditioned mixed media. In such cultures, there was no detectable difference in the overall length of the cartilages. Therefore, the negative regulatory factors in the mixed media do not overcompensate in the presence of the intact PC and PO (i.e., they do not produce regulation over and above that effected by the endogenous PC and PO). This indicates indirectly that when a certain level of factors exists (in this case, those from the intact PC/PO), additional factors (from the conditioned medium) have no effect.

Taken together, these results suggest that the most likely mechanism through which this negative regulation is achieved is one in which PC and PO cells secrete different factors and that these act cooperatively. If this interpretation is correct, it suggests a novel type of regulation in which separate factors produced by two different tissues (the PC and PO) act in the negative regulation of a third tissue (the endochondral cartilage).

This regulation by mixed media seems to compensate precisely for the normal regulation that occurs in the presence of intact PC and PO. Also, there appears to be an upper level of response to these factors above which no additional regulation occurs. This is suggested by two observations. One is that in cultures of intact tibiotarsi (with their PC and PO present), no additional negative regulation is observed with the PC/PO conditioned medium. The other is that little if any "overcompensation" of the negative regulation is observed in PC/PO-free tibiotarsal cultures when the quantities of factors from the PC and PO cell cultures are increased by lengthening time before the conditioned media are collected. Thus, the mechanism we have uncovered here seems to provide a unique means of regulating cartilage growth to the precise level that is normally seen in the intact tibiotarsi. As discussed below, this effect is not mimicked by other factors that have been previously suggested as negative regulators of cartilage growth.

Conceptually, the advantage of such a mechanism involving factors from both the PC and the PO (rather than from a single source) is that positional information *(34)* can be obtained vectorially from two sources. This can allow, for example, the spatial relationships of components within a structure to be determined by gradients of factors from opposing directions (e.g., by a double-gradient model; ref. *34*). In the case of the tibiotarsal growth cartilages *(35)* and most likely the growth cartilages of other long bones, the relative proportional sizes of the component zones (e.g., proliferative, maturation, and hypertrophy) remain similar throughout embryonic development. If a double-gradient is the type of mechanism employed in this system, factors secreted by the perichondrium and periosteum could be involved, for example, in determining the lengths of the proliferative and hypertrophic zones.

Cellular Parameters Affected by Perichondrial and Periosteal Regulation

The studies just described used as an assay overall cartilage length. This assay is highly advantageous in providing information concerning growth regulation, including the tissues involved, their interactions, and the factors they produce. However, it does not provide information concerning the cellular parameters that may be altered by these factors, such as cell number, cell size, and quantity of extracellular matrix.

To determine which of these parameters is altered upon removal of the PC and PO, we performed histology and morphometric analyses on the hypertrophic region of PC/PO-free cultures vs intact ones. We chose the hypertrophic region for these analyses because previous studies by Hunziker *(14)* showed that most changes affecting limb growth occurred in this region. Then, to determine whether the precise compensation of cartilage growth regulation effected by the factors in the PC/PO conditioned medium resulted from restoration of the same parameters to their state in the intact limbs, we also analyzed PC/PO-free cultures grown in PC/PO-conditioned medium.

The computerized image analysis that we wished to use in these studies required the following: (1) identification of the region of hypertrophy to ensure that all the measurements were made in this zone, (2) compensation for the cell shrinkage that occurs during fixation and embedding to ensure that we were measuring the original cell size, and (3) clear-cut histological staining differences between the extracellular cartilage matrix and the shrunken chondrocytes remaining within the lacunae. To demarcate the hypertrophic zone we used staining for type X collagen on serial cross sections along the length of the cartilage. To analyze cell size, we measured the lacunae (the areas occupied by cells in the cartilage extracellular matrix) rather than the cells themselves which, as stated above, undergo variable

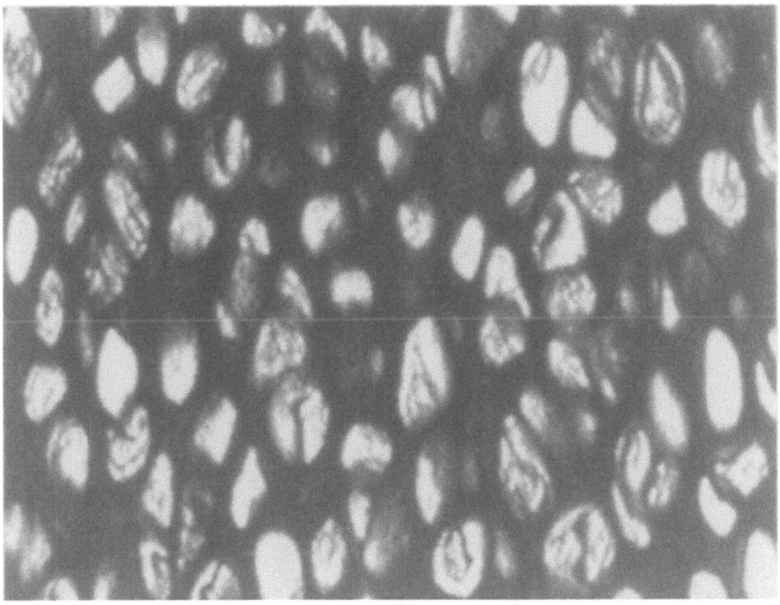

Fig. 7. Photomicrograph of a representative section of hypertrophic cartilage stained with toluidine blue to facilitate image analysis.

shrinkage. This had the added advantage that when the matrix is stained with toluidine blue, the borders of the lacunae are easily distinguished (*see* Fig. 7) by the image analysis program we use (Image Pro), both from the matrix and the shrunken chondrocytes, thus greatly facilitating the computerized analysis. Also, the toluidine blue staining of the proteoglycans in the matrix is more intense than that of the cellular components, allowing for computerized distinction and analysis of the matrix component.

Because the hypertrophic region of the cartilage is quite irregularly shaped, we found it difficult to obtain reliable data from sections cut longitudinally, even when examined serially. However, we determined that this could be alleviated by performing analyses on serial sections cut in cross section, starting with the tip of the cartilage adjacent to the marrow cavity and progressing through the entire zone of hypertrophy (as determined by staining for type X collagen).

In any given tissue section, the individual lacunae could be cut through regions that ranged from their middle (giving the largest cross-sectional area measurement) to an edge (giving the smallest measurement). To compensate for this, the cross-sectional measurements of the lacunae (indicative of cell size) were grouped in increments of 50 μm^2, giving the number of cells in each incremental area. Thus, in a graphic representation of the data, a shift of the profile to the right along the *x*-axis (Fig. 8) would indicate an increase in the cross-sectional area of the lacunae (i.e., cell sizes). From these data, we were also able to determine the total number of cells in the hypertrophic (type X collagen-positive) region, by summation of the cells in each of the incremental areas. Also, we could calculate the percentage of the hypertrophic zone represented by extracellular matrix, determined by subtracting the area occupied by the lacunae in each section from the total area of the section.

We first compared these three parameters in intact vs PC/PO-free cultures grown in control medium. The data showed that the increased extended growth we had observed in the PC/PO-free cultures resulted from both an increase in cell size, as evidenced by a shift in the size distribution to the right (Fig. 8, control medium), and an increase in the number of cells in the hypertrophic zone (Table 1, control medium). In addition, the increase in cell sizes was not uniform; instead, it occurred preferentially in

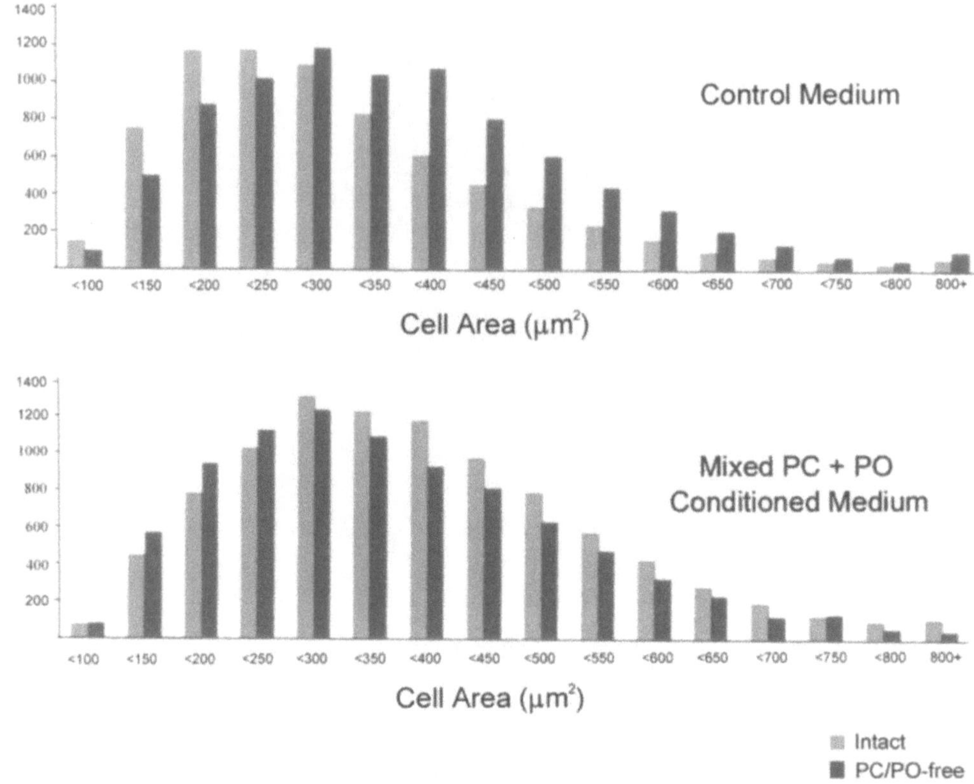

Fig. 8. Graphs representing the cross-sectional area of lacunae grouped as numbers of cells per increasing increment of area. Top graph represents organ culture pairs grown in plain serum-free medium. Bottom graph represents organ culture pair grown in PC/PO-conditioned medium.

the region of the newly formed hypertrophic chondrocytes. Conversely, removal of the PC and PO had no appreciable effect on the relative amount of extracellular matrix, with the PC/PO-free cultures showing, if anything, a slight decrease in this parameter (Table 2).

Then, we examined whether the negative regulatory factors secreted by the PC and PO acted the same as the endogenous PC and PO. For this, we examined whether the same cellular parameters that were increased in the hypertrophic zone of the PC/PO-free cultures grown in control medium (i.e., cell size and cell number) could be restored to their normal levels by culture in the mixed PC + PO conditioned medium. As can be seen in Fig. 8 (mixed PC + PO conditioned medium) and Table 2 (conditioned media), both of these parameters were now similar, if not identical, in both the intact and PC/PO-free cultures (as was also the area occupied by the extracellular matrix).

Thus, the factor(s) secreted by the PC and PO cells affect the same parameters as do the endogenous PC and PO of the intact tibiotarsus, further indicating that secretion of diffusible negative regulatory factors is one mechanism through which the perichondrium and periosteum regulate cartilage growth during normal limb development.

ADDITIONAL FACTORS THAT ACT THROUGH THE PERICHONDRIUM TO EFFECT NEGATIVE REGULATION OF CARTILAGE GROWTH

Previous studies by others had suggested that three factors, RA, FGF-2, or TGF-β1, could effect negative regulation of cartilage growth in intact limbs (refs. *23,26,30,36*; *see also* Introduction of this

Table 1
Analysis of the Number of Hypertrophic Chondrocytes

Medium	*Tibiotarsi*	*No. of cells in hypertrophic zone*	*Difference in no. of cells*
Control serum-free	Intact	7264	1084
	PC/PO free	8348	
Conditioned medium	Intact	7239	14
(mixed PC and PO)	PC/PO free	7253	

Table 2
Analysis of Hypertrophic Extracellular Matrix Area

Medium	*Tibiotarsi*	*% Area as ECM in hypertrophic region*	*% Increase in cell numbers*
Control serum-free	Intact	73.7	12.9
	PC/PO free	56.6	
Conditioned medium	Intact	44.1	0.02
(mixed PC and PO)	PC/PO free	44.5	

chapter). To determine whether negative regulation by any of these factors was consistent with that observed with the PC/PO-conditioned medium (i.e., whether any of them might be the negative regulator in the conditioned medium), we examined their effects when added to intact organ cultures versus PC/PO-free cultures. Using this method, the conclusions drawn from each experiment depended on whether the factor being tested showed negative regulation, and, if so, whether this regulation was observed in the PC/PO-free cultures, the intact cultures, or both. The conclusions also depend on whether the negative regulation is precise in that it compensates exactly for removal of the PC and PO, or whether the negative regulation overcompensates.

Overcompensation would be suggested if either of two results was observed. One would be a decrease in the PC/PO-free cultures of greater than 0.3 mm, which is the maximum negative regulation effected by the PC/PO-conditioned medium. The other would be any decrease at all in the intact cultures, as no concentration of PC/PO-conditioned medium we have been able to produce *(31)* had any detectible effect on the these cultures, most likely because of the endogenous PC and PO of the intact tibiotarsus producing the maximum negative regulation capable by this inherent mechanism.

Therefore, any factor that is a candidate for the PC/PO regulatory mechanism should effect precise compensation when added to the PC/PO-free cultures. Also, it should not produce overcompensation of negative growth. Overcompensation, if observed, would suggest that this factor, per se, was not responsible for the regulation observed with PC/PO-conditioned medium or, if it was involved, other factors and/or modulators would also be required to effect the precise regulation seen with the PC/PO-conditioned medium.

The results (presented next) showed that none of the three factors tested, FGF-2, RA, or TGF-β1, acted in a manner consistent with the PC/PO-conditioned medium. However, of potential importance, two of the factors (RA or TGF-β1), when added to cell cultures of PC cells, induced the PC cells to produce a factor(s) (detected in their conditioned medium) which, when added to the PC/PO-free organ cultures, effected precise negative regulation of growth *(32)*. Therefore, it seems that multiple mechanisms exist through which the perichondrium can affect precise growth control (later discussed in more detail; *see* RA and TGF-β1 sections).

FGF-2

FGF-2 produced negative regulation, which is consistent with previous studies on this factor (*see* Introduction). However, this occurred in both the intact cultures (Fig. 9A, PC/PO-intact) and the PC/PO-free ones (Fig, 9A,B, PC/PO-free) and the decrease in length was virtually identical for each (Fig. 9B). Thus, it worked directly on the cartilage, and, as far as we can tell, not at all through the PC or PO. The fact that FGF-2 negatively regulates cartilage growth of the intact cultures, whereas the PC/PO-conditioned medium does not, indicates that this molecule is not the factor active in the conditioned medium.

Even though these results eliminate FGF-2 as the component responsible for the negative regulation detected in the PC/PO-conditioned medium, they do show that this factor can function as a regulator, possibly serving in the role of an alternative, or redundant, mechanism . Therefore, we further investigated the action of this factor to determine whether its negative effect on cartilage growth was caused by a change in chondrocyte proliferation, hypertrophy, or both. The results of this analysis showed that both of these parameters are affected and that this occurred in both the PC/PO-intact and PC/PO-free cultures. It can be seen that the region of chondrocyte hypertrophy was reduced in FGF-2-treated cultures, as determined by immunohistochemistry for type X collagen (Fig. 9D). In addition, FGF-2 treatment resulted in almost a complete block of proliferation, as analyzed by BrdU incorporation (Fig. 9C). PC/PO-conditioned medium treatment, however, resulted in a decrease in proliferation of PC/PO-free cultures but did not abolish it as seen with FGF-2. Therefore, this factor is not that of the PC/PO conditioned medium.

RA

RA also produced negative regulation in both the PC/PO-free cultures and the intact cultures *(32)*. However, unlike the FGF-2, the reduction in cartilage length with RA was even greater for the intact cultures than for the PC/PO-free ones, suggesting multiple mechanisms of action for this factor.

In the PC/PO-free cultures, the cartilage length was reduced, showing that one action in the negative regulation by RA is directly on the cartilage. In the intact cultures, RA also produced a reduction in cartilage length, and this reduction was even greater than in the PC/PO-free cultures. This effect of RA on the intact cultures again represents an overcompensation of negative regulation, which, as described above, is not observed with the PC/PO-conditioned medium. Also, because the negative regulation in the intact cultures is greater than that observed in the PC/PO-free cultures, RA must have another mechanism of action in addition to its direct action on cartilage. Most likely this mechanism involves the PC and/or the PO. Both of these observations eliminate RA as the component in the PC/PO-conditioned medium.

At the cell and tissue levels, the most obvious effect of RA was a reduction in cellular proliferation, which was more pronounced in the intact cultures than in the PC/PO-free ones. The length of the hypertrophic zone, however, showed no difference between the RA-treated and the untreated cultures, and this was observed for both the intact cultures and the PC/PO-free ones. These results for RA differ from those of the PC/PO-conditioned medium, which acts both on proliferation and on hypertrophy.

The observation that the effect of RA on proliferation was more pronounced in the intact cultures than the PC/PO-free ones suggested that the negative regulation by RA, in addition to affecting the cartilage directly, is also mediated by a second mechanism, most likely involving the PC and/or the PO. One possibility we considered for this additional regulation was an additive effect of RA plus any endogenous negative regulatory factor(s) that might be inherently produced by the PC and the PO. However, experiments in which RA was added to various conditioned media suggested that this was not likely correct.

Alternatively, RA could act on the PC and/or the PO, altering the production of regulatory factors by these tissues, or possibly inducing the production of additional types of regulatory factors by these tissues. To test this possibility, PC and PO cell cultures were treated with RA and the conditioned medium

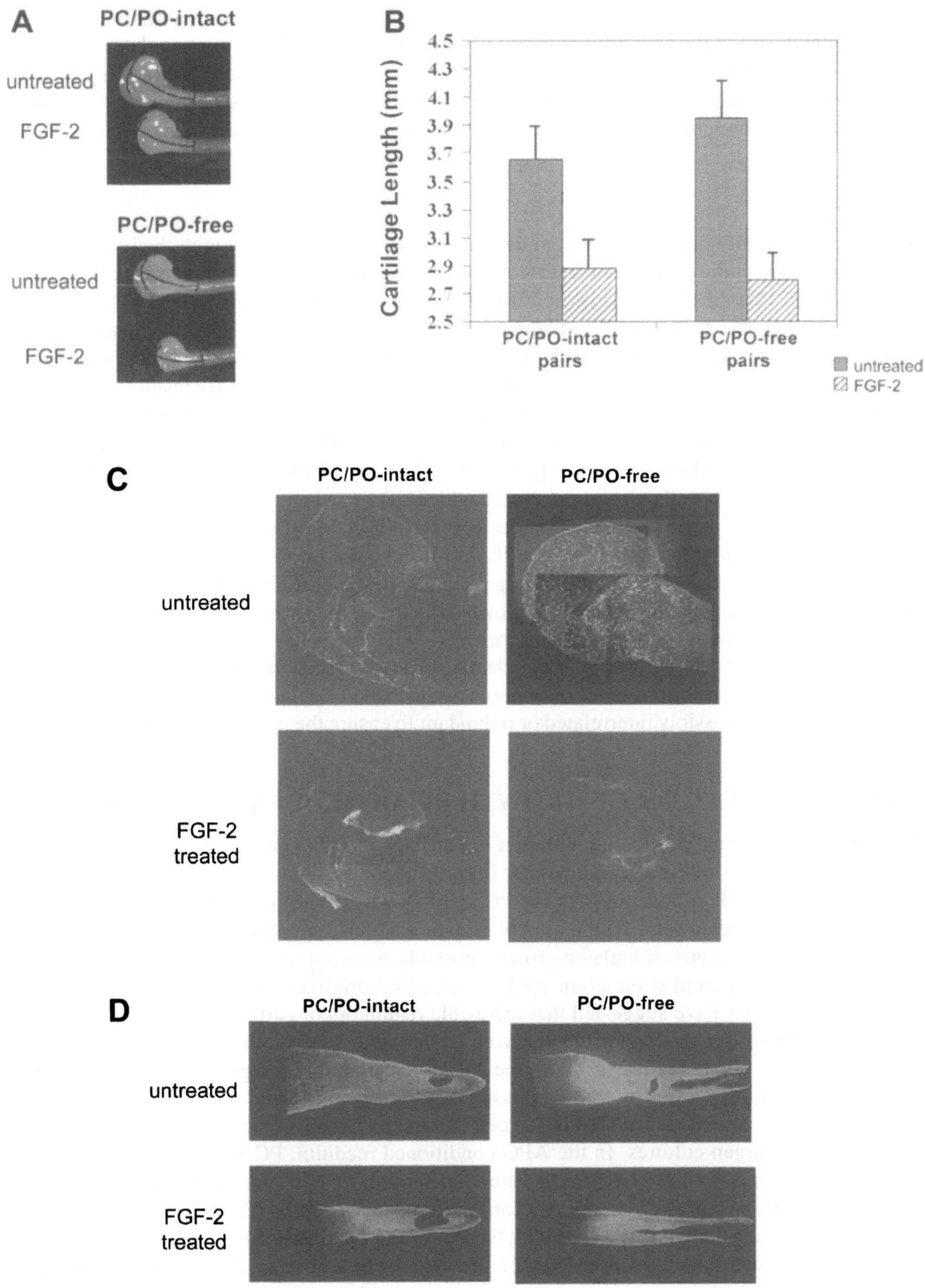

Fig. 9. A, Pairs of organ cultures consisting of two intact cultures or two PC/PO-free cultures, in which one member of each pair was treated with FGF-2. **B**, Bar graph showing the average cartilage length for the pairs of cultures shown in (A). **C**, BrdU incorporation in the zone of proliferation of cultures shown in (A). **D**, Type X collagen staining in the zone of hypertrophy of cultures shown in (A).

subsequently produced (after RA removal) was tested on the PC/PO-free organ cultures. This conditioned medium from the PC cells (but not the PO cells) now effected negative regulation that compensated precisely for the removal of the PC and PO. These data, when taken together, suggests that RA has at least two possible mechanisms of regulating cartilage growth, one by acting directly on the cartilage and another by acting indirectly through the PC. The PC in turn, produces and secretes factors that negatively regulate cartilage growth in a precise manner (*see* ref. *32*).

TGF-β1

TGF-β1 was the only factor that showed negative regulation exclusively with the intact cultures, with the PC/PO-free cultures showing no effect from the treatment *(32)*. This suggests that the action of TGF-β is on the PC or the PO, and also confirms a previous study using mouse metatarsal bones *(36)*. At the cellular level, this reduction in cartilage length results from decreases in both chondrocyte proliferation and hypertrophy (shown by BrdU incorporation and type X collagen staining, respectively).

As just described for RA, at least two possible mechanisms could explain these results with TGF-β1. As we found from experiments similar to those used for RA, the most likely explanation for TGF-β1 is that it acts on the PC, inducing the production of a new regulator(s), and that it is these regulators from the PC that act on the cartilage to regulate growth. Similar to results with RA, we observed that conditioned medium from PC cell cultures pretreated with TGF-β1, when added to PC/PO-free cultures, precisely compensated for the removal of the endogenous PC and PO, which resulted in almost identical cartilage lengths for both PC/PO-free and PC/PO-intact cultures. This suggests that TGF-β1, like RA, acts to regulate cartilage growth by eliciting a secondary signal from the PC (*see* ref. *32*).

Overall, the precise regulation of cartilage growth effected by the action of the perichondrial derived factor(s) elicited from perichondrial cells by treatment with either RA or TGF-β1, when combined with our previous results showing similar yet clearly different precise regulation by the PC/PO-conditioned medium, suggests the existence of multiple mechanisms of negative growth regulation involving the perichondrium possibly interrelated or redundant to ensure the proper growth of endochondral skeletal elements.

POSITIVE REGULATION OF GROWTH BY ARTICULAR PERICHONDRIUM

Last, we also examined positive stimulation of cartilage growth and obtained results suggesting that this does occur in a multifactorial manner *(31)*. As mentioned earlier, we observed that conditioned medium from cell cultures of both the PC and PO, when examined separately in the PC/PO-free organ cultures, effected some stimulation of growth. Likewise conditioned medium from cultures of hypertrophic chondrocytes stimulated growth, possibly in an autocrine manner.

However, the most potent stimulation we have observed originates from the articular perichondrium. Previous studies have suggested that diffusible regulators of cartilage, PTHrP *(8)* and Wnt4 *(37)*, are produced by the perichondrium covering the articular surface, the articular perichondrium (APC, shown in Fig. 10A). The proximity of the APC to the underlying region of proliferating chondrocytes also raised the possibility that this tissue is a source of positive regulation. Therefore, we examined the effect of conditioned medium of cell cultures derived from the articular perichondrium on the PC/PO-free organ cultures. In the APC-conditioned medium, PC/PO-free tibiotarsi showed extended growth that was almost two-fold greater than those grown in control medium, thus suggesting a role for the APC in positive regulation of cartilage growth (Fig. 10B). This is approximately three-fold greater stimulation than that observed with the PC- or PO-conditioned medium alone and approximately twofold greater than that observed with the hypertrophic chondrocyte conditioned medium.

CONCLUSIONS

Our work on the regulatory roles of the PC and PO suggests that multiple secreted factors are released from these tissues and are required for the precise regulation of cartilage growth This precise regula-

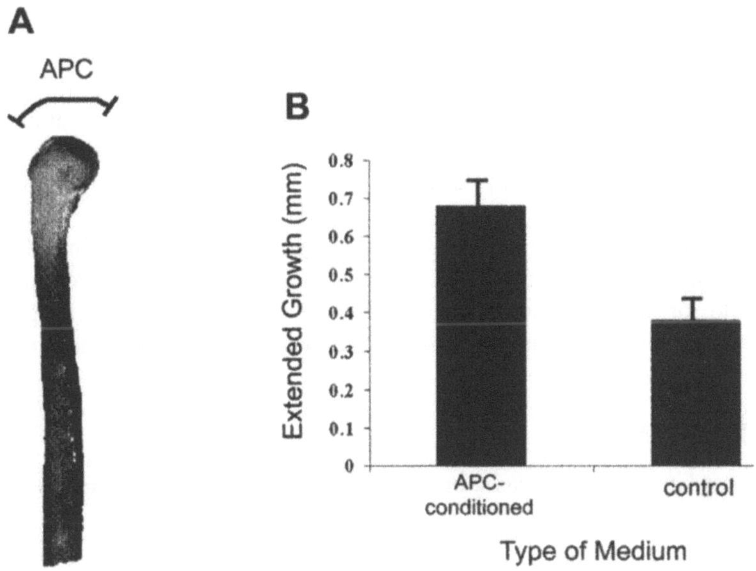

Fig. 10. A, Depiction of the region of the tibiotarsus used for cultures of articular perichondrium (APC cells). **B**, Bar graphs showing extended growth in control medium and APC-conditioned medium. Modified from Di Nino et al. *(31)*.

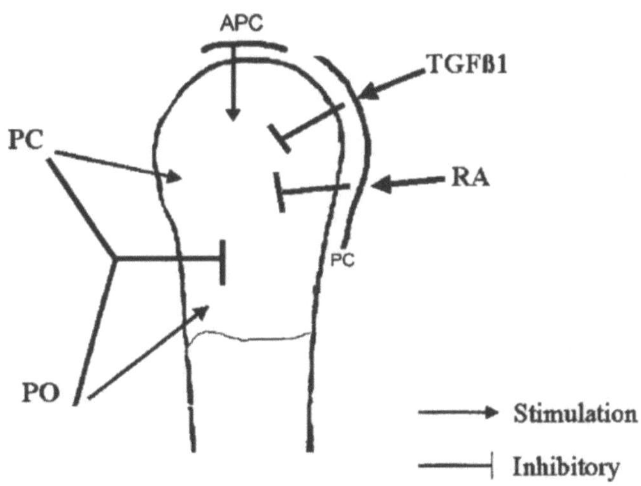

Fig. 11. A schematic diagram showing positive and negative regulation of cartilage growth by the perichondrium (PC), the periosteum (PO), and the articular perichondrium (APC). As shown on the left hand side of the figure, the PC and PO themselves each independently stimulate growth, as does the APC (shown at the top). However, when the PC and PO act together they effect precise negative regulation. As shown on the right, both TGF-β1 and RA act on the perichondrium, to induce this tissue to produce a factor (or factors) that also effect precise negative regulation. It seems likely that these different forms of negative regulation of growth predominate over the positive stimulation; however, this remains to be tested experimentally.

tion appears to involve both positive and negative factors that are secreted from the PC and PO (as shown schematically in Fig. 11). Stimulation of cartilage growth was observed when using conditioned medium from either PC or PO, and especially from the articular perichondrium. The factors contained in these types of medium caused an increase in the overall length of PC/PO-free cartilage, suggesting that they are effecting the positive regulation of cartilage growth. We observed multiple mechanisms of negative regulation of cartilage growth. The first and most novel involves cooperative action of factors that are independently secreted by the PC and PO. When PC/PO-free organ cultures are grown in the presence of both PC and PO conditioned medium, the result is complete compensation for PC/PO removal. These organ cultures grow to the same extent as their intact contralateral limbs. Additional negative regulatory roles for the PC were observed in response to RA and TGF-β1. When PC cells were exposed to either RA or TGF-β1, the conditioned media from these treated cells also resulted in the precise regulation of cartilage growth. The PC/PO-free cultures grown in these types of medium grew to similar lengths as their intact contralateral limbs. This suggests that RA and TGF-β1 elicit the production of a secondary signal from the PC. Taken together, this work illustrates three roles of the PC in negative regulation of cartilage growth. These multiple mechanisms may serve to provide redundancy in regulating cartilage growth to ensure proper formation of long bones.

ACKNOWLEDGMENTS

The work presented in this article was supported by National Institutes of Health Grant HD233681.

REFERENCES

1. Schmid, T. M. and Linsenmayer, T. F. (1985) Developmental acquisition of type X collagen in the embryonic chick tibiotarsus. *Dev. Biol.* **107,** 373–381.
2. Long, F. X. and Linsenmayer, T. F. (1998) Regulation of growth region cartilage proliferation and differentiation by perichondrium. *Development* **125,** 1067–1073.
3. Chen, Q., Gibney, E., Leach, R. M., and Linsenmayer, T. F. (1993) Chicken tibial dyschondroplasia: a limb mutant with two growth plates and possible defects in cartilage crosslinking. *Dev. Dyn.* **196,** 54–61.
4. Howlett, C. R. (1979) The fine structure of the proximal growth plate of the avian tibia. *J. Anat.* **128,** 377–399.
5. Nurminskaya, M., Magee, C., Nurminsky, D., and Linsenmayer, T. F. (1998) Plasma transglutaminase in hypertrophic chondrocytes: Expression and cell-specific intracellular activation produce cell death and externalization. *J. Cell Biol.* **142,** 1135–1144.
6. Bianco, P., Cancedda, F. D., Riminucci, M., and Cancedda, R. (1998) Bone formation via cartilage models: the "borderline" chondrocyte. *Matrix Biol.* **17,** 185–192.
7. Pathi, S., Rutenberg, J. B., Johnson, R. L., and Vortkamp, A. (1999) Interaction of Ihh and BMP Noggin signaling during cartilage differentiation. *Dev. Biol.* **209,** 239–253.
8. Vortkamp, A., Lee, K., Lanske, B., Segre, G. V., Kronenberg, H. M., and Tabin, C. J. (1996) Regulation of rate of cartilage differentiation by Indian hedgehog and PTH-related protein. *Science* **273,** 613–622.
9. Deng, C., Wynshaw-Boris, A., Zhou, F., Kuo, A., and Leder, P. (1996) Fibroblast growth factor receptor 3 is a negative regulator of bone growth. *Cell* **84,** 911–921.
10. Lanske, B., Karaplis, A. C., Lee, K., Luz, A., Vortkamp, A., Pirro, A., et al. (1996) PTH/PTHrP receptor in early development and Indian hedgehog- regulated bone growth. *Science* **273,** 663–666.
11. Marigo, V., Davey, R. A., Zuo, Y., Cunningham, J. M., and Tabin C. J. (1996) Biochemical evidence that patched is the Hedgehog receptor. *Nature* **384,** 176–179.
12. Karp, S. J., Schipani, E., St-Jaques, B., Hunzelman, J., Kronenberg, H., and McMahon, A. P. (2000) Indian hedgehog coordinates endochondral bone growth and morphogenesis via parathyroid hormone related-protein-dependent and -independent pathways. *Development* **127,** 543–548.
13. St-Jacques, B., Hammerschmidt, M., and McMahon, A. P. (1999) Indian hedgehog signaling regulates proliferation and differentiation of chondrocytes and is essential for bone formation. *Genes Dev.* **13,** 2072–2086.
14. Hunziker, E. H., Kapfinger, E., and Saager, C. (1999) Hypertrophy of growth plate chondrocytes in vivo is accompanied by modulations in the activity state and surface area of their cytoplasmic organelles. *Histochem. Cell Biol.* **112,** 115–123.
15. Kingsley, D. M. (1994) The TGF-beta superfamily: new members, new receptors and new genetic test of function in different organisms. *Genes Dev.* **8,** 133–146.
16. Wang, E. A., Rose, V., Cordes, P., Hewick, R. M., Kriz, M. J., Luxenberg, D. P., et al. (1988) Purification and characterization of other distinct bone-inducing factors. *Proc. Natl. Acad. Sci. USA* **85,** 9484–9488.
17. Bitgood, M. J. and McMahon, A. P. (1995) Hedgehog and Bmp genes are coexpresed at many diverse sites of cell-cell interaction in the mouse embryo. *Dev. Biol.* **172,** 126–138.
18. Macias, D., Ganan, Y., Sampath, T. K., Piedra, M. E., Ros, M. A., and Hurle, J. M. (1997) Role of BMP-2 and OP-1 (BMP-7) in programmed cell death and skeletogenesis during chick limb development. *Development* **124,** 1109–1117.
19. Zou, H., Wieser, R., Massague, J., and Niswander, L. (1997) Distinct roles of type I bone morphogenetic protein receptors in the formation and differentiation of cartilage. *Genes Dev.* **11,** 2191–2203.

20. Segev, O., Chumakov, I., Nevo, Z., Givol, D., Madar-Shapiro, L., Sheinin, U., et al. (2000) Restrained chondrocyte proliferation and maturation with abnormal growth plate vascularization and ossification in human FGFR-3^{G390R} transgenic mice. *Human Mol. Genet.* **9,** 249–258.
21. Shiang, R., Thompson, L. M., Zhu, Y. Z., Church, D. M., Fielder, T. J., Bocian, M., et al. (1994) Mutations in the transmembrane domain of FGFR3 cause the most common genetic form of dwarfism, achondroplasia. *Cell* **78,** 335–342.
22. Green, P. J., Walsh, F. S., and Doherty, P. (1996) Promiscuity of fibroblast growth factor receptors. *BioEssays* **18,** 639–646.
23. Mancilla, E. E., De Luca, F., Uyeda, J. A., Czerwiec, F. S., and Baron, J. (1998) Effects of fibroblast growth factor-2 on longitudinal bone growth. *Endocrinology* **139,** 2900–2904.
24. Pelton, R. W., Hogan, B. L., Miller, D. A., and Moses, H. L. (1990) Differential expression of genes encoding TGFs beta 1, beta 2, and beta 3 during murine palate formation. *Dev. Biol.* **141,** 456–460.
25. Serra, R., Johnson, M., Filvaroff, E. H., LaBorder, J., Sheehan, D. M., Derynck, R., et al. (1997) Expression of a truncated, kinase-defective TGF-β type II receptor in mouse skeletal tissue promotes terminal chondrocyte differentiation and osteoarthritis. *J. Cell Biol.* **139,** 541–552.
26. Serra, R., Karaplis, A., and Sohn, P. (1999) Parathyroid hormone-related peptide (PTHrP)-dependent and -independent effects of transforming growth factor β (TGF-β) on endochondral bone formation. *J. Cell Biol.* **145,** 783–794.
27. Howell, J. and Thompson, J. (1967) Observations on the lesions in vitamin A deficient adult fowls with particular reference to changes in bone and central nervous system. *Br. J. Exp. Pathol.* **48,** 450–454.
28. Koyama, E., Golden, E. B., Kirsch, T., Adams, S. L., Chandraratna, R. A. S., Michaille, J. J., et al. (1999) Retinoid signaling is required for chondrocyte maturation and endochondral bone formation during limb skeletogenesis. *Dev. Biol.* **208,** 375–391.
29. Smith, S. M., Kirstein, I. J., Wang, Z. S., Fallon, J. F., Kelley, J., and Bradshaw-Rouse, J. (1995) Differential expression of retinoic acid receptor-beta isoforms during chick limb ontogeny. *Dev. Dyn.* **202,** 54–66.
30. De Luca, F., Uyeda, J. A., Mericq, V., Mancilla, E. E., Yanovski, J. A., Barnes, K. M., et al. (2000) Retinoic acid is a potent regulator of growth plate chondrogenesis. *Endocrinology* **141,** 346–353.
31. Di Nino, D. L., Long, F., and Linsenmayer, T. F. (2001) Regulation of Edochondral Cartilage growth in the developing avian limb: cooperative involvement of perichondrium and periosteum. *Dev. Biol.* **240,** 433–442.
32. Di Nino, D. L., Crochiere, M. L., and Linsenmayer, T. F. (2002) Multiple mechanisms of perichondrial regulation of cartilage growth. *Dev. Dyn.* **225,** 250–259.
33. Lovitch, D. and Christianson, M. L. (1997) Mineralization is more reliable in periosteum explants from size-selected chicken embryos (letter). *In Vitro Cell. Dev. Biol. Animal* **33,** 234–235.
34. Wolpert, L. (1969) Positional information and the spatial pattern of cellular differentiation. *J. Theor. Biol.* **25,** 1–47.
35. Stocum, D. L., Davis, R. M., Leger, M., and Conrad, H. E. (1979) Development of the tibiotarsus in the chick embryo: biosynthetic activities of histologically distinct regions. *J. Embryol. Exp. Morphol.* **54,** 155–170.
36. Alvarez, J., Horton, J., Sohn, P., and Serra, R. (2001) The perichondrium plays an important role in mediating the effects of TGF-β1 on endochondral bone formation. *Dev. Dyn.* **221,** 311–321.
37. Hartmann, C. and Tabin, C. J. (2000) Dual roles of Wnt signaling during chondrogenesis in the chicken limb. *Development* **127,** 3141–3159.

17

Computer Simulations of Cancellous Bone Remodeling

Jacqueline C. van der Linden, Harrie Weinans, and Jan A. N. Verhaar

BONE REMODELING

The bone remodeling process is essential for the maintenance of our skeleton. It enables adaptation of the bone mass and architecture to changes in external loads *(1,2)*, and it prevents accumulation of damage *(3,4)*. Damage accumulation is prevented by a frequent turnover of the bone tissue by the bone remodeling process: old tissue is replaced by new tissue. Bone remodeling is performed by two types of cells: osteoclasts, which are multinucleated bone resorbing cells, and osteoblasts, which are bone-forming cells. Osteoclasts resorb packets of bone tissue, and osteoblasts replace the resorbed tissue with new mineralized bone tissue (*see* Fig. 1).

In the cortex, the outer shell of the bones, the bone-resorbing cells dig tunnels in the longitudinal direction, which are refilled with new bone tissue. The ends of the long bones are filled with cancellous bone, a very porous bone structure made of mineralized plates and struts, the trabeculae. This cancellous bone gives the bones a relatively low mass and a high stiffness. Cancellous bone is also found in the spine, in flat bones like the skull and the pelvis and in the hand and feet. In the cancellous bone, remodeling takes place at the surface of the trabeculae (*see* Fig. 1).

It is not exactly known how bone remodeling is regulated, but several hypotheses exist. Bone remodeling could be distributed randomly throughout the bone tissue, it could be targeted to repair damage, or it could be regulated by stresses or strains according to the mechanostat theory. These possibilities do not exclude each other; in vivo bone remodeling is probably a combination of these three types of bone remodeling. Numerous studies have investigated the reaction of bone cells to mechanical loading, changes in cancellous architecture with age, and the effects of damage in bone tissue *(4–6)*.

A healthy skeleton can withstand forces higher than the forces that act on the skeleton during normal daily loading *(7)*. However, even the normal daily loads cause some damage in the bone tissue *(8,9)*. This microdamage consists of small cracks in the bone tissue, which are far too small to cause failure of a whole bone or even a single trabecula. To prevent these cracks from growing and coalescing into bigger cracks, the damaged tissue must be replaced by new tissue.

It is possible that bone remodeling is targeted to repair microdamage, but damage could also be repaired just because most bone tissue is replaced by random remodeling. Several authors have tried to estimate the contribution of damage-targeted remodeling to the total bone turnover, with the estimated values varying widely from 30 to 100% *(10,11)*. In cancellous bone, no estimates of targeted and nontargeted remodeling exist. However, because of the high turnover rate of cancellous bone, it is likely that the rate of cancellous bone turnover is higher than needed for damage repair *(12)*.

From: *The Skeleton: Biochemical, Genetic, and Molecular Interactions in Development and Homeostasis*
Edited by: E. J. Massaro and J. M. Rogers © Humana Press Inc., Totowa, NJ

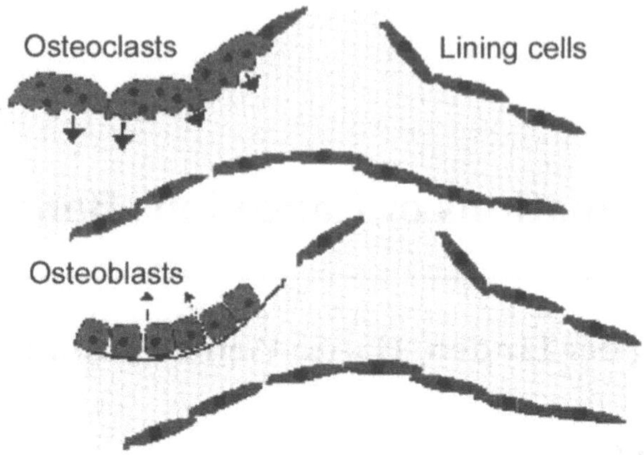

Fig. 1. Schematic representation of bone resorption by osteoclasts and bone formation by osteoblasts in cancellous bone.

The bone remodeling process also has negative effects on the skeleton: with aging, bone mass decreases slowly. This decrease is caused by the formation deficit: during remodeling, the amount of newly formed bone is slightly smaller than the amount of resorbed bone *(13)*. As a result of this, the porosity of the cortex increases, trabeculae become thinner, and plates in the cancellous bone are perforated. In addition, more bone may be lost because trabeculae that are breached by resorption cavities are probably not repaired *(14,15)*. This leads to loss of bone mass, strength, and stiffness and increases in fracture risk. In extreme cases, bone mass decreases rapidly and the skeleton becomes osteoporotic. Particularly because of these negative effects, a lot of research has been aimed to describe these mechanisms and to understand the bone loss with age.

Microcomputed tomography (CT) scanners have been used frequently to investigate the cancellous bone architecture and bone mass in young and old, healthy and diseased bone. These scanners make X-ray projection images of bone specimens from different directions. From these projection images, the three-dimensional architecture is calculated. In these studies the cancellous architecture and changes in this architecture with age have been investigated *(16–19)*. This technique gives detailed information about the cancellous architecture at a certain timepoint, although it does not give information on how the bone remodeling process changes the architecture. Using fluorochrome-labeling techniques, remodeling parameters, such as resorption, resting, and refill period, have been determined *(20)*. These labeling studies yield information about bone-remodeling parameters but not about the three-dimensional architecture of the cancellous bone. Examples of breached trabeculae and perforated plates have been shown in scanning electron microscopy studies of trabecular bone specimens, in which the three dimensional trabecular architecture is visualized *(15,21)*.

From these studies, it is known that bone is lost because of the formation deficit and breached trabeculae. However, the contributions of these mechanisms to the total bone loss are not known yet. The relation between the remodeling parameters and the changes in architecture and mechanical properties is unclear. Moreover, it is not known what is more important in preventing or reducing bone loss using antiresorptive treatment, such as bisphosphonates or selective estrogen receptor modulators (SERMs): reducing resorption depth or reducing the formation deficit. A large formation deficit leads to fast thinning of trabeculae, and a large resorption depth increases the chance of breaching of trabeculae. The changes in architecture and the subsequent changes in mechanical properties depend on a combination of parameters and cannot be predicted easily.

COMPUTER SIMULATIONS

Several studies have used computer models to gain more insight in the relation between bone remodeling and changes in the skeleton with age, during menopause, or in osteoporosis. The first models of cancellous bone treated the cancellous bone as a number of bone packages *(22)* or used trabeculae with a certain thickness distribution derived from published histomorphometric data *(23)*. In these models, the trabeculae were not connected to form a cancellous architecture.

Later models used two-dimensional networks to simulate the trabecular architecture. In these studies, trabeculae were removed or thinned to investigate the effect of aging and bone loss on strength and stiffness of the architecture *(24,25)*. The effects of thinning of trabeculae have also been investigated three dimensionally *(26)*. Both two-dimensional and three-dimensional studies found that loss of trabeculae has more drastic effects on the mechanical properties of cancellous bone than thinning of trabeculae.

In reality, the bone architecture changes during the remodeling cycle because of over- or underfilling of resorption cavities. If a resorption cavity breaches a trabecula, this trabecula is probably not repaired *(15)*. This last effect is ignored in simulations that mimic aging in cancellous bone by gradually thinning trabeculae.

For a close examination of the effects of bone remodeling on cancellous bone architecture and stiffness, models that simulate the whole remodeling cycle are needed. In these models, creation and refilling of resorption cavities should be mimicked in three dimensional cancellous bone models. Currently, two studies that simulate the bone remodeling cycle in cancellous bone in three dimensions are described in literature.

The first study used an artificial bar-plate model to simulate the cancellous bone *(27)*. In this model, resorption cavities were created in the middle of the bars that simulated the trabeculae. Using this model, the authors determined contributions of the formation deficit and breached trabeculae to the total bone loss. They found that breached trabeculae accounted for 20 to 40 % of the total bone loss, depending on remodeling rate.

We introduced another approach using detailed computer reconstructions made by micro-CT *(28)*. These micro-CT models have a resolution high enough to represent the individual trabeculae in the model. In this simulation model, bone resorption could be initiated everywhere on the surface of the trabeculae, mimicking in vivo bone remodeling. For the bone remodeling parameters such as resorption depth and formation deficit, values determined in bone histology studies were used. This second model is described in detail in this chapter.

These simulation models can be used to determine the contributions of the formation deficit, breached trabeculae, and loose fragments to the total bone loss. Changes in morphology caused by remodeling can be investigated and the effects of changes in remodeling parameters, for example, a larger resorption depth, on the architecture can be examined. The effects of these changes in architecture on the mechanical properties of the specimens can be determined.

SIMULATION OF BONE REMODELING IN HUMAN CANCELLOUS BONE

A computer model was developed by using micro-CT scans to simulate the bone remodeling cycle in models of human cancellous vertebral bone (*see* Fig. 2). In this model, bone formation was coupled to previous resorption.

To enable a simulation of months or years of bone remodeling within a reasonable amount of computing time, we must simplify the bone remodeling cycle. In reality, bone resorption as well as formation take a number of weeks. This gradual resorption and formation of bone tissue was discretized in the model: resorption cavities were made completely at a certain time point and refilled completely a later time point (a number of simulation cycles later).

Changes in architecture are caused by either the formation deficit or by the breaching of a trabecula by a resorption cavity during the remodeling cycle. Whether a trabecula is breached by a resorption

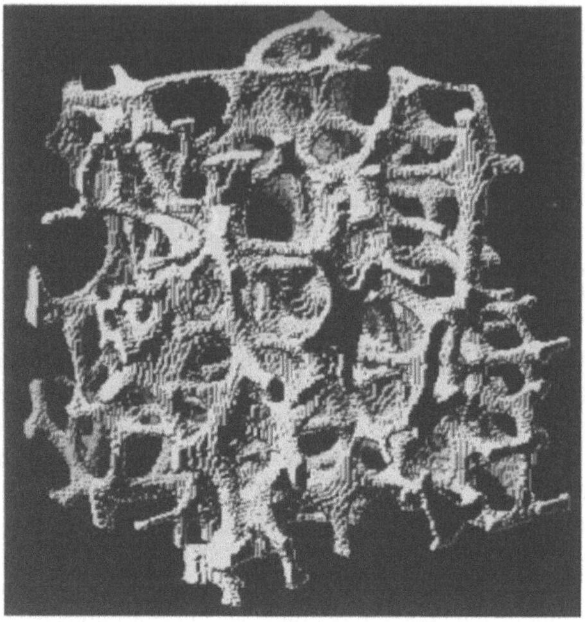

Fig. 2. Three-dimensional computer model of a cancellous bone specimen made by using a micro-CT scanner.

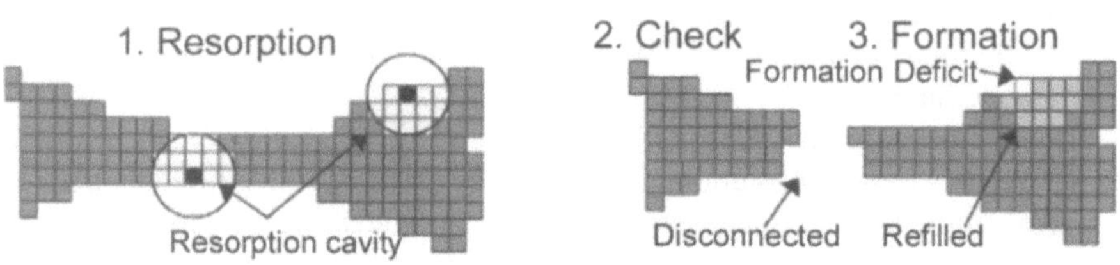

Fig. 3. Schematic representation in two dimensions of the simulation model of bone remodeling in cancellous bone in three dimensions. Reproduced from *J. Bone Miner. Res.* 2001;16:688–696, with permission of the American Society for Bone and Mineral Research.

cavity or not is only determined by the thickness of the trabecula and the maximal depth of the cavity. The bone loss resulting from the formation deficit is also independent of the duration of the resorption and formation period. Therefore, the discretization of the bone remodeling process in the simulation model does not affect the long-term effects of bone remodeling on the cancellous architecture.

The remodeling process was simulated in three steps: resorption of bone tissue to make resorption cavities, a resting period, and finally bone formation in the resorption cavities. The three steps in the bone remodeling model are illustrated in Fig. 3. In the first step, hemispherical resorption cavities were created, starting from elements in the surface of the trabeculae. These resorption cavities are distributed randomly over the surface of the trabeculae. The resorption depth of the cavities could be varied in the biologically relevant range.

In the second step, a check for breached trabeculae was performed. If a resorption cavity breached a trabecula, that cavity was not refilled; the trabecula was not repaired. This resulted in two remaining struts, which were connected to the main architecture, but not to each other anymore. If one of these remaining struts was breached again by a resorption cavity, this resulted in a loose fragment that was not connected to the main structure anymore. These loose fragments were removed from the model.

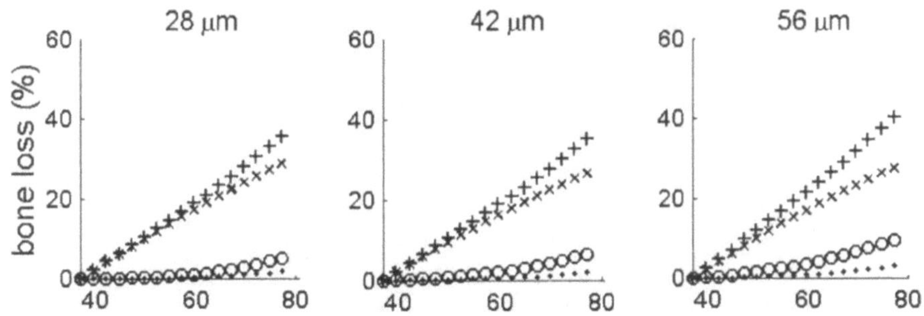

Fig. 4. Contributions of the bone loss mechanisms to this total bone loss, expressed as a percentage of the total bone volume, resulting from simulated remodeling with a resorption depth of 28, 42, or 56 μm. Total bone loss (+), formation deficit (x), breached trabeculae (open circles), and loose fragments (closed dots) are shown. Forty years of remodeling were simulated in a specimen from a 37-yr-old donor.

In the third step, all cavities that did not breach trabeculae were refilled. These cavities were not refilled completely to simulate the formation deficit. These three steps were repeated to simulate ongoing physiological remodeling. During each simulation cycle, new resorption cavities were created and old cavities were refilled.

In the simulation, each simulation cycle represented 1 mo in reality. In reality, new resorption cavities are made and old cavities are refilled each day. Instead of making a small number of resorption cavities each day in the simulation, a larger number of cavities was made each month.

Two more parameters could be chosen in the model: the remodeling space and the duration of the remodeling cycle. The duration of the remodeling cycle is the number of months between bone resorption and refilling of a cavity. The remodeling space is the percentage of the bone volume that is occupied by resorption cavities that still have to be refilled.

Simulations were performed in a number of computer models of human cancellous bone with varying resorption depth (28–56 mm) and formation deficit (2–5% of a cavity; ref. *28*). In these simulations, remodeling space and the duration of the remodeling cycle were kept constant. The duration of the remodeling cycle was assumed to be 3 mo, and the remodeling space was 4% of the bone volume in all simulations. This resulted in a turnover of 16% per year, which corresponds to values found in histological studies of human bone *(29)*. During the simulation, bone lost by the formation deficit, breached trabeculae, and loose fragments was determined each simulation cycle. The cancellous architecture was saved at specific time points to determine morphological and mechanical properties afterwards.

BONE LOSS

The formation deficit accounted for the major part of the bone loss in simulated age related remodeling. The contribution of breached trabeculae to the total bone loss increased with age, as the trabeculae became thinner and the probability of trabecula being breached by a resorption cavity increased. The contributions of breached trabeculae, formation deficit and loose fragments to the total bone loss are shown in Fig. 4.

According to this simulation model, the formation deficit accounted for 69–95% of the total bone loss, 1–21% of breached trabeculae, and 1–17% of loose fragments that were removed from the model *(28)*. The rate of bone loss varied between 0.3 and 1.1% per year, which is in the biologically relevant range *(30–32)*. The rate of bone loss increased with simulated age, as trabeculae became thinner and the chance of breached trabeculae increased.

The formation deficit had a larger influence on the rate of bone loss than the resorption depth. This was not unexpected because an increase in formation deficit results directly in more bone loss, whereas

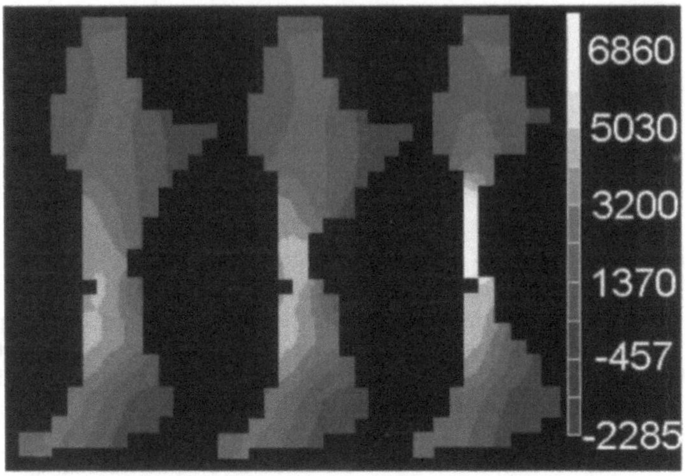

Fig. 5. Illustration of strain peaks below resorption cavities in cancellous bone. A resorption cavity was made in a trabecula aligned in the main load-bearing direction in a finite element model of a cancellous bone specimen. Resorption depth increases from 28 to 84 μm from left to right. The image shows the strain in the bone tissue, which increased with increasing resorption depth.

an increase in resorption depth has only indirect effects: trabeculae have a higher chance of being breached. As long as the resorption depth was much smaller than the trabecular thickness, the resorption depth had no effect on the rate of bone loss. An increase in resorption depth from 42 μm to 56 μm resulted in a 10% increase in the rate of bone loss. In preventing bone loss, restoring the balance between bone resorption and bone formation seems to be more important than reducing resorption depth.

However, deeper cavities resulted in a faster decrease of the stiffness of the cancellous architecture. This can be explained by the large strain peaks at the bottom of deep resorption cavities *(33)*. In Fig. 5, the strains in bone tissue below a resorption cavity are shown. These strains increase rapidly with increasing resorption depth. Although cavities of 56 μm resulted in only 10% faster bone loss than cavities of 42 μm, mechanical stiffness decreased 25 to 50% more. Decreasing the formation deficit helps to prevent bone loss, but reducing resorption depth is more effective in preventing loss of mechanical stiffness.

The rate of bone loss resulting from the bone remodeling process depends on the bone remodeling parameters. Some of these parameters can be determined directly from bone histology, but other parameters cannot be measured directly. Remodeling space, the formation deficit, and the duration of the remodeling cycle can only be estimated by derivation from other, measurable, parameters *(34, 35)*. On the one hand, this is a limitation for computer simulation models because estimated values must be used instead of directly measured values. On the other hand, this is exactly the power of this type of models: the estimated values can be incorporated in the simulation model, and by comparing the output of the model to changes observed in reality, it can be shown whether the parameter values were realistic. In this simulation model, we used biologically relevant values as input for the remodeling parameters and found rates of bone loss and changes in architecture similar to changes during life. This indicates that the remodeling parameters we used were in the biologically relevant range. The simulation model can be used to investigate the long-term effects of bone remodeling on cancellous bone. Effects of changes in e.g. resorption depth or formation deficit can be examined.

The strength and stiffness of cancellous bone depend on the three-dimensional architecture and the quality of the bone tissue. To describe the architecture of cancellous bone, a variety of parameters can be used. For example, trabecular thickness is a measure of the thickness of the rods and plates in the cancellous architecture, trabecular spacing of the distance between the trabeculae *(16)*.

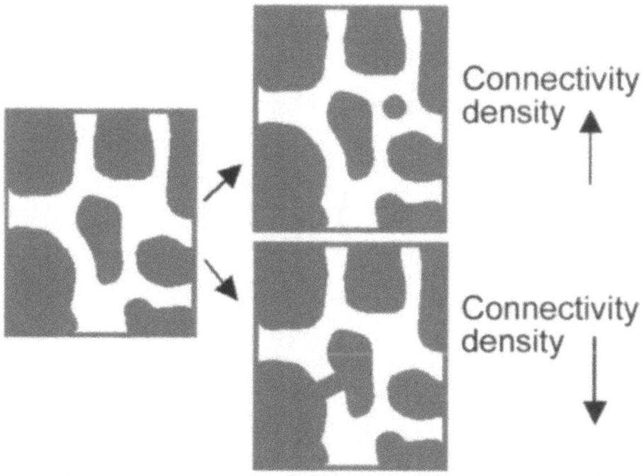

Fig. 6. Illustration of the possible effects of remodeling on cancellous bone architecture. Plates can be perforated, which increases connectivity density, and trabeculae can be breached, which decreases connectivity density.

The trabeculae in the cancellous bone form a multiply connected network: when a trabecula is cut through, the remaining struts are still connected to each other via other trabeculae. Connectivity density is used to determine how well connected the cancellous architecture is. Connectivity density can be determined by counting the number of trabeculae that can be cut through before the structure falls apart *(18)*.

The cancellous architecture has a preferred orientation: the architecture is aligned to the main in vivo load bearing direction *(2,36)*. The anisotropy of the architecture is a measure of the alignment of the architecture: the higher the anisotropy, the more aligned the cancellous architecture is. For example, the morphological anisotropy gives information over the distribution of the bone material: how much bone tissue is found in trabeculae in the main load bearing direction and how much in transversal directions (the transversal directions are perpendicular to the main load bearing direction). This morphological anisotropy can be determined in different ways *(17)*. The morphological alignment of cancellous bone is highly correlated to its mechanical alignment *(37)*.

CONNECTIVITY DENSITY

Bone remodeling can result in increases as well as in decreases in the connectivity density of cancellous bone. Trabeculae can be breached by resorption cavities, this decreases connectivity density. However, plates can be perforated by resorption cavities, which increases the connectivity density (*see* Fig. 6). These effects of remodeling both occur in vivo *(21)*. In vivo, the breaching of plates and the perforation of trabeculae results in a more or less constant connectivity density with age *(6)*.

Simulated remodeling resulted in increases or decreases in connectivity density, depending on resorption depth and formation deficit (*see* Fig. 7). The values for connectivity density in our simulation model were in the same range as in experimental studies using human trabecular bone specimens *(6,19)*. A small resorption depth resulted in gradual thinning of trabeculae, breaching of some thin trabeculae and a decrease in connectivity density. A large resorption depth resulted in perforation of plates and an increase in connectivity density.

Connectivity density alone cannot be used as an indicator of stiffness or strength of trabecular bone. However, it can give an indication of how much of the mechanical strength of trabecular bone can be regained after large amounts of bone have been lost *(38)*. If connectivity density is decreased as a result of bone loss, the number of trabeculae is decreased. If connectivity density is not decreased during bone loss, trabeculae will be thinner, but not breached. Loss of trabeculae is irreversible, while thin trabeculae can thicken again as a result of antiresorptive treatment or increased mechanical loads.

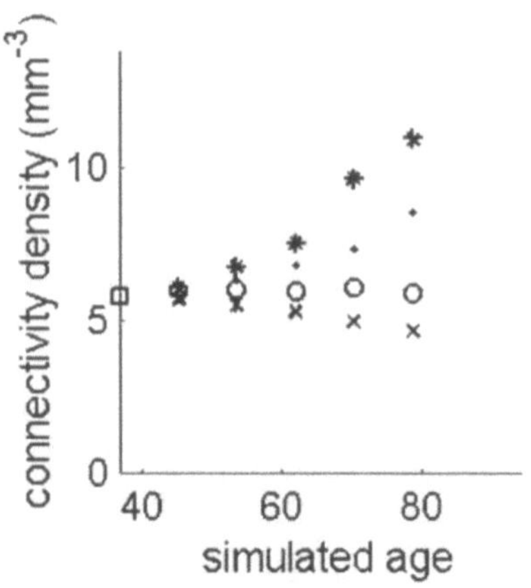

Fig. 7. Changes in connectivity density resulting from simulated remodeling. Small resorption depth and formation deficit resulted in a decrease of connectivity density, larger resorption depth, and/or formation deficit resulted in increased connectivity density (x, depth: 28 μm, formation deficit: 3.6% per cavity; open circles, 42 μm, 1.8%; closed diamond, 42 μm, 3.6%; asterisk, 42 μm, 5.4%).

MORPHOLOGICAL ANISOTROPY

The effect of the simulated bone remodeling on the morphological anisotropy was determined from the mean intercept length method, illustrated in Fig. 8. This method is described more extensively in the references *(17)*. The morphological anisotropy did not change much as a result of simulated remodeling, because the struts that remained as a trabecula was breached were not removed from the computer model.

MECHANICAL PROPERTIES

To fulfill its load bearing function, the strength and stiffness of the skeleton have to be high enough to withstand the forces applied to the bones in vivo. Because of this important function of the bone, the strength and stiffness of bone specimens have been determined in mechanical experiments in several studies. The stiffness of a material is a measure of its deformation under load and can be determined in a compression test. The stiffness is calculated as stress (force per unit of area) divided by strain (deformation in % of original size).

Alternatively, the stiffness of cancellous bone specimens can be determined by simulating mechanical tests in finite element computer models. By simulating six uniaxial strain tests, three compression and three shear tests *(39)*, the stiffness of the specimen can be calculated in all directions. The stiffness of a cancellous bone specimen is shown by the three-dimensional shape in Fig. 9. The stiffness in a certain direction is the distance from the origin of this shape to the surface in that direction, as illustrated by the white arrows in Fig. 9B.

The cancellous bone architecture is aligned to the external loads applied during normal daily loading. As a result of this, the stiffness will be maximal in the main in vivo load bearing direction. This can be seen in Fig. 9: the stiffness in the superior inferior direction is higher than the stiffness in transversal directions. From this information, the mechanical anisotropy of the cancellous bone can be determined: this is the maximum stiffness (in the main load bearing direction) divided by the minimal stiffness (in a transversal direction).

With aging, the stiffness and strength of cancellous bone both decrease. Because relatively more bone tissue is lost from transversal trabeculae, the anisotropy of the cancellous architecture increases with age *(6,40)*. The stiffness decreases in all directions, but more in the transversal directions than in the main load bearing direction. This results in a higher anisotropy: the cancellous bone architecture becomes more aligned with the main load bearing direction with increasing age.

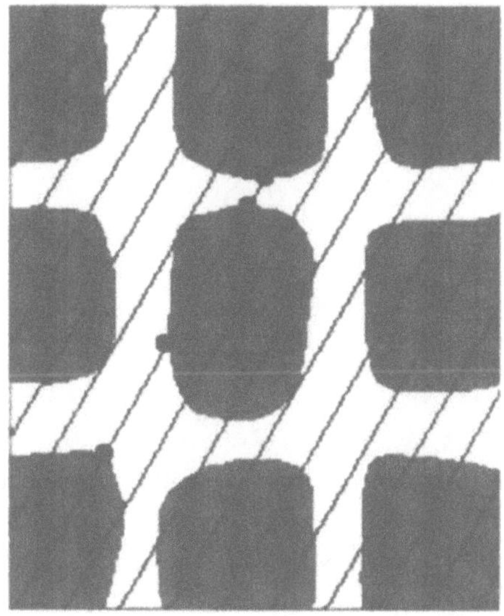

Fig. 8. Illustration of determination of morphological anisotropy using the mean intercept length (MIL) method. The number of bone marrow intercepts (black dots) is counted along each line, and the MIL is the total length of the lines divided by the number of intercepts. By rotating the grid, the mean intercept length can be determined in all directions.

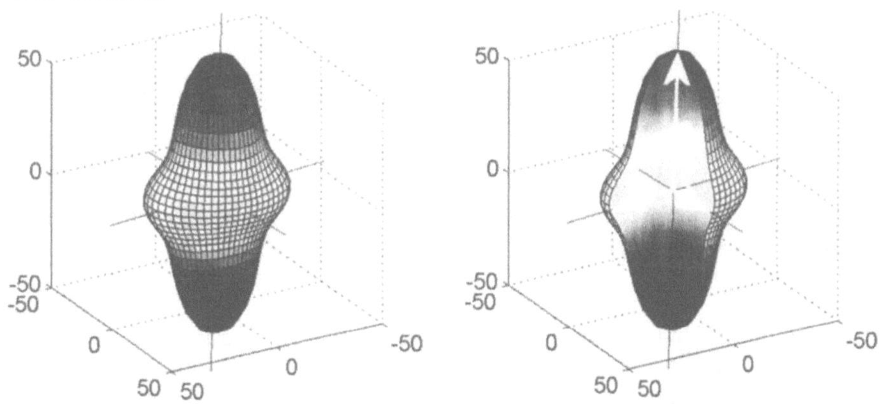

Fig. 9. Left panel, stiffness of a cancellous bone specimen, calculated in all directions. The stiffness in a certain direction is the distance from the origin to the surface, as shown by the white arrows (right panel). The main load-bearing direction (superior–inferior) corresponds to the top-down direction in the figure.

The changes in the cancellous bone architecture caused by simulated remodeling were similar to changes seen in vivo. Simulated remodeling resulted in decreases of the stiffness in all directions. Even though the remodeling sites in this simulation model are distributed randomly over the surface of the trabeculae, the anisotropy of the specimens increased. The decrease in stiffness was larger in transversal directions than in the main in vivo load bearing direction, which corresponds to changes in cancellous bone seen in vivo. This resulted in an increase in mechanical anisotropy, as can be seen by comparing Figs. 9 and 10. Figure 9 shows the stiffness of a cancellous bone specimen from a 37-yr-old donor. Figure 10 shows the stiffness of this same specimen after 50 yr of simulated remodeling. It can be seen that the stiffness is smaller in all directions, and that the shape is more anisotropic.

The increase in anisotropy during the simulated remodeling results from the existing anisotropy of the cancellous bone. In the specimens that were used as input for the simulation, the architecture was

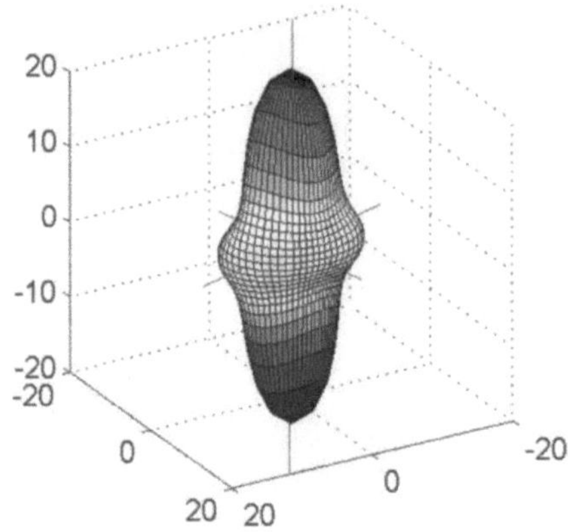

Fig. 10. Global stiffness of the same specimen in Fig. 9 after 50 yr of simulated remodeling. Note the decrease in stiffness and the increase in anisotropy.

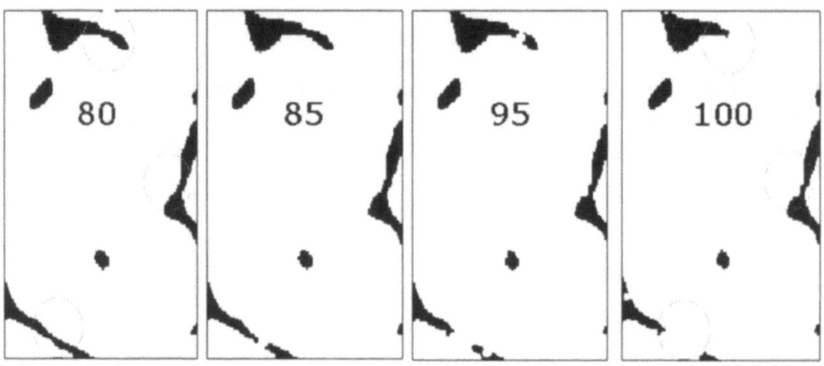

Fig. 11. One slice from a computer of a cancellous bone specimen. The images show bone loss caused by simulated remodeling. The simulated age is shown in the figure.

aligned to the main in vivo load bearing direction. Trabeculae aligned in the load bearing direction were somewhat thicker than the transversal trabeculae. During the simulation, the thinner horizontal trabeculae have a larger chance of becoming breached by resorption cavities. If a trabecula was breached during the simulation, this trabecula did not contribute to the load bearing in the simulated mechanical test. Therefore, the stiffness in transversal directions decreased more than the stiffness in the main load bearing direction.

The unloading of breached trabeculae is assumed to lead to a rapid resorption of the remaining struts in vivo *(15)*. In the simulation model, breached, and therefore unloaded trabeculae were not removed rapidly from the model. The remaining struts do not contribute to the stiffness of the specimen because no load is transferred though these struts. Therefore, this does not influence the changes in stiffness anisotropy resulting from the simulated remodeling. Furthermore, if a strut was cut through, the loose fragment that was created in this way was removed from the model, resulting in a fast removal of the remaining struts (*see* Fig. 11). Thus, although we did not include mechanical feedback to regulate bone remodeling like others did in two dimensions *(41)*, the simulation model enhances the existing anisotropy.

CONCLUSIONS AND FUTURE EXTENSIONS OF THE MODEL

The present simulation model provides a relation between bone loss caused by the remodeling process in trabecular bone and the remodeling parameters that describe this remodeling process. Although

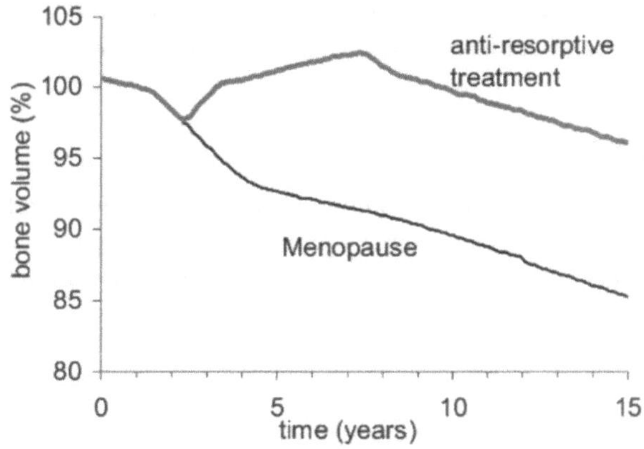

Fig. 12. Changes in bone volume during simulated menopause and 5 yr of antiresorptive treatment.

other computer studies of bone remodeling have been performed, this is the first model that uses detailed three dimensional models that represent the cancellous architecture.

An aspect that certainly plays a role in physiological remodeling and that was not taken into account in the present simulation is the role of mechanical loading. Numerous hypotheses exist about the way the loading influences the remodeling process. Disuse results in the resorption of bone matrix *(42)* and heavy use in the apposition of bone *(43)*. In the present simulation, the cavities were distributed randomly over the surface of the trabecula. No stress, strain or damage distribution in the trabeculae was taken into account. At the moment, a three-dimensional simulation of remodeling at the level of detail of the present study based on stress or strain criteria is unfeasible, but less detailed simulations have been performed *(41,44)*. As computer technology develops further, a detailed simulation that includes bone resorption and formation and mechanical loading of the cancellous bone will be possible in the future.

Architectures similar to cancellous bone can be created from artificial meshes in computer models in which mechanical feedback is incorporated *(41,44)*. In these models, adaptation of cancellous architectures to changes in external loads was also simulated. From these simulation models, it was concluded that modeling of cancellous bone architecture according to mechanical feedback is a feasible concept.

These models did not include resorption and formation, but they just added bone where needed, and removed unloaded tissue. The resulting changes in architecture are similar to changes that result from creating and refilling resorption cavities, where the local strains determine whether a cavity if filled for less or more than 100%. The difference is that resorption cavities can breach trabeculae and perforate plates, while adding or removing small amounts of bone at the trabecular surface has smaller effects on the architecture.

During, for example, fracture healing or when external loads change, this mechanical feedback probably plays a role. In an adult skeleton, where the architecture is adapted to more or less constant external loads this adaptive capacity is probably not used: random remodeling in our simulation resulted in changes in cancellous bone similar to in vivo changes.

In the simulations described in this chapter, the remodeling parameters were kept fixed during the simulation. No increased resorption depth or increased remodeling space was included in the model, to study changes in bone remodeling in, for example, menopause or Paget's disease. However, these changes can be incorporated in the model, by changing remodeling parameters at a certain simulated age. This way, the effect of, for example, menopause and antiresorptive treatment on bone mass and architecture can be investigated. In Fig. 12, an example of the changes in bone volume resulting from simulated menopause and anti-resorptive treatment is shown. As these models become more advanced, they might play a role in preclinical testing of e.g. anti-resorptive agents used in osteoporosis treatment in the future.

ACKNOWLEDGMENTS

J.C. van der Linden was supported by the Dutch Foundation for Research (NWO/MW), and the National Computing Facilities Foundation (NCF) provided computing time. The authors thank Prof. Peter Ruegsegger for providing the CT scan data from the European Union project "Assessment of Bone Quality in Osteoporosis."

REFERENCES

1. Frost, H. M. (1987) Bone "mass" and the "mechanostat": a proposal. *Anat. Rec.* **219,** 1–9.
2. Wolff, J. (1892) *Das gesetz der transformation der knochen* (translated as 'the law of bone remodeling' by P. Maquet and R. Furlong), 1986, Springer-Verlag, Berlin. Hirchwild.
3. Burr, D. B. (1993) Remodeling and the repair of fatigue damage. *Calcif. Tissue Int.* **53(Suppl 1),** S75–S80; discussion S80–S81.
4. Mori, S. and Burr, D. B. (1993) Increased intracortical remodeling following fatigue damage. *Bone* **14,** 103–109.
5. Klein-Nulend, J., et al. (2002) Donor age and mechanosensitivity of human bone cells. *Osteoporos. Int.* **13,** 137–146.
6. Ding, M., et al. (2002) Age-related variations in the microstructure of human tibial cancellous bone. *J. Orthop. Res.* **20,** 615–621.
7. Biewener, A. A. (1993) Safety factors in bone strength. *Calcif. Tissue Int.* **53(Suppl 1),** S68–S74.
8. Bentolila, V., et al. (1998) Intracortical remodeling in adult rat long bones after fatigue loading. *Bone* **23,** 275–281.
9. Burr, D. B., et al. (1985) Bone remodeling in response to in vivo fatigue microdamage. *J. Biomech.* **18,** 189–200.
10. Burr, D. B. (2002) Targeted and nontargeted remodeling. *Bone* **30,** 2–4.
11. Martin, R. B. (2002) Is all cortical bone remodeling initiated by microdamage? *Bone* **30,** 8–13.
12. Parfitt, A. M. (2002) Targeted and nontargeted bone remodeling: relationship to basic multicellular unit origination and progression. *Bone* **30,** 5–7.
13. Parfitt, A. M. (1984) The cellular basis of bone remodeling: the quantum concept reexamined in light of recent advances in the cell biology of bone. *Calcif. Tissue Int.* **36(Suppl 1),** S37–S45.
14. Parfitt, A. M. (1984) Age-related structural changes in trabecular and cortical bone: cellular mechanisms and biomechanical consequences. *Calcif. Tissue Int.* **36(Suppl 1),** S123–S128.
15. Mosekilde, L. (1990) Consequences of the remodelling process for vertebral trabecular bone structure: a scanning electron microscopy study (uncoupling of unloaded structures). *Bone Miner.* **10,** 13–35.
16. Hildebrand, T. and Ruegsegger, P. (1997) A new method for the model-independent assessment of thickness in three-dimensional images. *J. Microscopy* **185,** 67–75.
17. Odgaard, A. (1997) Three-dimensional methods for quantification of cancellous bone architecture. *Bone* **20,** 315–328.
18. Odgaard, A. and Gundersen, H. J. (1993) Quantification of connectivity in cancellous bone, with special emphasis on 3-D reconstructions. *Bone* **14,** 173–182.
19. Kabel, J., et al. (1999) Connectivity and the elastic properties of cancellous bone. *Bone* **24,** 115–120.
20. Eriksen, E. F., Melsen, F., and Mosekilde, L. (1984) Reconstruction of the resorptive site in iliac trabecular bone: a kinetic model for bone resorption in 20 normal individuals. *Metab. Bone Dis. Relat. Res.* **5,** 235–242.
21. Jayasinghe, J. A., Jones, S. J., and Boyde, A. (1993) Scanning electron microscopy of human lumbar vertebral trabecular bone surfaces. *Virchows. Arch. A Pathol. Anat. Histopathol.* **422,** 25–34.
22. Kimmel, D. B. (1985) A computer simulation of the mature skeleton. *Bone* **6,** 369–372.
23. Reeve, J. (1986) A stochastic analysis of iliac trabecular bone dynamics. *Clin. Orthop.* **213,** 264–278.
24. Silva, M. J. and Gibson, L. J. (1997) Modeling the mechanical behavior of vertebral trabecular bone: effects of age-related changes in microstructure. *Bone* **21,** 191–199.
25. Gunaratne, G. H., et al. (2002) Model for bone strength and osteoporotic fractures. *Phys. Rev. Lett.* **88,** 68–101.
26. Muller, R. and Ruegsegger, P. (1996) Analysis of mechanical properties of cancellous bone under conditions of simulated bone atrophy. *J. Biomech.* **29,** 1053–1060.
27. Tayyar, S., et al. (1999) Computer simulation of trabecular remodeling using a simplified structural model. *Bone* **25,** 733–739.
28. van der Linden, J. C., Verhaar, J. A., and Weinans, H. (2001) A three-dimensional simulation of age-related remodeling in trabecular bone. *J. Bone Miner. Res.* **16,** 688–696.
29. Han, Z. H., et al. (1997) Effects of ethnicity and age or menopause on the remodeling and turnover of iliac bone: implications for mechanisms of bone loss. *J. Bone Miner. Res.* **12,** 498–508.
30. Grote, H. J., et al. (1995) Intervertebral variation in trabecular microarchitecture throughout the normal spine in relation to age. *Bone* **16,** 301–308.

31. Majumdar, S., et al. (1997) Correlation of trabecular bone structure with age, bone mineral density, and osteoporotic status: in vivo studies in the distal radius using high resolution magnetic resonance imaging. *J. Bone Miner. Res.* **12,** 111–118.
32. Mosekilde, L. (1989) Sex differences in age-related loss of vertebral trabecular bone mass and structure—biomechanical consequences. *Bone* **10,** 425–432.
33. van der Linden, J. C., et al. (2001) Mechanical consequences of bone loss in cancellous bone. *J. Bone Miner. Res.* **16,** 457–465.
34. Frost, H. M. (1985), The pathomechanics of osteoporoses. *Clin. Orthop.* **200,** 198–225.
35. Parfitt, A. M. (1983) The physiological and clinical significance of bone histomorphometric data, in Bone Histomorphometry: Techniques and Interpretation. CRC Press: Boca Raton, FL, pp. 143–223.
36. Roux, W. (1881) *Der Kampf der Theile im Organismu.* Leipzig, Engelmann.
37. Odgaard, A., et al. (1997) Fabric and elastic principal directions of cancellous bone are closely related. *J. Biomech.* **30,** 487–495.
38. Kinney, J. H. and Ladd, A. J. (1998) The relationship between three-dimensional connectivity and the elastic properties of trabecular bone. *J. Bone Miner. Res.* **13,** 839–845.
39. Van Rietbergen, B., et al. (1996) Direct mechanics assessment of elastic symmetries and properties of trabecular bone architecture. *J. Biomech.* **29,** 1653–1657.
40. Thomsen, J. S., Ebbesen, E. N., and Mosekilde, L. (2002) Age-related differences between thinning of horizontal and vertical trabeculae in human lumbar bone as assessed by a new computerized method. *Bone* **31,** 136–142.
41. Huiskes, R., et al. (2000) Effects of mechanical forces on maintenance and adaptation of form in trabecular bone. *Nature* **405,** 704–706.
42. Holick, M. F. (1998) Perspective on the impact of weightlessness on calcium and bone metabolism. *Bone* **22,** 105S–111S.
43. Layne, J. E. and Nelson, M. E. (1999) The effects of progressive resistance training on bone density: a review. *Med. Sci. Sports Exerc.* **31,** 25–30.
44. Mullender, M., et al. (1998) Effect of mechanical set point of bone cells on mechanical control of trabecular bone architecture. *Bone* **22,** 125–131.

18

Effects of Microgravity on Skeletal Remodeling and Bone Cells

Pierre J. Marie

INTRODUCTION

The skeleton is a complex living tissue that serves multiple functions, such as mechanical support of the body, protection of the vital organs, and reservoir of minerals. Gravity and loading exert important effects on the skeleton because they control bone mass. Consistently, unloading and microgravity induce multiple alterations in bone cell function and skeletal structure. This chapter, summarizes the effects of microgravity on bone metabolism and the most recent informations on the cellular and molecular mechanisms that might be involved in the effects of loading and unloading on bone cells.

BONE REMODELING

To keep its mechanical competence, the skeleton is continuously renewed by a process called remodeling. Bone remodeling is required for the integrity of mechanical properties of the skeleton. This cyclic process is ensured by osteoclasts, which resorb the calcified matrix, and osteoblasts, which synthesize a new bone matrix. The remodeling sequence begins with a phase of osteoclast differentiation followed by a resorption phase, whereby osteoclasts resorb the old bone matrix. During the next phase, called reversal phase, osteoblast precursors are recruited and differentiate. Thereafter, mature osteoblasts fill up the resorption cavity during the formation phase, the last step of the remodeling cycle. The maintenance of bone mass is dependent on the adequate coupling between the resorption and formation phases and on the equilibrium between resorption and formation activities. These processes are governed by systemic hormones (calcitonin, parathyroid hormone, 1,25 dihydroxyvitamin D, sex hormones, glucocorticoids) as well as local factors (cytokines, growth factors, soluble molecules; ref. *1*).

The commitment of bone cells, their proliferation, and progressive differentiation are key processes controlling resorption of bone by osteoclasts and the formation of bone matrix by osteoblasts. Osteoclast precursors originating from the monocyte-macrophage lineage fuse under the control of 1,25(OH)2 vitamin D, M-CSF, and receptor activator of NF-κB ligand (RANKL; ref. *2*). Mature osteoclasts are large polarized multinucleated cells attached to the bone matrix during the resorbing process at the level of the sealing zone. Cell attachment through cytoskeletal–integrin–matrix interactions is essential for bone resorption. Once attached, osteoclasts can develop a specialized cell membrane called ruffled border, and bone degradation occurs in the microcompartment localized between the ruffled border and the bone matrix *(3)*. At the end of the resorption period, osteoclasts detach from the matrix and undergo apoptosis. Osteoblasts originate from multipotential undifferentiated mesenchymal

From: *The Skeleton: Biochemical, Genetic, and Molecular Interactions in Development and Homeostasis*
Edited by: E. J. Massaro and J. M. Rogers © Humana Press Inc., Totowa, NJ

stem cells that are able to give rise to chondroblasts, osteoblasts, or adipocytes under induction by hormonal or local factors. The early commitment of mesenchymal stem cells toward osteoblast involves the expression of transcription factors, such as Runx2/Cbfa1, which control numerous osteoblast genes *(4)*. Differentiation of committed osteoblasts is characterized by the expression of alkaline phosphatase, an early marker of osteoblast phenotype, followed by the synthesis and deposition of type I collagen, bone matrix proteins and glycosaminoglycans, and increased expression of osteocalcin and bone sialoprotein at the onset of mineralization *(5)*. Once the bone matrix synthesis has been deposited and calcified, most osteoblasts become flattened lining cells, approx 10% of osteoblasts are embedded within the matrix and become osteocytes, and the others die by apoptosis. As it will be discussed in the Bone Cell Response to Strain and Mechanical Forces section, osteoblasts, lining cells, and osteocytes may play a role in the transduction of mechanical forces into biological signals and skeletal adaptation to loading.

SKELETAL ADAPTATION TO LOADING

The skeleton changes considerably throughout its lifespan. These changes in bone mass are in line with maintenance of the structural integrity of the skeleton that is required to support body mass. Bone mass increases linearly during childhood, peaks at sexual maturity, and plateaus at 20–30 yr of age. Bone mass thereafter decreases mildly and linearly until the end of the life in men, whereas in women bone mass falls rapidly and transiently after menopause. The skeletal adaptation to external loading and unloading throughout life occurs through changes in bone architecture and mass in response to exercise, immobilization, and weightlessness. Increased strain applied on the skeleton increases bone formation, reduces bone resorption, and increases bone mass to optimize bone resistance and reduce fracture risks. Inversely, decreased skeletal strain reduces bone formation and increases bone resorption to optimize the bone structure with respect to mechanical strength. It has been proposed that changes in bone modeling and remodeling in response to loading and unloading are initiated by an internal mechanostat that is able to sense strain. In this view, changes in bone remodeling occur in response to decreased or increased strain to adjust bone mass to a level that is appropriate *(6)*. In addition to be determined by biomechanical strain, bone mass and mechanical quality of bone are genetically determined *(7)*. Several genetic determinants control bone density and may contribute to bone loss *(8)*. In addition, polymorphism of several genes have been linked to bone mass, bone quality, and risk of fractures in humans *(9,10)*.

Mechanical loading is essential for the maintenance of skeletal integrity. This is shown by the fact that reduction of mechanical loading induces bone loss, resulting from uncoupling between bone resorption and formation. This causes reduction in the density, spatial orientation, and connectivity of bone trabeculae, leading to reduced bone strength and increased risk of fractures. Therefore, both bone architecture and bone density play essential roles in skeletal strength resistance. The mechanisms that mediate the skeletal adaptation involve signals that activate or inhibit bone remodeling in a controlled way *(11)*. Although strain increases bone formation, only dynamic loading is effective *(12)*. Moreover, the nature and amplitude of strains are essential for efficiently stimulate bone formation and bone mass *(13)*. In humans, active exercise (weight lifting, rowing, jogging, walking, but not swimming) increases bone mass, although the effects differ between bone areas *(14)*. Thus, selective strain and loading play a role in the maintenance of the weight-bearing skeleton.

INFLUENCE OF MICROGRAVITY ON BONE

Effects of Space Flights on Bone

Consistent with the positive effect of loading on bone mass, loss of loading induced by microgravity affects bone metabolism. This is reflected by changes in mineral metabolism, hormonal status, bone cell activity, and bone mass during space flights *(15,16)*. However, the amplitude of bone loss depends on the type of bone because weight-bearing bones are more affected by microgravity than nonweight-bearing bones. In humans, prolonged flights in space result in decreased bone mass in vertebrae, spine, femur neck, trochanter, and pelvis, and up to 0.5% of bone mass can be lost per month *(16)*. Biochemical parameters of bone formation decrease whereas indices of bone resorption increase after flight *(17)*. Microgravity decreases bone formation, whereas bone resorption increases simultaneously and transiently *(18)*. This uncoupling between bone formation and resorption during space flights results in decreased metaphyseal bone mass associated with altered bone architecture and quality. However, bone formation can be improved after recovery on Earth, and partial recovery of cancellous bone mass may occur after space flights *(15,16)*.

Mechanisms of Bone Loss

The role of calcium-regulating hormones in bone response to microgravity is not established *(19)*. Sw abolish bone changes induced by space flights *(20)*. Serum parathyroid hormone (PTH) and 1,25$(OH)_2$ vitamin D levels decrease during flights in space, but this may be secondary events to increased serum calcium levels resulting from increased bone resorption *(19)*. In contrast, microgravity in space flights appears to affect directly bone formation and resorption through changes in the activity of bone cells *(21)*. Space flights increase osteoclastic bone resorption and reduce osteoblast differentiation *(21–23)*. Reduced osteoblast proliferation and increased apoptosis also were observed under simulated microgravity conditions *(24,25)*. Alterations in cell shape, proliferation, differentiation, and apoptolsis induced by microgravity are likely to be responsible for the decreased bone formation observed in microgravity, presumably to adapt the skeleton to unloading *(6)*.

EFFECTS OF SIMULATED MICROGRAVITY ON BONE

Bone Alterations Induced by Immobilization and Bed Rest

Because of the scarce possibilities of studying the effect of microgravity in space flights, ground models have been developed to mimic some of the effects of microgravity on the skeleton. Skeletal mobilization in animals results in trabecular bone loss, which is consistent with the effect of microgravity on bone mass *(26)*. As in space flights, bone loss in immobilized skeleton results from a rapid and transient surge in bone resorption followed by a sustained decrease in bone formation *(26)*. Thus, immobilization reproduces many skeletal alterations induced by microgravity, although the kinetics differ substantially. Bed rest is another model that mimics some of the alterations induced by microgravity*(27,28)*. The head-down-tilted position during continuous bed rest results in more than 1% bone loss per month. Bone mass decreases in the lower body and increases in the skull, suggesting that changes in fluid shifts and regional blood flows affect mineral accretion in different parts of the skeleton. Bone loss induced by bed rest results mainly from excessive bone resorption and in part from decreased bone formation *(29)*. This disequilibrium in bone remodeling results in reduced mechanical properties of affected bones (Fig. 1).

Bone Alterations Induced by Hind-Limb Suspension

Skeletal unloading induced by hind-limb suspension in tail-suspended rodents offers another model to study the effects of microgravity on long bones *(19,30)*. In this model, hypokinesis induces trabecular bone loss and impairs mechanical properties. Bone loss results mainly from reduced trabecular thickness and number and is reversed by reloading or treadmill training *(15,16)*. In the rat suspended model, bone resorption is transiently increased and is followed by decreased bone formation *(19)*. In tail-suspended mice, however, bone resorption is increased together with decreased bone formation *(31)*. We have shown that the decreased bone formation induced by skeletal unloading results from an impaired proliferation of osteoprogenitor cells and decreased function of mature osteoblasts *(32)*. This is associated with increased adipocyte differentiation in the bone marrow stroma *(33)*. A

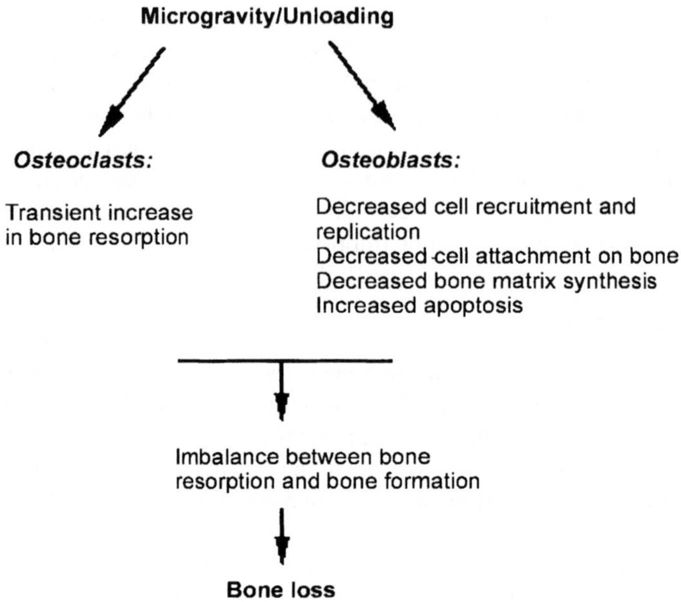

Fig. 1. General effects of microgravity/unloading on bone remodeling.

reduction in blood flow in long bones was also observed in hind-limb unloading in rats, which may affect bone cells *(34)*. Bone loss does not result from changes in serum corticosteroid, 25-hydroxy-vitamin D, or PTH levels *(19)*. In contrast, bone cell alterations in skeletal unloading may result from local changes in growth factor expression *(35)*. Indeed, skeletal unloading decreases insulin-like growth factor (IGF)-I expression in marrow stromal cells *(36)*. Space flight also alters IGF-I signaling in osteoblasts *(37)*. We have shown that IGF-I and IGF-I receptor mRNA levels fall during the first week of suspension, suggesting a role in IGF-I signaling in trabecular bone loss induced by unloading *(38)*. Accordingly, preventive treatment with recombinant IGF-I in unloaded rats increases osteoblastic cell proliferation and differentiation and partially corrects the defective bone formation and osteopenia *(39)*. Besides IGF-I, hind limb unloading also induces a rapid and transient fall in transforming growth factor-β (TGF-β) and TGF-β receptor II mRNA levels in bone *(33,37)*, which is reminiscent to space flights *(40)*. This may play a role in bone loss induced by unloading because TGF-β2 administration corrects the abnormal expression of Runx2/Cbfa1, osteocalcin, and collagen type I and reverses the altered bone formation and bone mass in skeletal unloaded rats *(41)*. In addition, TGF-β2 inhibits the increased adipocyte differentiation induced by unloading in the bone marrow stroma *(33)*. This effect results from downregulation of adipocyte-specific genes and reduction of the number and volume of adipocytes in unloaded bone *(33)*. Thus, TGF-β signaling may play an important role in the defective bone formation induced by skeletal unloading. Its absence leads the common precursor cell to promote its commitment in the adipocyte lineage at the expense of the osteoblastic lineage *(33)*. Besides growth factors, bone loss induced by skeletal unloading in rats can also be partly improved by the administration of PTH, which also promotes bone formation *(42)* or by agents that inhibit bone resorption such as bisphosphonates *(43)* or osteoprotegerin (OPG) *(44)*.

BONE CELL RESPONSE TO STRAIN AND MECHANICAL FORCES

Effects of Strain on Bone Cells

Given the marked effect of loading and unloading on bone formation, it has been proposed that bone cells are responsive to mechanical forces *(22)*. However, the response may be complex in nature because loading induces bending forces, mechanical stretch, and pressure, which drive fluid flow and stress at the cellular level *(45–47)*. Bone cells were found to be responsive to mechanical stress in various in vitro systems, such as hypotonic swelling, stretching or bending of the cell substratum, fluid shear stress, hypergravity, and dynamic strain *(22)*. However, it is unknown whether these effects reflect a physiological stress *(47)*. In osteoblasts, the immediate changes in cell shape induced by gravity are associated with alterations in focal contacts and cytoskeleton protein organization *(48)*. In addition, mechanical forces induce multiple effects on osteoblast replication, differentiation and apoptosis in vitro *(49–53)*. However, these effects depend on the magnitude and frequency of the strain applied. High strain levels appear to increase cell proliferation and decrease osteoblast marker expression, whereas low strain affects mature osteoblasts by decreasing cell proliferation and increasing cell differentiation *(47)*. One important question is to identify bone cells that may be responsive to strain and mechanical forces. Only cells from normally loaded bones respond to mechanical stress *(54)*. Osteoblasts, osteocytes, and lining cells are in close proximity with the bone matrix and the extracellular fluid and may perhaps sense compression forces exerted on the matrix *(22,55)*. In addition, the fluid flow induced by strain may affect osteoblasts/osteocytes through the osteocytic canalicular system *(55)*. However, the bone cell response may vary with the stage of maturation, with young cells being more responsive to biomechanical stress in vitro than old cells *(55,56)*. It is therefore possible that mechanical forces may exert multiple effects on bone cells, depending on their location and stage of maturation.

Transduction of Mechanical Signals in Bone Cells

Although it is still unknown whether bone cells are directly sensitive to physiological loading *(47)*, several mechanisms have been proposed to mediate the transduction of mechanical signals in bone cells. This may involve a cascade of events starting by mechanosensing through putative membrane mechanoreceptors leading to activation of signal transduction within bone cells resulting in activation of transcription factors and change in gene expression.

The Integrin–Cytoskeleton Pathway

Integrins are transmembrane proteins that link extracellular matrix proteins to the cytoskeleton and control cell deformation, focal adhesion, and cell adherence to the matrix. It has been proposed that the integrin–cytoskeleton system may play a role in the transmission of signals in lining cells, osteoblasts, or osteocytes *(57)*. This is supported by several arguments. First, integrin-mediated binding is necessary for resistance to strain in human osteoblastic cells *(58)*, and both mechanical perturbation and cell adhesion stimulate the expression of integrins in osteoblasts *(59)*. Second, osteoblasts appear to be able to sense locally applied stress on the cell surface via integrins *(60)*. Also, the transduction of mechanical signals in bone cells requires cytoskeleton integrity: both microtubules and actin filaments appear to be involved in the cellular response to strain *(61)*. Finally, mechanical stimulation in osteoblasts alters focal contacts and cytoskeleton and induces tyrosine phosphorylation of several proteins linked to the cytoskeleton, including focal adhesion kinase (FAK), which leads to early gene transcription *(62)*. The final observation that integrin function plays a role in the signal transduction process of cell attachment and mechanical stimulation *(63,64)* suggests that the extracellular matrix–integrins–cytoskeletal axis may be involved in the signal transduction of mechanical strain in bone cells.

Mechanosensitive Membrane Channels and Receptors

Besides the integrin–cytoskeletal system, several membrane proteins may be responsive to strain and mechanical forces. Long-lasting (L-type) voltage-sensitive channels are involved in the influx of Ca^{2+} into bone cells and may trigger molecular signals involved in mechanotransduction *(65)*. Stretch-sensitive channels responsive to mechanical perturbation are present in various cell types *(66)* and are upregulated by chronic intermittent strain in osteoblasts. Chronic cyclic mechanical strain increases the whole cell conductance in response to cell stretch via these mechanosensitive channels, which may

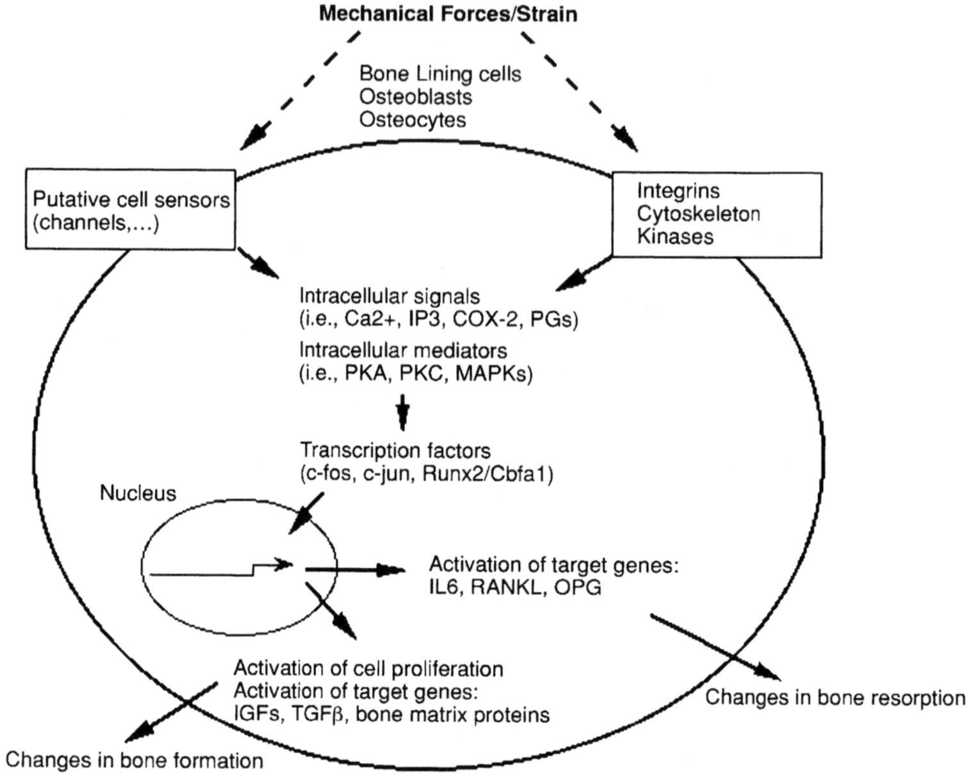

Fig. 2. Proposed cascade of events induced by mechanical forces in osteoblastic cells.

act as a signal transducer for mechanical strain on osteoblastic cells *(67)*. Glutamate receptors that are present in osteoblasts, osteocytes, and osteoclasts also may be involved in the effects of strain in bone cells *(68)*. Moreover, mechanical stretch was found to enhance gap junctional communications between osteoblastic cells by modulating intracellular localization of connexin connexin 43, a protein involved in cell–cell communication *(69)*. Thus, mechanical forces may perhaps increase metabolic coupling between bone cells through various channels and cell–cell adhesion molecules (Fig. 2).

Estrogen receptors are likely to interact with mechanical strain and modify the skeletal response to mechanical unloading. This is supported by several studies. First, space flights result in greater bone loss induced by estrogen deficiency in ovariectomized rats *(70)*. In addition, mechanical loading and estrogens in combination have more than additive effects on cell division and collagen synthesis in organ culture, showing interactions between strain and estrogen receptors *(71)*. Moreover, strain activation of cell proliferation in rat osteoblastic cells is dependent on estrogen receptor *(72)*. In rat osteoblasts, estrogen-related proliferation occurs through IGF-I receptor whereas mechanical strain stimulates cell proliferation through IGF-II production. In human osteoblasts, the proliferative response to strain and estrogens is mediated by the estrogen receptor and IGF-I signaling *(73)*. Finally, mechanical strain activates estrogen response elements in bone cells transfected with estrogen receptor alpha *(74)*. Recent data support the obligatory involvement of this receptor in the early responses to mechanical strain in vivo *(75)*. A reduction in estrogen receptor alpha expression or function following estrogen withdrawal may contribute to postmenopausal osteoporosis *(75)*. This strongly suggests that estrogens may modulate the response to microgravity and loading and that mechanical forces may modulate the response to estrogen.

Intracellular Mediators of Mechanotransduction

Multiple signaling pathways and intracellular molecules were suggested to mediate the bone cell response to strain and mechanical forces. Strain induces activation of extracellular signal-related kinase (ERK)-1/2, c-jun N-terminal kinase (JNK), phospholipase C and protein kinase C, and intracellular calcium mobilization *(76–79)*. This results in the release of soluble molecules that modulate bone cell metabolism. For example, activation of ERK-1/2 is involved in mechanical strain inhibition of RANKL *(77)*. Prostaglandins may play an important role as a local mediator of the anabolic effects of mechanical strain or microgravity in osteoblastic cells *(22)*. In vitro, stretch, strain, compressive forces, pulsating fluid flow, and intermittent hydrostatic compression induce PGE2 release in bone cells *(22,80)*. The release of prostaglandin E2 (PGE2) is essential for the induction of gap junctions between osteocytes-like cells in response to mechanical strain *(81)*. As a result of increased PGE2 release, strain induces cAMP and cGMP levels *(82)*. In addition to prostaglandins, fluid flow induces a rapid and transient increase in nitric oxide *(83)*. Nitric oxide (NO) is produced by osteoblasts in response to mechanical stimulation and is a mediator of mechanical effects in bone cells, leading to increased PGE2 release in osteocytes *(84)*. Fluid flow or strain also induces the expression of inducible cycloxygenase COX-2 in osteoblasts and osteocytes *(85)*. This effect is dependent on cytoskeleton–integrin interactions *(62)* and occurs via an ERK-signaling pathway in osteoblasts *(85)*. The fluid shear stress-induced COX-2 expression is mediated by C/EBP beta, cAMP-response element binding-proteins, and activator protein-1 (AP-1) in osteoblastic cells *(86)*. Inhibition of COX-2, the key enzyme in the formation of prostaglandins, prevents mechanically induced bone formation in vivo, suggesting a major role of COX-2 and prostaglandins in maintaining skeletal integrity. Strain also increases intracellular levels of inositol triphosphate. This effect is partly dependent on prostaglandin synthesis. The inositol phosphate pathway appears to be involved in the mechanical strain-induced proliferation of bone cells *(87)*. Overall, the transduction of stimulus into a biochemical response in response to mechanical strain in bone cells appears to involve a rise in calcium levels, which precedes activation of protein kinase A, protein kinase C, and increased inositol triphosphate, activates *c-fos*, COX-2 transcription, resulting in the production of PGE2, intracellular cAMP levels, and downstream target molecules, such as IGF-I and osteocalcin in osteoblasts (Fig. 3; refs. *47,88*). Because multiple pathways may be used for the transmission of a mechanical signal in osteoblast–lining cells–osteocytes, the actual intracellular signaling pathways that are activated by mechanical loading in physiological strain conditions remain to be identified.

MECHANORESPONSIVE GENES IN BONE CELLS

The final response to mechanical stimulus in bone cells resides in the expression of target genes that include transcription factors, growth factors, matrix proteins, and soluble molecules.

Transcription Factors

Several transcription factors that are affected by strain in vitro have been identified. Elements, including AP-1 sites, cAMP response elements and shear stress response elements were found in the promoter of several genes regulated by mechanical stress *(89)*. Several data indicate that AP-1 proteins are involved in the transduction of mechanical stress to biological effect. Mechanical loading increases the expression of the early proto-oncogene *c-fos* in bone cells through the ERK pathway *(90,91)*. *c-fos* and *c-jun*, which are components of the AP-1 transcription factor are early key effectors of mechanical stress mediated by ERK and p38 MAPK or src kinases in osteoblastic cells *(92,93)*. Actin polymerization is required for *c-fos* translocation in the nucleus *(62)*, which provides a mechanism by which cytoskeleton organization cooperates with transcription factor activation to transduce mechanical signaling into metabolic changes in osteoblasts. Activation of *c-fos* and *c-jun* may in turn modulate osteoblast and osteoclast replication or differentiation through activation of target genes whose promoters present functional AP-1 sites.

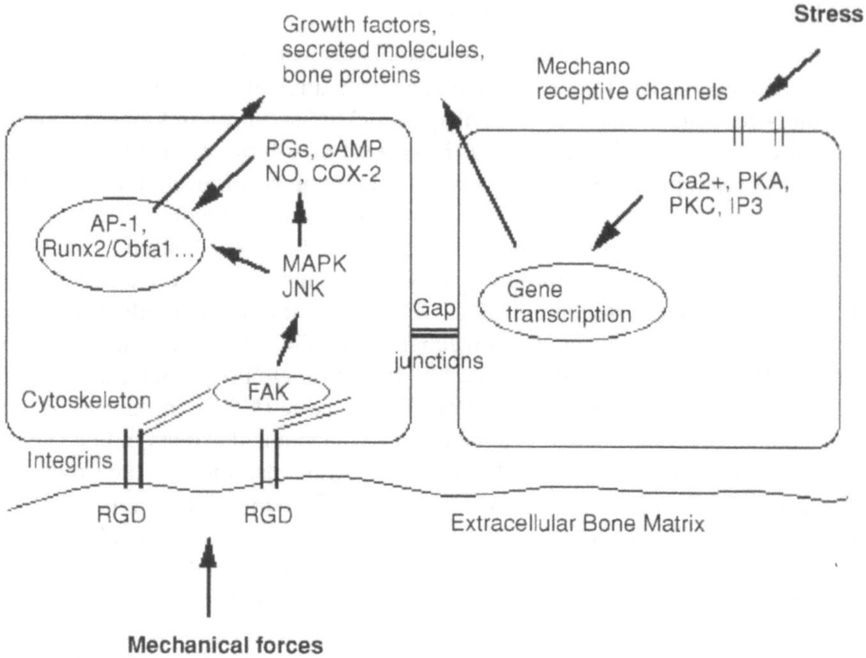

Fig. 3. Proposed signaling mechantransduction pathways in response to mechanical forces and stress in osteoblasts–lining cells–osteocytes.

Strain induces increased expression of other transcription factors, such as egr-1, junB, junD, Fra-1, and Fra-2 *(88,89)*, which are all important modulators of osteoblasts and osteoclasts. p53 is another important modulator of cell cycling and apoptosis. Interestingly, skeletal unloading does not induce bone loss in p53-deficient mice, suggesting that it mediates osteoblast/osteoclast apoptosis in skeletal unloading *(94)*. Recent data indicate that mechanical deformation by stretching upregulates the expression and DNA binding of the osteoblast transcription factor Runx2/Cbfa1. Mechanostressing activates ERK MAPK, which phosphorylates Cbfa1, providing a link between mechanostressing and osteoblast differentiation *(95)*. Moreover, simulated microgravity suppresses Runx2 levels and osteoblast phenotype *(96)*. Thus, changes in early transcription factors (*c-fos*, *c-jun*, etc) in response to mechanical forces may affect cell proliferation in osteoblasts, whereas changes in Runx2/Cbfa1 induced by loading may in turn affect differentiation genes that are Cbfa1 dependent. The overall resulting effect is changes in cell growth and differentiation that are required to adapt bone formation to loading (Fig. 3).

Soluble Factors

Some growth factors are also target genes that are modulated by microgravity and mechanical forces in osteoblastic cells. Microgravity affects TGF-β expression in the hind-limb *(97)*. Consistent with this, mechanical stimulation of cultured osteoblasts increases the expression of TGF-β transcripts *(98)* via the cation channel function *(99)*, which promotes cell proliferation *(100)*. Because IGFs and TGF-β are potent anabolic agents for bone, these factors may mediate part of the effects of loading and unloading on osteoblasts and bone formation *(35)*.

Microgravity and mechanical forces also alter the expression of soluble factors that modulate osteoclastogenesis. Besides prostaglandins, microgravity increases the expression by osteoblasts of interleukin-6, which in turn activates osteoclast formation *(101)*. Hind-limb suspension also results in increased interleukin-6 secretion, which may enhance osteoclastogenesis *(102)*. However, studies using a clinostat showed that vector-averaged environment induces a cAMP-dependent elevation of RANKL and a decrease in OPG expression in marrow stromal cells *(103)*, which may in turn stimulate osteoclastogenesis. Consistently, the administration of OPG reduces bone loss by inhibiting bone resorption in tail-suspended mice *(44)*. Moreover, mechanical loading inhibits the expression of RANKL by osteoblasts, causing reduction in osteoclast formation *(104)*. Thus, modulation of these molecules by loading and unloading may be involved in the alterations of osteoclast formation and bone resorption induced by unloading (Fig. 2).

Bone Matrix Proteins

Space flights *(105–107)* and skeletal unloading *(37,38,41)* reduce type I collagen expression and osteocalcin synthesis in rats. Microgravity also affects the expression of bone matrix proteins in cultured bone cells *(23,108)*. Consistently, mechanical forces induces type I collagen expression by osteoblasts *(23,109)*. Mechanical forces may promote bone matrix protein expression through AP-1 sites, cAMP or Runx2/Cbfa1 response elements that are present in the promoter region of mechanical stress-response genes *(89)*. Alternatively, the release of growth factors in response to stress may in turn enhance type I collagen and osteocalcin expression in osteoblasts (Fig. 3).

Osteopontin is another gene that is target for mechanical forces. Mechanical stimuli increase osteopontin expression in cultured osteoblasts and in vivo *(36,109–112)*. Induction of osteopontin expression by mechanical stimuli is protein kinase A dependent and is mediated through integrin receptors *(113)* and microfilaments *(62)*. Osteopontin gene regulation by oscillatory fluid flow occurs via intracellular mobilization and activation of ERK and p38 MAPK in osteoblasts *(79)*. Consistently, skeletal unloading reduces osteopontin expression in vivo *(110)*. Interestingly, the presence of osteopontin is required for the effect of mechanical strain on bone because osteopontin-deficient mice do not show reduce bone mass in response to unloading, which may be due to the role of osteopontin in osteoclastic bone resorption *(114)*. Although osteopontin may be critical in mechanotransduction in bone cells, it is likely that other genes are modulated by loading or unloading. The availability of genetically modified mice may allow in the future to identify specific genes involved in the effect of microgravity and loading on bone mass.

CONCLUSIONS AND PERSPECTIVES

The skeleton adapts to microgravity, unloading, and loading by changes in bone mass and architecture. Several changes in osteoblast and osteoclast recruitment and function and in bone formation and resorption in response to loading or unloading have been identified. The mechanisms by which mechanical strain may be transduced into cellular biochemical signals begin to be understood. It has been proposed that selected bone cells may respond to mechanical forces through multiple putative mechanoreceptors that are responsive to changes in the mechanical environment. Transduction of mechanical forces to biochemical signals may involve the coordination of multiple pathways, including integrins, cytoskeletal proteins, and activation of kinases, resulting in the release of signaling molecules, changes in cell proliferation, and gene expression in bone cells. Some key signaling molecules and transcription factors controlling bone cells in response to mechanical forces have been identified. However, multiple signals may play a role as recipients and generators of signaling information in response to mechanical forces or microgravity. Moreover, the sequence of events involved in the physiological bone response to mechanical forces and microgravity remains unknown. Future cell biology prospects on cell–substrate adhesion molecules, cytoskeleton, intracellular signaling pathways, transcription factors, and target genes induced by mechanical forces may lead to identify the mechanisms involved in the physiological response of bone cells to loading, strain or microgravity. The identification of these mechanisms that are influenced by mechanical forces in the skeleton may contribute to the development of novel therapeutic strategies for bone loss in long term space flight programs as well as in disuse osteoporosis on Earth.

ACKNOWLEDGMENTS

Because of space limitations, only a selected number of references on the subject could be quoted. The reader is invited to read the indicated reviews for a larger selection of papers related to the subject. The author's work on microgravity was in part supported by grants from the CNES (France).

REFERENCES

1. de Vernejoul, M. C. and Marie, P. J. (2001) New aspects of bone biology, in *Spectrum of Renal Osteodystrophy* (Drueke, T. and Salusky, I. B., eds.), Oxford University Press, Oxford, pp. 3–22.
2. Suda, T., Takahashi, N., Udagawa, N., Jimi, E., Gillespie, M. T., and Martin, T. J. (1999) Modulation of osteoclast differentiation and function by the new members of the tumor necrosis factor receptor and ligand families. *Endocr. Rev.* **20,** 345–357.
3. Baron, R. (1996) Molecular mechanisms of bone resorption: therapeutic implications. *Rev. Rhum. Engl. Ed.* **63,** 633–638.
4. Karsenty, G. (2001) Minireview: transcriptional control of osteoblast differentiation. *Endocrinology* **142,** 2731–2733.
5. Marie, P. J. (1999) Osteoblasts and bone formation, in *Advances in Organ Biology: Molecular and Cellular Biology of Bone* Vol. 5B (Zaidi, M., ed.), JAI Press, Stamford, CT, pp. 401–427.
6. Frost, H. M., Ferretti, J. L., and Jee, W. S. (1998) Perspectives: some roles of mechanical usage, muscle strength, and the mechanostat in skeletal physiology, disease, and research. *Calcif. Tissue Int.* **62,** 1–7.
7. Sheng, M. H., Baylink, D. J., Beamer, W. G., Donahue, L. R., Rosen, C. J., Lau, K. H., et al. (1999) Histomorphometric studies show that bone formation and bone mineral apposition rates are greater in C3H/HeJ (high-density) than C57BL/6J (low-density) mice during growth. *Bone* **25,** 421–429.
8. Marie, P. J. (2001) The molecular genetics of bone formation: implications for therapeutic interventions in bone disorders. *Am. J. Pharmacogenomics* **1,** 175–187.
9. Eisman, J. A. (1999) Genetics of osteoporosis. *Endocr. Rev.* **20,** 788–804.
10. Ralston, S. H. (2001) Genetics of osteoporosis. *Rev. Endocr. Metab. Disord.* **2,** 13–21.
11. Landis, W. J. (1999) An overview of vertebrate mineralization with emphasis on collagen-mineral interaction. *Gravit. Space Biol. Bull.* **12,** 15–26.
12. Robling, A. G., Duijvelaar, K. M., Geevers, J. V., Ohashi, N., and Turner, C. H. (2001) Modulation of appositional and longitudinal bone growth in the rat ulna by applied static and dynamic force. *Bone* **29,** 105–113.
13. Rubin, C., Turner, A. S., Bain, S., Mallinckrodt, C., and McLeod, K. (2001) Anabolism. Low mechanical signals strengthen long bones. *Nature* **412,** 603–604.
14. Krall, E. A. and Dawson-Hughes, B. (1994) Walking is related to bone density and rates of bone loss. *Am. J. Med.* **96,** 20–26.
15. Zerath, E. (1998) Effects of microgravity on bone and calcium homeostasis. *Adv. Space Res.* **21,** 1049–1058.
16. Vico, L. M., Hinsenkamp, D., Jones Marie, P. J., Zallone, A., and Cancedda, R. (2001) Osteobiology, strain and microgravity. Part II: studies at the tissue level. *Calcif. Tissue Int.* **68,** 1–10.
17. Smith, S. M., Nillen, J. L., Leblanc, A., Lipton, A., Demers, L. M., Lane, H. W., et al. (1998) Collagen cross-link excretion during space flight and bed rest. *J. Clin. Endocrinol. Metab.* **83,** 3584–3591.
18. Caillot-Augusseau, A., Lafage-Proust, M. H., Soler, C., Pernod, J., Dubois, F., and Alexandre, C. (1998) Bone formation and resorption biological markers in cosmonauts during and after a 180-day space flight (Euromir 95). *Clin. Chem.* **44,** 578–585.
19. Morey-Holton, E. R. and Globus, R. K. (1998) Hindlimb unloading of growing rats: a model for predicting skeletal changes during space flight. *Bone* **22,** 83S–88S.
20. Zerath, E., Holy, X., Roberts, S. G., Andre, C., Renault, S., Hott, M., et al. (2000) Spaceflight inhibits bone formation independent of corticosteroid status in growing rats. *J. Bone Miner. Res.* **15,** 1310–1320.
21. Marie, P. J., Jones, D., Vico, L., Zallone, A., Hinsenkamp, M., and Cancedda, R. (2000) Osteobiology, strain, and microgravity: part, I. Studies at the cellular level. *Calcif. Tissue Int.* **67,** 2–9.
22. Burger, E. H. and Klein-Nulend, J. (1998) Microgravity and bone cell mechanosensitivity. *Bone* **22,** 127S–130S.
23. Landis, W. J., Hodgens, K. J., Block, D., Toma, C. D., and Gerstenfeld, L. C. (2000) Spaceflight effects on cultured embryonic chick bone cells. *J. Bone Miner. Res.* **15,** 1099–1112.
24. Guignandon, A., Usson, Y., Laroche, N., Lafage-Proust, M. H., Sabido, O., Alexandre, C., et al. (1997) Effects of intermittent or continuous gravitational stresses on cell-matrix adhesion: quantitative analysis of focal contacts in osteoblastic ROS 17/2.8 cells. *Exp. Cell Res.* **236,** 66–75.
25. Rucci, N., Migliaccio, S., Zani, B. M., Taranta, A., and Teti, A. (2002) Characterization of the osteoblast-like cell phenotype under microgravity conditions in the NASA-approved Rotating Wall Vessel bioreactor (RWV). *J. Cell. Biochem.* **85,** 167–179.
26. Jee, W. S. and Ma, Y. (1999) Animal models of immobilization osteopenia. *Morphologie* **83,** 25–34.
27. Zerwekh, J. E., Ruml, L. A., Gottschalk, F., and Pak, C. Y. (1998) The effects of twelve weeks of bed rest on bone histology, biochemical markers of bone turnover, and calcium homeostasis in eleven normal subjects. *J. Bone Miner. Res.* **13,** 1594–1601.

28. Inoue, M., Tanaka, H., Moriwake, T., Oka, M., Sekiguchi, C., and Seino, Y. (2000) Altered biochemical markers of bone turnover in humans during 120 days of bed rest. *Bone* **26,** 281–286.
29. Palle, S., Vico, L., Bourrin, S., and Alexandre, C. (1992) Bone tissue response to four-month antiorthostatic bedrest: a bone histomorphometric study. *Calcif. Tissue Int.* **51,** 189–194.
30. Wronski, T. J. and Morey-Holton, E. R. (1987) Skeletal response to simulated weightlessness: a comparison of suspension techniques. *Aviat. Space Environ. Med.* **58,** 63–68.
31. Sakata, T., Sakai, A., Tsurukami, H., Okimoto, N., Okazaki, Y., Ikeda, S., et al. (1999) Trabecular bone turnover and bone marrow cell development in tail-suspended mice. *J. Bone Miner. Res.* **14,** 1596–1604.
32. Machwate, M., Zerath, E., Holy, X., Hott, M., Modrowski, D., Malouvier, A., et al. (1993) Skeletal unloading in rat decreases proliferation of rat bone and marrow-derived osteoblastic cells. *Am. J. Physiol.* **264,** E790–E799.
33. Ahdjoudj, S., Lasmoles, F., Holy, X., Zerath, E., and Marie, P. J. (2002) Transforming growth factor beta2 inhibits adipocyte differentiation induced by skeletal unloading in rat bone marrow stroma. *J. Bone Miner. Res.* **17,** 668–677.
34. Colleran, P. N., Wilkerson, M. K., Bloomfield, S. A., Suva, L. J., Turner, R. T., and Delp, M. D. (2000) Alterations in skeletal perfusion with simulated microgravity: a possible mechanism for bone remodeling. *J. Appl. Physiol.* **89,** 1046–1054.
35. Marie, P. J. and Zerath, E. (2000) Role of growth factors in osteoblast alterations induced by skeletal unloading in rats. *Growth Factors* **18,** 1–10.
36. Zhang, R., Supowit, S. C., Klein, G. L., Lu, Z., Christensen, M. D., Lozano, R., et al. (1995) Rat tail suspension reduces messenger RNA level for growth factors and osteopontin and decreases the osteoblastic bone differentiation of bone marrow stromal cells. *J. Bone Miner. Res.* **10,** 415–423.
37. Kumei, Y., Nakamura, H., Morita, S., Akiyama, H., Hirano, M., Ohya, K., et al. (2002) Space flight and insulin-like growth factor-I signaling in rat osteoblasts. *Ann. NY Acad. Sci.* **973,** 75–78.
38. Drissi, H., Lomri, A., Lasmoles, F., Holy, X., Zerath, E., and Marie, P. J. (1999) Skeletal unloading induces biphasic changes in insulin-like growth factor-I mRNA levels and osteoblast activity. *Exp. Cell Res.* **251,** 275–284.
39. Machwate, M., Zerath, E., Holy, X., Pastoureau, P., and Marie, P. J. (1994) Insulin-like growth factor-I increases trabecular bone formation and osteoblastic cell proliferation in unloaded rats. *Endocrinology* **134,** 1031–1038.
40. Westerlind, K. C. and Turner, R. T. (1995) The skeletal effects of spaceflight in growing rats: tissue-specific alterations in mRNA levels for TGF-beta. *J. Bone Miner. Res.* **10,** 843–848.
41. Machwate, M., Zerath, E., Holy, X., Hott, M., Godet, D., Lomri, A., and Marie, P. J. (1995) Systemic administration of transforming growth factor-beta 2 prevents the impaired bone formation and osteopenia induced by unloading in rats. *J. Clin. Invest.* **96,** 1245–1253.
42. Turner, R. L., Evans, G. L., Cavolina, J. M., Halloran, B., and Morey-Holton, E. (1998) Programmed administration of parathyroid hormone increases bone formation and reduces bone loss in hindlimb-unloaded ovariectomized rats. *Endocrinology* **139,** 4086–4091.
43. Kodama, Y., Nakayama, K., Fuse, H., Fukumoto, S., Kawahara, H., Takahashi, H., et al. (1997) Inhibition of bone resorption by pamidronate cannot restore normal gain in cortical bone mass and strength in tail-suspended rapidly growing rats. *J. Bone Miner. Res.* **12,** 1058–1067.
44. Bateman, T. A., Dunstan, C. R., Ferguson, V. L., Lacey, D. L., Ayers, R. A., and Simske, S. J. (2000) Osteoprotegerin mitigates tail suspension-induced osteopenia. *Bone* **26,** 443–449.
45. Duncan, R. L. and Turner, C. H. (1995) Mechanotransduction and the functional response of bone to mechanical strain. *Calcif. Tissue Int.* **57,** 344–358.
46. Cowin, S. C. (1998) On mechanosensation in bone under microgravity. *Bone* **22,** 119S–125S.
47. Jones, D., Leivseth, G., and Tenbosch, J. (1995) Mechano-reception in osteoblast-like cells. *Biochem. Cell Biol.* **73,** 525–534.
48. Guignandon, A., Usson, Y., Laroche, N., Lafage-Proust, M. H., Sabido, O., Alexandre, C., and Vico, L. (1997) Effects of intermittent or continuous gravitational stresses on cell-matrix adhesion: quantitative analysis of focal contacts in osteoblastic ROS 17/2.8 cells. *Exp. Cell Res.* **236,** 66–75.
49. Hasegawa, S., Sato, S., Saito, S., Suzuki, Y., and Brunette, D. M. (1985) Mechanical stretching increases the number of cultured bone cells synthesizing DNA and alters their pattern of protein synthesis. *Calcif. Tissue Int.* **37,** 431–436.
50. Ozawa, H., Imamura, K., Abe, E., Takahashi, N., Hiraide, T., Shibasaki, Y., et al. (1990) Effect of a continuously applied compressive pressure on mouse osteoblast-like cells (MC3T3-E1) in vitro. *J. Cell Physiol.* **142,** 177–185.
51. Raab-Cullen, D. M., Thiede, M. A., Petersen, D. N., Kimmel, D. B., and Recker, R. R. (1994) Mechanical loading stimulates rapid changes in periosteal gene expression. *Calcif. Tissue Int.* **55,** 473–478.
52. Harter, L. V., Hruska, K. A., and Duncan, R. L. (1995) Human osteoblast-like cells respond to mechanical strain with increased bone matrix protein production independent of hormonal regulation. *Endocrinology* **136,** 528–535.
53. Sarkar, D., Nagaya, T., Koga, K., Nomura, Y., Gruener, R., and Seo, H. (2000) Culture in vector-averaged gravity under clinostat rotation results in apoptosis of osteoblastic ROS 17/2.8 cells. *J. Bone Miner. Res.* **15,** 489–498.
54. Rawlinson, S. C., Mosley, J. R., Suswillo, R. F., Pitsillides, A. A., and Lanyon, L. E. (1995) Calvarial and limb bone cells in organ and monolayer culture do not show the same early responses to dynamic mechanical strain. *J. Bone Miner. Res.* **10,** 1225–1232.
55. Burger, E. H., Klein-Nulend, J., van der Plas, A., and Nijweide, P. J. (1995) Function of osteocytes in bone—their role in mechanotransduction. *J. Nutr.* **125(7 Suppl),** 2020S–2023S.

56. Burger, E. H. and Klein-Nulend, J. (1999) Mechanotransduction in bone—role of the lacuno-canalicular network. *FASEB J.* **13(Suppl),** S101–S112.
57. Chen, K. D., Li, Y. S., Kim, M., Li, S., Yuan, S., Chien, S., and Shyy, J. Y. (1999) Mechanotransduction in response to shear stress. Roles of receptor tyrosine kinases, integrins, and Shc. *J. Biol. Chem.* **274,** 18393–18400.
58. Lacouture, M. E., Schaffer, J. L., and Klickstein, L. B. (2002) A comparison of type I collagen, fibronectin, and vitronectin in supporting adhesion of mechanically strained osteoblasts. *J. Bone Miner. Res.* **17,** 481–492.
59. Carvalho, R. S., Bumann, A., Schaffer, J. L., and Gerstenfeld, L. C. (2002) Predominant integrin ligands expressed by osteoblasts show preferential regulation in response to both cell adhesion and mechanical perturbation. *J. Cell Biochem.* **84,** 497–508.
60. Pommerenke, H., Schmidt, C., Durr, F., Nebe, B., Luthen, F., Muller, P., and Rychly, J. (2002) The mode of mechanical integrin stressing controls intracellular signaling in osteoblasts. *J. Bone Miner. Res.* **17,** 603–611.
61. Ajubi, N. E., Klein-Nulend, J., Alblas, M. J., Burger, E. H., and Nijweide, P. J. (1999) Signal transduction pathways involved in fluid flow-induced PGE2 production by cultured osteocytes. *Am. J. Physiol.* **276(1 Pt 1),** E171–E178.
62. Pavalko, F. M., Chen, N. X., Turner, C. H., Burr, D. B., Atkinson, S., Hsieh, Y. F., et al. (1998) Fluid shear-induced mechanical signaling in MC3T3-E1 osteoblasts requires cytoskeleton-integrin interactions. *Am. J. Physiol.* **275(6 Pt 1),** C1591–C1601.
63. Salter, D. M., Robb, J. E., and Wright, M. O. (1997) Electrophysiological responses of human bone cells to mechanical stimulation: evidence for specific integrin function in mechanotransduction. *J. Bone Miner. Res.* **12,** 1133–1141.
64. Carvalho, R. S., Schaffer, J. L., and Gerstenfeld, L. C. (1998) Osteoblasts induce osteopontin expression in response to attachment on fibronectin: demonstration of a common role for integrin receptors in the signal transduction processes of cell attachment and mechanical stimulation. *J. Cell. Biochem.* **70,** 376–390.
65. Li, J., Duncan, R. L., Burr, D. B., and Turner, C. H. (2002) L-type calcium channels mediate mechanically induced bone formation in vivo. *J. Bone Miner. Res.* **17,** 1795–1800.
66. Sackin, H. (1995) Stretch-activated ion channels. *Kidney Int.* **48,** 1134–1147.
67. Duncan, R. L. and Hruska, K. A. (1994) Chronic, intermittent loading alters mechanosensitive channel characteristics in osteoblast-like cells. *Am. J. Physiol.* **267,** F909–F916.
68. Mason, D. J., Suva, L. J., Genever, P. G., Patton, A. J., Steuckle, S., Hillam, R. A., and Skerry, T. M. (1997) Mechanically regulated expression of a neural glutamate transporter in bone: a role for excitatory amino acids as osteotropic agents? *Bone* **20,** 199–205.
69. Ziambaras, K., Lecanda, F., Steinberg, T. H., and Civitelli, R. (1998) Cyclic stretch enhances gap junctional communication between osteoblastic cells. *J. Bone Miner. Res.* **13,** 218–228.
70. Westerlind, K. C., Wronski, T. J., Ritman, E. L., Luo, Z. P., An, K. N., Bell, N. H., et al. (1997) Estrogen regulates the rate of bone turnover but bone balance in ovariectomized rats is modulated by prevailing mechanical strain. *Proc. Natl. Acad. Sci. USA* **94,** 4199–4204.
71. Cheng, M. Z., Zaman, G., and Lanyon, L. E. (1994) Estrogen enhances the stimulation of bone collagen synthesis by loading and exogenous prostacyclin, but not prostaglandin E2, in organ cultures of rat ulnae. *J. Bone Miner. Res.* **9,** 805–816.
72. Zaman, G., Cheng, M. Z., Jessop, H. L., White, R., and Lanyon, L. E. (2000) Mechanical strain activates estrogen response elements in bone cells. *Bone* **27,** 233–239.
73. Cheng, M. Z., Rawlinson, S. C., Pitsillides, A. A., Zaman, G., Mohan, S., Baylink, D. J., et al. (2002) Human osteoblasts' proliferative responses to strain and 17beta-estradiol are mediated by the estrogen receptor and the receptor for insulin-like growth factor, I. *J. Bone Miner. Res.* **17,** 593–602.
74. Jessop, H. L., Sjoberg, M., Cheng, M. Z., Zaman, G., Wheeler-Jones, C. P., and Lanyon, L. E. (2001) Mechanical strain and estrogen activate estrogen receptor alpha in bone cells. *J. Bone Miner. Res.* **16,** 1045–1055.
75. Lee, K., Jessop, H., Suswillo, R., Zaman, G., and Lanyon, L. (2003) Endocrinology: bone adaptation requires oestrogen receptor-alpha. *Nature* **424,** 389.
76. Carvalho, R. S., Scott, J. E., Suga, D. M., and Yen, E. H. (1994) Stimulation of signal transduction pathways in osteoblasts by mechanical strain potentiated by parathyroid hormone. *J. Bone Miner. Res.* **9,** 999–1011.
77. Rubin, J., Murphy, T. C., Fan, X., Goldschmidt, M., and Taylor, W. R. (2002) Activation of extracellular signal-regulated kinase is involved in mechanical strain inhibition of RANKL expression in bone stromal cells. *J. Bone Miner. Res.* **17,** 1452–1460.
78. Geng, W. D., Boskovic, G., Fultz, M. E., Li, C., Niles, R. M., Ohno, S., and Wright, G. L. (2001) Regulation of expression and activity of four PKC isozymes in confluent and mechanically stimulated UMR-108 osteoblastic cells. *J. Cell Physiol.* **189,** 216–228.
79. You, J., Reilly, G. C., Zhen, X., Yellowley, C. E., Chen, Q., Donahue, H. J., and Jacobs, C. R. (2001) Osteopontin gene regulation by oscillatory fluid flow via intracellular calcium mobilization and activation of mitogen-activated protein kinase in MC3T3-E1 osteoblasts. *J. Biol. Chem.* **276,** 13365–13371.
80. Klein-Nulend, J., Burger, E. H., Semeins, C. M., Raisz, L. G., and Pilbeam, C. C. (1997) Pulsating fluid flow stimulates prostaglandin release and inducible prostaglandin G/H synthase mRNA expression in primary mouse bone cells. *J. Bone Miner. Res.* **12,** 45–51.
81. Cheng, B., Kato, Y., Zhao, S., Luo, J., Sprague, E., Bonewald, L. F., and Jiang, J. X. (2001) PGE(2) is essential for gap junction-mediated intercellular communication between osteocyte-like MLO-Y4 cells in response to mechanical strain. *Endocrinology* **142,** 3464–3473.

82. Binderman, I., Shimshoni, Z., and Somjen, D. (1984) Biochemical pathways involved in the translation of physical stimulus into biological message. *Calcif. Tissue Int.* **36(Suppl 1),** S82–S85.
83. van't Hof, R. J. and Ralston, S. H. (2001) Nitric oxide and bone. *Immunology* **103,** 255–261.
84. Klein-Nulend, J., Semeins, C. M., Ajubi, N. E., Nijweide, P. J., and Burger, E. H. (1995) Pulsating fluid flow increases nitric oxide (NO) synthesis by osteocytes but not periosteal fibroblasts—correlation with prostaglandin upregulation. *Biochem. Biophys. Res. Commun.* **217,** 640–648.
85. Wadhwa, S., Godwin, S. L., Peterson, D. R., Epstein, M. A., Raisz, L. G., and Pilbeam, C. C. (2002) Fluid flow induction of cyclo-oxygenase 2 gene expression in osteoblasts is dependent on an extracellular signal-regulated kinase signaling pathway. *J. Bone Miner. Res.* **17,** 266–274.
86. Ogasawara, A., Arakawa, T., Kaneda, T., Takuma, T., Sato, T., Kaneko, H., et al. (2001) Fluid shear stress-induced cyclooxygenase-2 expression is mediated by C/EBP beta, cAMP-response element-binding protein, and AP-1 in osteoblastic MC3T3-E1 cells. *J. Biol. Chem.* **276,** 7048–7054.
87. Reich, K. M. and Frangos, J. A. (1991) Effect of flow on prostaglandin E2 and inositol trisphosphate levels in osteoblasts. *Am. J. Physiol.* **261,** C428–C432.
88. Kawata, A. and Mikuni-Takagaki, Y. (1998) Mechanotransduction in stretched osteocytes—temporal expression of immediate early and other genes. *Biochem. Biophys. Res. Commun.* **246,** 404–408.
89. Nomura, S. and Takano-Yamamoto, T. (2000) Molecular events caused by mechanical stress in bone. *Matrix Biol.* **19,** 91–96.
90. Peake, M. A., Cooling, L. M., Magnay, J. L., Thomas, P. B., and El Haj, A. J. (2000) Selected contribution: regulatory pathways involved in mechanical induction of c-fos gene expression in bone cells. *J. Appl. Physiol.* **89,** 2498–2507.
91. Mikuni-Takagaki, Y. (1999) Mechanical responses and signal transduction pathways in stretched osteocytes. *J. Bone Miner. Metab.* **17,** 57–60.
92. Kletsas, D., Basdra, E. K., and Papavassiliou, A. G. (2002) Effect of protein kinase inhibitors on the stretch-elicited c-Fos and c-Jun up-regulation in human PDL osteoblast-like cells. *J. Cell Physiol.* **190,** 313–321.
93. Granet, C., Vico, A. G., Alexandre, C., and Lafage-Proust, M. H. (2002) MAP and src kinases control the induction of AP-1 members in response to changes in mechanical environment in osteoblastic cells. *Cell Signal.* **14,** 679–688.
94. Sakai, A., Sakata, T., Tanaka, S., Okazaki, R., Kunugita, N., Norimura, T., and Nakamura, T. (2002) Disruption of the p53 gene results in preserved trabecular bone mass and bone formation after mechanical unloading. *J. Bone Miner. Res.* **17,** 119–127.
95. Ziros, P. G., Gil, A. P., Georgakopoulos, T., Habeos, I., Kletsas, D., Basdra, E. K., et al. (2002) The bone-specific transcriptional regulator Cbfa1 is a target of mechanical signals in osteoblastic cells. *J. Biol. Chem.* **277,** 23934–23941.
96. Ontiveros, C., and McCabe, L. R. (2003) Simulated microgravity suppresses osteoblast phenotype, Runx2 levels and AP-1 transactivation. *J. Cell Biochem.* **88,** 427–437.
97. Westerlind, K. C., Morey-Holton, E., Evans, G. L., Tanner, S. J., and Turner, R. T. (1996) TGF-β may help couple mechanical strain and bone cell activity in vivo. *J. Bone Miner. Res.* **11,** S:377.
98. Klein-Nulend, J., Roelofsen, J., Sterck, J. G., Semeins, C. M., and Burger, E. H. (1995) Mechanical loading stimulates the release of transforming growth factor- beta activity by cultured mouse calvariae and periosteal cells. *J. Cell Physiol.* **163,** 115–119.
99. Sakai, K., Mohtai, M., and Iwamoto, Y. (1998) Fluid shear stress increases transforming growth factor beta 1 expression in human osteoblast-like cells: modulation by cation channel blockades. *Tissue Int.* **63,** 515–520.
100. Zhuang, H., Wang, W., Tahernia, A. D., Levitz, C. L., Luchetti, W. T., and Brighton, C. T. (1996) Mechanical strain-induced proliferation of osteoblastic cells parallels increased TGF-beta 1 mRNA. *Biochem. Biophys. Res. Commun.* **229,** 449–453.
101. Kumei, Y., Shimokawa, H., Katano, H., Hara, E., Akiyama, H., Hirano, M., et al. (1996) Microgravity induces prostaglandin E2 and interleukin-6 production in normal rat osteoblasts: role in bone demineralization. *J. Biotechnol.* **47,** 313–324.
102. Grano, M., Mori, G., Minielli, V., Barou, O., Colucci, S., Giannelli, G., et al. (2002) Rat hindlimb unloading by tail suspension reduces osteoblast differentiation, induces IL-6 secretion, and increases bone resorption in ex vivo cultures. *Tissue Int.* **70,** 176–185.
103. Kanematsu, M., Yoshimura, K., Takaoki, M., and Sato, A. (2002) Vector-averaged gravity regulates gene expression of receptor activator of NF-kappaB (RANK) ligand and osteoprotegerin in bone marrow stromal cells via cyclic AMP/protein kinase A pathway. *Bone* **30,** 553–558.
104. Rubin, J., Murphy, T., Nanes, M. S., and Fan, X. (2000) Mechanical strain inhibits expression of osteoclast differentiation factor by murine stromal cells. *Am. J. Physiol. Cell Physiol.* **278,** C1126–C1132.
105. Backup, P., Westerlind, K., Harris, S., Spelsberg, T., Kline, B., and Turner, R. (1994) Spaceflight results in reduced mRNA levels for tissue-specific proteins in the musculoskeletal system. *Am. J. Physiol.* **266,** E567–E573.
106. Bikle, D. D., Harris, J., Halloran, B. P., and Morey-Holton, E. (1994) Altered skeletal pattern of gene expression in response to spaceflight and hindlimb elevation. *Am. J. Physiol.* **267,** E822–E827.
107. Cavolina, J. M., Evans, G. L., Harris, S. A., Zhang, M., Westerlind, K. C., and Turner, R. T. (1997) The effects of orbital spaceflight on bone histomorphometry and messenger ribonucleic acid levels for bone matrix proteins and skeletal signaling peptides in ovariectomized growing rats. *Endocrinology* **138,** 1567–1576.
108. Carmeliet, G., Nys, G., and Bouillon, R. (1997) Microgravity reduces the differentiation of human osteoblastic MG-63 cells. *J. Bone Miner. Res.* **12,** 786–794.

109. Harter, L. V., Hruska, K. A., and Duncan, R. L. (1995) Human osteoblast-like cells respond to mechanical strain with increased bone matrix protein production independent of hormonal regulation. *Endocrinology* **136,** 528–535.
110. Toma, C. D., Ashkar, S., Gray, M. L., Schaffer, J. L., and Gerstenfeld, L. C. (1997) Signal transduction of mechanical stimuli is dependent on microfilament integrity: identification of osteopontin as a mechanically induced gene in osteoblasts. *J. Bone Miner. Res.* **12,** 1626–1636.
111. Terai, K., Takano-Yamamoto, T., Ohba, Y., Hiura, K., Sugimoto, M., Sato, M., et al. (1999) Role of osteopontin in bone remodeling caused by mechanical stress. *J. Bone Miner. Res.* **14,** 839–849.
112. Morinobu, M., Ishijima, M., Rittling, S. R., Tsuji, K., Yamamoto, H., Nifuji, A., et al. (2003) Osteopontin expression in osteoblasts and osteocytes during bone formation under mechanical stress in the calvarial suture in vivo. *J. Bone Miner. Res.* **18,** 706–715.
113. Carvalho, R. S., Bumann, A., Schaffer, J. L., and Gerstenfeld, L. C. (2002) Predominant integrin ligands expressed by osteoblasts show preferential regulation in response to both cell adhesion and mechanical perturbation. *J. Cell Biochem.* **84,** 497–508.
114. Ishijima, M., Rittling, S. R., Yamashita, T., Tsuji, K., Kurosawa, H., Nifuji, A., Denhardt, D. T., and Noda, M. (2001) Enhancement of osteoclastic bone resorption and suppression of osteoblastic bone formation in response to reduced mechanical stress do not occur in the absence of osteopontin. *J. Exp. Med.* **193,** 399–404.

V
Bone Mineralization

19

Quantitative Analyses of the Development of Different Hard Tissues

Siegfried Arnold, Hans J. Höhling, and Ulrich Plate

INTRODUCTION

The mineral apatite is the inorganic base element of hard tissues and its main configuration is the hexagonal hydroxyapatite. The physical and chemical characteristics are defined by the orientation of the crystals at the organic matrix. The formation of such hard tissues is a multistep process in which crystal formation and crystal growth are the final steps. This chapter will discuss these final steps from the first appearing crystallites and their further arrangement and structural orientation.

According to morphological and structural analyses of the crystal formations of different hard tissues, the primary crystallites are chains composed of nanometer-sized apatitic particles (islands) *(1–5)*. These chains of islands coalesce rapidly in longitudinal direction to needle-like crystallites, which further coalesce laterally to ribbon-like crystallites *(1–7)*. This crystal growth of hard tissue is similar to the crystallization of inorganic apatite, which also shows a first crystallization parallel to the c-axis direction, forming needle-like crystallites and afterwards a lateral crystallisation *(8–11)*.

Crystallites in developing hard tissues and calcium-phosphate pharmaceuticals, for example, dibasic calcium phosphate dihydrate, have structurally an intermediate state between amorphous and fully crystalline, which can be analysed by x-ray diffraction and electron diffraction *(12–23)*. Early crystallites in hard tissues like dentine and bone exhibit structurally already an apatitic character with lattice distortions. The degree of crystallinity of these calcium phosphate crystallites increases during tissue maturation, but even in the mature stage, lattice distortions of the apatite crystallites still exist. The lattice distortions of the apatitic crystallites of developing bone, circumpulpal dentine, and of synthetic Calcium-phosphate pharmaceuticals can be resolved quantitatively using the theory of paracrystals of Hosemann and Bagchi *(16,20,23–25)*. Paracrystals are characterized by the fact that their lattice bricks have different sizes and shapes and are mixed statistically. This means that paracrystals describe structurally an intermediate state between amorphous and fully crystalline.

This chapter describes the differences and similarities of the structural aspects of crystal formation and crystal growth of three different hard tissues. As collagen-rich hard tissues, the continuously growing dentine and the calvaria bone are analyzed and as collagen-free hard tissue, the developing enamel is analyzed at early biomineralization stages and at mature stages. By the use of energy-filtering selected area electron diffraction (SAED) and the theory of paracrystals, the interesting stages of crystal formation can be analyzed quantitatively for developing dentine, bone, and enamel and could be compared with the results for pure inorganic apatite. These paracrystalline parameters of the three

From: *The Skeleton: Biochemical, Genetic, and Molecular Interactions in Development and Homeostasis*
Edited by: E. J. Massaro and J. M. Rogers © Humana Press Inc., Totowa, NJ

different hard tissues can be compared with their composition of organic and inorganic substance, which change during the process of biomineralization.

MATERIALS AND METHODS

Preparation

Young Sprague–Dawley rats (60–70 g) and young Wistar rats (50–90 g) were anesthetized, and the upper and lower incisors and the calvaria bone of the suture were rapidly dissected and transferred to liquid nitrogen-cooled propane. The time for tissue preparation was approx 1–3 min. These shockfrozen specimens were freeze-dried at –80°C. After slowly warming up to room temperature in vacuum, they were vacuum embedded in epoxy resin, avoiding a rehydration or redistribution of the mineralized particles. Ultrathin sections were cut transversal to the longitudinal axis of the incisor with an ultramicrotome to a thickness of less than 80 nm. The time of water contact in the microtome trough was minimized to avoid crystal dissolution and the water kept at neutral pH *(26)*.

The inorganic apatite was crushed and embedded in epoxy resin at the same conditions as for the hard-tissue specimens. After polymerization of the resin, ultrathin sections were also cut with the ultramicrotome to a thickness of less than 80 nm.

About 30 different specimens at different mineralization stages of enamel, dentine, and calvaria bone were analyzed. Additionally, the mineralization of the whole dentine was analyzed by SAED patterns recorded in lateral steps of about 2 μm from the predentine–dentine to the dentine–enamel border.

Energy-Filtering Electron Microscope

Elastically (zero-loss)-filtered SAED patterns were taken in an energy-filtering transmission electron microscope (Zeiss EM902) at an acceleration voltage of 80 keV. Using zero-loss filtering, the background of the inelastically scattered electrons decreases and faint Debye Scherrer rings became visible, which could not have been observed in unfiltered diffraction patterns *(27,28)*. Line scans of these patterns were obtained by a scintillator–photomultiplier combination under the final screen of the energy-filtering transmission electron microscope, whereby the zero-loss-filtered SAED patterns were shifted sequentially over the detector by scanning coils *(3,5,29)*.

The morphological investigations were conducted in the electron spectroscopic imaging mode. This mode uses the zero-loss filtering to enhance the contrast by decreasing the background of the inelastically scattered electrons *(28)*.

Theory of Paracrystals

According to the theory of Hosemann et al. *(24,30,31)* the lattice of a paracrystal is characterized by the fact that the periodically arranged atoms fluctuate around their mean atomic distance in all directions. If lattice bricks have different sizes and shapes and are mixed statistically, their mutual distances fluctuate, and they build a paracrystalline lattice *(30,32)*. This fluctuation of the lattice planes can be characterised by the fluctuation factor g_{hkl} with hkl as the Miller indices. This fluctuation factor g_{hkl} and the paracrystal size L, which corresponds to the size of coherent diffraction domains, are related to the integral breadth δb of the corresponding electron diffraction profile, by Eq. 1:

$$\delta b = \frac{1}{L} + \frac{(\pi\, g_{khl})^2}{\bar{d}_{hkl}} h^2 \tag{1}$$

(31,32), where d_{hkl} is the mean lattice plane distance of the hkl lattice planes, and h represents the successive orders of the obtained Bragg-reflections. The integral breadth δb is the integral under the recorded diffraction profile above the background divided by the amplitude of the profile without background and it is corrected by the Wagner method *(33)*:

$$\delta b = \delta b_{obs} - \frac{(\delta b_{inst})^2}{\delta b_{obs}} \tag{2}$$

with δb_{obs} as the observed and δb_{inst} as the integral breadth of the instrumental broadening profile.

The limit of the number N_{hkl} of lattice planes and the restriction of crystal growth is explained in the paracrystalline theory by the fluctuation of lattice distances, described by the empirical α^*-relation expressed by Eq. 3:

$$\sqrt{N_{hkl}}\, g_{hkl} = \alpha^* = 0.15 \pm 0.05 \tag{3}$$

This means that the surface lattice planes of paracrystals have a statistical distance fluctuation of about 15% and this implies a limit of the number N_{hkl} of lattice planes and restricts the growth of the paracrystal *(30–32)*.

CRYSTAL FORMATION

Circumpulpal Dentine

Crystal Growth

Structural analyses of the crystallization process in the circumpulpal dentine (Fig. 1) performed by zero-loss filtered SAED with selected areas of 1 μm have shown that at the mineralization front the first-appearing Bragg reflection has a lattice spacing value d = 0.388 nm. Its intensity decreases with maturation of dentine. The maximum of its intensity directly at the mineralization front might suggest that it reflects aspects of the structural organization of the just stable nanometer sized particles with a diameter in the range of 1–2 nm. Therefore, it was assumed that it represents the (111) apatite lattice plane *(5)*. However, an octacalcium phosphate reflection also lies in this range as a possible precursor of apatite. The next-appearing reflections are reflections of the lattice planes perpendicular to the bipolar *c*-axis of apatite (002), (004), (006; Fig. 3A; refs. *4,5,21,22*). These reflections represent the primary crystallites, which are chains composed of nanometer-sized apatitic particles (islands) along the bipolar *c*-axis (Fig. 2; refs. *1–4,21, 22*). These chains of apatitic islands coalesce rapidly in longitudinal direction to needle-like crystallites, which further coalesce laterally to ribbon-like crystallites. This is shown by appearing (300) and (210) apatite reflections in the SAED patterns (Fig. 3B).

In the mature stage of dentine mineralization, the microfibrils are arranged parallel along the c-axis, which can be shown by the only appearing texture of the (002) reflections (Fig. 3C). This texture disappears in SAED patterns of selected areas of 3 μm, which represent a statistical arrangement of mircofibril groups *(5,22)*. In all mature mineralization stages, the line scans of these SAED patterns exhibit Debye Scherrer rings of all appearing reflections of biological apatite. The (002) reflection intensity is even higher than that of the (300) reflection at the mineralization front, which corresponds to the c-axis orientation of the first crystallites *(5)*. This described crystal growth is supported by the decrease of the net-signal intensity ratio of the (002) to (300) reflection, which has its maximum at the mineralization front (Fig. 4). Analyses of the whole dentine zone proceeding in steps of 1.5 to 2 μm from the mineralization front up to the enamel/dentine border show a further peak of this intensity ratio again in a lateral distance of about 6 to 12 μm from the mineralization front, however, with decreasing height. This process of increase and decrease of the (002) to (300) net-signal intensity ratio repeats about four to five times in distances of about 8 to 16 μm, proceeding through the whole dentine zone (Fig. 4). The mean value of the distances between such intensity-ratio maxima lies in the range of 9 to 14 μm (Fig. 4) *(4)*. This corresponds to the distances of the well-known incremental lines, von-Ebner lines, which were analyzed morphologically by light microscopical investigations *(34–38)*. The distances between these incremental lines in rat incisor dentine would correspond to the measured daily rate of mineral apposition, that is, about 16 μm/d with a variation of about 50% because of the topographical

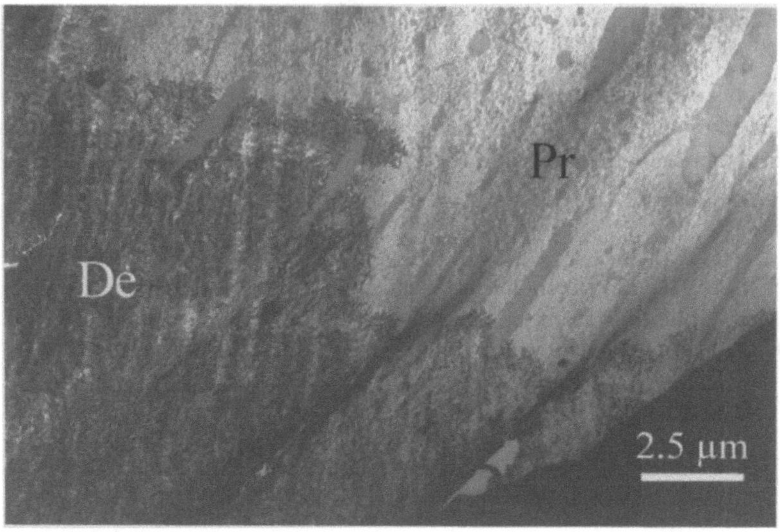

Fig. 1. Zero-loss filtered electron micrograph of circumpulpal dentine at the dentine (De)/predentine (Pr) border.

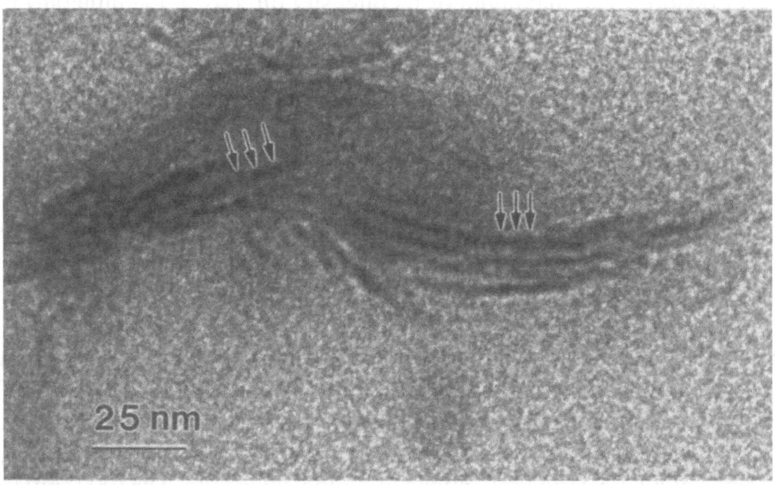

Fig. 2. Zero-loss filtered ESI micrograph of dentine crystallites at the beginning stage of dentine mineralization. (Arrows: chains of nanometer-sized particles along collagen fibrils (1) inside and (2) at the surface of the collagen fibrils.)

location and the lifecycle of the odontoblasts *(36,37,39)*. The incremental lines are built by the periodical growth of the circumpulpal dentine. They represent the actual formation phase of dentine and possibly earlier mineralization fronts *(5)*.

Crystal Structure

About 30 zero-loss-filtered SAED patterns with the corresponding linescans were taken for each specimen in the mineralized circumpulpal dentine near the mineralization front (Fig. 1; about 10 μm behind the predentine/dentine border) up to the region approx 5 μm before the dentine/enamel border. In crystallites, without any lattice distortion, the integral breadth δb of the Bragg reflection is propor-

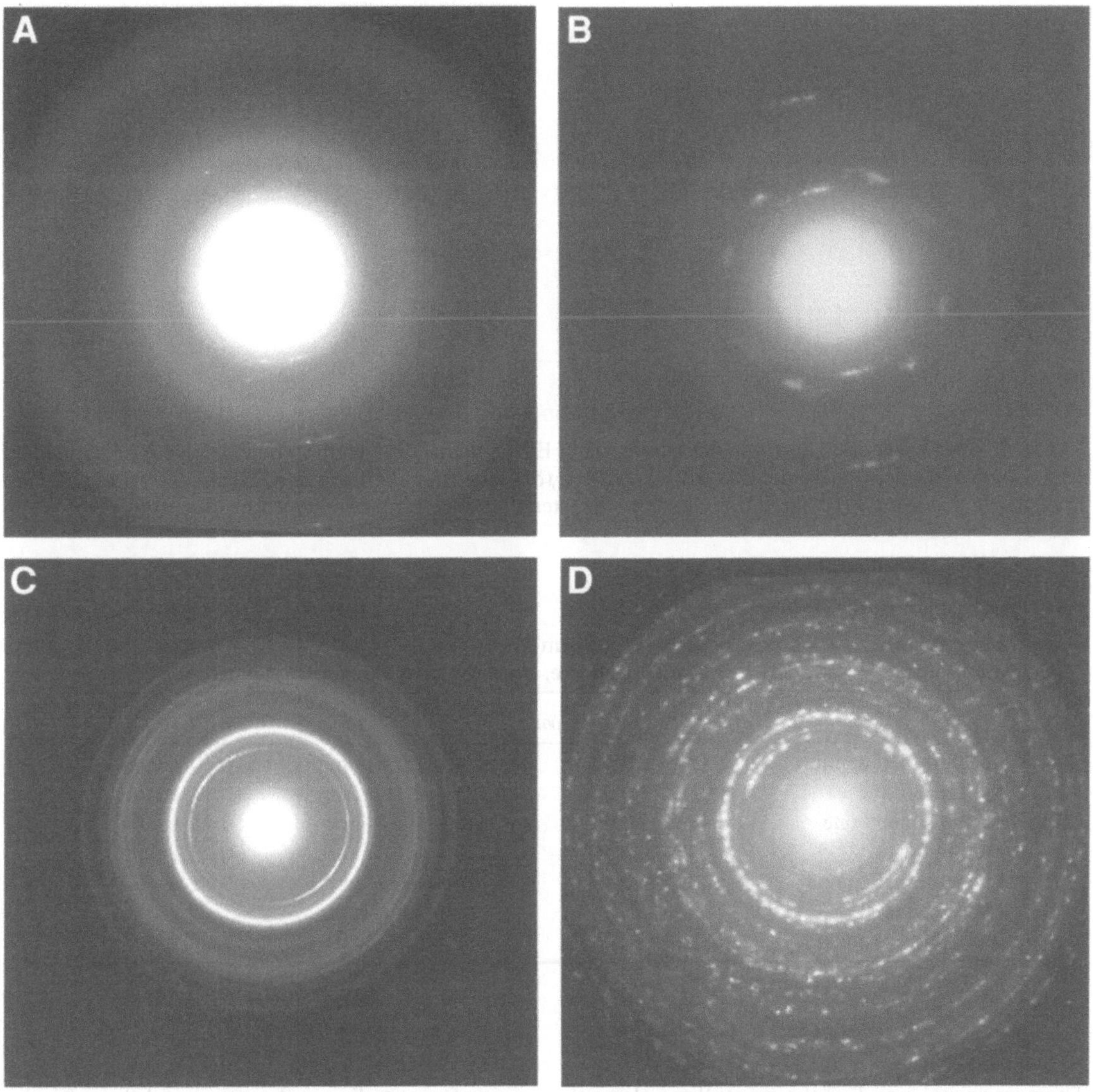

Fig. 3. Zero-loss filtered ESD patterns of a selected area of 1 µm in dentine (**A**) directly at the mineralization front, (**B**) in a distance of about 1 µm from the mineralization front, (**C**) in mature dentine, and (**D**) at the dentine–enamel border.

tional to the reciprocal crystal size *L*. In paracrystalline formations, δb is also a function of the lattice fluctuation *g (31)*. Fig. 9C shows two plots of δb against the successive orders h^2 of Bragg reflections one for the early and one for the mature mineralization stage, determined from the linescans. All plots of the integral breadth increase linearly; and this indicates the paracrystalline character of the apatitic crystallites for these mineralization stages in the circumpulpal dentine *(21,22)*.

The paracrystalline fluctuation factor *g* of early formed and mature crystallites (Table 1) shows that the apatitic crystallites in the circumpulpal dentine of rat incisors have lattice fluctuations during the whole mineralization process. In the early stage of mineralization, a fluctuation of about 3.4% exists, and for the mature stages a fluctuation of approx 2.3% of the mean atom lattice distances *(21,22)*.

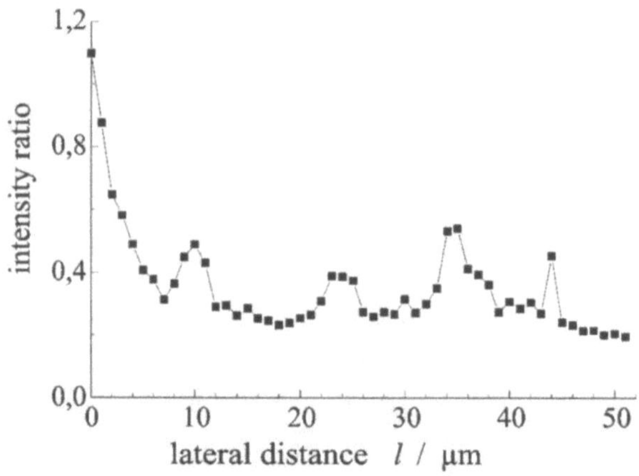

Fig. 4. Mean value of 50 line scan measurements of ESD patterns through the whole dentine zone. Graphical presentation of the net signal-intensity-ratio $I_{002}(\delta)/I_{3000}(\delta)$ of the Bragg reflections (002) and (300) (width of the Bragg angle window δ = 1.5 mrad) in relation to the lateral distance *l* from the mineralization front.

Table 1
Paracrystalline Parameters of Newly Formed and Mature Crystallites of Dentine, Bone, Enamel, and Inorganic Apatite

	Fluctuation factor g_{001}	*Crystal size* L_{00l}	$\alpha^* = \sqrt{L/\bar{d}_{001}}\, g_{001}$
Early formed dentine	3.5% ± 0.4%	(4.8 ± 0.9) nm	0.10 ± 0.02
Mature dentine	2.3% ± 0.3%	(21.1 ± 1.4) nm	0.14 ± 0.03
Early formed bone	4.4% ± 0.5%	(6.0 ± 1.2) nm	0.15 ± 0.04
Mature bone	3.7% ± 0.5%	(25.2 ± 1.8) nm	0.20 ± 0.05
Early formed enamel	3.5% ± 0.4%	(6.5 ± 0.7) nm	0.11 ± 0.02
Mature enamel		No paracrystal	
Inorganic apatite		No paracrystal	

d_{hkl}, interplanar spacing *(22,23)*.

The paracrystal size *L* of the crystallites along the c-axis of apatite lies in the range of 4.8 nm for the early mineralization stage, approx 10 µm behind the predentine/dentine border, and 21 nm for the mature mineralization stage in dentine, in a distance of approx 5 µm from the enamel/dentine border (Table 1; refs. *21,22*).

Calvaria Bone

The earliest crystal formations in bone build mineral chains of nanometer-sized particles along the collagen matrix *(40–42)*. These first crystallizations are arranged along the bipolar *c*-axis of apatite *(22,40,42)*. The SAED patterns of a selected area of 1 µm of the first minerals show only textures of the apatite *c*-axis (002) (Fig. 5A; refs. *22,42*). These primary crystallites are chains composed of nanometer-sized apatitic particles (dots) along the bipolar *c*-axis *(22,41,42)*. These chains of apatitic dots coalesce rapidly in longitudinal direction to needle-like crystallites, which further coalesce laterally to ribbon-like crystallites. This is shown by the appearing (300) and (210) apatite reflections in the SAED patterns (Fig. 5B; refs. *22,42*). In the mature stage of bone mineralization, the only texture that appears is the texture of the (002) reflection (Fig. 5C) resulting by the parallel arrangement of the collagen microfibrils.

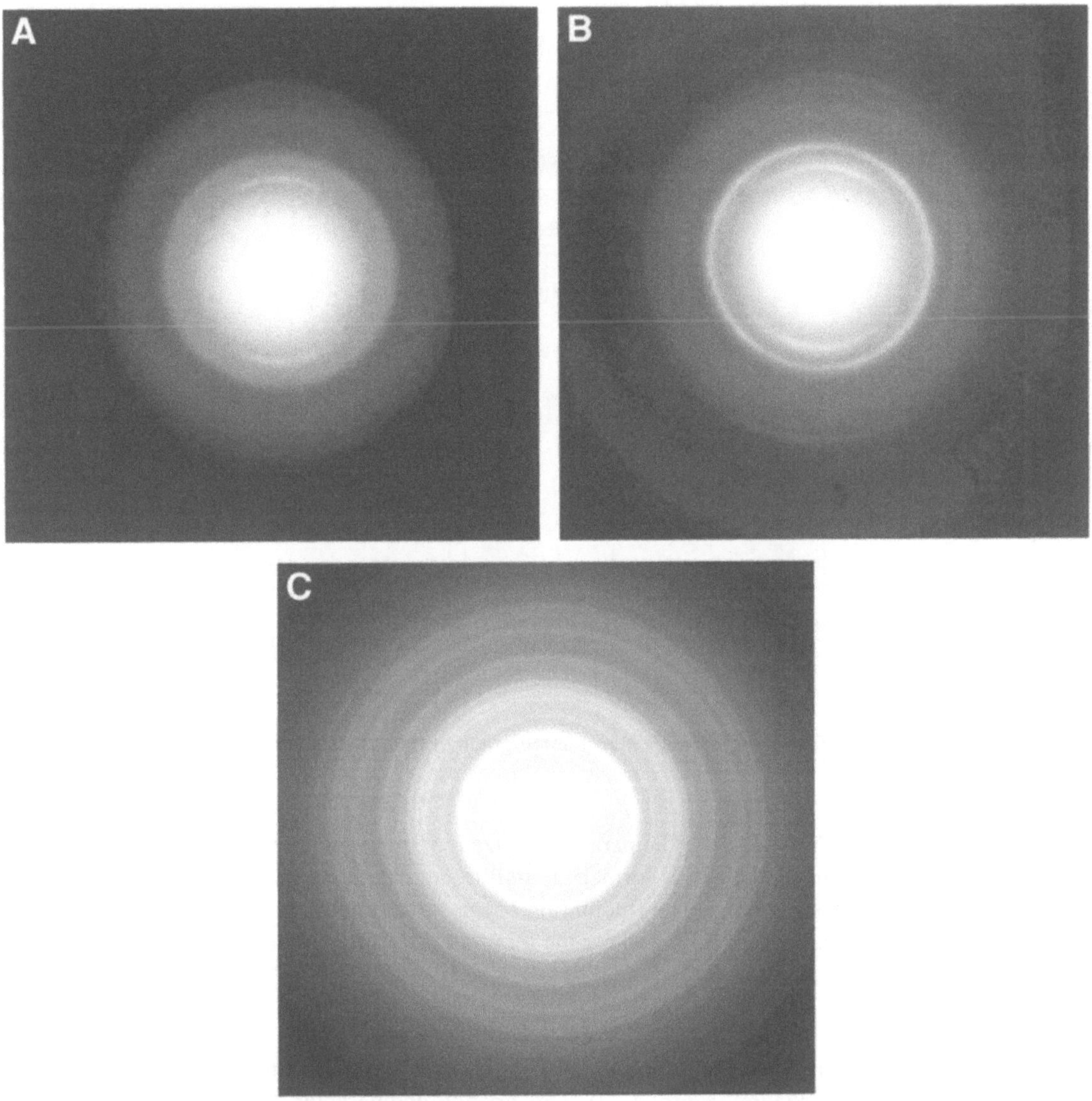

Fig. 5. Zero-loss filtered ESD patterns of a selected area of 1 μm in calvaria bone (**A**) of matrix vesicles, (**B**) at the bone mineralization front, and (**C**) in mature bone.

Zero-loss filtered SAED patterns and their corresponding linescans of about 30 different tissue specimens were taken in the just mineralized calvaria bone near the matrix vesicles and in the region of mature crystalline tissue (Fig. 6). The integral breadths δb of the reflections at the crystal lattice planes in *c*-axis direction, corrected with Eq. 2, are plotted against the square of the order of successive reflections h^2 (Fig. 9A). In all stages of mineralization, these plots of the integral breadths increase linearly. This behavior of the plots indicates the paracrystalline character of the apatitic crystallites for these stages of mineralization in the calvaria bone *(22,23)*.

According to Eq. 1 and the plots of the integral breadths δb against the order of the reflections the apatitic crystallites of the calvaria bone show during the whole mineralization process lattice fluctuations in *c*-axis direction with a fluctuation factor $g_{001} > 0$ (Table 1). In the early stage a fluctuation of about $g_{001} = 4.4\%$ and for the mature stage of about $g_{001} = 3.7\%$ of the mean atomic distances in *c*-axis

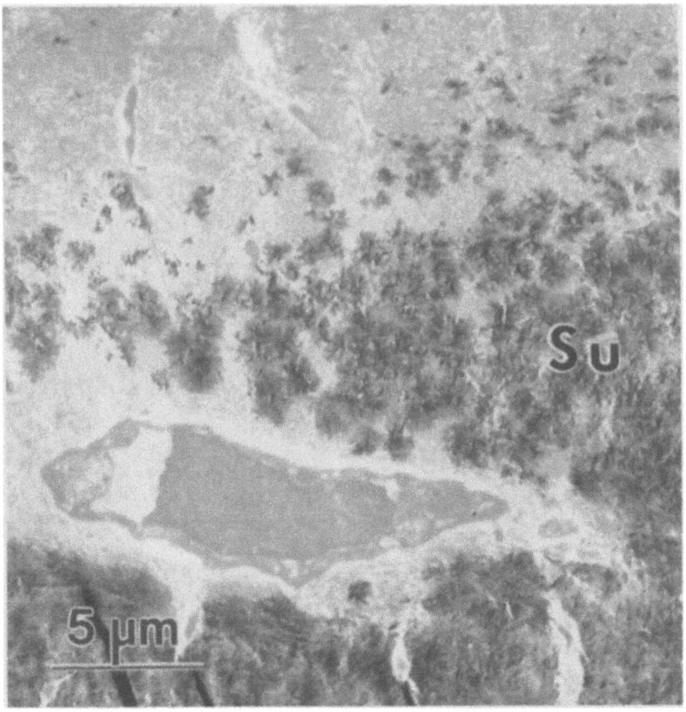

Fig. 6. Zero-loss-filtered electron micrograph of the calvaria bone (Su).

direction exists (Table. 1; refs. *22,23*). The paracrystal size *L* of the crystallites along the *c*-axis of apatite is in the region of 6 nm for the newly formed crystallites and of about 25 nm for the fully mineralized crystallites in developing bone. The fluctuation of the surface netplanes (α^*) lies for the newly formed crystallites in the range of 15% and for the mature crystallites in the range of 20% (Table 1; refs. *22,23*).

Enamel

The earliest crystal formations build up mineral chains of dots (nanometer-sized particles) along the enamel matrix proteins (Fig. 7; refs. *4,43*). This crystalline character of such mineral chains of nanometer-sized particles was analyzed by zero-loss filtered SAED patterns (Fig. 8). Textures of the 002 reflections of apatite appear in the primary stage of mineralization, whereby the 002 reflection is the first-appearing Bragg-reflection (Fig. 8A; refs. *4,22,43*). The dots in the mineral chains coalesce rapidly in longitudinal direction along the matrix proteins and build needles in which the nanometer-sized particles are no longer visible *(4,43)*. In a next step these needles coalesce rapidly in lateral directions to form ribbon-like crystallites. The development of such thicker crystallites of apatite can be described by the appearance of corresponding reflections with texture in the zero-loss filtered electron spectroscopic diffraction (ESD) patterns (Fig. 8C); first, the 300 and the 210 reflections in addition to the 004 and the primary 002 reflections *(4,22,43)*. The ribbon-like crystallites coalesce further to much thicker apatitic crystals than in dentine, which is supported by the existence of other textures of corresponding reflections (Figs. 8D and 3D; refs. *4,43*).

Zero-loss filtered SAED patterns of a selected area of 3 µm and their corresponding line scans of about 30 different tissue specimens were taken in the early mineralized enamel regions (Fig. 7) and in regions of mature enamel, near the dentine/enamel border. The corrected integral breadths δb of the reflections of the line scan in *c*-axis direction according to the Wagner method *(2)* are plotted against

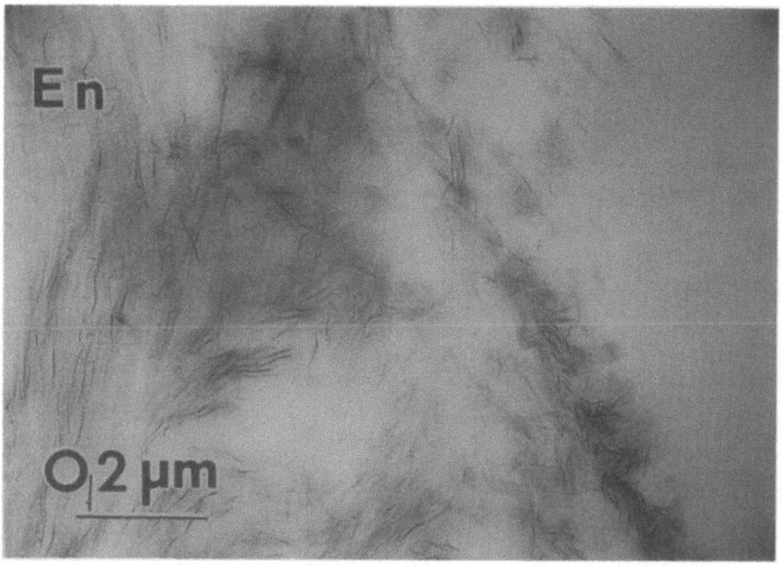

Fig. 7. Zero-loss-filtered electron micrograph of early mineralizing enamel (En).

the square of the order of successive reflections h^2 (Fig. 9B, top). In the case of the newly formed crystallites, the plots of the integral breadth increase linearly, indicating the paracrystalline character of the apatitic crystallites for this mineralization stage *(22,23)*. The integral breadths of the mature crystallites show parallel plots to the order of the reflections (Fig. 9B, bottom). This indicates that the mature crystallites of enamel have no more a paracrystalline character; they are fully crystalline *(22,23)*.

According to Eq. 1 and the plots of the integral breadths against the order of the reflections, the newly formed crystallites of enamel have a lattice fluctuation factor of about $g_{001}l = 3.5\%$ (Table 1). The paracrystal size *L* of the newly formed crystallites along the c-axis of apatite is in the region of 6.5 nm and the fluctuation of the surface net planes α^* is in the range of 11% (Table 1; refs. *22,23*).

Inorganic Apatite

Zero-loss filtered SAED patterns and their corresponding line scans were taken of ultrathin sections of pure apatite, which was crushed and embedded in epoxy resin. The corrected integral breadths δb of the reflections of the line scan in the *c*-axis direction according to the Wagner method *(2)* were plotted against the square of the order of successive reflections h^2. The integral breadths show only parallel plots to the order of the reflection h^2 (Fig. 9D). This indicates that pure inorganic apatite has no paracrystalline character and that it is fully crystalline *(22,23)*.

Comparison of the Different Apatitic Mineralization

According to the morphological and structural analyses of the earliest crystal formations of the discussed different hard tissues, the primary crystallites are chains composed of nanometer sized apatitic particles (islands; Figs. 2 and 10; refs. *1–5*). These chains of apatitic crystallites already are orientated parallel to the bipolar *c*-axis, and their further growth would be equal for both directions of this *c*-axis. The center-to-center distances between these first apatitic nanometer islands along the chains would reflect the distances between the nucleating sites along the acidic clusters of noncollagenous immobile proteins bound to collagen (Fig. 10; refs. *2,5,22)*. These chains of apatitic islands coalesce rapidly in longitudinal direction to needle-like crystallites, which further coalesce laterally to ribbon-like crystallites *(1–7)*. The in vitro crystallisation of inorganic apatite shows also a first

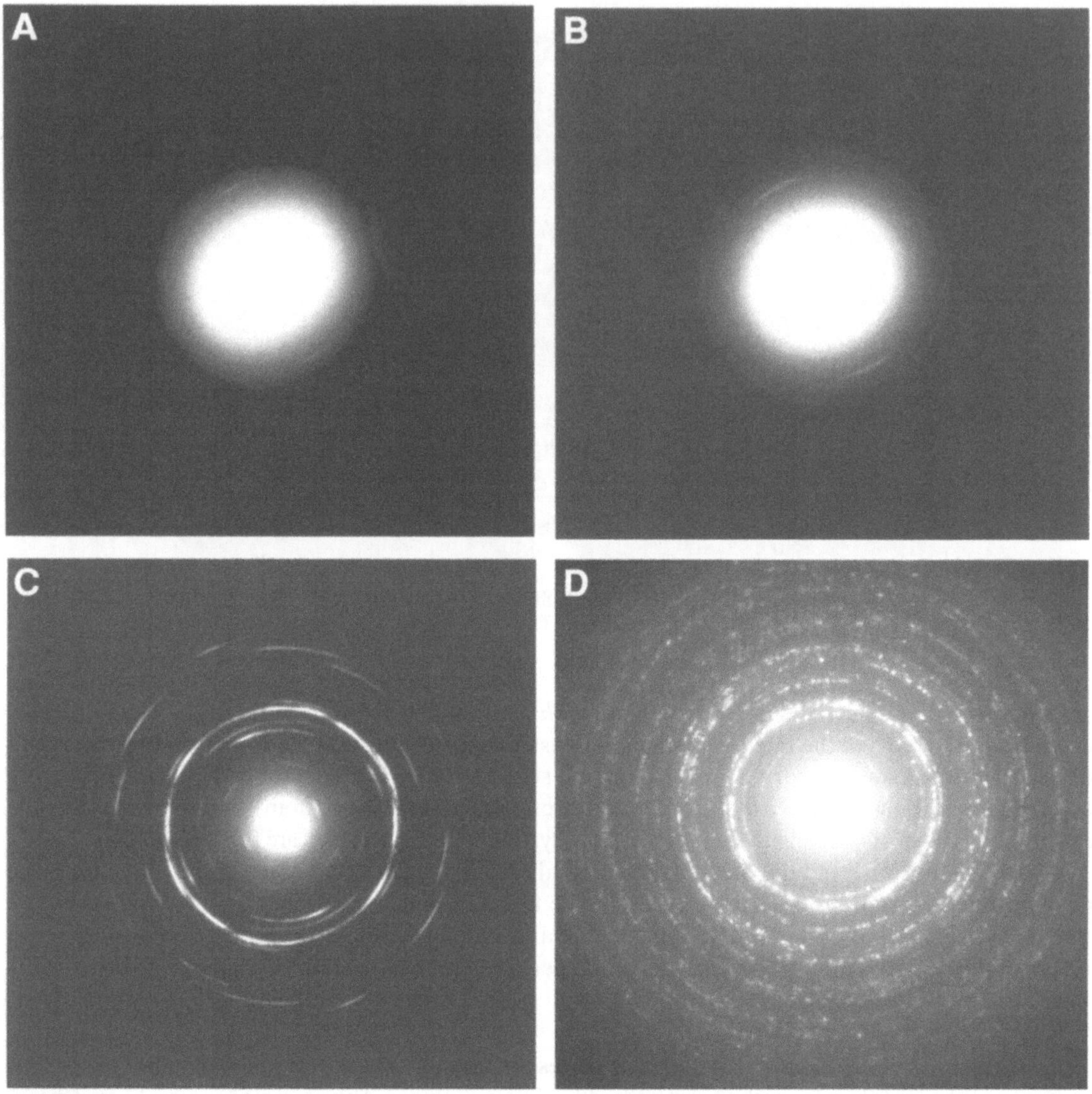

Fig. 8. Zero-loss filtered ESD patterns of a selected area of 1 µm in enamel (**A**) of the first crystallites, (**B**) in a distance of about 1 µm, (**C**) in mature enamel, and (**D**) in a distance of about 2 µm from the dentine–enamel border.

nucleation and crystal growth along the *c*-axis direction with formation of needle-like crystallites which afterwards coalesce in lateral direction *(8–11)*.

The limit of the number N_{hkl} of lattice planes and the restriction of crystal growth is explained in the paracrystalline theory by the fluctuation of the distances of lattice bricks in the surface, described by the empirical α^*-relation *(3)*. The surface lattice planes of paracrystals have a statistical distance fluctuation of about 15%, and this implies a limit of the number N_{hkl} of lattice planes and would restrict the growth of the paracrystal *(31)*. The value of α^* during the whole apatitic biomineralisation in circumpulpal dentine, calvaria bone and newly formed enamel lies between 0.10 and 0.20 (Table 1) *(23)*. These values lie in the same range as calcium phosphate formations of other authors *(16,20)* and those for other paracrystals, for example, molten metals, SiO_2 glasses, and polymers *(31,32)*.

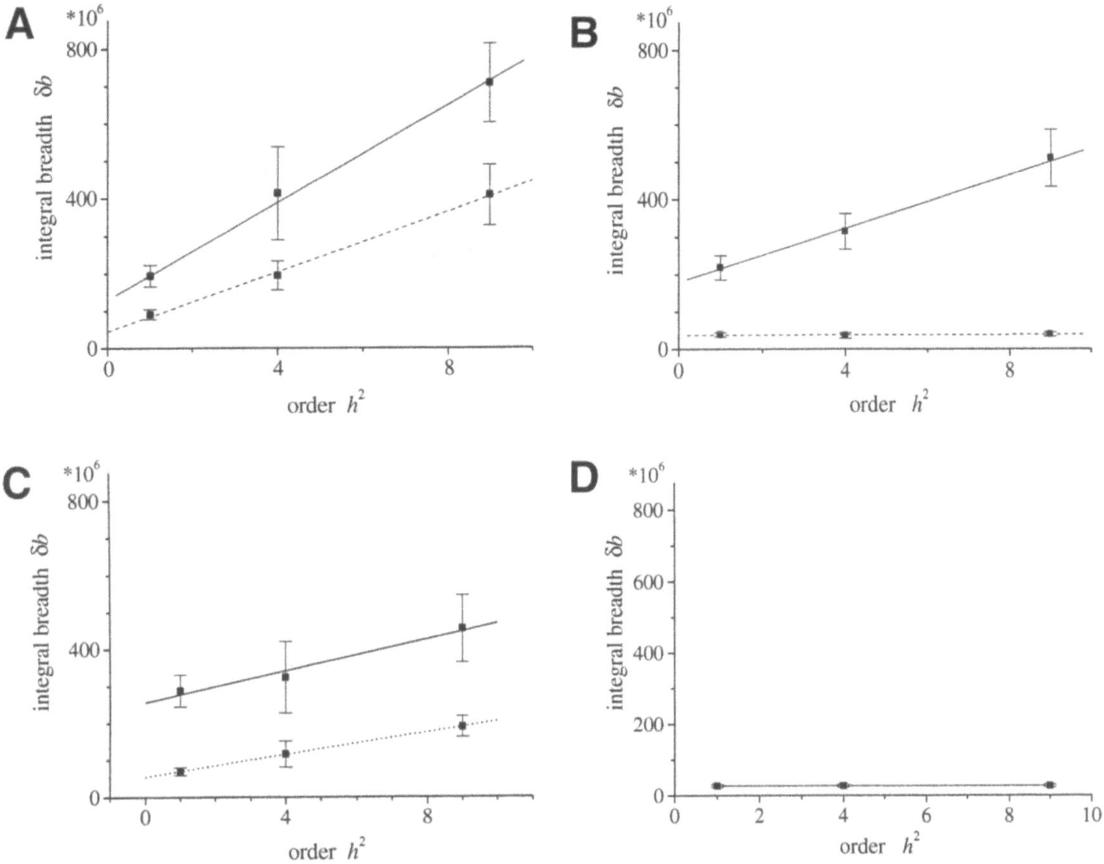

Fig. 9. Integral breadth δb against the successive orders h^2 of the reflections (002), (004), and (006) derived from the line scans of SAED patterns of newly formed and mature crystallites of (**A**) bone, (**B**) enamel, (**C**) dentine, and (**D**) inorganic apatite.

The integral breadth δb plotted against the square of the reflection order h^2 shows for all newly formed crystallites in the different developing hard tissues a linear increase (Fig. 9), which demonstrates the paracrystalline character of these early formed crystallites *(22,23)*. With maturation of the hard tissues, the lattice fluctuation of the paracrystals of all developing hard tissues decreases (Fig. 9; Table 1). In the early stage of biomineralization, the apatitic crystallites of all developing hard tissues have lattice fluctuations between $3\% < g_{001}l < 5\%$ (Table 1). The values of the lattice fluctuation of the mature crystallites decline with obviously different degree for the different hard tissues. The values of the mature calvaria bone lie in the range of $g_{001} = 3.7\%$, in mature dentine in the range of $g_{001} = 2.3\%$ and in mature enamel the crystallites show no lattice fluctuations like in inorganic apatite (Table 1; *22,23*).

The results of the radial distribution function analyses in developing bone *(17–19)* are in agreement with these results of the paracrystalline character of developing hard tissue crystallites. The radial distribution function analyses also have led to the conclusion that the apatitic crystal formations in bone are poorly crystalline hydroxyapatite, also with a decreasing lattice disorder during maturation, whereby the crystal lattice order would not reach the fully crystalline state.

The composition of tissue water, inorganic, and organic substance differs between the different hard tissues and changes during the process of biomineralization (Table 2; refs. *44,45*). The chemistry of the enamel apatitic crystallites changes quite dramatically in comparison to the bone and dentine crystallites during maturation. The total increase of inorganic mineral substance corresponds to the decrease of

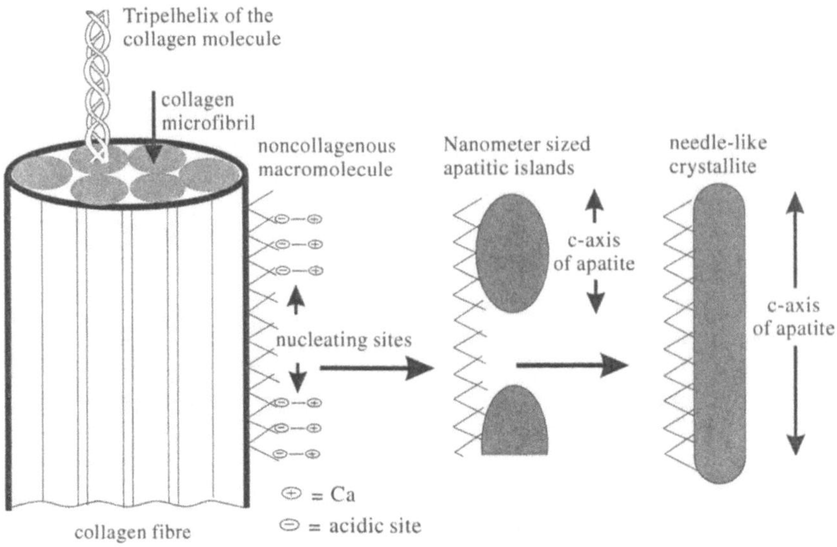

Fig. 10. Rough scheme of a linear Ca binding to acidic sites of a noncollagenous protein bound to collagen and a subsequent nucleation and development of chains of nanometer-sized apatitic crystallites.

Table 2
Composition of Inorganic and Organic Substance of Different Hard Tissues *(44,45)*

	Inorganic substance (%)	*Organic substance (%)*	*Water (%)*
Early bone	48	25	27
Bone	62	25	13
Dentine	69.3	17.5	13.2
Early enamel	≈60	≈20	≈20
Enamel	96	1.7	2.3

the lattice fluctuations of the crystallites in the developing hard tissues. The higher lattice fluctuations in the developing crystallites of the calvaria bone compared with those in dentine and enamel might be correlated to higher proportions of the organic matrix in bone *(22,23)*. However, it is not known whether this is the main reason for the differences in lattice fluctuation, but a loss of carbonate and magnesium results in an increase of crystalline disorder. In the mature stage the organic matrix of enamel has only a proportion of 1.7%, which is nearly comparable with the matrix-free inorganic apatite; both show no measurable lattice distortions according to the paracrystalline analyses *(22,23)*.

With energy filtered SAED, quantitative analyses for the crystal lattice distortions in developing dentine *(21)*, calvaria bone *(23)*, and collagen-free enamel *(23)* could be conducted on the basis of the paracrystalline theory. Applying the theory of paracrystals, often used for polymers and crystals of other fields of material science, different biomineralization stages of three different developing hard tissues have been compared quantitatively with their inorganic elements. However, all these analyses of complex biological systems are not able to answer whether the statistical distance fluctuation of the atoms at the surface restrict the growth of the paracrystals or whether the growth in the collagen-rich hard tissues is mainly determined by the surrounding organic matrix and their composition of organic and inorganic substance.

ACKNOWLEDGMENTS

Financial support by the DFG (Deutsche Forschungsgesellschaft) is gratefully acknowledged.

REFERENCES

1. Höhling, H. J., Barckhaus, R. H., Krefting, E. R., Althoff, J., and Quint, P. (1990) Collagen mineralization: aspects of the structural relationship between collagen and the apatitic crystallites, in *Ultrastructure of skeletal tissue* (Bonucci, E. and Motta, P. M., eds.), Kluwer, Boston Dordrecht London, pp. 41–62.
2. Höhling, H. J., Arnold, S., Barckhaus, R. H., Plate, U., and Wiesmann, H. P. (1995) Structural relationship between the primary crystal formations and the matrix macromolecules in different hard tissues. Discussion of a general principle. *Connect Tissue Res.* **33,** 493–500.
3. Plate, U., Arnold, S., Reimer, L., Höhling, H. J., and Boyde, A. (1994) Investigation of the early mineralization on collagen in dentine of rat incisors by quantitative electron spectroscopic diffraction (ESD). *Cell Tissue Res.* **278,** 543–547.
4. Plate, U., Arnold, S., Stratmann, U., Wiesmann, H. P., and Höhling, H. J. (1998) General principle of ordered apatitic crystal formation in enamel and collagen rich hard tissues. *Connect Tissue Res.* **38,** 149–157.
5. Arnold, S., Plate, U., Wiesmann, H. P., Kohl, H., and Höhling, H. J. (1997) Quantitative electron-spectroscopic diffraction (ESD) and electron spectroscopic imaging (ESI) analyses of dentine mineralisation in rat incisors. *Cell Tissue Res.* **288,** 185–190.
6. Fratzl, P., Schreiber, S., and Boyde, A. (1996) Characterization of bone mineral crystals in horse radius by small-angle x-ray scattering. *Calcif. Tissue Int.* **58,** 341–346.
7. Fratzl, P., Paris, O., Klaushofer, K., and Landis, W. J. (1996b) Bone mineralization in an osteogenesis imperfect mouse model studied by small-angle x-ray scattering. *J. Clin. Invest.* **97,** 396–402.
8. Koutsoukos, P. G. and Nancollas, G. H. (1981) The morphology of hydroxyapatite crystals grown in aqueous solution at 37°C. *J. Crystal Growth* **55,** 369–375.
9. Abbona, F. and Baronnet, A. (1996) A XRD and TEM study on the transformation of amorphous calcium phosphate in the presence of magnesium. *J. Crystal Growth* **165,** 98–105.
10. Graham, S. and Brown, P. W. (1996) Reactions of octacalcium phosphate to form hydroxyapatite. *J. Crystal Growth* **165,** 106–115.
11. Ma, C. L., Lu, H. B., Wang R. Z., Zhou, L. F., Cui, F. Z., and Qian, F. (1997) Comparison of controlled crystallization of calcium phosphates under three kinds of monolayers. *J. Crystal Growth* **173,** 141–149.
12. Höhling, H. J. (1966) *Die Bauelemente von Zahnschmelz und Dentin aus morphologischer, chemischer und struktureller Sicht.* Carl Hanser, München.
13. Höhling, H. J. (1989) Special aspects of biomineralisation of dental tissues, in *Teeth. Handbook of microscopic anatomy* Vol. V/6 (Oksche, A. and Vollrath, L., eds.), Springer, Berlin, pp. 475–524.
14. Posner, A. S. (1969) Crystal chemistry of bone mineral. *Physiol. Rev.* **49,** 760–792.
15. Posner, A. S., Betts, F., and Blumenthal, N. C. (1980) Formation and structure of synthetic and bone hydroxyapatites. *Prog. Crystal Growth Charact.* **3,** 49–64.
16. Wheeler, E. J. and Lewis, D. (1977) An x-ray study of the paracrystalline nature of bone apatite. *Calcif. Tissue Res.* **24,** 243–248.
17. Grynpas, M. D., Bonar, L. C., and Glimsher, M. J. (1984) Failure to detect an amorphous calcium-phosphate solid phase in bone mineral: a radial distribution function study. *Calcif. Tissue Int.* **36,** 291–301.
18. Bonar, L. C., Grynpas, M. D., Roberts, J. E., Griffin, R. G., and Glimcher, M. J. (1985) Physical and chemical characterisation of the development and maturation of bone mineral, in *The chemistry and biology of mineralized tissues* (Butler, W. T., ed.), Ebsca Media, Birmingham, pp. 226–233.
19. Glimcher, M. J. (1992) The nature of the mineral component of bone and the mechanism of calcification, in *Disorders of bone and mineral metabolism* (Coe, F. L. and Favus, M. J., eds.), Raven Press, New York, pp. 265–286.
20. Fukuoka, E., Terada, K., Makita, M., and Yamamura, S. (1995) Paracrystalline lattice distortion in crystalline pharmaceuticals determination of paracrystalline lattice distortion by powder x-ray diffraction. *Chem. Pharm. Bull.* **43,** 671–676.
21. Arnold, S., Plate, U., Wiesmann, H. P., Kohl, H., and Höhling, H. J. (1999) Quantitative electron spectroscopic diffraction analyses of the crystal formation in dentine. *J. Microsc.* **195,** 58–63.
22. Arnold, S. (1999) Quantitative Strukturuntersuchungen der Biomineralisation des hexagonalen Minerals Apatit mit Methoden der energiefilternden Elektronenmikroskopie. PhD thesis, Department of Physics, University of Münster.
23. Arnold, S., Plate, U., Wiesmann, H. P., Stratmann, U., Kohl, H., and Höhling, H. J. (2001) Quantitative analyses of the biomineralisation of different hard tissues. *J. Microsc.* **202,** 488–494.
24. Hosemann, R. and Bagchi, S. N. (1962) *Direct analysis of diffraction by matter.* North-Holland Publishing Company, Amsterdam.
25. Yamamura, S., Momose, Y., Terada, K., and Fukuoka, E. (1996) Evaluation of paracrystalline lattice distortion by profile analysis using a single x-ray diffraction peak. *Int. J. Pharm.* **133,** 117–125.
26. Plate, U., Höhling, H. J., Reimer, L., Barckhkaus, R. H., Wienecke, R., Wiesmann, H. P., and Boyde, A. (1992) Analyses of the calcium distribution in predentine by EELS and the early crystal formation in dentine by ESI and ESD. *J. Microsc.* **166,** 329–341.

27. Reimer, L., Fromm, I., Hirsch, P., Plate, U., and Rennekamp, R. (1992) Combination of EELS modes and electron spectroscopic imaging and diffraction in an energy-filtering electron microscope. *Ultramicroscopy* **46,** 335–347.
28. Reimer, L. (ed.) (1995) *Energy-filtering transmission electron microscopy*. Springer, Berlin.
29. Hülk, C. (1994) Energiefilterung der Debye-Scherrer-Ringe von polykristallincn Aufdampfschichten. Diplom-thesis in Physics, Münster.
30. Hindeleh, A. M. and Hosemann, R. (1991) Microparacrystals: the intermediate state between crystalline and amorphous. *J. Mater. Sci.* **26,** 5127–5133.
31. Hosemann, R. and Hindeleh, A. M. (1995) Structure of crystalline and paracrystalline condensed matter. *J. Macromol. Sci. Phys.* **B34,** 327–356.
32. Hosemann, R., Hentschel, M. P., Balta-Calleja, F. J., and Hindeleh, A. M. (1985) Evaluation of the alpha-constant in polymers, biopolymers and catalysts. *Exp. Tech. Phys.* **33,** 135–148.
33. Wagner, C. N. J. (1966) Analyses of the broadening and changes in position of peaks in an X-ray powder pattern, in *Local atomic arrangements studied by X-ray diffraction* (Cohen, J. B. and Hilliard, J. E., eds.), Gordon and Breach Science Publishers, New York, pp. 219–268.
34. Schour, I. and Hoffman, M. M. (1939) Studies in tooth development I. The 16 microns calcification rhythm in the enamel and dentine from fish to man. *J. Dent. Res.* **18,** 91–102.
35. Schour, I. and Hoffman, M. M. (1939) Studies in tooth development II. The rate of apposition of enamel and dentine in man and other mammals. *J. Dent. Res.* **18,** 161–175.
36. Kawasaki, K., Tanaka, S., and Ishikawa, T. (1977) On the incremental lines in human dentine as revealed by tetracycline labelling. *J. Anat.* **123,** 427–436.
37. Kawasaki, K., Tanaka, S., and Ishikawa, T. (1980) On the daily incremental lines in human dentine. *Arch. Oral Biol.* **24,** 939–943.
38. Mishima, H., Sakae, T., Kozawa, Y., and Hirai, G. (1988) Structural variations in labial dentine and lingual dentine in the rat incisor. *J. Nihon Univ. Sch. Dent.* **30,** 1–10.
39. Schour, I. and Steadman, S. R. (1935) The growth and daily rhythm of the incisor of the rat. *Anat. Rec.* **63,** 325–332.
40. Wiesmann, H. P., Arnold, S., Plate, U., Stratmann, U., Tkotz, Th., Höhling, H. J., et al. (1997) Microstructure and micro composition of sutural mineralization in rat calvaria. *Bone* **20,** 116S.
41. Wiesmann, H. P., Chi, L., Stratmann, U., Tkotz, Th., Höhling, H. J., and Joss, U. (1998) Sutural mineralization of rat calvaria characterized by atomic-force microscopy and transmission electron microscopy. *Cell Tissue Res.* **294,** 93–97.
42. Wiesmann, H. P., Arnold, S., Meyer, U., and Joos, U. (1999) Mineral crystal structure of rat calvaria. A comparison of mineral formation and bone resorption. *Calcif. Tissue Int.* **64,** S108.
43. Plate, U. and Höhling, H. J. (1994) Morphological and structural studies of early mineral formation in enamel of rat incisors by electron spectroscopic imaging (ESI) and electron spectroscopic diffraction (ESD). *Cell Tissue Res.* **277,** 151–158.
44. Deutsch, D. and Pe´er, E. (1982) Development of enamel in human fetal teeth. *J. Dent. Res.* **61,** 1543.
45. Leonhardt, H. (1990) *Histologie, Zytologie und Mikroanatomie des Menschen*. Thieme-Verlag, Stuttgart, New York, 8. Auflage.

20

Fetal Mineral Homeostasis and Skeletal Mineralization

Christopher S. Kovacs

FETAL ADAPTIVE GOALS

Fetal mineral and bone metabolism has been uniquely adapted to meet the specific needs of this developmental period, including the requirement to provide sufficient mineral to the skeleton and the requirement to maintain extracellular levels of minerals that are physiologically appropriate (i.e., for cell membrane stability, blood coagulation, etc). This chapter will review what is known about fetal mineral homeostasis and skeletal mineralization, with the emphasis on recent work from my laboratory. More detailed references are available in a recent but lengthier review *(1)*.

MINERALS AND CALCITROPIC HORMONES

Calcium

The total and ionized calcium concentration of the fetal circulation is higher than the maternal level during late gestation in mammals *(2)*, but the physiological importance of this is not known. A calcium level equal to the maternal calcium concentration (and not above it) appears to be sufficient for ensuring adequate mineralization of the fetal skeleton (*see* Fetal Skeleton section), and fetal survival to term is unaffected by extremes of hypocalcemia in *Pthrp*-null *(3)*, *Hoxa3*-null (aparathyroid; ref. *4*), and *Hoxa3/Pthrp* double-mutant fetuses *(5)*.

The fetus has a remarkable ability to maintain this higher level of blood calcium despite chronic, severe maternal hypocalcemia and appears to be relatively protected against acute changes in maternal calcium concentration *(2)*. As one example, mice lacking the gene that encodes the vitamin D receptor (*Vdr* null) have severe hypocalcemia and are prone to tetany as adults *(6)*, but *Vdr*-null fetuses have normal calcium concentrations *(7)*. Both parathyroid hormone (PTH) and parathyroid hormone-related peptide (PTHrP) are required to maintain the normal blood calcium level of the fetus (*see* sections Fetal Parathyroids and Blood Calcium Regulation; refs. *3,4,8*).

Phosphate

Serum phosphate levels are higher in the fetus than the mother in mammals *(1)*, which may indicate that phosphate is actively transported across the placenta; however, the regulators of phosphate transport are unknown. Both PTHrP and PTH are needed because the serum phosphate level is increased in *Pthrp*-null and *Hoxa3*-null (aparathyroid) fetuses (unpublished data; ref. *4*). 1,25-D has been suggested to play a role in placental phosphate transfer *(9)*; however, in *Vdr*-null fetuses, the serum phosphate levels and skeletal mineral content are normal *(7)*.

From: *The Skeleton: Biochemical, Genetic, and Molecular Interactions in Development and Homeostasis*
Edited by: E. J. Massaro and J. M. Rogers © Humana Press Inc., Totowa, NJ

Magnesium

Fetal magnesium metabolism has not been extensively studied, but the fetal magnesium level is at most slightly higher than the maternal magnesium concentration in most studies *(1)*. Although absence of PTHrP in the *Pthrp*-null fetuses does not affect serum magnesium (unpublished data), the absence of parathyroids and PTH (*Hoxa3* null) results in hypomagnesemia *(4)* and reduced skeletal magnesium content *(5)*. The absence of calcitonin (*Ct*-null fetuses) results in a selective, stepwise decrease in the serum magnesium concentration from wt to $Ct^{+/-}$ to *Ct*-null fetuses, indicating that calcitonin may regulate magnesium homeostasis *(10)*.

PTH

In fetal humans and other mammals, immunoreactive PTH blood levels are much lower than maternal PTH levels near the end of gestation *(1,2)*. It is unknown whether fetal PTH levels are low throughout gestation after the formation of the parathyroids or only in late gestation. PTH may be suppressed by a normal CaSR in response to the increased fetal blood calcium *(8)*. In the absence of PTHrP (*Pthrp*-null fetuses), the circulating PTH level rises *(5)* and serves to maintain the fetal blood calcium at the level that is normally set by the CaSR in adult mice *(3)*. The low level of PTH is critically important for maintaining the fetal blood calcium concentration because fetal mice lacking parathyroids and PTH (*Hoxa3*-null fetuses) have marked hypocalcemia (*see* sections Fetal Parathyroids and Blood Calcium Regulation; ref. *4*). The role of PTH in skeletal mineralization is discussed in the Fetal Skeleton section.

1,25-Dihydroxyvitamin D and Vitamin D

Circulating 1,25-D levels are lower than the maternal level in late gestation and appear to be largely if not completely derived from fetal sources *(1,2)*. The low circulating levels of 1,25-D in the fetus may be a response to the high serum phosphate and suppressed PTH levels in late gestation. The 1α-hydroxylase is responsive to PTH *in utero* as evidenced by study of $Casr^{+/-}$ and *Casr*-null fetuses, which have a step-wise increase in PTH and 1,25-D levels *(8)*. However, the high 1,25-D levels attained in *Casr*-null fetuses remain lower than that normally observed in adult wild-type mice (unpublished data).

1,25-D may not be essential for normal calcium and bone homeostasis in the fetus. In pregnant rats, sheep, and pigs that were hypocalcemic as a result of experimentally induced severe vitamin D deficiency, the fetuses maintained completely normal blood calcium and phosphate levels and had fully mineralized skeletons at term, as determined by total weight, ash weight, and calcium content of femurs *(1)*. Similarly, in hypocalcemic 1α-hydroxylase-deficient Hannover pigs, the fetuses maintained completely normal blood calcium and phosphate levels and fully mineralized their skeletons *(11)*. We have observed that *Vdr*-null fetal mice have normal calcium, magnesium, and phosphate levels and fully mineralized skeletons as determined by quantitative analysis (atomic absorption spectroscopy) of the ashed skeletal residue (unpublished data; ref. *7*). It is only after weaning that *Vdr*-null neonates develop hypocalcemia and rickets *(6)*.

Calcitonin

Fetal calcitonin levels are higher levels than maternal levels and are thought to reflect increased synthesis of the hormone *(1)*. There has been little convincing evidence of a role for calcitonin in fetal calcium homeostasis. On the one hand, infusion of calcitonin antiserum to fetal rats at day 21.5 of gestation slightly increased the fetal blood calcium 1 h later *(12)*, whereas fetal injection of calcitonin caused hypocalcemia and hypophosphatemia *(13)*. However, fetal thyroidectomy with subsequent thyroxine replacement did not affect the fetal blood calcium in sheep, indicating that fetal thyroidal C cells alone may not affect the regulation of the blood calcium level *(14)*.

More recently, examination of *Ct*-null fetuses *(15)* has confirmed that calcitonin is not required for normal fetal calcium homeostasis. Ionized calcium levels and skeletal calcium content were normal in *Ct*-null fetuses *(16)*. As noted (in the section entitled Magnesium), serum magnesium levels were reduced in *Ct*-null fetuses, suggesting that calcitonin might play a selective role in fetal magnesium homeostasis *(10)*.

PTH-Related Protein

In human umbilical cord blood, PTHrP levels are up to 15-fold higher than that of PTH *(1,2)*, unlike in the adult, wherein PTHrP is usually not detectable in the circulation. These and other observations led to the study of the role of PTHrP in fetal calcium homeostasis. PTHrP is a prohormone that is processed into separate circulating fragments, each of which may have different functional roles and receptors. PTHrP is produced in many sites throughout the developing embryo and fetus and plays multiple roles during embryonic and fetal development *(17)*, including the regulation of mineral and skeletal homeostasis. *Pthrp*-null fetuses have abnormalities of chondrocyte differentiation and skeletal development *(18)*, modest hypocalcemia *(3)*, and reduced placental calcium transfer (*see* section entitled Fetal Regulation). Because *Pthrp*-null fetuses have increased PTH levels *(5)* but still remain modestly hypocalcemic, it is clear that PTH cannot fully make up for lack of PTHrP in maintaining a normal calcium concentration in the blood.

Other Hormones and Factors

The role (if any) of the sex steroids in fetal skeletal development and mineral accretion is unknown, largely because the relevant analyses have not been performed. Estrogen receptor alpha and beta knockout mice have been shown to have altered skeletal metabolisms that develop postnatally, but the fetal skeleton has not been examined in detail *(1)*. Similarly, postnatal skeletal roles of receptor activator of NF-κB, receptor activator of NF-κB ligand, and osteoprotegerin have been demonstrated in relevant knockout mice *(1)*, but the role that this system plays in fetal bone metabolism and mineral accretion is not yet known.

PLACENTAL CALCIUM TRANSPORT

The bulk of placental calcium transfer occurs late in gestation, such that 80% occurs in the third trimester in humans, whereas 96% occurs in the last 5 d of gestation in the rat *(2)*. Active transport of calcium across the placenta is necessary for the fetal calcium requirement to be met. Analogous to calcium transfer across the intestinal mucosa, it has been theorized that calcium diffuses into calcium-transporting cells through maternal-facing basement membranes, is carried across these cells by calcium binding proteins, and is actively extruded at the fetal-facing basement membranes by Ca^{2+}-ATPase.

Maternal Regulation

Maternal hormones might influence fetal–placental calcium transport by raising or lowering the ambient maternal calcium level and by direct effects on the placenta. However, at least in animal models, a normal rate of maternal-to-fetal calcium transfer can usually be maintained despite the presence of maternal hypocalcemia or hormone deficiencies. Whether the same is true for human pregnancies is less certain. As examples, maternal hypocalcemia caused by parathyroidectomy or dietary calcium restriction did not affect the rate of fetal–placental calcium transfer as directly assessed in placental perfusion experiments in sheep *(19)*. Similarly, in *Vdr*-null fetal mice, placental calcium transfer was normal even though the *Vdr*-null mothers were severely hypocalcemic (unpublished data; ref. *7*). However, a normal rate of maternal–fetal calcium transfer does not necessarily imply that the fetus is unaffected by the maternal hypocalcemia. The fetal–placental unit must be working harder to extract the normal amount of calcium required from maternal blood that has a lower calcium concentration than normal.

Fetal Regulation

The contribution of the parathyroids to placental calcium transfer has been examined by studying the results of thyroparathyroidectomy in fetal lambs and decapitation (to approximate parathyroidectomy) in fetal rats *(1)*. When these surgically altered fetuses were removed so that the placentas could be artificially perfused *in situ*, active transport of calcium was found to be reduced *(14,20)*, indicating that parathyroid glands are required for active transport of calcium. Although administration of parathyroid hormone was without effect, synthetic PTHrP molecules of amino acid lengths 1–141, 1–86, and 67–86 were found to stimulate placental calcium transport in these experimentally perfused placentas *(21,22)*. These results suggested that PTHrP, perhaps produced by the parathyroid glands, stimulates active transport of calcium across the placenta. *Pthrp*-null fetal mice also have reduced placental calcium transport that can be stimulated by treatment with PTHrP 1–86 or PTHrP 67–86 but not by PTHrP 1–34 or intact PTH *(3)*.

The studies in fetal lambs and *Pthrp*-null fetuses both demonstrated that midmolecular forms of PTHrP (containing amino acids 67–86) stimulated placental calcium transfer, and that amino-terminal forms of PTHrP and PTH did not. More recently, additional studies in fetal lambs demonstrated that PTHrP 38–94, considered to be the true mid-molecular form of PTHrP, also stimulated placental calcium transfer *(23)*. These findings indicate that fetal PTHrP regulates placental calcium transfer through a receptor that has yet to be cloned. In *Pthr1*-null fetuses that lack the PTH/PTHrP receptor, placental calcium transfer is increased to 150% of the wild-type sibling value, perhaps due to the observed 11-fold upregulation of the plasma PTHrP level in the presence of a normal midmolecule receptor *(3,4)*.

The experimental findings in surgically altered lambs and in *Pthrp*-null fetuses are consistent in demonstrating a role for PTHrP in placental calcium transfer, but the relevant tissue source of this PTHrP remains uncertain. *Hoxa3*-null fetuses lack parathyroid glands and PTH but have a normal plasma PTHrP level and a normal rate of placental calcium transfer *(4)*. This observation suggests that, unlike in fetal lambs, fetal parathyroids do not contribute importantly to the plasma PTHrP level or the rate of placental calcium transfer. In *Pthr1*-null fetuses that have an 11-fold upregulation of the plasma PTHrP level, it is not the neck region but the placenta and liver that show upregulation of PTHrP mRNA and molecule, suggesting that these may be the tissue sources that contribute to the circulating PTHrP level in mice *(4)*.

PLACENTAL TRANSPORT OF MAGNESIUM AND PHOSPHATE

Although less well studied, it is evident that magnesium and phosphate are also actively transported across the placenta *(1)*. Midmolecular fragments of PTHrP stimulated magnesium transport across *in situ*-perfused placentas of fetal lambs *(22)* but not rats *(24)*. PTHrP and PTH do not stimulate placental transport of phosphate in sheep *(25)*; the regulators of phosphate transport are unknown.

FETAL PARATHYROIDS

The evidence is consistent across species that intact parathyroid glands are required for maintenance of a normal fetal calcium level as demonstrated in the studies of fetal lambs (thyroparathyroidectomy), rats (decapitation), and mice (loss of parathyroids through ablation of *Hoxa3*). Recent studies in genetically engineered mice have served to demonstrate that the parathyroids (and PTH) have a greater impact on blood calcium regulation than PTHrP *(4,5)*. The *Pthrp* and *Hoxa3* gene deletions were placed into the same colony, such that *Pthrp*-null, *Hoxa3*-null, and *Hoxa3/Pthrp* double mutants would be present within the same litter. In this controlled situation, single mutant *Pthrp*-null fetuses had a modestly reduced blood calcium (equal to the maternal calcium concentration), single mutant *Hoxa3*-null fetuses had a markedly reduced blood calcium (below the maternal calcium concentration), and *Hoxa3/Pthrp* double mutants had the lowest blood calcium *(5)*. Thus, lack of PTH

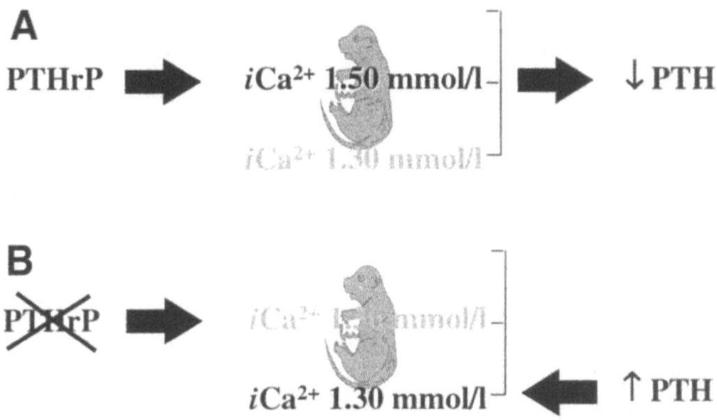

Fig. 1. Fetal blood calcium regulation. **A**, Normal high fetal calcium level, which is dependent on PTHrP, activates the parathyroid CaSR, and PTH is suppressed. **B**, In the absence of PTHrP, the fetal calcium level falls to a level that is now set by the parathyroid CaSR; PTH is stimulated to maintain the ionized calcium at the normal adult level (= maternal). Reproduced with permission from ref. *1*.

had a greater impact on the fetal blood calcium than lack of PTHrP; the combined loss of both PTH and PTHrP resulted in the lowest blood calcium level, a level that is equal to that observed in fetal mice lacking the PTH/PTHrP receptor (*Pthr1*-null fetuses) in the same genetic background.

Fetal parathyroids also are required for normal regulation of serum magnesium and phosphate concentrations, as observed in thyroparathyroidectomized fetal lambs that had a reduced serum magnesium concentration *(26)* and an increase in the serum phosphate level *(27)*. Similarly, absence of PTH and parathyroids in *Hoxa3*-null fetuses also causes hypomagnesemia and hyperphosphatemia *(4)*. Absence of PTHrP alone causes hyperphosphatemia, but the serum magnesium concentration is unaltered (unpublished data; ref. *4*).

Although a *Pth*-null model has now been published, the effects of lack of PTH on fetal calcium, phosphate or magnesium concentrations has not been reported *(28)*.

As discussed (*see* section titled Fetal Regulation), there is consistent evidence that PTHrP regulates placental calcium transfer, but conflicting evidence between sheep and mouse models that parathyroids are required for this process or that parathyroids make PTHrP. A detailed examination of normal fetal rat parathyroids found no detectable PTHrP mRNA by *in situ* hybridization or rt-PCR, and no detectable PTHrP by immunohistochemistry *(29)*. The fetal parathyroids are required for normal accretion of mineral by the fetal skeleton, as discussed in section entitled Fetal Skeleton.

CALCIUM-SENSING RECEPTOR

Postnatally, the CaSR sets the ionized calcium concentration in the peripheral circulation through its actions to regulate PTH. Homozygous ablation of the CaSR results in severe hyperparathyroidism and hypercalcemia *(30)*, analogous to the human condition of neonatal severe primary hyperparathyroidism. However, in fetal life, the role of the CaSR is less clearly established. The normal elevation of the fetal serum calcium above the maternal calcium concentration is dependent on PTHrP but not the CaSR; instead, the CaSR is likely suppressing PTH in response to the elevated fetal serum calcium concentration (Fig. 1A). In the absence of PTHrP (*Pthrp*-null fetuses), the fetal serum calcium falls to the normal adult level and the serum PTH is increased, likely indicating the responsiveness of the CaSR to this situation (Fig. 1B). The serum calcium increases above the normal fetal level in response to ablation of the CaSR in fetal life, and the serum PTH increases in a stepwise fashion from wt to $Casr^{+/-}$ to *Casr* null *(8)*. However, the serum calcium of *Casr*-null fetuses is no higher than that of the heterozygous (*Casr*$^{+/-}$) siblings *(8)*, indicating that (unlike in postnatal life) some aspect of the intrauterine environment prevents *Casr*-null fetuses from achieving a higher blood calcium level. The CaSR is clearly dependent on PTH but not PTHrP in order to contribute to the regulation of the fetal blood calcium level. Loss of PTHrP does not impair the effect of ablation of the CaSR to increase the fetal calcium level (*Casr/Pthrp* double mutant; ref. *8*). However, if the effect of PTH is blocked by simultaneous deletion of the PTH/PTHrP receptor (*Casr/Pthr1* double mutant), then ablation of the CaSR does not affect the fetal blood calcium level *(8)*. Similarly, in the absence of PTH (*Hoxa*-null), ablation of the CaSR has no effect on the fetal blood calcium (*Casr/Hoxa3* double mutant; ref. *4*).

Ablation of the CaSR has also been noted to decrease the rate of transfer of calcium across the placenta *(8)*, and we have noted that the CaSR is expressed in murine placenta *(31)*. The reduction in placental calcium transfer may be a consequence of the loss of calcium sensing capability within the placenta; alternatively, it may be that downregulation of calcium transfer is in response to the elevated serum calcium concentration or the elevated PTH concentrations that occur in these null mice.

In addition to raising the blood calcium and increasing PTH secretion, ablation of the CaSR would be expected to decrease renal calcium clearance as it does in the adult *(30)*. However, *Casr*$^{+/-}$ and *Casr*-null fetal mice have increased amniotic fluid calcium levels, suggesting that renal calcium excretion is increased in proportion to the raised serum calcium concentration *(8)*. The discrepancy between adult and fetal effects of CaSR ablation on renal calcium handling may be explained by the observation that the kidneys express very low levels of CaSR mRNA until the first postnatal day *(32)*.

THYMUS

PTH is not solely produced in the parathyroids; *Gcm2*-null mice lack the two parathyroids that are normally present in mice but have parathyroid tissue in the thymus that produces relatively normal amounts of PTH *(33)*. In contrast, *Hoxa3*-null mice lack parathyroids and thymus and have completely absent PTH *(4)*. Whether thymic PTH normally contributes to fetal calcium metabolism has not been determined. Rats and mice have two parathyroid glands, in contrast to humans, who have four (and occasionally more than four). Whether thymic parathyroid tissue in mice is the evolutionary equivalent of the lower parathyroids of humans has not been determined.

FETAL KIDNEYS AND AMNIOTIC FLUID

Fetal kidneys may partly regulate calcium homeostasis by adjusting the relative reabsorption and excretion of calcium, magnesium, and phosphate by the renal tubules in response to the filtered load and other factors, such as PTHrP and/or PTH *(1)*. The fetal kidneys may also participate by synthesizing 1,25-D, but because absence of VDR in fetal mice does not impair fetal calcium homeostasis or placental calcium transfer *(7)*, it appears likely that renal production of 1,25-D is relatively unimportant for fetal calcium homeostasis.

Renal calcium handling in fetal life may be less important as compared with the adult for the regulation of calcium homeostasis because calcium excreted by the kidneys is not permanently lost to the fetus. Fetal urine is the major source of fluid and solute in the amniotic fluid, and fetal swallowing of amniotic fluid is a pathway by which excreted calcium can be made available again to the fetus.

FETAL SKELETON

The skeleton must undergo substantial growth and be sufficiently mineralized by the end of gestation to support the organism, but as in the adult, the fetal skeleton participates in the regulation of mineral homeostasis. Calcium accreted by the fetal skeleton may be subsequently resorbed to help maintain the concentration of calcium in the blood, as indicated by several lines of evidence. Maternal hypocalcemia caused by thyroparathyroidectomy or calcitonin infusion increases the basal level of bone resorption in subsequently cultured fetal rat bones *(34,35)*. These effects were blocked by previous fetal decapitation, which is thought to mimic the effects of thyroparathyroidectomy *(34,35)*; thus, fetal hyperparathyroidism mobilized calcium from the skeleton. Further, in response to maternal hypocalcemia, fetal rat parathyroid glands enlarge *(36,37)*, and fetal femur length and mineral ash content are reduced *(38)*. Several recent observations in genetically engineered mice also support a role for the skeleton in fetal calcium homeostasis. The ionized calcium of PTH/PTHrP receptor-ablated fetal mice (*Pthr1*-null) is lower than that of *Pthrp*-null fetal mice despite the fact that placental calcium transport is supranormal in *Pthr1*-null fetuses and subnormal in *Pthrp*-null fetuses *(3)*. Lack of bone responsiveness to the amino-terminal portion of PTH and PTHrP may well, therefore, contribute to the hypocalcemia in mice without PTH/PTHrP receptors. Placement of a constitutively active PTH/PTHrP receptor into the growth plates of *Pthrp*-null fetuses not only reverses the chondrodysplasia *(39)* but results in a higher fetal blood calcium level (unpublished data). *Casr*-null fetuses have a higher ionized calcium than normal, and this is maintained at least in part through increased PTH-stimulated bone resorption *(8)*. As a consequence of this increased resorption, the skeletal calcium and magnesium content of *Casr*-null skeletons is significantly depleted as compared to their siblings (unpublished observations; ref. *8*).

Functioning fetal parathyroid glands are needed for normal skeletal mineral accretion because thyroparathyroidectomy in fetal lambs caused decreased skeletal calcium content and rachitic changes *(40,41)*. These effects could be partly reversed or prevented by fetal calcium and phosphate infusions; thus, much of the effect of fetal parathyroidectomy was caused by a decrease in blood levels of calcium and phosphate *(41)*. Recent examination of the skeletons of the aparathyroid *Hoxa3*-null fetuses are consistent with these observations in fetal lambs because, despite a normal rate of placental calcium transfer, *Hoxa3*-null fetuses have skeletons that have accreted less calcium and magnesium by the end of gestation *(5)*.

Further comparative study of *Pthrp*-null, *Pthr1*-null, and *Hoxa3*-null fetuses has clarified the relative role of PTH and PTHrP in regulation of the development and mineralization of the fetal skeleton. PTHrP produced locally in the growth plate directs the development of the cartilaginous scaffold that is later broken down and transformed into endochondral bone *(42)*, whereas PTH controls the mineralization of bone through its contribution to maintaining the fetal blood calcium and magnesium *(5)*. In the absence of PTHrP, a severe chondrodysplasia results *(18)*, but the fetal skeleton is fully mineralized *(5)*. In the absence of parathyroids and PTH (*Hoxa3*-null), endochondral bone forms normally but is significantly undermineralized *(5)*. Because the blood calcium and magnesium were also significantly reduced in *Hoxa3*-null fetuses, the effect of lack of PTH on bone may have been through its effect on maintaining the blood calcium and magnesium. That is, by impairing the amount of mineral presented to the skeletal surface and to osteoblasts, lack of PTH thereby impaired mineral accretion by the skeleton. When both PTH and PTHrP are deleted (*Hoxa3/Pthrp* double-mutants), the typical *Pthrp*-null chondrodysplasia results but the skeleton is smaller and contains less mineral *(5)*. Similarly, in the absence of the PTH/PTHrP receptor, *Pthr1*-null skeletons are significantly undermineralized *(5)*. Therefore, functioning fetal parathyroids are required for normal mineralization of the skeleton; the specific contribution may be through PTH alone. Whether that contribution is through direct actions of PTH on osteoblasts, or indirect through the actions of PTH to maintain the fetal blood calcium, remains to be clarified.

Apart from undermineralization of the skeleton, the lengths of the long bones and the growth plates of the *Hoxa3*-null were normal at both the gross and microscopic level, and the expression of several osteoblast and osteoclast specific genes was unaltered by loss of parathyroids and PTH *(5)*. In other words, loss of PTH did not appear to affect the development of the cartilaginous scaffold or of the bone matrix that replaced it, but loss of PTH did impair the final mineralization of that bone matrix. It is, therefore, unlikely that abnormal osteoblast function can explain the reduced mineralization of *Hoxa3*-null bones. However, it is clear that the PTH1 receptor influences osteoblast function in the fetal growth plate because *Pthr1*-null growth plates show a defect in osteoblast function and reduced expression of osteopontin, osteocalcin, and interstitial collagenase *(43,44)*. Because PTHrP is produced locally in the growth plate and periosteum it is likely the ligand that normally acts on the PTH1 receptor to regulate these genes. However, because the expression of osteopontin, osteocalcin, and interstitial collagenase is not reduced in the *Pthrp*-null fetus *(43)* and there is no evidence of impaired osteoblast function *(44)*, PTH may be able to penetrate the relatively avascular growth plate and compensate for the absence of PTHrP. The elevated PTH levels observed in the *Pthrp*-null fetus are compatible with this observation *(5)*. Therefore, osteopontin, osteocalcin, and interstitial collagenase may be downregulated in the *Pthr1*-null fetus because neither PTH nor PTHrP can act in the absence of the PTH1 receptor; these genes are not downregulated by absence of PTH or PTHrP alone. Because only *Pthr1*-null shows evidence of impaired osteoblast function *(44)* but both the *Hoxa3* null and the *Pthr1* null show a similar degree of reduced mineralization *(5)*, the undermineralization of both null phenotypes may be the result of the reduced availability of mineral presented to the osteoblast surface (i.e., the reduced blood calcium and magnesium level in both phenotypes); the availability of mineral is dependent on the action of PTH.

The recently reported *Pth*-null mice also have undermineralized skeletons, but they differ from the phenotype of *Hoxa3*-null mice in that the long bones of the *Pth*-null mice are modestly shortened, and there is evidence of reduced osteoblast number and function in studies that were not been performed on *Hoxa3*-null mice *(28)*. The *Pth*-null and *Hoxa3*-null models will need to be compared within the same genetic background to be certain which aspects of the respective phenotypes are caused by the loss of PTH and which might be caused by other confounding effects (e.g., aparathyroid and athymic in *Hoxa3*-null mice, marked parathyroid hyperplasia in *Pth*-null mice, lower blood calcium in C57BL6 background of studied *Pth*-null mice vs higher blood calcium in Black Swiss background of studied *Hoxa3*-null mice, etc).

In summary, normal mineralization of the fetal skeleton requires intact fetal parathyroid glands and adequate delivery of calcium to the fetal circulation. Although both PTH and PTHrP are involved, PTH plays the more critical role in ensuring full mineralization of the skeleton before term.

MATERNAL SKELETON

The maternal skeleton may accrete mineral early in gestation in preparation for the peak fetal demand later in pregnancy, such that the maternal skeleton contributes to the mineral ultimately accreted by the fetal skeleton (reviewed in detail in refs. *2* and *45*). The contribution during pregnancy is much more modest than the 5–10% decline in bone density that occurs during lactation in humans and the 30% or greater decrease in maternal skeletal mineral content during lactation in rodents *(2,45)*. Experimental calcitonin deficiency induced by thyroidectomy worsened the maternal calcium losses (reviewed in refs. *1* and *2*), a finding that prompted the hypothesis that calcitonin normally protects the maternal skeleton from excessive resorption during pregnancy and lactation. The decline in bone mineral content that occurs during pregnancy and (especially) lactation is normally reversed after weaning.

FETAL RESPONSE TO MATERNAL HYPERPARATHYROIDISM

In humans, maternal primary hyperparathyroidism has been associated in the literature with adverse fetal outcomes, including spontaneous abortion, stillbirth, and tetany *(2)*. These adverse fetal outcomes are thought to result from suppression of the fetal parathyroid glands; because PTH cannot cross the placenta, the fetal parathyroid suppression may result from increased calcium flux across the placenta to the fetus, facilitated by the maternal hypercalcemia. Similar suppression of the fetal parathyroids occurs when the mother has hypercalcemia because of familial hypocalciuric hypercalcemia *(2)*. Chronic elevation of the maternal serum calcium in *Casr*$^{+/-}$ mice (the equivalent of familial hypocalciuric hypercalcemia in humans) results in suppression of the fetal PTH level as compared with fetuses obtained from wild-type sibling mothers *(8)*, but fetal outcome is not notably affected by this.

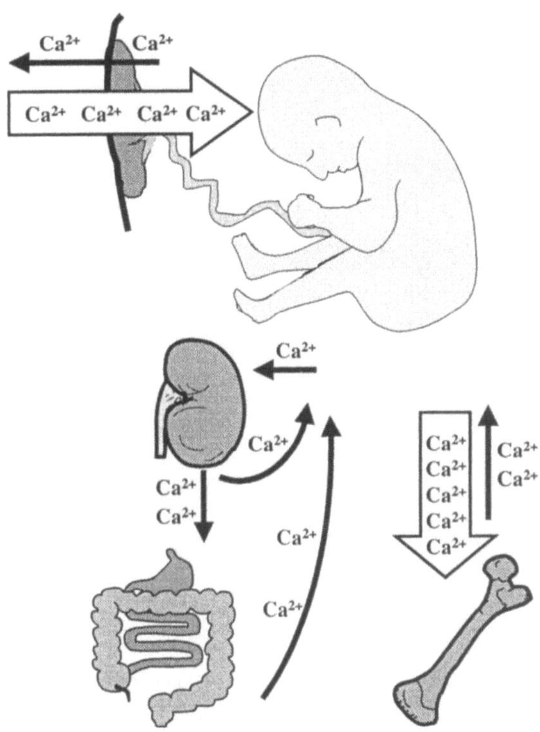

Fig. 2. Calcium sources in fetal life. Reproduced with permission from ref. *1*.

FETAL RESPONSE TO MATERNAL HYPOPARATHYROIDISM

Maternal hypoparathyroidism in human pregnancy has been associated with the development of intrauterine, fetal hyperparathyroidism. This condition is characterized by fetal parathyroid gland hyperplasia, generalized skeletal demineralization, subperiosteal bone resorption, bowing of the long bones, osteitis fibrosa cystica, rib and limb fractures, low birth weight, spontaneous abortion, stillbirth, and neonatal death *(2)*. Similar skeletal findings have been reported in the fetuses and neonates of women with pseudohypoparathyroidism, renal tubular acidosis, and chronic renal failure *(2)*. These changes in human skeletons differ from what has been found in animal models of maternal hypocalcemia (discussed previously), in which the fetal skeleton and the blood calcium is generally normal.

INTEGRATED FETAL CALCIUM HOMEOSTASIS

The evidence discussed in the preceding sections suggests the following summary models.

Calcium Sources

The main flux of calcium (and other minerals) is across the placenta and into fetal bone, but calcium is also made available to the fetal circulation through several routes (Fig. 2). Some calcium filtered by the kidneys is reabsorbed into the circulation; calcium that is excreted by the kidneys into the urine and amniotic fluid may be swallowed and absorbed by the intestine; calcium is also resorbed from the developing skeleton to maintain the circulating calcium concentration. Some calcium also returns to the maternal circulation (backflux). The maternal skeleton is a critical source of mineral (in addition to maternal dietary intake), and the maternal skeleton is compromised in maternal dietary deficiency states in order to provide to the fetus.

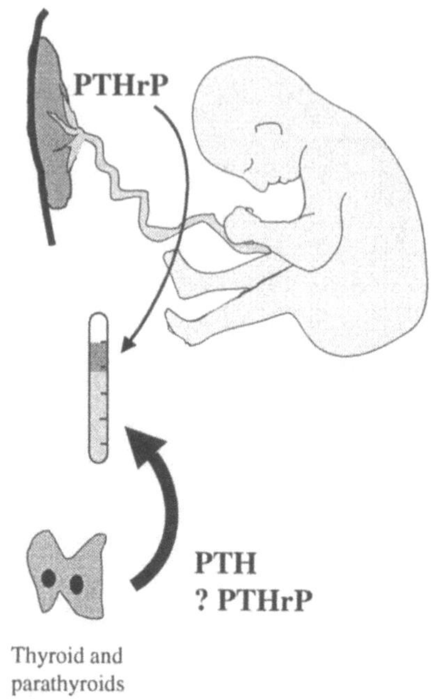

Fig. 3. Fetal blood calcium regulation. PTH has a more dominant effect on fetal blood calcium regulation than PTHrP, with blood calcium represented schematically as a thermometer (light gray = contribution of PTH; dark gray = contribution of PTHrP). In the absence of PTHrP, the blood calcium falls to the maternal level. In the absence of PTH (*Hoxa3*-null that has absent PTH but normal circulating PTHrP levels), the blood calcium falls well below the maternal calcium concentration. In the absence of both PTHrP and PTH (*Hoxa3/Pthrp* double mutant) the blood calcium falls even further than in the absence of PTH alone. Reproduced with permission from ref. *1*.

Blood Calcium Regulation

The fetal blood calcium is set at a level higher than maternal through the actions of PTHrP and PTH acting in concert (among other potential factors; Fig. 3). Although the parathyroid CaSR appears to respond appropriately to this increased level of calcium by suppressing PTH, the low level of PTH is critically required for maintaining a normal blood calcium and normal mineral accretion by the skeleton. 1,25-D synthesis and secretion are, in turn, suppressed due to the effects of low PTH, and high blood calcium and phosphate. The parathyroids may play a central role by producing PTH and PTHrP, or may produce PTH alone whereas PTHrP is produced by the placenta and other fetal tissues.

PTH and PTHrP, both present in the fetal circulation, independently and additively regulate the fetal blood calcium, with PTH having the greater effect. Neither hormone can make up for absence of the other: if one is missing, the blood calcium is reduced, and if both are missing, the blood calcium is reduced even further. How the PTH/PTHrP (PTH1) receptor can mediate the actions of these two ligands in the circulation, simultaneously and independently, is not clear. The contribution of PTHrP to the fetal blood calcium may not be through the PTH1 receptor at all, but perhaps only through the actions of mid-molecular PTHrP to regulate placental transfer of calcium (a process which has been shown to be independent of the PTH1 receptor). Thus, PTH may contribute to the blood calcium through actions on the PTH1 receptor in classic target tissues (kidney, bone), whereas PTHrP might contribute through placental calcium transfer and actions on other (non-PTH) receptors.

The normal elevation of the fetal blood calcium above the maternal calcium concentration was historically considered as the first evidence that placental calcium transfer was largely an active pro-

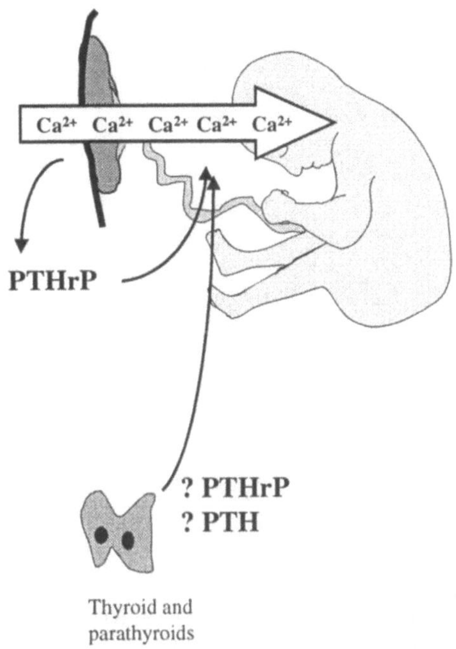

Fig. 4. Placental calcium transfer is regulated by PTHrP but not by PTH. Whether the parathyroids produce PTHrP or not is uncertain; experiments in *Hoxa3*-null mice indicate that absence of parathyroids does not impair placental calcium transfer. Reproduced with permission from ref. *1*.

cess. However, the fetal blood calcium level is not simply determined by the rate of placental calcium transfer because placental calcium transfer is normal in *Hoxa3*-null and increased in *Pthr1*-null mice, but both null phenotypes have significantly reduced blood calcium levels *(3,4)*. Also, *Casr*-null fetuses have reduced placental calcium transfer but markedly increased blood calcium levels *(8)*.

Placental Calcium Transfer

Placental calcium transfer is regulated by PTHrP but not by PTH (Fig. 4). Although the exact tissue source(s) of PTHrP that are relevant for placental calcium transfer remain uncertain, the placenta is one proven source of PTHrP that is likely involved in calcium transfer. Whether the parathyroids produce PTHrP or not is uncertain; in contrast to fetal lambs, experiments in *Hoxa3*-null mice indicate that absence of parathyroids does not impair placental calcium transfer*(4)*.

Skeletal Mineralization

PTH and PTHrP have separate roles with respect to skeletal development and mineralization (Fig. 5). PTH normally acts systemically (i.e., outside of bone) to direct the mineralization of the bone matrix by maintaining the blood calcium at the adult level, and possibly by direct actions on osteoblasts within the bone matrix. PTH is capable of directing certain aspects of endochondral bone development in the absence of PTHrP (e.g., regulation of expression of osteocalcin, osteopontin, interstitial collagenase within the growth plate; ref. *5*). In contrast, PTHrP acts both locally within the growth plate to direct endochondral bone development, and outside of bone to affect skeletal development and mineralization by contributing to the regulation of the blood calcium and placental calcium transfer. PTH has the more critical role in maintaining skeletal mineral accretion as compared to PTHrP.

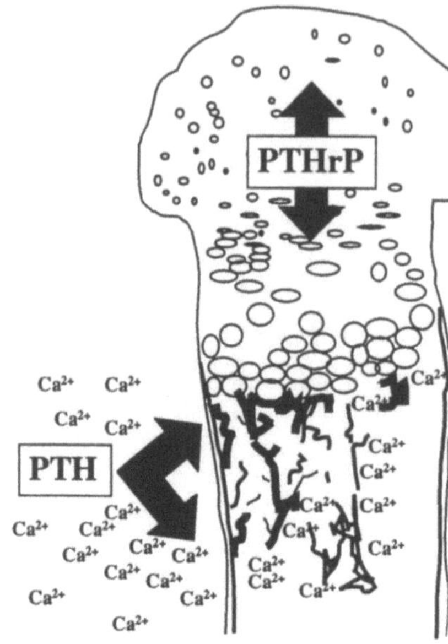

Fig. 5. Schematic model of the relative contribution of PTH and PTHrP to endochondral bone formation and skeletal mineralization. PTHrP is produced within the cartilaginous growth plate and directs the development of this scaffold that will later be broken down and replaced by bone. In the absence of PTHrP (*Pthrp*-null), a severe chondrodysplasia results but the skeleton is normally mineralized. PTH reaches the skeleton systemically from the parathyroids and directs the accretion of mineral by the developing bone matrix. In the absence of PTH (*Hoxa3*-null fetus), the bones form normally but are severely undermineralized. Reproduced with permission from ref. *1*.

The rate of placental calcium transfer has been historically considered to be the rate-limiting step for skeletal mineral accretion. However, it is now possible to conclude that the rate of placental calcium transfer is not the rate limiting step for skeletal mineralization since the accretion of mineral was reduced in the presence of normal placental calcium transfer (*Hoxa3*-null) and increased placental calcium transfer (*Pthr1*-null mice; ref. *5*). Furthermore, *Pthrp*-null fetuses showed normal skeletal mineral content in the presence of reduced placental calcium transfer and a modestly reduced blood calcium *(5)*. The rate-limiting step for skeletal mineralization appears to be the blood calcium level, which in turn is largely determined by PTH. The level of blood calcium achieved in the *Pthrp*-null—that is, the normal adult level of blood calcium—is sufficient to allow normal skeletal accretion of mineral, whereas lower levels of blood calcium (*Hoxa3*-null, *Pthr1*-null, and *Hoxa3/Pthrp* double-mutant mice) impair the rate of mineral accretion.

ACKNOWLEDGMENTS

Supported by a Scholarship and Operating Grants from the Canadian Institutes for Health Research (formerly Medical Research Council of Canada), in addition to support from Memorial University of Newfoundland. I gratefully acknowledge the support and advice of Dr. Henry M. Kronenberg, my collaborators (Drs. Marie Demay, James Friel, Robert Gagel, Andrew Karaplis, Gerard Karsenty, Nancy Manley, Jack Martin, Jane Moseley, Ernestina Schipani, and Peter Wookey), my research assistant Neva Fudge, and my students.

REFERENCES

1. Kovacs, C. S. (2003) Fetal mineral homeostasis, Chapter 11, in Pediatric Bone: Biology and Diseases (Glorieux, F. H., Pettifor, J. M., and Jüppner, H., eds.), Academic Press, San Diego, CA, pp. 271–302.

2. Kovacs, C. S. and Kronenberg, H. M. (1997) Maternal-fetal calcium and bone metabolism during pregnancy, puerperium and lactation. *Endocr. Rev.* **18,** 832–872.
3. Kovacs, C. S., Lanske, B., Hunzelman, J. L., Guo, J., Karaplis, A. C., and Kronenberg, H. M. (1996) Parathyroid hormone-related peptide (PTHrP) regulates fetal-placental calcium transport through a receptor distinct from the PTH/PTHrP receptor. *Proc. Natl. Acad. Sci. USA* **93,** 15233–15238.
4. Kovacs, C. S., Manley, N. R., Moseley, J. M., Martin, T. J., and Kronenberg, H. M. (2001) Fetal parathyroids are not required to maintain placental calcium transport. *J. Clin. Invest.* **107,** 1007–1015.
5. Kovacs, C. S., Chafe, L. L., Fudge, N. J., Friel, J. K., and Manley, N. R. (2001) PTH regulates fetal blood calcium and skeletal mineralization independently of PTHrP. *Endocrinology* **142,** 4983–4993.
6. Li, Y. C., Pirro, A. E., Amling, M., Delling, G., Baron, R., Bronson, R., and Demay, M. B. (1997) Targeted ablation of the vitamin D receptor: an animal model of vitamin D dependent rickets type II with alopecia. *Proc. Natl. Acad. Sci. USA* **94,** 9831–9835.
7. Woodland, M. L., Chafe, L. L., McDonald, K. R., Demay, M. B., and Kovacs, C. S. (2000) Ablation of the VDR minimally affects fetal-placental calcium metabolism and placental calcitropic gene expression [abstract]. *J. Bone Miner. Res.* **15(Suppl 1),** S181.
8. Kovacs, C. S., Ho-Pao, C. L., Hunzelman, J. L., Lanske, B., Fox, J., Seidman, J. G., et al. (1998) Regulation of murine fetal-placental calcium metabolism by the calcium-sensing receptor. *J. Clin. Invest.* **101,** 2812–2820.
9. Moore, E. S., Langman, C. B., Favus, M. J., and Coe, F. L. (1985) Role of fetal 1,25-dihydroxyvitamin D production in intrauterine phosphorus and calcium homeostasis. *Pediatr. Res.* **19,** 566–569.
10. McDonald, K. R., Woodland, M. L., Chafe, L. L., Friel, J. K., Hoff, A. O., Cote, G. J., et al. (2001) Analysis of calcitonin null mice reveals a selective defect in fetal magnesium but not calcium metabolism, in *Program & Abstracts Book of ENDO2001*, the 83rd Annual Meeting of the Endocrine Society, Denver, Colorado, June 20–23, 2001, Endocrine Society, Bethesda, MD, pp. 255.
11. Lachenmaier-Currle, U. and Harmeyer, J. (1989) Placental transport of calcium and phosphorus in pigs. *J. Perinat. Med.* **17,** 127–136.
12. Garel, J. M. and Barlet, J. P. (1978) Calcitonin in the mother, fetus and newborn. *Ann. Biol. Anim. Biochim. Biophys.* **18,** 53–68.
13. Garel, J. M., Milhaud, G., and Jost, A. (1968) [Hypocalcemic and hypophosphatemic action of thyrocalcitonin in fetal rats]. *C. R. Acad. Sci. Hebd. Seances. Acad. Sci. D.* **267,** 344–347.
14. Care, A. D., Caple, I. W., Abbas, S. K., and Pickard, D. W. (1986) The effect of fetal thyroparathyroidectomy on the transport of calcium across the ovine placenta to the fetus. *Placenta* **7,** 417–424.
15. Hoff, A. O., Thomas, P. M., Cote, G. J., Qiu, H., Bain, S., Puerner, D., et al. (1998) Generation of a calcitonin knockout mouse model. *Bone* **23(suppl 5),** S164.
16. McDonald, K. R., Woodland, M. L., Chafe, L. L., Hoff, A. O., Cote, G. J., Gagel, R. F., et al. (2000) Effects of calcitonin gene deletion on fetal-placental calcium metabolism and maternal fertility. *J. Bone Miner. Res.* **15(Suppl 1),** S251.
17. Philbrick, W. M., Wysolmerski, J. J., Galbraith, S., Holt, E., Orloff, J. J., Yang, K. H., et al. (1996) Defining the roles of parathyroid hormone-related protein in normal physiology. *Physiol. Rev.* **76,** 127–173.
18. Karaplis, A. C., Luz, A., Glowacki, J., Bronson, R. T., Tybulewicz, V. L., Kronenberg, H. M., et al. (1994) Lethal skeletal dysplasia from targeted disruption of the parathyroid hormone-related peptide gene. *Genes Dev.* **8,** 277–289.
19. Weatherley, A. J., Ross, R., Pickard, D. W., and Care, A. D. (1983) The transfer of calcium during perfusion of the placenta and intact and thyroparathyroidectomized sheep. *Placenta* **4,** 271–277.
20. Robinson, N. R., Sibley, C. P., Mughal, M. Z., and Boyd, R. D. (1989) Fetal control of calcium transport across the rat placenta. *Pediatr. Res.* **26,** 109–115.
21. Rodda, C. P., Kubota, M., Heath, J. A., Ebeling, P. R., Moseley, J. M., Care, A. D., et al. (1988) Evidence for a novel parathyroid hormone-related protein in fetal lamb parathyroid glands and sheep placenta: comparisons with a similar protein implicated in humoral hypercalcaemia of malignancy. *J. Endocrinol.* **117,** 261–271.
22. Care, A. D., Abbas, S. K., Pickard, D. W., Barri, M., Drinkhill, M., Findlay, J. B., et al. (1990) Stimulation of ovine placental transport of calcium and magnesium by mid-molecule fragments of human parathyroid hormone-related protein. *Exp. Physiol.* **75,** 605–608.
23. Wu, T. L., Vasavada, R. C., Yang, K., Massfelder, T., Ganz, M., Abbas, S. K., et al. (1996) Structural and physiologic characterization of the mid-region secretory species of parathyroid hormone-related protein. *J. Biol. Chem.* **271,** 24371–24381.
24. Shaw, A. J., Mughal, M. Z., Maresh, M. J., and Sibley, C. P. (1991) Effects of two synthetic parathyroid hormone-related protein fragments on maternofetal transfer of calcium and magnesium and release of cyclic AMP by the in-situ perfused rat placenta. *J. Endocrinol.* **129,** 399–404.
25. Barlet, J. P., Davicco, M. J., Rouffet, J., Coxam, V., and Lefaivre, J. (1994) Short communication: parathyroid hormone-related peptide does not stimulate phosphate placental transport. *Placenta* **15,** 441–444.
26. Barri, M., Abbas, S. K., Pickard, D. W., Hammonds, R. G., Wood, W. I., Caple, I. W., Martin, T. J., and Care, A. D. (1990) Fetal magnesium homeostasis in the sheep. *Exp. Physiol.* **75,** 681–688.
27. MacIsaac, R. J., Horne, R. S., Caple, I. W., Martin, T. J., and Wintour, E. M. (1993) Effects of thyroparathyroidectomy, parathyroid hormone, and PTHrP on kidneys of ovine fetuses. *Am. J. Physiol.* **264,** E37–E44.
28. Miao, D., He, B., Karaplis, A. C., and Goltzman, D. (2002) Parathyroid hormone is essential for normal fetal bone formation. *J. Clin. Invest.* **109,** 1173–1182.

29. Tucci, J., Russell, A., Senior, P. V., Fernley, R., Ferraro, T., and Beck, F. (1996) The expression of parathyroid hormone and parathyroid hormone-related protein in developing rat parathyroid glands. *J. Mol. Endocrinol.* **17,** 149–157.
30. Ho, C., Conner, D. A., Pollak, M. R., Ladd, D. J., Kifor, O., Warren, H. B., et al. (1995) A mouse model of human familial hypocalciuric hypercalcemia and neonatal severe hyperparathyroidism. *Nat. Genet.* **11,** 389–394.
31. Kovacs, C. S., Chafe, L. L., Woodland, M. L., McDonald, K. R., Fudge, N. J., and Wookey, P. J. (2002) Calcitropic gene expression suggests a role for intraplacental yolk sac in maternal-fetal calcium exchange. *Am. J. Physiol. Endocrinol. Metab.* **282,** E721–E732.
32. Chattopadhyay, N., Baum, N., Bai, M., Riccardi, D., Hebert, S. C., Harris, E. W., et al. (1996) Ontogeny of the extracellular calcium-sensing receptor in rat kidney. *Am. J. Physiol.* **271,** F736–F743.
33. Günther, T., Chen, Z. F., Kim, J., Priemel, M., Rueger, J. M., Amling, M., et al. (2000) Genetic ablation of parathyroid glands reveals another source of parathyroid hormone. *Nature* **406,** 199–203.
34. Rebut-Bonneton, C., Garel, J. M., and Delbarre, F. (1983) Parathyroid hormone, calcitonin, 1,25-dihydroxycholecalciferol, and basal bone resorption in the rat fetus. *Calcif. Tissue Int.* **35,** 183–189.
35. Rebut-Bonneton, C., Demignon, J., Amor, B., and Miravet, L. (1983) Effect of calcitonin in pregnant rats on bone resorption in fetuses. *J. Endocrinol.* **99,** 347–353.
36. Sinclair, J. G. (1942) Fetal rat parathyroids as affected by changes in maternal serum calcium and phosphorus through parathyroidectomy and dietary control. *J. Nutr.* **23,** 141–152.
37. Garel, J. M. and Geloso-Meyer, A. (1971) [Fetal hyperparathyroidism in rats following maternal hypoparathyroidism]. *Rev. Eur. Etud. Clin. Biol.* **16,** 174–178.
38. Chalon, S. and Garel, J. M. (1985) Plasma calcium control in the rat fetus. I. Influence of maternal hormones. *Biol. Neonate* **48,** 313–322.
39. Schipani, E., Lanske, B., Hunzelman, J., Luz, A., Kovacs, C. S., Lee, K., et al. (1997) Targeted expression of constitutively active PTH/PTHrP receptors delays endochondral bone formation and rescues PTHrP-less mice. *Proc. Natl. Acad. Sci. USA* **94,** 13689–13694.
40. Aaron, J. E., Makins, N. B., Caple, I. W., Abbas, S. K., Pickard, D. W., and Care, A. D. (1989) The parathyroid glands in the skeletal development of the ovine foetus. *Bone Miner.* **7,** 13–22.
41. Aaron, J. E., Abbas, S. K., Colwell, A., Eastell, R., Oakley, B. A., Russell, R. G., and Care, A. D. (1992) Parathyroid gland hormones in the skeletal development of the ovine foetus: the effect of parathyroidectomy with calcium and phosphate infusion. *Bone Miner.* **16,** 121–129.
42. Karsenty, G. (2001) Chondrogenesis just ain't what it used to be. *J. Clin. Invest.* **107,** 405–407.
43. Lanske, B., Divieti, P., Kovacs, C. S., Pirro, A., Landis, W. J., Krane, S. M., et al. (1998) The parathyroid hormone/parathyroid hormone-related peptide receptor mediates actions of both ligands in murine bone. *Endocrinology* **139,** 5192–5204.
44. Lanske, B., Amling, M., Neff, L., Guiducci, J., Baron, R., and Kronenberg, H. M. (1999) Ablation of the PTHrP gene or the PTH/PTHrP receptor gene leads to distinct abnormalities in bone development. *J. Clin. Invest.* **104,** 399–407.
45. Kovacs, C. S. (2001) Calcium and bone metabolism in pregnancy and lactation. *J. Clin. Endocrinol. Metab.* **86,** 2344–2348.

21

Control of Osteoblast Function and Bone Extracellular Matrix Mineralization by Vitamin D

Johannes P. T. M. van Leeuwen, Marjolein van Driel, and Hulbert A. P. Pols

INTRODUCTION: VITAMIN D

Vitamin D is the major regulator of calcium homeostasis and protects the organism from calcium deficiency via effects on the intestine, kidney, parathyroid gland, and bone. Disturbances in the vitamin D endocrine system, for example, vitamin D-dependent rickets type I and type II, result in profound effects on the mineralization of bone. Also, recent studies with vitamin D receptor (VDR) knockout mice show effects on bone. It is questioned whether vitamin D has a direct effect on bone formation and mineralization. In rickets and in particular vitamin D receptor knockout mice, calcium supplementation restores bone mineralization. However, the vitamin D receptor (*see* Vitamin D Receptor section) is present in osteoblasts, and vitamin D affects the expression of various genes in osteoblasts (*see* Introduction: Osteoblasts and Effects of Vitamin D on Osteoblast Function and Mineralization sections). Vitamin D regulates the expression of genes and osteoblast activity not in an independent manner but often in interaction with other hormones and/or growth factors (*see* section titled Interaction of Vitamin D with Other Factors).

The most biologically active vitamin D molecule is 1,25-dihydroxyvitamin D3 (1,25-$(OH)_2D_3$), which is formed after two consecutive hydroxylations in the liver (C-25 position) and kidney (C-1α position) of skin-derived vitamin D_3 (cholecalciferol). The vitamin D_3 molecule can also be hydroxylated at the C-24 position resulting in 24,25-$(OH)_2D_3$ or 1,24,25-$(OH)_3D_3$. The 24-hydroxylation was generally considered the first step in the degradation cascade of vitamin D_3. However, over the years data have accumulated that also metabolites formed in the C-24 hydroxylation cascade have biological activity (*see* Metabolism: 24-Hydroxylase Activity section).

VITAMIN D AND BONE

The relationship between vitamin D and bone is, among others, illustrated by the treatment of osteoporosis with vitamin D, which has been studied and discussed in various studies *(1,2)*. In addition, a reduction of fracture risk by treatment with vitamin D has been reported *(3–6)*. Last year, an overview of all randomized trials studying vitamin D treatment in elderly men or women with involutional or postmenopausal osteoporosis has been published *(7)*. However, the effects on calcium and phosphate homeostasis make it difficult to identify whether vitamin D is directly involved in control of bone metabolism. The bone abnormalities in hypo- and hypervitamin D states mostly result of indirect effects because of changes in concentrations of serum calcium and phosphate. For example, studies

From: *The Skeleton: Biochemical, Genetic, and Molecular Interactions in Development and Homeostasis*
Edited by: E. J. Massaro and J. M. Rogers © Humana Press Inc., Totowa, NJ

with patients with hereditary vitamin D-resistant rickets showed that normal mineralization can be achieved by intravenous supplementation of calcium *(8–11)*. Also in mice lacking the VDR, skeletal homeostasis could be preserved in mice with normal mineral ion homeostasis and not in hypocalcemic VDR-null mice *(12)*.

Albeit, during the last years a couple of in vivo studies with rats provided evidence for a direct anabolic effect of 1,25-$(OH)_2D_3$ on bone. Both chronic treatment with 1,25-$(OH)_2D_3$ *(13)* and short-term treatment *(14)* increased bone formation. Both treatment schemes increased the number of bone-forming cells (osteoblasts) or osteoblast precursor cells, which may underlie the increased bone formation. However, Amling et al. reported an increased osteoblast number, and osteoid volume in the hypocalcemic VDR-null mice *(12)*. Whether this is mouse-specific is not clear because direct bone anabolic effects of 1,25-$(OH)_2D_3$ in osteopenic ovariectomized rats also have been described *(15)*. A direct effect of vitamin D on bone is also suggested as the VDR is present in osteoblasts and precursors of the bone-resorbing cells (osteoclasts) and has more recently been identified in mature osteoclasts by reverse transcription polymerase chain reaction analysis and immunohistochemistry *(16–18)*. A recent study using mice transgenic for VDR under control of an osteoblast-specific (osteocalcin) promoter also indicated the bone anabolic effects of vitamin D by demonstrating a 20% increased trabecular bone volume and increased bone strength and reduced bone resorption surface in mice with enhanced osteoblast VDR levels *(19)*.

1,25-$(OH)_2D_3$ is involved in keeping the balance between bone formation and resorption by direct and indirect effects on both the osteoblasts and the osteoclasts. In the current review, we will discuss the direct effects of 1,25-$(OH)_2D_3$ on osteoblast function and mineralization.

INTRODUCTION: OSTEOBLASTS

Osteoblasts are the bone-forming cells and originate, like fibroblasts, adipocytes, and chondrocytes, from mesenchymal stem cells. The control of and switches in gene expression during proliferation and differentiation of osteoblasts have been extensively studied and described in detail for rat osteoblasts *(20)*. Comparable differentiation profiles have been described for mouse *(21,22)*, chicken *(23)*, and human osteoblasts *(24,25)*. In general, it can be concluded that osteoblasts proceed through a well-defined differentiation process, controlled by lineage specific factors, resulting in mineralization of the extracellular matrix formed and finally in the matrix-embedded osteocyte (for reviews, *see* refs. *20* and *26*). However, the available data show differences in details of expression of the osteoblast phenotype, which may be attributed to various causes like differences between species or origin of the osteoblast (i.e., site in the skeleton: e.g., long bone or calvaria derived). This may also be related to presence or absence of hormones, cytokines, mechanical loading, etc., thereby representing different metabolic stages or different culture conditions *(27)*. In view of these osteoblast characteristics, it is important to appreciate that not only hormonal responses but also other regulatory processes may be different depending on the differentiation status, origin, and in vitro culture conditions of the osteoblasts. In relation to this, the various osteosarcoma cell lines with osteoblastic characteristics used in research (e.g., UMR106, ROS 17/2.8, MG63, SaOS cells) are most likely to represent particular, different differentiation stages of the osteoblast and may show different qualitative and quantitative responses. These aspects will be more exemplified in relation to 1,25-$(OH)_2D_3$ responses in the next section.

EFFECTS OF VITAMIN D ON OSTEOBLAST FUNCTION AND MINERALIZATION

Osteoblasts are derived from multipotential progenitor cells within the bone marrow stroma that can also differentiate into cells of other mesenchymal lineages. 1,25-$(OH)_2D_3$ plays a role in the regulation of these early stages of human osteoblast differentiation by promoting an osteogenic differentiation (in human bone marrow stromal cell cultures; *[28]* and in clonal cell lines derived from human trabecular bone) although the induction of both osteogenic and adipocytic pathways have been described as well *(29,30)*. In bone marrow stromal cultures from species other than human (rat and mouse), 1,25-$(OH)_2D_3$ was clearly found to favor the differentiation into the osteoblastic instead of the adipocytic lineage *(31–35)*. However, it has been reported that in primary rat calvaria cells, 1,25-$(OH)_2D_3$ stimulated differentiation into adipocytes *(36)*. 1,25-$(OH)_2D_3$ has been shown to regulate the expression of genes and proteins involved in the developmental control and regulation of differentiation, cbfa1 *(37,38)*, I-mfa (inhibitor of the MyoD family; ref. *39*), and Notch *(40)*.

In vitro studies using osteoblast-like cells of various origin demonstrated clear effects of 1,25-$(OH)_2D_3$ on mRNA and protein expression and on enzyme activities. However, some contradictory effects have been described, for example, stimulation as well as inhibition of osteocalcin *(41–43)* and cbfa1 expression *(37,38)*. This can be attributed to various causes among other species differences, which will be discussed here with primary focus on data obtained with human osteoblasts. Initially, the effects on alkaline phosphatase, mineralization, apoptosis, and proliferation and next the effects of 1,25-$(OH)_2D_3$ on the regulation of collagen type I and various noncollagenous proteins, plasminogen, prostaglandins, and growth factors will be discussed.

Alkaline Phosphatase

Alkaline phosphatase activity, an important biochemical marker of bone formation *(44)* with a possible role in mineralization because of the hypophosphatasia observed in alkaline phosphate knockout mice, is shown in many in vitro osteoblast studies to be regulated by 1,25-$(OH)_2D_3$.

In human osteoblasts, 1,25-$(OH)_2D_3$ has been reported to stimulate the alkaline phosphatase activity *(45)*, alkaline phosphatase mRNA, and protein expression *(30)* during both proliferation and differentiation stages. But the stimulatory effect of 1,25-$(OH)_2D_3$ on alkaline phosphatase protein expression was not always found in late-stage postconfluental cultures *(46)*. Other studies, particularly on mature human osteoblasts, described synergistic effects of 1,25-$(OH)_2D_3$ and transforming growth factor (TGF)-β on alkaline phosphatase activity *(47–50)*.

1,25-$(OH)_2D_3$ treatment also was found to stimulate alkaline phosphatase activity in rat osteoblasts *(51,52)*. When different differentiation stages of rat osteoblasts were compared, acute 1,25-$(OH)_2D_3$ treatment inhibited alkaline phosphatase mRNA expression during the highest basal expression levels (early phase) but stimulated expression at the lowest basal expression levels (during the mineralization period of the cells; ref. *53*).

In contrast, in mouse osteoblastic cells, alkaline phosphatase activity was stimulated by 1,25-$(OH)_2D_3$ in the early phase of differentiation, and no effect was found during the late phase when mineralization occurs *(54)* or when alkaline phosphatase activity was reduced by 1,25-$(OH)_2D_3$ during confluency *(55)*.

Mineralization

Alkaline phosphatase activity is important for mineralization of bone and even of other tissues *(56,57)*. Speculations have been made that a stimulatory effect of 1,25-$(OH)_2D_3$ on the alkaline phosphatase activity of osteoblasts indicates a direct involvement of 1,25-$(OH)_2D_3$ in bone mineralization *(51)*. In rat bone, the cells with the highest alkaline phosphatase activity and the highest intracellular calcium content (regulated by 1,25-$(OH)_2D_3$) were the cells closest to the forming bone *(58)*. Electron microscopy showed that the origin of alkaline phosphatase-positive bone matrix vesicles was polarized to the mineral-facing side of osteoblasts *(59)*. In contrast, it has also been reported that when alkaline phosphatase activity is repressed, mouse osteoblasts still differentiate to a mineral-secreting phenotype *(60)*.

In human cultured osteoblasts, 1,25-$(OH)_2D_3$ has been reported to stimulate mineralization of the extracellular matrix, which was promoted by vitamin K *(61)*, and increased with advancing donor age *(62)*.The relation with multipotent stem cell differentiation is demonstrated by the vitamin D enhancement of extracellular mineralization by cells derived from adipose tissue *(63)*. Low doses of 1,25-$(OH)_2D_3$

stimulated the activity of ecto-NTP pyrophosphatase, that is involved in the regulation of mineralization in bone, whereas higher doses had no effect *(64)* or have even been reported to inhibit the mineralization of human osteoblasts *(65)*.

In rats, it has been found that 1,25-$(OH)_2D_3$ may stimulate bone mineralization by a direct effect on osteoblasts, stimulating phosphatidylserine synthesis, which is thought to be important for apatite formation and bone mineralization by binding calcium and phosphate to form calcium–phosphatidylserin–phosphate complexes *(66)*. Furthermore 1,25-$(OH)_2D_3$ is proposed to have a role in calcium transport from osteoblasts towards sites of active bone mineralization via the stimulation of calbindin-D9K synthesis *(67)*. However, it has been found that a 1,25-$(OH)_2D_3$-induced upregulation of alkaline phosphatase and osteocalcin genes in rat osteoblasts cultured on a collagen matrix was accompanied by an inhibited mineralization *(68)*.

In mouse osteoblast-like MC3T3 cells, treatment with 1,25-$(OH)_2D_3$ stimulated calcium accumulation during the mineralization stage of the cell culture *(54)*, and this could be blocked by constitutive calreticulin expression, which negatively interacts with the VDR *(69)*. However, it also has been shown that 1,25-$(OH)_2D_3$ downregulates mineralization in primary mouse osteoblast cultures, together with downregulation of Phex mRNA and protein, which are shown to be involved in cell differentiation and β-glycerophosphate-induced mineralization *(70)*. Also in mice with impaired function of the 25-hydroxyvitamin D-24-hydroxylase enzyme and therefore elevated levels of 1,25-$(OH)_2D_3$, deficient mineralization of intramembranous bone was detected *(71)*. These differences could possibly be explained by the necessity of an interplay with 24,25-$(OH)_2D_3$ or 1,24,25-$(OH)_2D_3$ for optimal mineralization of bone *(72)*.

In addition to bone, vitamin D may also be involved in the calcification of other tissues as has been recently shown for the aorta and the femoral, mesenteric, hepatic, renal, and carotid arteries *(73)*. Interestingly, these authors demonstrated that the osteoclast inhibitor osteoprotegerin completely blocked calcification in each of these arteries and reduced the levels of calcium and phosphate in the abdominal aorta to control levels.

Apoptosis

The process of mineralization has been shown to be associated with apoptosis of osteoblast/osteocyte-like cells from fetal rat calvaria *(74)*. Apoptosis was found to be related to the differentiative response of rat osteoblasts in fracture healing *(75)* and has been associated with differentiation (collagen I expression and mineralization) in mouse craniosynostosis *(76)*, although others have reported differently *(77)*.

In human osteoblastic cells 1,25-$(OH)_2D_3$ and several of its analogs has no clear effect on apoptosis; however, induction of apoptosis by camptothecin and staurosporin is strongly reduced by 1,25-$(OH)_2D_3$ *(78)*. In contrast, 1,25-$(OH)_2D_3$ has been reported to induce tumor necrosis factor-α–mediated apoptosis in parallel to an increased cell differentiation, shown by a stimulation of osteocalcin and alkaline phosphatase *(79)*. Also in canine osteosarcoma cells, 1,25-$(OH)_2D_3$, was involved in the induction of apoptosis and cell differentiation *(80,81)*.

Proliferation

In relation to the effects of 1,25-$(OH)_2D_3$ on the induction of apoptosis are the studies that show an inhibition of osteoblast proliferation after treatment with 1,25-$(OH)_2D_3$. Proliferation of human osteoblast-like cells (MG63) was found to be inhibited by 1,25-$(OH)_2D_3$ *(41)*. Effects on human osteoblast proliferation, however, can be dependent on the concentration of 1,25-$(OH)_2D_3$: high doses (5×10^{-9} to 5×10^{-6} *M*) showed a decreased proliferation, and low doses (5×10^{-12} *M*) showed an increased proliferation *(82)*.

In rat osteoblasts, differences have been reported in the regulation of proliferation either inhibition *(83,84)* or stimulation *(41)* by 1,25-$(OH)_2D_3$. The stage of differentiation of the osteoblasts might be important because it has been reported that 1,25-$(OH)_2D_3$ treatment increased the amount of p57(Kip2), a member of the cyclin-dependent kinase inhibitors in rat calvarial primary osteoblasts in the transit from proliferation toward differentiation *(85)*.

In mouse osteoblasts, inhibitory actions of 1,25-$(OH)_2D_3$ on the proliferation of osteoblasts have been described *(83,86,87)*. However, studies with mouse osteoblasts have shown that cell proliferation rate can determine the cellular responses to 1,25-$(OH)_2D_3$ via a change in receptor levels *(88)*.

Collagen Type I

The effect of 1,25-$(OH)_2D_3$ on collagen I, the major component of the extracellular matrix formed by osteoblasts, is investigated by numerous studies. Collagen I consists of a triple-helix formation, containing two identical Iα1 chains and a structurally similar, but genetically different, Iα2 chain. Collagens are synthesized as procollagen molecules with an extracellular removal of their N- and C-propeptides. These propeptides can be detected as byproducts of collagen synthesis and are clinically used as markers of bone formation.

1,25-$(OH)_2D_3$ has been described to stimulate the synthesis of type I collagen in human osteoblasts (MG-63 osteosarcoma cells), both the Iα1 and Iα2 components *(89)*. This positive effect of 1,25-$(OH)_2D_3$ on type I collagen has also been shown in other human osteoblast culture systems, both at the mRNA *(90)* and protein level *(30)* after long-term 1,25-$(OH)_2D_3$ treatment. The effect of 1,25-$(OH)_2D_3$3 could be enhanced by coincubation with TGF-β *(48)* or sodium fluoride *(91)*. However, some studies did not find any effect of 1,25-$(OH)_2D_3$ on collagen synthesis in human osteoblasts *(30, 46,49)* mainly after short-term treatment. Osteoblasts do not only synthesize collagen type I but also collagenases that allow the initiation of bone resorption by generating collagen fragments that activate osteoclasts *(92)*. With 1,25-$(OH)_2D_3$, an upregulation of collagenase was found in human osteoblasts *(93)*. This may reflect the dual role of osteoblasts in bone metabolism, on the one hand bone formation, and on the other hand bone resorption via control of osteoclast formation and activity.

In rat osteoblastic cells, 1,25-$(OH)_2D_3$ has been shown to reduce type I collagen synthesis and procollagen mRNA, and this reduction is even stronger in the presence of dexamethasone *(94,95)*. These 1,25-$(OH)_2D_3$ effects in rat osteoblasts on collagen I synthesis have been shown to be dependent on differentiation and duration of 1,25-$(OH)_2D_3$ treatment: an inhibitory effect during proliferation (high basal levels), and stimulatory effect during the mineralization period (low basal levels) after acute hormone treatment *(53)*.

In mouse osteoblasts, 1,25-$(OH)_2D_3$ inhibited the collagen Iα1 promoter activity *(96)*. 1,25-$(OH)_2D_3$ also inhibited the collagen I synthesis in mouse calvarial osteoblasts grown on collagen I coatings; this was accompanied by an increased collagenase and gelatinase secretion and a reduction in free tissue inhibitor of metalloproteinases (ref. *97*; although this effect was not observed when serum-free medium was used without plasminogen; ref. *98*). In contrast, it has also been reported that 1,25-$(OH)_2D_3$ could inhibit collagenolysis in mouse osteoblasts, with a reduction in collagenase activity and increase in free tissue Inhibitor of metalloproteinases *(99)*. These different effects of 1,25-$(OH)_2D_3$ might again be to the result of different differentiation stages of the mouse osteoblasts, because in early phase MC3T3-E1 cells, 1,25-$(OH)_2D_3$ has been found to stimulate collagen synthesis, whereas in late phase osteoblasts, no effects were found *(54)*.

OSTEOCALCIN

Osteocalcin is the most abundant noncollagenous protein in bone, produced by osteoblasts but also released during degradation of osteoclasts *(100)*. Vitamin K facilitates the carboxylation of the osteocalcin molecule and recently it has been shown that 1,25-$(OH)_2D_3$ stimulates vitamin K2 metabolism to epoxide in osteoblasts, which acts as a cofactor of gamma-glutamyl carboxylase *(101)*. These gamma-carboxyglutamyl residues have a highly specific affinity to the calcium ion of the hydroxyapatite molecule *(102)*. Osteocalcin-deficient mice have a higher bone mass and bones of improved functional quality because of an increase in bone formation without impairing bone resorption and mineralization *(103)*. Through the years several studies have reported the strong induction of osteocalcin production by 1,25-$(OH)_2D_3$ in human osteoblast cultures *(30,45,49,82,104,105)*. During differentiation of primary human osteoblasts, 1,25-$(OH)_2D_3$ has been found to stimulate osteocalcin secretion and mRNA expression to the same absolute level at all different stages *(46)*, but it has also been described that the 1,25-$(OH)_2D_3$–induced stimulation of osteocalcin in culture supernatant decreases towards the mineralization stage of human osteoblasts because of a concurrent accumulation of osteocalcin in the extracellular matrix *(106)*. Another described pattern is that in the human osteosarcoma cell line MG-63, 1,25-$(OH)_2D_3$ induces osteocalcin secretion in nonconfluent cell cultures, this stimulation reaches peak values in subconfluent cultures, and then decreases again in confluent cultures. Interestingly, a similar expression profile has been observed for the 1,25-$(OH)_2D_3$receptor *(107)*.

Also, in osteoblasts from other species, the effects of 1,25-$(OH)_2D_3$ in the regulation of osteocalcin expression seem to depend very much on the different cell culture situations. In studies with rat osteoblasts, the osteocalcin gene expression was stimulated by 1,25-$(OH)_2D_3$ both at the transcriptional and posttranscriptional level *(108,109)*. Osteocalcin mRNA expression was found to be upregulated by 1,25-$(OH)_2D_3$ in mature rat calvaria cells *(110)* or after the onset of mineralization *(53)*. Because of the occupancy of the activating protein-1 sites (*see* section entitled Vitamin D Receptor) in the osteocalcin box (CCAAT-containing proximal promoter element) overlapping the vitamin D response element (VDRE) of the osteocalcin gene, the osteocalcin expression is suppressed before the onset of mineralization *(111–113)*. However, more recently, also in the early stages of osteoblast differentiation in cultures of fetal rat calvarial-derived osteoblasts, 1,25-$(OH)_2D_3$ has been reported to enhance osteocalcin transcription. The effect of 1,25-$(OH)_2D_3$ induction on osteocalcin mRNA levels declined during maturation, probably because of the increase of basal osteocalcin mRNA expression during osteoblast differentiation *(114)*.

In contrast to this role of 1,25-$(OH)_2D_3$ as a positive regulator of osteocalcin expression (although differences exist in the maturation stages of the osteoblasts), in murine osteoblasts there is evidence for 1,25-$(OH)_2D_3$ as a negative regulator *(115)*. It is supposed that 1,25-$(OH)_2D_3$ either indirectly *(116)* or directly *(43)* inhibits osteocalcin gene expression in mice. However, in neonatal murine calvarial osteoblasts 1,25-$(OH)_2D_3$ was also found to stimulate osteocalcin secretion *(117)*.

A negative regulation of osteocalcin by 1,25-$(OH)_2D_3$also was seen in chicken embryonic osteoblasts: osteocalcin mRNA and protein accumulation were inhibited during differentiation when 1,25-$(OH)_2D_3$ treatment was initiated *(118)*.

Matrix Gla Protein (MGP)

MGP is like osteocalcin (Bone Gla protein), a member of the vitamin K-dependent gamma-carboxyglutamic acid (Gla) proteins, and is synthesized by osteoblasts *(119,120)*. MGP is a possible regulator of extracellular matrix calcification because MGP-deficient mice exhibit spontaneous calcification of various cartilages and arteries *(121)*.

To our knowledge, no data on the effect of 1,25-$(OH)_2D_3$ on human osteoblasts are available, although possible VDR binding sites have been described in the promoter of the human MGP gene *(122)*. MGP regulation by 1,25-$(OH)_2D_3$ has been studied in rat osteoblasts. 1,25-$(OH)_2D_3$ treatment rapidly and dramatically increased MGP mRNA and secretion by UMR 106-01 cells *(123)* and induced MGP mRNA expression and secretion by ROS 17/2 cells *(124)*. This positive regulatory effect occurred throughout osteoblast growth and differentiation *(125)*, although MGP remained stimulated to a lesser degree by 1,25-$(OH)_2D_3$ at the last stages of rat osteoblast differentiation, either after acute or chronic 1,25-$(OH)_2D_3$ incubation *(53)*.

Osteopontin

Osteopontin is an abundant noncollagenous sialoprotein in the bone matrix produced by osteoblasts that has a role in osteoclast attachment *(126)* and resorption *(127)*. The early effect of 1,25-

$(OH)_2D_3$ in stimulating osteogenic differentiation was reflected in an increased osteopontin mRNA expression in secondary human bone marrow cultures *(28)*; in addition, a 1,25-$(OH)_2D_3$-induced upregulation of osteopontin was observed in human osteoblast-like MG-63 cells *(128)*.

Osteopontin expression is shown to be regulated by 1,25-$(OH)_2D_3$ in several osteoblastic cells of rat origin. After treatment with 1,25-$(OH)_2D_3$, the osteopontin secretion into the culture medium was increased in ROS 17/2.8 cells *(129)* and osteopontin mRNA was increased in cultured rat bone tissues *(130)*. This 1,25-$(OH)_2D_3$-induced enhancement of osteopontin expression in rat osteoblasts is modulated by a helix-loop–helix-type transcription factor *(131)*. Because different levels of osteopontin were observed in rat calvaria cells in different stages of differentiation, the 1,25-$(OH)_2D_3$ effect may selectively affect mature osteoblasts *(110)*. However, it has also been shown that acute 1,25-$(OH)_2D_3$ treatment stimulated osteopontin mRNA expression in rat osteoblasts during the proliferation period and to a lesser extent in the later periods (though higher levels were found in these periods). Chronic treatment with 1,25-$(OH)_2D_3$ did even show a partial inhibition of the osteopontin mRNA expression in these cultures during the last stages of development *(53)*.

In mice, it has been reported that 1,25-$(OH)_2D_3$ induced the synthesis of osteopontin mRNA in both osteoblastic cell lines (MC3T3-E1) and mouse primary osteoblast-like cells *(132)*.

Bone Sialoprotein (BSP)

BSP is like osteopontin, another sialoprotein that is present in the matrix of osteoblasts and may have a role as a nucleator of hydroxyapatite crystal formation and cell attachment *(133)*. In human bone marrow stromal cells, the addition of 1,25-$(OH)_2D_3$ alone had no significant effect on BSP mRNA expression, but high levels of BSP were observed in dexamethasone-treated cultures to which 1,25-$(OH)_2D_3$ had been added *(28)*.

In rat osteoblasts, 1,25-$(OH)_2D_3$ suppressed BSP mRNA expression *(130)* via a VDRE that overlaps a unique inverted TATA box in the rat BSP gene *(134)*. BSP mRNA was found to be downregulated by 1,25-$(OH)_2D_3$ in rat osteoblasts during all stages of differentiation *(110)*, and a dexamethasone-induced increase in BSP was inhibited by 1,25-$(OH)_2D_3$ *(135)*.

Osteonectin

Osteonectin is a noncollagenous bone matrix protein that is involved in cell attachment *(136)*. It supports bone remodeling and the maintenance of bone mass in vertebrates, as is shown by osteonectin-deficient mice *(137)*. So far not many studies have evaluated the effect of 1,25-$(OH)_2D_3$ on osteonectin expression in osteoblasts. In human MG-63 osteoblasts grown on collagen I, 1,25-$(OH)_2D_3$ incubation had no effect on osteonectin secretion *(47)*.

Plasminogen

Osteonectin may also act as an anchor for plasminogen on collagen matrices *(138)*. The regulated production of plasmin (serine protease) by plasminogen activators is a potentially important regulatory system in bone remodeling. Osteoblasts produce two types of plasminogen activators, tissue-type (tPA) and urokinase-type (uPA), and a plasminogen activator inhibitor. An increased PA activity facilitates bone resorption *(139,140)*.

In human osteoblasts, it has been reported that 1,25-$(OH)_2D_3$ increased the production of both PAs *(141)*, and two VDREs were found in the human tPA enhancer *(142)*. However, 1,25-$(OH)_2D_3$ also has been found to increase the expression of thrombomodulin in human osteoblasts, which inhibits uPA *(143)*. This points to a complicated role of 1,25-$(OH)_2D_3$ in bone remodeling. As in human osteoblasts, 1,25-$(OH)_2D_3$incubation was found to stimulate PA activity in rat osteoblasts *(141,144,145)*. Also matrix metalloproteinases (MMPs) are targets for regulation by vitamin D. MMP-13 is upregulated by 1,25-$(OH)_2D_3$3 in mouse osteoblasts and was postulated to play a role in stimulation of bone resorption *(146,147)*. A recent study showed that 1,25-$(OH)_2D_3$ as well as the 1,25-$(OH)_2D_3$ analog EB1089 enhance MMP-9 mRNA and protein expression as well as vascular endothelial growth factor expression, which coincides with the stimulation of angiogenesis during endochondral bone formation. It also demonstrates and additional role for 1,25-$(OH)_2D_3$ in the development of bone, that is, regulation of vascularization *(148)*.

Prostaglandins

Prostaglandins (enzymatically oxygenated derivatives of free arachidonic acid) are strong stimulators of bone formation and resorption but may also have inhibitory effects on fully differentiated osteoblasts and osteoclasts *(149)*.

In human osteoblasts, 1,25-$(OH)_2D_3$ has been found to decrease prostaglandin E (PGE) biosynthesis, both under normal and cytokine-stimulated incubation conditions *(150)*. Basal PGE_2 levels might be important because 1,25-$(OH)_2D_3$ increased low PGE_2 levels in high proliferative osteoblasts and decreased the production in low proliferative cells with higher basal PGE_2 levels *(151)*. In a study using osteoblasts from different origins, 1,25-$(OH)_2D_3$ did not stimulate the production of PGE_2 and E_2 in human and rat osteoblasts, only in mouse osteoblasts *(152)*.

Growth Factors

TGF-β

TGF-β is one of the most abundant growth factors secreted by bone cells and its regulation is crucial for bone development and growth. The inhibitory effect of 1,25-$(OH)_2D_3$ on cell growth could be related to an induction of TGF-β synthesis *(153)*. VDREs have been identified in the human TGF-β gene *(154)*, and 1,25-$(OH)_2D_3$ has been found to increase TGF-β2 mRNA and TGF-β2 concentration in culture supernatant of human osteoblasts, as well as TGF-β receptor type I and II synthesis *(155)*. 1,25-$(OH)_2D_3$ increased the release of TGF-β in cultured bone cells from patients with isolated growth hormone deficiency and normal controls but not in cells from patients with multiple pituitary hormone deficiencies *(156)*. Recently it has also been shown that 1,25-$(OH)_2D_3$ increases the expression of both TGF-β type I and II receptors on human osteoblasts and a coupling has been made with the growth regulatory effects of 1,25-$(OH)_2D_3$*(157)*.

Also in osteoblasts from murine origin, 1,25-$(OH)_2D_3$ has been reported to stimulate the production of TGF-β *(158)*, with a stronger effect on cells derived from older mice, who had lower TGF-β mRNA expression compared with younger mice *(159)*. The effect of the interaction of 1,25-$(OH)_2D_3$ and TGF-β will be discussed in detail in the section Interaction of Vitamin D with Other Factors.

Bone Morphogenetic Proteins (BMPs)

BMPs are members of the TGF-β superfamily and play an important role in the induction of ectopic bone formation *(160)*. In human osteoblasts, 1,25-$(OH)_2D_3$ was found to downregulate BMP-2 and BMP-4 mRNA expression *(161)* but to stimulate BMP-3 mRNA expression *(162)*.

Insulin-Like Growth Factor

Osteoblasts produce insulin-like growth factors (IGF) I and II. IGFs promote cell proliferation and matrix synthesis, and IGF-I has been considered a mediator of growth hormone activity in bone *(163, 164)*. The activity of IGFs is regulated by binding to a family of IGF-binding proteins (IGFBPs), which are controlled by proteolytic processing via IGFBP proteases *(165,164)*.

Several studies have focussed on 1,25-$(OH)_2D_3$ regulation of IGF-I in bone cells and cultured bone tissue. 1,25-$(OH)_2D_3$ increased IGF-I levels in human bone cell supernatants *(166)* and caused a small but not significant increase in the release of IGF-I in the supernatant of rat osteoblast-like cells *(167)*. However, 1,25-$(OH)_2D_3$ inhibited production of IGF-I in mouse osteoblasts and mouse calvaria *(168)*.

It has been shown that 1,25-$(OH)_2D_3$ had no effect on IGF-II mRNA expression and secretion in the culture supernatant of fetal rat osteoblast cultures *(169)*. In mouse calvaria, 1,25-$(OH)_2D_3$ was found to stimulate IGF-II release *(170)*.

Some studies focused on the IGFBPs. 1,25-$(OH)_2D_3$ could enhance the amount of IGFBP-2 secreted in culture by rat osteoblasts *(171)*. In human osteoblasts, 1,25-$(OH)_2D_3$ was found to increase IGFBP-3 secretion and mRNA expression *(172,173)*. Both in human and mouse osteoblasts, 1,25-$(OH)_2D_3$ has been reported to stimulate IGFBP-4 mRNA expression and secretion *(168,172)*. Another study also showed at mRNA and protein level the stimulation of IGFBP-2, -3, and -4 but not -5 and -6 by 1,25-$(OH)_2D_3$ in human bone marrow cells with potential to differentiate into osteoblasts *(174)*. In rat osteoblasts, 1,25-$(OH)_2D_3$ has been shown to increase IGFBP-5 mRNA expression *(175,176)*.

Effects of 1,25-$(OH)_2D_3$ on other growth factors produced by osteoblast are listed in Table 1. This table also contains a summary of other target molecules for 1,25-$(OH)_2D_3$ action in osteoblasts. In the near future the number of genes regulated by vitamin D in bone cells but also in other cell types will definitely increase as a consequence of the application of microarray techniques *(177,178)*.

VITAMIN D RECEPTOR

The VDR plays a central role in the biological activities of 1,25-$(OH)_2D_3$, as is illustrated by the observed hypocalcemia, hypophosphatemia, hyperparathyroidism, and severely impaired bone formation in VDR knockout mice *(179,180)*. The presence of a functional VDR seems to be essential to observe effects of 1,25-$(OH)_2D_3$ on bone metabolism and cell proliferation *(41,181–183)*. Furthermore, in osteoblasts the VDR is essential for 1,25-$(OH)_2D_3$-stimulated osteoclast formation. This was illustrated by studies using cocultures of osteoblasts from VDR knockout mice and wild-type spleen cells (as a source of osteoclast progenitors) showing that 1,25-$(OH)_2D_3$-mediated osteoclast formation was abolished *(183)*.

A study using an in vitro model of cellular senescence indicated that both VDR mRNA and protein does not change with the aging of the osteoblasts *(184)*; however, a study on osteoblasts derived from donors who were different ages showed a decrease in VDR mRNA expression with aging *(185)*. Obviously, more detailed studies are needed to assess a relation between VDR level and ageing and altered 1,25-$(OH)_2D_3$ activity and osteoblast function. 1,25-$(OH)_2D_3$ is able to upregulate its own receptor level, both in vivo *(186,187)*, and in vitro *(187–189)*. Homologous receptor upregulation might be part of the mechanism by which 1,25-$(OH)_2D_3$-mediated gene transcription is regulated, as is suggested by several studies showing a relationship between VDR levels and the biological response to 1,25-$(OH)_2D_3$ *(88,190–193)*. Also, as discussed in the section Metabolism: 24-Hydroxylase Activity, it is coupled to the induction of 24-hydroxylase activity and initiation of the C24 oxidation pathway.

1,25-$(OH)_2D_3$ also exerts effects that do not seem to be mediated via an interaction of the VDR with the genome *(194–196)*. These nongenomic processes include the rapid changes in intracellular calcium *(197,198)*, and the rapid stimulation of Ca^{2+} transport in the intestine (transcaltachia; ref. *199*). Furthermore, 1,25-$(OH)_2D_3$ can rapidly stimulate phosphoinositide metabolism *(200,201)*, leading to activation of protein kinase C *(202)*, an important regulator of cell proliferation and differentiation *(203)*. In chondrocytes *(204)* and, more recently, in osteoblasts *(205,206)* and in the cells, ameloblasts and odontoblasts, which are involved in the formation of mineralized dental tissue, a membrane-associated VDR has been detected *(206)*. In addition, for 1,25-$(OH)_2D_3$, a specific membrane receptor also seems to exist *(205,207)*. The discovery of membrane receptors is challenging their importance in other nongenomic effects of vitamin D metabolites. However, so far the genes for these membrane receptors have not been cloned and the way these membrane receptors might interact with the nuclear VDR-mediated pathway remains to be established *(208)*.

In addition to the classical nuclear VDR and the increase in data on a membrane receptor for 1,25-$(OH)_2D_3$, a new class of 1,25-$(OH)_2D_3$ regulatory proteins has been identified: intracellular vitamin

Table 1
1,25-(OH)2D3 Effects on Growth Factors and Other Osteoblast-Related Molecules

Factor	*1,25-(OH)2D3 effect*	*Source*	*Species*	*Reference*
Aromatase	↑	mRNA	Human	*(293)*
	↑	mRNA + protein	Human	*(294)*
Cbfa1	↓	mRNA	Rat	*(37)*
	↓(1 h) ↑ (48 h)	mRNA	Human	*(38)*
EGFR	↑	Protein	Rat	*(295)*
	↑	mRNA	Rat	*(296)*
ETRA	↑	mRNA	Human	*(297)*
HCYR61	↑	mRNA	Human	*(298)*
HLA-DR	↑	Protein	Human	*(299)*
GM-CSF	→	Protein	Mouse	*(300)*
IL-1	↑	mRNA	Mouse	*(301)*
IL-1R I	↑	mRNA + protein	Mouse	*(302)*
IL-1R II	→	mRNA + protein	Mouse	*(302)*
IL-IR[a]	→	Protein	Mouse	*(303)*
IL-4R	↑	mRNA + protein	Mouse	*(304)*
IL-6	↑	Protein	Mouse, rat	*(305)*
	↓	Protein	Mouse	*(257)*
	→	Protein	Mouse, rat	*(306)*
	→	Protein	Rat	*(307)*
	→	mRNA + protein	Human	*(307)*
IL-6R	→	mRNA	Human	*(307)*
IL-11	↑	Protein	Mouse	*(308)*
IL-11R	→	mRNA	Mouse	*(308)*
I-mfa	↑	mRNA + protein	Mouse, rat	*(39)*
IP3R	↓	mRNA	Rat	*(309)*
M-CSF	↑	Protein	Mouse	*(310)*
	↑	mRNA + protein	Mouse	*(87)*
MMP-9	↑	mRNA + protein	Mouse, rat	*(148)*
MMP-13	↑	mRNA	Mouse	*(146,147)*
Na^+-Ca^{2+} exchange	↓	Protein	Rat	*(311,312)*
NGF	↑	mRNA	Rat	*(313)*
	↑	Protein	Rat	*(314)*
Notch 1 and 2	↓	mRNA	Human	*(40)*
Notch 4	↑	mRNA	Human	*(40)*
NPR-C	↑	mRNA + protein	Mouse	*(315)*
ODF	↑	mRNA	Mouse	*(316)*
OPG	↑[b]	mRNA + protein	Human	*(317)*
	↑	mRNA	Mouse	*(316)*
OPGL	↑	mRNA	Mouse	*(318)*
PDGF	↑	Protein	Human	*(319)*
PTHrP	↓	mRNA	Rat	*(320)*
VEGF	↑	mRNA + protein	Human	*(321)*
	↑	mRNA + protein	Human	*(322)*
	↑	Protein	Human	*(323)*
	↑	mRNA	Mouse,rat	*(148)*

[a]IL-1 receptor subtype not specified.
[b]Effect not seen in preosteoblastic cells.

Abbrevations: EGFR, epidermal growth factor receptor; ETRA, endothelin-1; IP3R: inositol trisphosphate receptor; HLA-DR, human leukocyte antigen receptor ligand; HCYR61, cysteine-rich protein 61; I-mfa, inhibitor of the MyoD family; M-CSF, macrophage colony-stimulating factor; MMP, matrix metalloproteinase; NGF, nerve growth factor; NPR-C, natriuretic peptide; OPG, osteoprotegerin; ODF, osteoclast differentiation factor; PDGF, platelet-derived growth factor; PTHrP, parathyroid hormone-related peptide; VEGF, vascular endothelial growth factor.

D binding proteins (IDBPs; refs. *209–211*). These IDBPs may interfere at different levels in the intracellular life of 1,25-$(OH)_2D_3$. They may regulate the metabolism of 1,25-$(OH)_2D_3$ by controlling the delivery to the 1α- and 24-hydroxylase activity (211) or interfere with the binding of VDR to DNA. Future research will definitively provide knowledge on IBDPs in bone cells and delineate their role in 1,25-$(OH)_2D_3$ regulation of bone metabolism.

METABOLISM: 24-HYDROXYLASE ACTIVITY

A final aspect to be discussed, in particular in relation to heterologous regulation of VDR, is the significance of 24-hydroxylase (24-OHase, CYP24). As discussed previously, an increase in VDR level is not always followed by an increase in biological response of 1,25-$(OH)_2D_3$. However, up to now the alterations in VDR level are always closely coupled to a change in the same direction in 1,25-$(OH)_2D_3$ induction of the enzyme 24-OHase *(88,128,212,213)*. 24-OHase is induced by 1,25-$(OH)_2D_3$ in all target tissues studied so far. 24-OHase mediates the conversion of 1,25-$(OH)_2D_3$ into 1,24,25-$(OH)_3D_3$, which is actually the initial step in a more extensive C24 and C23 oxidation of the side chain and ultimately results in the production of calcitroic acid. In other words, the self-induced metabolism of 1,25-$(OH)_2D_3$ may provide a means to regulate its concentration at the level of target tissues and thereby limit its activity. Previously, this concept has been shown to be valid as 24-OHase activity limited biological activity in osteoblasts *(188)*. Inhibition of 24-OHase activity by ketoconazole enhanced homologous upregulation of VDR. The significance of 24-OHase activity for the biological activity of 1,25-$(OH)_2D_3$ is also very nicely shown in prostate cancer cells. The growth inhibition of a panel of prostate cancer cells by 1,25-$(OH)_2D_3$ was inversely related to the 24-OHase activity of these cell lines *(214)*. Moreover, an aggressive human prostate cancer cell line, DU145, appeared to be insensitive to 1,25-$(OH)_2D_3$for growth inhibition while the VDR was present. Inhibition of 24-hydroxylase activity by liarozole resulted in growth inhibition of the DU145 prostate cancer cell line by 1,25-$(OH)_2D_3$ *(215)*. Together, these observations emphasize the significance of VDR levels and 24-OHase activity for the eventual biological response of 1,25-$(OH)_2D_3$. VDR level has been shown to change in relation to cell density and osteoblast differentiation *(114,216*, our own unpublished observations), it is therefore conceivable that also 24-OHase may vary accordingly and thereby modulate 1,25-$(OH)_2D_3$ activity differentiation stage-dependent.

What can be the overall significance of the tight control by 1,25-$(OH)_2D_3$ of its own catabolism and the relation with VDR level? As a consequence of VDR upregulation 1,25-$(OH)_2D_3$ responses may initially be enhanced. At the same time the 24-OHase activity is induced and the degradation of 1,25-$(OH)_2D_3$ and thereby long-term 1,25-$(OH)_2D_3$ activity or over-stimulation by 1,25-$(OH)_2D_3$ is prevented. Why should this be so effectively regulated for 1,25-$(OH)_2D_3$? One reason may be the important role of vitamin D in the control of serum calcium. Prolonged stimulation by 1,25-$(OH)_2D_3$ might then lead to hypercalcemia, which is a important disadvantageous and potentially life-threatening effect.

The 24-oxidation pathway eventually leads to the degradation and production of calcitroic acid; however, it is becoming clear that intermediate products, in particular the 24-hydroxylated forms of 1,25-$(OH)D_3$ and 1,25-$(OH)_2D_3$ can have direct effects on osteoblasts *(216)*. Recently, a specific membrane receptor for 24,25-$(OH)_2D_3$ in osteoblasts has been indicated *(205)*. These direct effects of 24,25-$(OH)_2D_3$ are not new and osteoblast-specific because they have been studied and described more extensively for chondrocytes *(217–219)*.

In addition to the 24-hydroxylase pathway, more recently target tissue-specific metabolites of 1,25-$(OH)_2D_3$, 3-epi metabolites, with biological activity have been described *(220,221)*. Also, in rat osteoblast-like cells 24,25-$(OH)_2D_3$ can be processed to 3 epi metabolites; however, so far no biological activity has been demonstrated *(222)*. Thus, besides 24-hydroxylation, 3-epimerization may play an important role in modulating the concentration and the biological activity of these two major vitamin D3 metabolites in target tissues *(222)*.

INTERACTION OF VITAMIN D WITH OTHER FACTORS

As mentioned in the Introduction: Osteoblasts section, differentiation of osteoblasts may vary depending on the presence and absence of hormones, growth factors, and so on. In relation to this, it is conceivable that the presence and absence of these factors may significantly modulate the action of vitamin D. Several examples from in vitro studies are present to support the assumption that 1,25-$(OH)_2D_3$ does not act independently but regulates osteoblast activity via interaction with multiple factors. These include local factors, that is, growth factors and cytokines produced in the vicinity of bone, and other hormones such as parathyroid hormone (PTH) and estradiol.

Ample attention has been paid to regulation of the VDR expression. Aside from homologous upregulation by 1,25-$(OH)_2D_3$ itself, VDR is regulated by a wide variety of factors acting via cAMP, for instance, PTH *(189,223–227)*, PTH-related peptide *(189,223,224)*, forskolin *(228)*, and PGE_2 *(229)*. A recent study demonstrated that the inducible cAMP early repressor plays a regulatory role in the upregulation of VDR via cAMP *(229)*. VDR expression may also be regulated via other signaling pathways as shown by the effects of growth hormone *(230)*, glucocorticoids *(190,231)* epidermal growth factor *(232)*, TGF-β *(233)*, phorbol esters *(234,235)*, retinoic acid *(212,231,236,237)*, ER ligands *(230,238–241)*, androgen receptor ligands *(239)*, progesterone receptor ligands *(231)*, and phosphorus *(242)*. However, the significance of changes in abundance of the VDR for the ultimate biological activity of 1,25-$(OH)_2D_3$ is not always obvious. In the past several studies demonstrated that increase or decrease of VDR level by various treatments is paralleled by an increase or decrease in vitamin D activity, respectively *(190,243,244)*. For dexamethasone and vitamin D, Chen et al. showed that an increase in VDR was coupled to an enhancement of 1,25-$(OH)_2D_3$-induced osteocalcin synthesis *(190)*. However, Shaloub et al. recently reported an increase in VDR mRNA by dexamethasone in long-term rat osteoblast cultures, which was paralleled by a decrease in transcriptional activation of the osteocalcin gene and osteocalcin mRNA expression in the early phase of culture *(114)*. They demonstrated that in the later phases of culture, that is, in differentiated osteoblasts, dexamethasone enhanced 1,25-$(OH)_2D_3$-induced increase in osteocalcin mRNA whereas osteocalcin gene transcription remained inhibited, implicating an effect on mRNA stability. Irrespective of differences between these studies, which might be attributed to differences in osteoblast differentiation, the latter study by Shaloub et al. demonstrated a dissociation between VDR mRNA and a 1,25-$(OH)_2D_3$-induced biological response. Interestingly, in view of the relationship between VDR level and 24-OHase activity, it was recently shown that dexamethasone also enhances 1,25-$(OH)_2D_3$ induced 24-OHase activity *(245)*.

Unfortunately, Shaloub et al. did not provide VDR protein data but a comparable dissociation between regulation of VDR protein levels and 1,25-$(OH)_2D_3$ activity has been shown before. We have shown that upregulation of the VDR by TGF-β was not followed by an increased induction of both osteocalcin and osteopontin mRNA expression and osteocalcin protein synthesis. In contrast, the upregulation of VDR by TGF-β is coupled to a strong inhibition of osteocalcin and osteopontin expression *(233)*. This inhibition was the result of a TGF-β–induced block of the VDR–retinoid X receptor complex binding to the VDRE in the osteocalcin and osteopontin gene *(42)*. Furthermore, in relation to the TGF-β and 1,25-$(OH)_2D_3$ interaction, Yanagisawa et al. showed in transfection studies using the nonbone COS-1 cells that SMAD3, one of the SMADs in the intracellular TGF-β signaling pathway, enhanced VDR-mediated action of 1,25-$(OH)_2D_3$ *(246)*. Recently, they showed that the inhibitory SMAD7 abrogated the SMAD3-mediated enhancement of VDR function *(247)*. Although the authors did not show TGF-β regulation of neither SMAD7 nor SMAD3 in bone cells, these studies underscore the interaction between TGF-β and 1,25-$(OH)_2D_3$ and provide a mechanism to override increases in VDR level (for an overview on the interaction between 1,25-(OH)2D3 and TGF-β, *see* ref. *248*). This example of interaction with TGF-β demonstrates three important aspects regarding the action of 1,25-$(OH)_2D_3$: first, that the presence of a target tissue-derived factor may dramatically modify the response to 1,25-$(OH)_2D_3$; second, that the balance of negative and positive components of intracellular signaling pathways of these factors is of importance. This may differ between different stages of differentiation and between cell types and thereby form the basis of differentiation-dependent and cell type-specific interactions between growth factors and vitamin D. In relation to this TGF-β has also been shown to modulate the profile of nuclear matrix proteins during osteoblast differentiation *(250)*. Third, it is demonstrated that the level of VDR is not the ultimate determinant of the eventual biological activity of 1,25-$(OH)_2D_3$.

In addition, interaction of multiple other factors with 1,25-$(OH)_2D_3$ in the control of its biological activity have been described. Although it is beyond the scope of this review to discuss all these interactions in detail, two other examples will be mentioned shortly: PTH and IGF-I. In addition to 1,25-$(OH)_2D_3$, PTH is the other major calciotropic hormone, and interactions between this peptide and the secosteroid hormone have been described. 1,25-$(OH)_2D_3$ and PTH mutually regulate each others' synthesis in a feedback loop manner. PTH stimulates 1,25-$(OH)_2D_3$synthesis whereas in return 1,25-$(OH)_2D_3$ inhibits PTH synthesis and secretion. Also at the bone and osteoblast level PTH and 1,25-$(OH)_2D_3$ act in an interrelated manner. 1,25-$(OH)_2D_3$ inhibited PTH stimulation of cAMP production whereas, as mentioned above, PTH upregulated VDR in osteoblasts and modulated 1,25-$(OH)_2D_3$ activity *(189,223,224,227,250,251)*. PTH and 1,25-$(OH)_2D_3$ regulate bone resorption in an interrelated manner in which prostaglandins appear to be involved *(252)*. This observation on interaction PTH between 1,25-$(OH)_2D_3$ in stimulating bone resorption has recently been confirmed and it was extended by showing the significance of 1,25-$(OH)_2D_3$-induced rises in intracellular calcium *(253)*. Studies on mouse osteoblasts provided additional data on interaction between prostaglandins and 1,25-$(OH)_2D_3$. 1,25-$(OH)_2D_3$ inhibited PGE_2-induced cAMP and inositol trisphosphate accumulation *(254)* and calcium influx *(255)*, PGF_2 α-induced PGE_2 synthesis *(256)*, and $PGF_2\alpha$ or PGE_1- induced interleukin-6 synthesis *(257)*.

As is TGF-β, IGF-I is abundantly present in bone. It is synthesized by osteoblasts and osteocytes, stored in the bone matrix, and has anabolic effects on bone. At the kidney level interactions have been demonstrated as IGF-I has been shown to stimulate 1,25-$(OH)_2D_3$synthesis *(258–260)*. Besides interactions at the level of IGF-I synthesis in bone cells, a functional interplay of 1,25-$(OH)_2D_3$ and IGF-I in the regulation of bone and bone cell metabolism also has been described *(261–263)*. With respect to bone resorption, IGF-I inhibited 1,25-$(OH)_2D_3$- as well as PTH-stimulated bone resorption *(115)*. This is in contrast to TGF-β, which specifically inhibited 1,25-$(OH)_2D_3$-stimulated bone resorption *(115)*, demonstrating growth factor-specific interactions.

At present, the interactions described above are the ones most extensively studied, but it is not limited to these factors and interactions of 1,25-$(OH)_2D_3$, with multiple other factors are being reported. However, yet these are generally limited to one or two observations but knowledge will definitively increase over the coming years. Some interesting interactions are with estradiol *(264,265)*, BMP *(266)*, and hepatocyte growth factor *(267)* but also with metal ions like cobalt, present in orthopedic implants *(268)* ,and mechanical loading *(269)*.

VITAMIN D ANALOGS

Throughout the last decades multiple analogs of 1,25-$(OH)_2D_3$ have been synthesized *(270)*. Initially, these analogs were predominantly developed to have low calcemic and bone resorbing activity and to be applied in areas like immunology, dermatology, and oncology. As a consequence of data coming up on positive effects of vitamin D on bone metabolism, more recently also the development of vitamin D analogs with bone anabolic effects has come into focus *(271)*. A few recent examples are ED-71 *(272,273)*, RO-26-9228 *(274)*, 26,27-hexafluoro-1,25-(OH)2D3 *(275)*, and 2-methylene-19-nor-(20S)1,25-$(OH)_2D_3$ *(276)*. However, as knowledge about response- and target tissue-specific actions of steroid hormones and in particular vitamin D increases, this number of synthetic analogs will certainly increase in the coming future.

Although not a real synthetic analog, it must be mentioned that also vitamin D_2 is studied in relation to bone anabolic actions. Already, in 1981, it was shown that vitamin D_2 prevented the inhibitory effect of hydrocortisone on mineral apposition *(277)*, and effects on osteoblasts have been described *(278)*. The metabolite 19-nor-1,25-$(OH)_2D_2$ also has been shown to have similar effects as 1,25-$(OH)_2D_3$ on human osteoblasts *(279)*. Based on these data and those on intestinal calcium absorption, it is interesting to pursue the effects of vitamin D2 and its metabolites on bone in more detail.

CONCLUSION

Combining all data discussed in this review on 1,25-$(OH)_2D_3$ and osteoblasts together it can be concluded that 1,25-$(OH)_2D_3$ has direct effects on osteoblasts and is involved in osteoblast differentiation, control of osteoblast activity, bone formation, and in bone resorption. However, the interpretation of the different studies is dependent on many factors that influence the data obtained, like the difference among species *(116,117,152,280,281)*, differentiation stage *(54,110,282,283)*, basal levels of gene expression *(53)*, heterogeneity of the population *(284)*, interaction with other factors *(285)*, the use of glucocorticosteroids (dexamethasone; ref. *83*), the use of cell lines or primary cells, the different skeletal site of origin of bone biopsies *(286)*, the age differences of donors *(286)*, early or late passages of cell culture *(84)*, cell density *(251,287)*, culture conditions *(288)*, acute or chronic vitamin D treatment *(30,53)*, dosage of 1,25-$(OH)_2D_3$ *(64,70)*, additives (ascorbate, β-glycerophosphate; refs. *289* and *290*), and extracellular calcium concentration *(291,292)*. Taking all these factors into consideration will clarify the differences between studies and will add to the knowledge about the pleiotropic functions of 1,25-$(OH)_2D_3$ in osteoblast differentiation and bone formation. Moreover, in light of the differences in action in mice, rat an men it is for the development of new drugs based on vitamin D action desirable to focus mainly on human systems. Finally, the vast knowledge on vitamin D analogs and target tissue-specific actions obtained throughout the last decade holds promise for further development and specific application in bone and bone-related diseases.

REFERENCES

1. Fujita, T. (1992) Vitamin D in the treatment of osteoporosis. *Proc. Soc. Exp. Biol. Med.* **199,** 394–399.
2. Fujita, T. (1996) Vitamin D in the treatment of osteoporosis revisited. *Proc. Soc. Exp. Biol. Med.* **212,** 110–115.
3. Gallagher, J. C., Riggs, B. L., Recker, R. R., and Goldgar, D. (1989) The effect of calcitriol on patients with postmenopausal osteoporosis with special reference to fracture frequency. *Proc. Soc. Exp. Biol. Med.* **191,** 287–292.
4. Tilyard, M. W., Spears, G. F., Thomson, J., and Dovey, S. (1992) Treatment of postmenopausal osteoporosis with calcitriol or calcium (see comments). *N. Engl. J. Med.* **326,** 357–362.
5. Chapuy, M. C., Arlot, M. E., Duboeuf, F., Brun, J., Crouzet, B., Arnaud, S., et al. (1992) Vitamin D3 and calcium to prevent hip fractures in the elderly women. *N. Engl. J. Med.* **327,** 1637–1642.
6. Francis, R. M. (1997) Is there a differential response to alfacalcidol and vitamin D in the treatment of osteoporosis? *Calcif. Tissue Int.* **60,** 111–114.
7. Gillespie, W. J., Avenell, A., Henry, D. A., O'Connell, D. L., and Robertson, J. (2001) Vitamin D and vitamin D analogues for preventing fractures associated with involutional and post-menopausal osteoporosis. *Cochrane. Database. Syst. Rev.* CD000227–
8. Balsan, S., Garabedian, M., Larchet, M., Gorski, A. M., Cournot, G., Tau, C., et al. (1986) Long-term nocturnal calcium infusions can cure rickets and promote normal mineralization in hereditary resistance to 1,25-dihydroxyvitamin D. *J. Clin. Invest.* **77,** 1661–1667.
9. Weisman, Y., Bab, I., Gazit, D., Spirer, Z., Jaffe, M., and Hochberg, Z. (1987) Long-term intracaval calcium infusion therapy in end-organ resistance to 1,25-dihydroxyvitamin D. *Am. J. Med.* **83,** 984–990.
10. Bliziotes, M., Yergey, A. L., Nanes, M. S., Muenzer, J., Begley, M. G., Vieira, N. E., et al. (1988) Absent intestinal response to calciferols in hereditary resistance to 1,25-dihydroxyvitamin D: documentation and effective therapy with high dose intravenous calcium infusions. *J. Clin. Endocrinol. Metab.* **66,** 294–300.
11. al Aqeel, A., Ozand, P., Sobki, S., Sewairi, W., and Marx, S. (1993) The combined use of intravenous and oral calcium for the treatment of vitamin D dependent rickets type II (VDDRII). *Clin. Endocrinol. (Oxf.)* **39,** 229–237.
12. Amling, M., Priemel, M., Holzmann, T., Chapin, K., Rueger, J. M., Baron, R., et al. (1999) Rescue of the skeletal phenotype of vitamin D receptor-ablated mice in the setting of normal mineral ion homeostasis: formal histomorphometric and biomechanical analyses. *Endocrinology* **140,** 4982–4987.
13. Wronski, T. J., Halloran, B. P., Bikle, D. D., Globus, R. K., and Morey-Holton, E. R. (1986) Chronic administration of 1,25-dihydroxyvitamin D3: increased bone but impaired mineralization. *Endocrinology* **119,** 2580–2585.
14. Erben, R. G., Scutt, A. M., Miao, D., Kollenkirchen, U., and Haberey, M. (1997) Short-term treatment of rats with high dose 1,25-dihydroxyvitamin D3 stimulates bone formation and increases the number of osteoblast precursor cells in bone marrow. *Endocrinology* **138,** 4629–4635.

15. Erben, R. G., Bromm, S., and Stangassinger, M. (1998) Therapeutic efficacy of 1alpha,25-dihydroxyvitamin D3 and calcium in osteopenic ovariectomized rats: evidence for a direct anabolic effect of 1alpha,25-dihydroxyvitamin D3 on bone. *Endocrinology* **139,** 4319–4328.
16. Johnson, J. A., Grande, J. P., Roche, P. C., and Kumar, R. (1996) Ontogeny of the 1,25-dihydroxyvitamin D3 receptor in fetal rat bone. *J. Bone Miner. Res.* **11,** 56–61.
17. Mee, A. P., Hoyland, J. A., Braidman, I. P., Freemont, A. J., Davies, M., and Mawer, E. B. (1996) Demonstration of vitamin D receptor transcripts in actively resorbing osteoclasts in bone sections. *Bone* **18,** 295–299.
18. Langub, M. C., Reinhardt, T. A., Horst, R. L., Malluche, H. H., and Koszewski, N. J. (2000) Characterization of vitamin D receptor immunoreactivity in human bone cells. *Bone* **27,** 383–387.
19. Gardiner, E. M., Baldock, P. A., Thomas, G. P., Sims, N. A., Henderson, N. K., Hollis, B., et al. (2000) Increased formation and decreased resorption of bone in mice with elevated vitamin D receptor in mature cells of the osteoblastic lineage. *FASEB J.* **14,** 1908–1916.
20. Stein, G. S., Lian, J. B., Stein, J. L., Van Wijnen, A. J., and Montecino, M. (1996) Transcriptional control of osteoblast growth and differentiation. *Physiol. Rev.* **76,** 593–629.
21. Quarles, L. D., Yohay, D. A., Lever, L. W., Caton, R., and Wenstrup, R. J. (1992) Distinct proliferative and differentiated stages of murine MC3T3-E1 cells in culture: an in vitro model of osteoblast development. *J. Bone Miner. Res.* **7,** 683–692.
22. Choi, J. Y., Lee, B. H., Song, K. B., Park, R. W., Kim, I. S., Sohn, K. Y., et al. (1996) Expression patterns of bone-related proteins during osteoblastic differentiation in MC3T3-E1 cells. *J. Cell Biochem.* **61,** 609–618.
23. Gerstenfeld, L. C., Chipman, S. D., Glowacki, J., and Lian, J. B. (1987) Expression of differentiated function by mineralizing cultures of chicken osteoblasts. *Dev. Biol.* **122,** 49–60.
24. Cheng, S. L., Yang, J. W., Rifas, L., Zhang, S. F., and Avioli, L. V. (1994) Differentiation of human bone marrow osteogenic stromal cells in vitro: induction of the osteoblast phenotype by dexamethasone. *Endocrinology* **134,** 277–286.
25. Siggelkow, H., Rebenstorff, K., Kurre, W., Niedhart, C., Engel, I., Schulz, H., et al. (1999) Development of the osteoblast phenotype in primary human osteoblasts in culture: comparison with rat calvarial cells in osteoblast differentiation. *J. Cell Biochem.* **75,** 22–35.
26. Ducy, P., Schinke, T., and Karsenty, G. (2000) The osteoblast: a sophisticated fibroblast under central surveillance. *Science* **289,** 1501–1504.
27. Aubin, J. E., Candeliere, G. A., and Bonnelye, E. (1999) The heterogeneity of the osteoblast phenotype. *The Endocrinologist* **9,** 25–31.
28. Beresford, J. N., Joyner, C. J., Devlin, C., and Triffitt, J. T. (1994) The effects of dexamethasone and 1,25-dihydroxyvitamin D3 on osteogenic differentiation of human marrow stromal cells in vitro. *Arch. Oral Biol.* **39,** 941–947.
29. Nuttall, M. E., Patton, A. J., Olivera, D. L., Nadeau, D. P., and Gowen, M. (1998) Human trabecular bone cells are able to express both osteoblastic and adipocytic phenotype: implications for osteopenic disorders. *J. Bone Miner. Res.* **13,** 371–382.
30. Hicok, K. C., Thomas, T., Gori, F., Rickard, D. J., Spelsberg, T. C., and Riggs, B. L. (1998) Development and characterization of conditionally immortalized osteoblast precursor cell lines from human bone marrow stroma. *J. Bone Miner. Res.* **13,** 205–217.
31. Beresford, J. N., Bennett, J. H., Devlin, C., Leboy, P. S., and Owen, M. E. (1992) Evidence for an inverse relationship between the differentiation of adipocytic and osteogenic cells in rat marrow stromal cell cultures. *J. Cell Sci.* **102, (Pt 2),** 341–351.
32. Shionome, M., Shinki, T., Takahashi, N., Hasegawa, K., and Suda, T. (1992) 1 alpha,25-dihydroxyvitamin D3 modulation in lipid metabolism in established bone marrow-derived stromal cells, MC3T3-G2/PA6. *J. Cell Biochem.* **48,** 424–430.
33. Rickard, D. J., Kazhdan, I., and Leboy, P. S. (1995) Importance of 1,25-dihydroxyvitamin D3 and the nonadherent cells of marrow for osteoblast differentiation from rat marrow stromal cells. *Bone* **16,** 671–678.
34. Kelly, K. A. and Gimble, J. M. (1998) 1,25-Dihydroxy vitamin D3 inhibits adipocyte differentiation and gene expression in murine bone marrow stromal cell clones and primary cultures. *Endocrinology* **139,** 2622–2628.
35. Okazaki, R., Toriumi, M., Fukumoto, S., Miyamoto, M., Fujita, T., Tanaka, K., et al. (1999) Thiazolidinediones inhibit osteoclast-like cell formation and bone resorption in vitro. *Endocrinology* **140,** 5060–5065.
36. Bellows, C. G., Wang, Y. H., Heersche, J. N., and Aubin, J. E. (1994) 1,25-dihydroxyvitamin D3 stimulates adipocyte differentiation in cultures of fetal rat calvaria cells: comparison with the effects of dexamethasone. *Endocrinology* **134,** 2221–2229.
37. Drissi, H., Pouliot, A., Koolloos, C., Stein, J. L., Lian, J. B., Stein, G. S., et al. (2002) 1,25-(OH)2-vitamin D3 suppresses the bone-related Runx2/Cbfa1 gene promoter. *Exp. Cell Res.* **274,** 323–333.
38. Viereck, V., Siggelkow, H., Tauber, S., Raddatz, D., Schutze, N., and Hufner, M. (2002) Differential regulation of Cbfa1/Runx2 and osteocalcin gene expression by vitamin-D3, dexamethasone, and local growth factors in primary human osteoblasts. *J. Cell Biochem.* **86,** 348–356.
39. Tsuji, K., Kraut, N., Groudine, M., and Noda, M. (2001) Vitamin D(3) enhances the expression of I-mfa, an inhibitor of the MyoD family, in osteoblasts. *Biochim. Biophys. Acta* **1539,** 122–130.
40. Schnabel, M., Fichtel, I., Gotzen, L., and Schlegel, J. (2002) Differential expression of Notch genes in human osteoblastic cells. *Int. J. Mol. Med.* **9,** 229–232.
41. Van Den Bemd, G. J., Pols, H. A., Birkenhager, J. C., Kleinekoort, W. M., and Van Leeuwen, J. P. (1995) Differential effects of 1,25-dihydroxyvitamin D3-analogs on osteoblast-like cells and on in vitro bone resorption. *J. Steroid Biochem. Mol. Biol.* **55,** 337–346.

42. Staal, A., Van Wijnen, A. J., Desai, R. K., Pols, H. A., Birkenhager, J. C., DeLuca, H. F., et al. (1996) Antagonistic effects of transforming growth factor-beta on vitamin D3 enhancement of osteocalcin and osteopontin transcription: reduced interactions of vitamin D receptor/retinoid X receptor complexes with vitamin E response elements. *Endocrinology* **137,** 2001–2011.
43. Lian, J. B., Shalhoub, V., Aslam, F., Frenkel, B., Green, J., Hamrah, M., et al. (1997) Species-specific glucocorticoid and 1,25-dihydroxyvitamin D responsiveness in mouse MC3T3-E1 osteoblasts: dexamethasone inhibits osteoblast differentiation and vitamin D down-regulates osteocalcin gene expression. *Endocrinology* **138,** 2117–2127.
44. Watts, N. B. (1999) Clinical utility of biochemical markers of bone remodeling. *Clin. Chem.* **45,** 1359–1368.
45. Bodine, P. V., Vernon, S. K., and Komm, B. S. (1996) Establishment and hormonal regulation of a conditionally transformed preosteocytic cell line from adult human bone. *Endocrinology* **137,** 4592–4604.
46. Siggelkow, H., Schulz, H., Kaesler, S., Benzler, K., Atkinson, M. J., and Hufner, M. (1999) 1,25 dihydroxyvitamin-D3 attenuates the confluence-dependent differences in the osteoblast characteristic proteins alkaline phosphatase, procollagen I peptide, and osteocalcin. *Calcif. Tissue Int.* **64,** 414–421.
47. Andrianarivo, A. G., Robinson, J. A., Mann, K. G., and Tracy, R. P. (1992) Growth on type I collagen promotes expression of the osteoblastic phenotype in human osteosarcoma MG-63 cells. *J. Cell Physiol.* **153,** 256–265.
48. Wergedal, J. E., Matsuyama, T., and Strong, D. D. (1992) Differentiation of normal human bone cells by transforming growth factor-beta and 1,25(OH)2 vitamin D3. *Metabolism* **41,** 42–48.
49. Ingram, R. T., Bonde, S. K., Riggs, B. L., and Fitzpatrick, L. A. (1994) Effects of transforming growth factor beta (TGF beta) and 1,25 dihydroxyvitamin D3 on the function, cytochemistry and morphology of normal human osteoblast-like cells. *Differentiation* **55,** 153–163.
50. Kassem, M., Kveiborg, M., and Eriksen, E. F. (2000) Production and action of transforming growth factor-beta in human osteoblast cultures: dependence on cell differentiation and modulation by calcitriol. *Eur. J. Clin. Invest.* **30,** 429–437.
51. Manolagas, S. C., Burton, D. W., and Deftos, L. J. (1981) 1,25-Dihydroxyvitamin D3 stimulates the alkaline phosphatase activity of osteoblast-like cells. *J. Biol. Chem.* **256,** 7115–7117.
52. Halstead, L. R., Scott, M. J., Rifas, L., and Avioli, L. V. (1992) Characterization of osteoblast-like cells from normal adult rat femoral trabecular bone. *Calcif. Tissue Int.* **50,** 93–95.
53. Owen, T. A., Aronow, M. S., Barone, L. M., Bettencourt, B., Stein, G. S., and Lian, J. B. (1991) Pleiotropic effects of vitamin D on osteoblast gene expression are related to the proliferative and differentiated state of the bone cell phenotype: dependency upon basal levels of gene expression, duration of exposure, and bone matrix competency in normal rat osteoblast cultures. *Endocrinology* **128,** 1496–1504.
54. Matsumoto, T., Igarashi, C., Takeuchi, Y., Harada, S., Kikuchi, T., Yamato, H., et al. (1991) Stimulation by 1,25-dihydroxyvitamin D3 of in vitro mineralization induced by osteoblast-like MC3T3-E1 cells. *Bone* **12,** 27–32.
55. Lomri, A., Marie, P. J., Tran, P. V., and Hott, M. (1988) Characterization of endosteal osteoblastic cells isolated from mouse caudal vertebrae. *Bone* **9,** 165–175.
56. Narisawa, S., Frohlander, N., and Millan, J. L. (1997) Inactivation of two mouse alkaline phosphatase genes and establishment of a model of infantile hypophosphatasia. *Dev. Dyn.* **208,** 432–446.
57. Hui, M. and Tenenbaum, H. C. (1998) New face of an old enzyme: alkaline phosphatase may contribute to human tissue aging by inducing tissue hardening and calcification. *Anat. Rec.* **253,** 91–94.
58. Imai, K., Neuman, M. W., Kawase, T., and Saito, S. (1992) Calcium in osteoblast-enriched bone cells. *Bone* **13,** 217–223.
59. Anderson, H. C. (1989) Mechanism of mineral formation in bone. *Lab. Invest.* **60,** 320–330.
60. Beck, G. R. Jr., Sullivan, E. C., Moran, E., and Zerler, B. (1998) Relationship between alkaline phosphatase levels, osteopontin expression, and mineralization in differentiating MC3T3-E1 osteoblasts. *J. Cell Biochem.* **68,** 269–280.
61. Koshihara, Y., Hoshi, K., Ishibashi, H., and Shiraki, M. (1996) Vitamin K2 promotes 1alpha,25(OH)2 vitamin D3-induced mineralization in human periosteal osteoblasts. *Calcif. Tissue Int.* **59,** 466–473.
62. Koshihara, Y., Hirano, M., Kawamura, M., Oda, H., and Higaki, S. (1991) Mineralization ability of cultured human osteoblast-like periosteal cells does not decline with aging. *J. Gerontol.* **46,** B201–B206.
63. Halvorsen, Y. D., Franklin, D., Bond, A. L., Hitt, D. C., Auchter, C., Boskey, A. L., et al. (2001) Extracellular matrix mineralization and osteoblast gene expression by human adipose tissue-derived stromal cells. *Tissue Eng.* **7,** 729–741.
64. Oyajobi, B. O., Russell, R. G., and Caswell, A. M. (1994) Modulation of ecto-nucleoside triphosphate pyrophosphatase activity of human osteoblast-like bone cells by 1 alpha,25-dihydroxyvitamin D3, 24R,25-dihydroxyvitamin D3, parathyroid hormone, and dexamethasone. *J. Bone Miner. Res.* **9,** 1259–1266.
65. Slater, M., Patava, J., and Mason, R. S. (1994) Role of chondroitin sulfate glycosaminoglycans in mineralizing osteoblast-like cells: effects of hormonal manipulation. *J. Bone Miner. Res.* **9,** 161–169.
66. Matsumoto, T., Kawanobe, Y., Morita, K., and Ogata, E. (1985) Effect of 1,25-dihydroxyvitamin D3 on phospholipid metabolism in a clonal osteoblast-like rat osteogenic sarcoma cell line. *J. Biol. Chem.* **260,** 13704–13709.
67. Balmain, N., Berdal, A., Hotton, D., Cuisinier-Gleizes, P., and Mathieu, H. (1989) Calbindin-D9K immunolocalization and vitamin D-dependence in the bone of growing and adult rats. *Histochemistry* **92,** 359–365.
68. Lynch, M. P., Stein, J. L., Stein, G. S., and Lian, J. B. (1995) The influence of type I collagen on the development and maintenance of the osteoblast phenotype in primary and passaged rat calvarial osteoblasts: modification of expression of genes supporting cell growth, adhesion, and extracellular matrix mineralization. *Exp. Cell Res.* **216,** 35–45.
69. St. Arnaud, R., Prud'homme, J., Leung-Hagesteijn, C., and Dedhar, S. (1995) Constitutive expression of calreticulin in osteoblasts inhibits mineralization. *J. Cell Biol.* **131,** 1351–1359.

70. Ecarot, B. and Desbarats, M. (1999) 1,25-(OH)2D3 down-regulates expression of Phex, a marker of the mature osteoblast. *Endocrinology* **140,** 1192–1199.
71. St. Arnaud, R., Arabian, A., Travers, R., Barletta, F., Raval-Pandya, M., Chapin, K., et al. (2000) Deficient mineralization of intramembranous bone in vitamin D-24-hydroxylase-ablated mice is due to elevated 1,25-dihydroxyvitamin D and not to the absence of 24,25-dihydroxyvitamin D. *Endocrinology* **141,** 2658–2666.
72. van Leeuwen, J. P. T. M., van den Bemd, G. J. C. M., van Driel, M., Buurman, C. J., and Pols, H. A. P. (2001) 24,25-Dihydroxyvitamin D3 and bone metabolism. *Steroids* **66,** 375–380.
73. Price, P. A., June, H. H., Buckley, J. R., and Williamson, M. K. (2001) Osteoprotegerin inhibits artery calcification induced by warfarin and by vitamin D. *Arterioscler. Thromb. Vasc. Biol.* **21,** 1610–1616.
74. Lynch, M. P., Capparelli, C., Stein, J. L., Stein, G. S., and Lian, J. B. (1998) Apoptosis during bone-like tissue development in vitro. *J. Cell Biochem.* **68,** 31–49.
75. Landry, P., Sadasivan, K., Marino, A., and Albright, J. (1997) Apoptosis is coordinately regulated with osteoblast formation during bone healing. *Tissue Cell* **29,** 413–419.
76. Mathijssen, I. M. J., van Leeuwen, J. P. T. M., and Vermeij-Keers, C. (2000) Simultaneous induction of apoptosis, collagen type I expression and mineralization in the developing coronal suture following FGF4 and FGF2 application. *J. Craniofacial Genet. Devel. Biol.* **20,** 127–136.
77. Mansukhani, A., Bellosta, P., Sahni, M., and Basilico, C. (2000) Signaling by fibroblast growth factors (FGF) and fibroblast growth factor receptor 2 (FGFR2)-activating mutations blocks mineralization and induces apoptosis in osteoblasts. *J. Cell Biol.* **149,** 1297–1308.
78. Hansen, C. M., Hansen, D., Holm, P. K., and Binderup, L. (2001) Vitamin D compounds exert anti-apoptotic effects in human osteosarcoma cells in vitro. *J. Steroid Biochem. Mol. Biol.* **77,** 1–11.
79. Pascher, E., Perniok, A., Becker, A., and Feldkamp, J. (1999) Effect of 1alpha,25(OH)2-vitamin D3 on TNF alpha-mediated apoptosis of human primary osteoblast-like cells in vitro. *Horm. Metab. Res.* **31,** 653–656.
80. Nozaki, K., Kadosawa, T., Nishimura, R., Mochizuki, M., Takahashi, K., and Sasaki, N. (1999) 1,25-Dihydroxyvitamin D3, recombinant human transforming growth factor- beta 1, and recombinant human bone morphogenetic protein-2 induce in vitro differentiation of canine osteosarcoma cells. *J. Vet. Med. Sci.* **61,** 649–656.
81. Nozaki, K., Kadosawa, T., Nishimura, R., Mochizuki, M., Takahashi, K., and Sasaki, N. (1999) 1,25-Dihydroxyvitamin D3, recombinant human transforming growth factor- beta 1, and recombinant human bone morphogenetic protein-2 induce in vitro differentiation of canine osteosarcoma cells. *J. Vet. Med. Sci.* **61,** 649–656.
82. Skjodt, H., Gallagher, J. A., Beresford, J. N., Couch, M., Poser, J. W., and Russell, R. G. (1985) Vitamin D metabolites regulate osteocalcin synthesis and proliferation of human bone cells in vitro. *J. Endocrinol.* **105,** 391–396.
83. Chen, T. L., Cone, C. M., and Feldman, D. (1983) Effects of 1 alpha,25-dihydroxyvitamin D3 and glucocorticoids on the growth of rat and mouse osteoblast-like bone cells. *Calcif. Tissue Int.* **35,** 806–811.
84. Murray, S., Glackin, C., and Murray, E. (1993) Variation in 1,25-dihydroxyvitamin D3 regulation of proliferation and alkaline phosphatase activity in late-passage rat osteoblastic cell lines. *J. Steroid Biochem. Mol. Biol.* **46,** 227–233.
85. Urano, T., Hosoi, T., Shiraki, M., Toyoshima, H., Ouchi, Y., and Inoue, S. (2000) Possible involvement of the p57 (Kip2) gene in bone metabolism. *Biochem. Biophys. Res. Commun.* **269,** 422–426.
86. Kanatani, M., Sugimoto, T., Fukase, M., and Chihara, K. (1993) Effect of 1,25-dihydroxyvitamin D3 on the proliferation of osteoblastic MC3T3-E1 cells by modulating the release of local regulators from monocytes. *Biochem. Biophys. Res. Commun.* **190,** 529–535.
87. Rubin, J., Fan, X., Thornton, D., Bryant, R., and Biskobing, D. (1996) Regulation of murine osteoblast macrophage colony-stimulating factor production by 1,25(OH)2D3. *Calcif. Tissue Int.* **59,** 291–296.
88. Chen, T. L., Li, J. M., Ye, T. V., Cone, C. M., and Feldman, D. (1986) Hormonal responses to 1,25-dihydroxyvitamin D3 in cultured mouse osteoblast-like cells—modulation by changes in receptor level. *J. Cell Physiol.* **126,** 21–28.
89. Franceschi, R. T., Romano, P. R., and Park, K. Y. (1988) Regulation of type I collagen synthesis by 1,25-dihydroxyvitamin D3 in human osteosarcoma cells. *J. Biol. Chem.* **263,** 18938–18945.
90. Tasaki, Y., Takamori, R., and Koshihara, Y. (1991) Prostaglandin D2 metabolite stimulates collagen synthesis by human osteoblasts during calcification. *Prostaglandins* **41,** 303–313.
91. Kassem, M., Mosekilde, L., and Eriksen, E. F. (1993) 1,25-dihydroxyvitamin D3 potentiates fluoride-stimulated collagen type I production in cultures of human bone marrow stromal osteoblast-like cells. *J. Bone Miner. Res.* **8,** 1453–1458.
92. Holliday, L. S., Welgus, H. G., Fliszar, C. J., Veith, G. M., Jeffrey, J. J., and Gluck, S. L. (1997) Initiation of osteoclast bone resorption by interstitial collagenase. *J. Biol. Chem.* **272,** 22053–22058.
93. Meikle, M. C., Bord, S., Hembry, R. M., Compston, J., Croucher, P. I., and Reynolds, J. J. (1992) Human osteoblasts in culture synthesize collagenase and other matrix metalloproteinases in response to osteotropic hormones and cytokines. *J. Cell Sci.* **103(Pt 4),** 1093–1099.
94. Harrison, J. R., Petersen, D. N., Lichtler, A. C., Mador, A. T., Rowe, D. W., and Kream, B. E. (1989) 1,25-Dihydroxyvitamin D3 inhibits transcription of type I collagen genes in the rat osteosarcoma cell line ROS 17/2.8. *Endocrinology* **125,** 327–333.
95. Kim, H. T. and Chen, T. L. (1989) 1,25-Dihydroxyvitamin D3 interaction with dexamethasone and retinoic acid: effects on procollagen messenger ribonucleic acid levels in rat osteoblast-like cells. *Mol. Endocrinol.* **3,** 97–104.
96. Bedalov, A., Salvatori, R., Dodig, M., Kapural, B., Pavlin, D., Kream, B. E., et al. (1998) 1,25-Dihydroxyvitamin D3 inhibition of col1a1 promoter expression in calvariae from neonatal transgenic mice. *Biochim. Biophys. Acta* **1398,** 285–293.

97. Thomson, B. M., Atkinson, S. J., Reynolds, J. J., and Meikle, M. C. (1987) Degradation of type I collagen films by mouse osteoblasts is stimulated by 1,25 dihydroxyvitamin D3 and inhibited by human recombinant TIMP (tissue inhibitor of metalloproteinases). *Biochem. Biophys. Res. Commun.* **148,** 596–602.
98. Thomson, B. M., Atkinson, S. J., McGarrity, A. M., Hembry, R. M., Reynolds, J. J., and Meikle, M. C. (1989) Type I collagen degradation by mouse calvarial osteoblasts stimulated with 1,25-dihydroxyvitamin D-3: evidence for a plasminogen-plasmin-metalloproteinase activation cascade. *Biochim. Biophys. Acta* **1014,** 125–132.
99. Meikle, M. C., McGarrity, A. M., Thomson, B. M., and Reynolds, J. J. (1991) Bone-derived growth factors modulate collagenase and TIMP (tissue inhibitor of metalloproteinases) activity and type I collagen degradation by mouse calvarial osteoblasts. *Bone Miner.* **12,** 41–55.
100. Christenson, R. H. (1997) Biochemical markers of bone metabolism: an overview. *Clin. Biochem.* **30,** 573–593.
101. Miyake, N., Hoshi, K., Sano, Y., Kikuchi, K., Tadano, K., and Koshihara, Y. (2001) 1,25-Dihydroxyvitamin D3 promotes vitamin K2 metabolism in human osteoblasts. *Osteoporos. Int.* **12,** 680–687.
102. Weber, P. (1997) Management of osteoporosis: is there a role for vitamin K? *Int. J. Vitam. Nutr. Res.* **67,** 350–356.
103. Ducy, P., Desbois, C., Boyce, B., Pinero, G., Story, B., Dunstan, C., et al. (1996) Increased bone formation in osteocalcin-deficient mice. *Nature* **382,** 448–452.
104. Beresford, J. N., Gallagher, J. A., Poser, J. W., and Russell, R. G. (1984) Production of osteocalcin by human bone cells in vitro. Effects of 1,25(OH)2D3, 24,25(OH)2D3, parathyroid hormone, and glucocorticoids. *Metab. Bone Dis. Relat. Res.* **5,** 229–234.
105. Lajeunesse, D., Kiebzak, G. M., Frondoza, C., and Sacktor, B. (1991) Regulation of osteocalcin secretion by human primary bone cells and by the human osteosarcoma cell line MG-63. *Bone Miner.* **14,** 237–250.
106. Hosoda, K., Kanzaki, S., Eguchi, H., Kiyoki, M., Yamaji, T., Koshihara, Y., et al. (1993) Secretion of osteocalcin and its propeptide from human osteoblastic cells: dissociation of the secretory patterns of osteocalcin and its propeptide. *J. Bone Miner. Res.* **8,** 553–565.
107. Lajeunesse, D., Frondoza, C., Schoffield, B., and Sacktor, B. (1990) Osteocalcin secretion by the human osteosarcoma cell line MG-63. *J. Bone Miner. Res.* **5,** 915–922.
108. Lian, J., Stewart, C., Puchacz, E., Mackowiak, S., Shalhoub, V., Collart, D., et al. (1989) Structure of the rat osteocalcin gene and regulation of vitamin D-dependent expression. *Proc. Natl. Acad. Sci. USA* **86,** 1143–1147.
109. Mosavin, R. and Mellon, W. S. (1996) Posttranscriptional regulation of osteocalcin mRNA in clonal osteoblast cells by 1,25-dihydroxyvitamin D3. *Arch. Biochem. Biophys.* **332,** 142–152.
110. Bellows, C. G., Reimers, S. M., and Heersche, J. N. (1999) Expression of mRNAs for type-I collagen, bone sialoprotein, osteocalcin, and osteopontin at different stages of osteoblastic differentiation and their regulation by 1,25 dihydroxyvitamin D3. *Cell Tissue Res.* **297,** 249–259.
111. Stein, G. S., Lian, J. B., and Owen, T. A. (1990) Bone cell differentiation: a functionally coupled relationship between expression of cell-gr. *Curr. Opin. Cell Biol.* **2,** 1018–1027.
112. Owen, T. A., Bortell, R., Yocum, S. A., Smock, S. L. , Zhang, M., Abate, C., et al. (1990) Coordinate occupancy of AP-1 sites in the vitamin D-responsive and CCAAT box elements by Fos-Jun in the osteocalcin gene: model for phenotype suppression of transcription. *Proc. Natl. Acad. Sci. USA* **87,** 9990–9994.
113. Stein, G. S. and Lian, J. B. (1993) Molecular mechanisms mediating proliferation/differentiation interrelationships during progressive development of the osteoblast phenotype. *Endocr. Rev.* **14,** 424–442.
114. Shalhoub, V., Aslam, F., Breen, E., van Wijnen, A., Bortell, R., Stein, G. S., et al. (1998) Multiple levels of steroid hormone-dependent control of osteocalcin during osteoblast differentiation: glucocorticoid regulation of basal and vitamin D stimulated gene expression. *J. Cell Biochem.* **69,** 154–168.
115. Staal, A., Geertsma-Kleinekoort, W. M., Van Den Bemd, G. J., Buurman, C. J., Birkenhager, J. C., Pols, H. A., et al. (1998) Regulation of osteocalcin production and bone resorption by 1,25-dihydroxyvitamin D3 in mouse long bones: interaction with the bone-derived growth factors TGF-beta and IGF-I. *J. Bone Miner. Res.* **13,** 36–43.
116. Zhang, R., Ducy, P., and Karsenty, G. (1997) 1,25-dihydroxyvitamin D3 inhibits Osteocalcin expression in mouse through an indirect mechanism. *J. Biol. Chem.* **272,** 110–116.
117. Chen, T. L. and Fry, D. (1999) Hormonal regulation of the osteoblastic phenotype expression in neonatal murine calvarial cells. *Calcif. Tissue Int.* **64,** 304–309.
118. Broess, M., Riva, A., and Gerstenfeld, L. C. (1995) Inhibitory effects of 1,25(OH)2 vitamin D3 on collagen type I, osteopontin, and osteocalcin gene expression in chicken osteoblasts. *J. Cell Biochem.* **57,** 440–451.
119. Price, P. A. (1989) Gla-containing proteins of bone. *Connect. Tissue Res.* **21,** 51–57.
120. Shearer, M. J. (2000) Role of vitamin K and gla proteins in the pathophysiology of osteoporosis and vascular calcification. *Curr. Opin. Clin. Nutr. Metab. Care* **3,** 433–438.
121. Luo, G., Ducy, P., McKee, M. D., Pinero, G. J., Loyer, E., Behringer, R. R., et al. (1997) Spontaneous calcification of arteries and cartilage in mice lacking matrix GLA protein. *Nature* **386,** 78–81.
122. Cancela, L., Hsieh, C. L., Francke, U., and Price, P. A. (1990) Molecular structure, chromosome assignment, and promoter organization of the human matrix Gla protein gene. *J. Biol. Chem.* **265,** 15040–15048.
123. Fraser, J. D., Otawara, Y., and Price, P. A. (1988) 1,25-Dihydroxyvitamin D3 stimulates the synthesis of matrix gamma-carboxyglutamic acid protein by osteosarcoma cells. Mutually exclusive expression of vitamin K-dependent bone proteins by clonal osteoblastic cell lines. *J. Biol. Chem.* **263,** 911–916.
124. Fraser, J. D. and Price, P. A. (1990) Induction of matrix Gla protein synthesis during prolonged 1,25-dihydroxyvitamin D3 treatment of osteosarcoma cells. *Calcif. Tissue Int.* **46,** 270–279.

125. Barone, L. M., Owen, T. A., Tassinari, M. S., Bortell, R., Stein, G. S., and Lian, J. B. (1991) Developmental expression and hormonal regulation of the rat matrix Gla protein (MGP) gene in chondrogenesis and osteogenesis. *J. Cell Biochem.* **46,** 351–365.
126. Reinholt, F. P., Hultenby, K., Oldberg, A., and Heinegard, D. (1990) Osteopontin—a possible anchor of osteoclasts to bone. *Proc. Natl. Acad. Sci. USA* **87,** 4473–4475.
127. Yoshitake, H., Rittling, S. R., Denhardt, D. T., and Noda, M. (1999) Osteopontin-deficient mice are resistant to ovariectomy-induced bone resorption (published erratum appears in *Proc. Natl. Acad. Sci. USA* 1999 Sep 14;**96(19),** 10944). *Proc. Natl. Acad. Sci. USA* **96,** 8156–8160.
128. Staal, A., Van Den Bemd, G. J., Birkenhager, J. C., Pols, H. A., and Van Leeuwen, J. P. (1997) Consequences of vitamin D receptor regulation for the 1,25-dihydroxyvitamin D3-induced 24-hydroxylase activity in osteoblast-like cells: initiation of the C24-oxidation pathway. *Bone* **20,** 237–243.
129. Prince, C. W. and Butler, W. T. (1987) 1,25-Dihydroxyvitamin D3 regulates the biosynthesis of osteopontin, a bone-derived cell attachment protein, in clonal osteoblast-like osteosarcoma cells. *Coll. Relat. Res.* **7,** 305–313.
130. Chen, J., Thomas, H. F., and Sodek, J. (1996) Regulation of bone sialoprotein and osteopontin mRNA expression by dexamethasone and 1,25-dihydroxyvitamin D3 in rat bone organ cultures. *Connect. Tissue Res.* **34,** 41–51.
131. Matsue, M., Kageyama, R., Denhardt, D. T., and Noda, M. (1997) Helix-loop-helix-type transcription factor (HES-1) is expressed in osteoblastic cells, suppressed by 1,25(OH)2 vitamin D3, and modulates 1,25(OH)2 vitamin D3 enhancement of osteopontin gene expression. *Bone* **20,** 329–334.
132. Jin, C. H., Miyaura, C., Ishimi, Y., Hong, M. H., Sato, T., Abe, E., et al. (1990) Interleukin 1 regulates the expression of osteopontin mRNA by osteoblasts. *Mol. Cell Endocrinol.* **74,** 221–228.
133. Ganss, B., Kim, R. H., and Sodek, J. (1999) Bone sialoprotein. *Crit. Rev. Oral Biol. Med.* **10,** 79–98.
134. Kim, R. H., Li, J. J., Ogata, Y., Yamauchi, M., Freedman, L. P., and Sodek, J. (1996) Identification of a vitamin D3-response element that overlaps a unique inverted TATA box in the rat bone sialoprotein gene. *Biochem. J.* **318,** 219–226.
135. Oldberg, A., Jirskog-Hed, B., Axelsson, S., and Heinegard, D. (1989) Regulation of bone sialoprotein mRNA by steroid hormones. *J. Cell Biol.* **109,** 3183–3186.
136. Young, M. F., Kerr, J. M., Ibaraki, K., Heegaard, A. M., and Robey, P. G. (1992) Structure, expression, and regulation of the major noncollagenous matrix proteins of bone. *Clin. Orthop.* 275–294.
137. Delany, A. M., Amling, M., Priemel, M., Howe, C., Baron, R., and Canalis, E. (2000) Osteopenia and decreased bone formation in osteonectin-deficient mice (published erratum appears in *J. Clin. Invest.* 2000 May;**105(9),** 1325). *J. Clin. Invest.* **105,** 915–923.
138. Kelm, R. J. Jr., Swords, N. A., Orfeo, T., and Mann, K. G. (1994) Osteonectin in matrix remodeling. A plasminogen-osteonectin-collagen complex. *J. Biol. Chem.* **269,** 30147–30153.
139. Martin, T. J., Allan, E. H., and Fukumoto, S. (1993) The plasminogen activator and inhibitor system in bone remodeling. *Growth Regul.* **3,** 209–214.
140. Allan, E. H. and Martin, T. J. (1995) The plasminogen activator inhibitor system in bone cell function. *Clin. Orthop.* **313,** 54–63.
141. Hoekman, K., Lowik, C. W., Ruit, M., Bijvoet, O. L., Verheijen, J. H., and Papapoulos, S. E. (1991) Regulation of the production of plasminogen activators by bone resorption enhancing and inhibiting factors in three types of osteoblast-like cells. *Bone Miner.* **14,** 189–204.
142. Merchiers, P., Bulens, F., Stockmans, I., De Vriese, A., Convents, R., Bouillon, R., et al. (1999) 1,25-Dihydroxyvitamin D(3) induction of the tissue-type plasminogen activator gene is mediated through its multihormone-responsive enhancer. *FEBS Lett.* **460,** 289–296.
143. Maillard, C., Berruyer, M., Serre, C. M., Amiral, J., Dechavanne, M., and Delmas, P. D. (1993) Thrombomodulin is synthesized by osteoblasts, stimulated by 1,25-(OH)2D3 and activates protein C at their cell membrane. *Endocrinology* **133,** 668 -674.
144. Hamilton, J. A., Lingelbach, S. R., Partridge, N. C., and Martin, T. J. (1984) Stimulation of plasminogen activator in osteoblast-like cells by bone-resorbing hormones. *Biochem. Biophys. Res. Commun.* **122,** 230–236.
145. Hamilton, J. A., Lingelbach, S., Partridge, N. C., and Martin, T. J. (1985) Regulation of plasminogen activator production by bone-resorbing hormones in normal and malignant osteoblasts. *Endocrinology* **116,** 2186–2191.
146. Uchida, M., Shima, M., Shimoaka, T., Fujieda, A., Obara, K., Suzuki, H., Nagai, Y., Ikeda, T., Yamato, H., and Kawaguchi, H. (2000) Regulation of matrix metalloproteinases (MMPs) and tissue inhibitors of metalloproteinases (TIMPs) by bone resorptive factors in osteoblastic cells. *J. Cell Physiol.* **185,** 207–214.
147. Uchida, M., Shima, M., Chikazu, D., Fujieda, A., Obara, K., Suzuki, H., et al. (2001) Transcriptional induction of matrix metalloproteinase-13 (collagenase-3) by 1alpha,25-dihydroxyvitamin D3 in mouse osteoblastic MC3T3-E1 cells. *J. Bone Miner. Res.* **16,** 221–230.
148. Lin, R., Amizuka, N., Sasaki, T., Aarts, M. M., Ozawa, H., Goltzman, D., et al. (2002) 1Alpha,25-dihydroxyvitamin D3 promotes vascularization of the chondro-osseous junction by stimulating expression of vascular endothelial growth factor and matrix metalloproteinase 9. *J. Bone Miner. Res.* **17,** 1604–1612.
149. Raisz, L. G. (1999) Prostaglandins and bone: physiology and pathophysiology. Osteoarthritis. Cartilage. **7,** 419–421.
150. Keeting, P. E., Li, C. H., Whipkey, D. L., Thweatt, R., Xu, J., Murty, M., Blaha, J. D., et al. (1998) 1,25-Dihydroxyvitamin D3 pretreatment limits prostaglandin biosynthesis by cytokine-stimulated adult human osteoblast-like cells. *J. Cell Biochem.* **68,** 237–246.

151. Marie, P. J., Hott, M., Launay, J. M., Graulet, A. M., and Gueris, J. (1993) In vitro production of cytokines by bone surface-derived osteoblastic cells in normal and osteoporotic postmenopausal women: relationship with cell proliferation. *J. Clin. Endocrinol. Metab.* **77,** 824–830.
152. Schwartz, Z., Dennis, R., Bonewald, L., Swain, L., Gomez, R., and Boyan, B. D. (1992) Differential regulation of prostaglandin E2 synthesis and phospholipase A2 activity by 1,25-(OH)2D3 in three osteoblast-like cell lines (MC-3T3-E1, ROS 17/2.8, and MG-63). *Bone* **13,** 51–58.
153. Heberden, C., Denis, I., Pointillart, A., and Mercier, T. (1998) TGF-beta and calcitriol. *Gen. Pharmacol.* **30,** 145–151.
154. Wu, Y., Craig, T. A., Lutz, W. H., and Kumar, R. (1999) Identification of 1 alpha,25-dihydroxyvitamin D3 response elements in the human transforming growth factor beta 2 gene. *Biochemistry* **38,** 2654–2660.
155. Wu, Y., Haugen, J. D., Zinsmeister, A. R., and Kumar, R. (1997) 1 alpha,25-Dihydroxyvitamin D3 increases transforming growth factor and transforming growth factor receptor type I and II synthesis in human bone cells. *Biochem. Biophys. Res. Commun.* **239,** 734–739.
156. Sterck, J. G., Klein-Nulend, J., Burger, E. H., and Lips, P. (1996) 1,25-dihydroxyvitamin D3-mediated transforming growth factor-beta release is impaired in cultured osteoblasts from patients with multiple pituitary hormone deficiencies. *J. Bone Miner. Res.* **11,** 367–376.
157. Nagel, D. and Kumar, R. (2002) 1 alpha,25-dihydroxyvitamin D3 increases TGF beta 1 binding to human osteoblasts. *Biochem. Biophys. Res. Commun.* **290,** 1558–1563.
158. Finkelman, R. D., Linkhart, T. A., Mohan, S., Lau, K. H., Baylink, D. J., and Bell, N. H. (1991) Vitamin D deficiency causes a selective reduction in deposition of transforming growth factor beta in rat bone: possible mechanism for impaired osteoinduction. *Proc. Natl. Acad. Sci. USA* **88,** 3657–3660.
159. Wang, X., Schwartz, Z., Yaffe, P., and Ornoy, A. (1999) The expression of transforming growth factor-beta and interleukin-1beta mRNA and the response to 1,25(OH)2D3' 17 beta-estradiol, and testosterone is age dependent in primary cultures of mouse-derived osteoblasts in vitro. *Endocrine* **11,** 13–22.
160. Wang, E. A., Rosen, V., D'Alessandro, J. S., Bauduy, M., Cordes, P., Harada, T., et al. (1990) Recombinant human bone morphogenetic protein induces bone formation. *Proc. Natl. Acad. Sci. USA* **87,** 2220–2224.
161. Virdi, A. S., Cook, L. J., Oreffo, R. O., and Triffitt, J. T. (1998) Modulation of bone morphogenetic protein-2 and bone morphogenetic protein-4 gene expression in osteoblastic cell lines. *Cell Mol. Biol. (Noisy.-le-grand)* **44,** 1237–1246.
162. Faucheux, C., Bareille, R., Amedee, J., and Triffitt, J. T. (1999) Effect of 1,25(OH)2D3 on bone morphogenetic protein-3 mRNA expression. *J. Cell Biochem.* **73,** 11–19.
163. Trippel, S. B. (1998) Potential role of insulinlike growth factors in fracture healing. *Clin. Orthop.* **355**(Suppl.), S301–S313.
164. Rosen, C. J. (1999) Serum insulin-like growth factors and insulin-like growth factor-binding proteins: clinical implications. *Clin. Chem.* **45,** 1384–1390.
165. Conover, C. A. (1995) Insulin-like growth factor binding protein proteolysis in bone cell models. *Prog. Growth Factor Res.* **6,** 301–309.
166. Chenu, C., Valentin-Opran, A., Chavassieux, P., Saez, S., Meunier, P. J., and Delmas, P. D. (1990) Insulin like growth factor I hormonal regulation by growth hormone and by 1,25(OH)2D3 and activity on human osteoblast-like cells in short-term cultures. *Bone* **11,** 81–86.
167. Chen, T. L., Mallory, J. B., and Hintz, R. L. (1991) Dexamethasone and 1,25(OH)2 vitamin D3 modulate the synthesis of insulin-like growth factor-I in osteoblast-like cells. *Calcif. Tissue Int.* **48,** 278–282.
168. Scharla, S. H., Strong, D. D., Mohan, S., Baylink, D. J., and Linkhart, T. A. (1991) 1,25-Dihydroxyvitamin D3 differentially regulates the production of insulin-like growth factor I (IGF-I) and IGF-binding protein-4 in mouse osteoblasts. *Endocrinology* **129,** 3139–3146.
169. McCarthy, T. L., Centrella, M., and Canalis, E. (1992) Constitutive synthesis of insulin-like growth factor-II by primary osteoblast-enriched cultures from fetal rat calvariae. *Endocrinology* **130,** 1303–1308.
170. Linkhart, T. A. and Keffer, M. J. (1991) Differential regulation of insulin-like growth factor-I (IGF-I) and IGF-II release from cultured neonatal mouse calvaria by parathyroid hormone, transforming growth factor-beta, and 1,25-dihydroxyvitamin D3. *Endocrinology* **128,** 1511–1518.
171. Chen, T. L., Chang, L. Y., Bates, R. L., and Perlman, A. J. (1991) Dexamethasone and 1,25-dihydroxyvitamin D3 modulation of insulin-like growth factor-binding proteins in rat osteoblast-like cell cultures. *Endocrinology* **128,** 73–80.
172. Scharla, S. H., Strong, D. D., Rosen, C., Mohan, S., Holick, M., Baylink, D. J. and Linkhart, T. A. (1993) 1,25-Dihydroxyvitamin D3 increases secretion of insulin-like growth factor binding protein-4 (IGFBP-4) by human osteoblast-like cells in vitro and elevates IGFBP-4 serum levels in vivo. *J. Clin. Endocrinol. Metab.* **77,** 1190–1197.
173. Nakao, Y., Hilliker, S., Baylink, D. J., and Mohan, S. (1994) Studies on the regulation of insulin-like growth factor binding protein 3 secretion in human osteosarcoma cells in vitro. *J. Bone Miner. Res.* **9,** 865–872.
174. Kveiborg, M., Flyvbjerg, A., Eriksen, E. F., and Kassem, M. (2001) 1,25-Dihydroxyvitamin D3 stimulates the production of insulin-like growth factor-binding proteins-2, -3 and -4 in human bone marrow stromal cells. *Eur. J. Endocrinol.* **144,** 549–557.
175. Schmid, C., Schlapfer, I., Gosteli-Peter, M. A., Hauri, C., Froesch, E. R., and Zapf, J. (1996) 1 alpha,25-dihydroxyvitamin D3 increases IGF binding protein-5 expression in cultured osteoblasts. *FEBS Lett.* **392,** 21–24.
176. Nasu, M., Sugimoto, T., and Chihara, K. (1997) Stimulatory effects of parathyroid hormone and 1,25-dihydroxyvitamin D3 on insulin-like growth factor-binding protein-5 mRNA expression in osteoblastic UMR-106 cells: the difference between transient and continuous treatments. *FEBS Lett.* **409,** 63–66.

177. Akutsu, N., Lin, R., Bastien, Y., Bestawros, A., Enepekides, D. J., Black, M. J., et al. (2001) Regulation of gene Expression by 1alpha,25-dihydroxyvitamin D3 and Its analog EB1089 under growth-inhibitory conditions in squamous carcinoma cells. *Mol. Endocrinol.* **15,** 1127–1139.
178. Farach-Carson, M. C. and Xu, Y. (2002) Microarray detection of gene expression changes induced by 1,25(OH)(2)D(3) and a Ca(2+) influx-activating analog in osteoblastic ROS 17/2.8 cells. *Steroids* **67,** 467–470.
179. Li, Y. C., Pirro, A. E., Amling, M., Delling, G., Baron, R., Bronson, R., et al. (1997) Targeted ablation of the vitamin D receptor: an animal model of vitamin D-dependent rickets type II with alopeci. *Proc. Natl. Acad. Sci. USA* **94,** 9831–9835.
180. Yoshizawa, T., Handa, Y., Uematsu, Y., Takeda, S., Sekine, K., Yoshihara, Y., et al. (1997) Mice lacking the vitamin D receptor exhibit impaired bone formation, uterine hypoplasia and growth retardation after weaning. *Nat. Genet.* **16,** 391–396.
181. Hedlund, T. E., Moffatt, K. A., and Miller, G. J. (1996) Vitamin D receptor expression is required for growth modulation by 1 alpha,25-dihydroxyvitamin D3 in the human prostatic carcinoma cell line ALVA-31. *J. Steroid Biochem. Mol. Biol.* **58,** 277–288.
182. Zhuang, S. H., Schwartz, G. G., Cameron, D., and Burnstein, K. L. (1997) Vitamin D receptor content and transcriptional activity do not fully predict antiproliferative effects of vitamin D in human prostate cancer cell lines. *Mol. Cell Endocrinol.* **126,** 83–90.
183. Takeda, S., Yoshizawa, T., Nagai, Y., Yamato, H., Fukumoto, S., Sekine, K., et al. (1999) Stimulation of osteoclast formation by 1,25-dihydroxyvitamin D requires its binding to vitamin D receptor (VDR) in osteoblastic cells: studies using VDR knockout mic. *Endocrinology* **140,** 1005–1008.
184. Kveiborg, M., Rattan, S. I., Clark, B. F., Eriksen, E. F., and Kassem, M. (2001) Treatment with 1,25-dihydroxyvitamin D3 reduces impairment of human osteoblast functions during cellular aging in culture. *J. Cell Physiol.* **186,** 298–306.
185. Martinez, P., Moreno, I., De Miguel, F., Vila, V., Esbrit, P., and Martinez, M. E. (2001) Changes in osteocalcin response to 1,25-dihydroxyvitamin D(3) stimulation and basal vitamin D receptor expression in human osteoblastic cells according to donor age and skeletal origin. *Bone* **29,** 35–41.
186. Costa, E. M. and Feldman, D. (1986) Homologous up-regulation of the 1,25 (OH)2 vitamin D3 receptor in rats. *Biochem. Biophys. Res. Commun.* **137,** 742–747.
187. Li, X. Y., Boudjelal, M., Xiao, J. H., Peng, Z. H., Asuru, A., Kang, S., et al. (1999) 1,25-Dihydroxyvitamin D3 increases nuclear vitamin D3 receptors by blocking ubiquitin/proteasome-mediated degradation in human skin. *Mol. Endocrinol.* **13,** 1686–1694.
188. Pols, H. A., Birkenhager, J. C., Schilte, J. P., and Visser, T. J. (1988) Evidence that the self-induced metabolism of 1,25-dihydroxyvitamin D-3 limits the homologous up-regulation of its receptor in rat osteosarcoma cells. *Biochim. Biophys. Acta* **970,** 122–129.
189. Van Leeuwen, J. P., Birkenhager, J. C., van den Bemd, G. C., and Pols, H. A. (1996) Evidence for coordinated regulation of osteoblast function by 1,25-dihydroxyvitamin D3 and parathyroid hormone. *Biochim. Biophys. Acta* **1312,** 54–62.
190. Chen, T. L., Hauschka, P. V., and Feldman, D. (1986) Dexamethasone increases 1,25-dihydroxyvitamin D3 receptor levels and augments bioresponses in rat osteoblast-like cells. *Endocrinology* **118,** 1119–1126.
191. Li, X. Q., Tembe, V., Horwitz, G. M., Bushinsky, D. A., and Favus, M. J. (1993) Increased intestinal vitamin D receptor in genetic hypercalciuric rats. A cause of intestinal calcium hyperabsorption. *J. Clin. Invest* **91,** 661–667.
192. Krieger, N. S., Stathopoulos, V. M., and Bushinsky, D. A. (1996) Increased sensitivity to 1,25(OH)2D3 in bone from genetic hypercalciuric rats. *Am. J. Physiol.* **271,** C130–C135.
193. Gensure, R. C., Antrobus, S. D., Fox, J., Okwueze, M., Talton, S. Y., and Walters, M. R. (1998) Homologous upregulation of vitamin D receptors is tissue specific in the rat. *J. Bone Miner. Res.* **13,** 454–463.
194. Cancela, L., Nemere, I., and Norman, A. W. (1988) 1 alpha,25(OH)2 vitamin D3: a steroid hormone capable of producing pleiotropic receptor-mediated biological responses by both genomic and nongenomic mechanisms. *J. Steroid Biochem.* **30,** 33–39.
195. Baran, D. T. (1994) Nongenomic actions of the steroid hormone 1 alpha,25-dihydroxyvitamin D3. *J. Cell Biochem.* **56,** 303–306.
196. Baran, D. T., Ray, R., Sorensen, A. M., Honeyman, T., and Holick, M. F. (1994) Binding characteristics of a membrane receptor that recognizes 1 alpha,25-dihydroxyvitamin D3 and its epimer, 1 beta,25-dihydroxyvitamin D3. *J. Cell Biochem.* **56,** 510–517.
197. Lieberherr, M. (1987) Effects of vitamin D3 metabolites on cytosolic free calcium in confluent mouse osteoblasts. *J. Biol. Chem.* **262,** 13168–13173.
198. Nakagawa, K., Tsugawa, N., Okamoto, T., Kishi, T., Ono, T., Kubodera, N., and Okano, T. (1999) Rapid control of transmembrane calcium influx by 1alpha,25-dihydroxyvitamin D3 and its analogues in rat osteoblast-like cells. *Biol. Pharm. Bull.* **22,** 1058–1063.
199. de Boland, A. R. and Norman, A. W. (1990) Influx of extracellular calcium mediates 1,25-dihydroxyvitamin D3-dependent transcaltachia (the rapid stimulation of duodenal Ca2+ transport). *Endocrinology* **127,** 2475–2480.
200. Lieberherr, M., Grosse, B., Duchambon, P., and Drueke, T. (1989) A functional cell surface type receptor is required for the early action of 1,25-dihydroxyvitamin D3 on the phosphoinositide metabolism in rat enterocytes. *J. Biol. Chem.* **264,** 20403–20406.
201. Civitelli, R., Kim, Y. S., Gunsten, S. L., Fujimori, A., Huskey, M., Avioli, L. V., et al. (1990) Nongenomic activation of the calcium message system by vitamin D metabolites in osteoblast-like cells. *Endocrinology* **127,** 2253–2262.

202. Wali, R. K., Baum, C. L., Sitrin, M. D., and Brasitus, T. A. (1990) 1,25(OH)2 vitamin D3 stimulates membrane phosphoinositide turnover, activates protein kinase C, and increases cytosolic calcium in rat colonic epithelium. *J. Clin. Invest.* **85,** 1296–1303.
203. Farago, A. and Nishizuka, Y. (1990) Protein kinase C in transmembrane signaling. *FEBS Lett.* **268,** 350–354.
204. Nemere, I., Schwartz, Z., Pedrozo, H., Sylvia, V. L., Dean, D. D., and Boyan, B. D. (1998) Identification of a membrane receptor for 1,25-dihydroxyvitamin D3 which mediates rapid activation of protein kinase C. *J. Bone Miner. Res.* **13,** 1353–1359.
205. Boyan, B. D., Bonewald, L. F., Sylvia, V. L., Nemere, I., Larsson, D., Norman, A. W., et al. (2002) Evidence for distinct membrane receptors for 1 alpha,25-(OH)(2)D(3) and 24R,25-(OH)(2)D(3) in osteoblasts. *Steroids* **67,** 235–246.
206. Mesbah, M., Nemere, I., Papagerakis, P., Nefussi, J. R., Orestes-Cardoso, S., Nessmann, C., et al. (2002) Expression of a 1,25-dihydroxyvitamin D3 membrane-associated rapid-response steroid binding protein during human tooth and bone development and biomineralization. *J. Bone Miner. Res.* **17,** 1588–1596.
207. Pedrozo, H. A., Schwartz, Z., Rimes, S., Sylvia, V. L., Nemere, I., Posner, G. H., et al. (1999) Physiological importance of the 1,25(OH)2D3 membrane receptor and evidence for a membrane receptor specific for 24,25(OH)2D3. *J. Bone Miner. Res.* **14,** 856–867.
208. Fleet, J. C. (1999) Vitamin D receptors: not just in the nucleus anymore. *Nutr. Rev.* **57,** 60–62.
209. Wu, S., Ren, S., Chen, H., Chun, R. F., Gacad, M. A., and Adams, J. S. (2000) Intracellular vitamin D binding proteins: novel facilitators of vitamin D-directed transactivation. *Mol. Endocrinol.* **14,** 1387–1397.
210. Chun, R. F., Chen, H., Boldrick, L., Sweet, C., and Adams, J. S. (2001) Cloning, sequencing, and functional characterization of the vitamin D receptor in vitamin D-resistant New World primates. *Am. J. Primatol.* **54,** 107–118.
211. Wu, S., Chun, R., Gacad, M. A., Ren, S., Chen, H., and Adams, J. S. (2002) Regulation of 1,25-dihydroxyvitamin D synthesis by intracellular vitamin d binding protein-1. *Endocrinology* **143,** 4135–4138.
212. Chen, T. L. and Feldman, D. (1985) Retinoic acid modulation of 1,25(OH)2 vitamin D3 receptors and bioresponse in bone cells: species differences between rat and mouse. *Biochem. Biophys. Res. Commun.* **132,** 74–80.
213. Chen, T. L., Hauschka, P. V., Cabrales, S., and Feldman, D. (1986) The effects of 1,25-dihydroxyvitamin D3 and dexamethasone on rat osteoblast-like primary cell cultures: receptor occupancy and functional expression patterns for three different bioresponses. *Endocrinology* **118,** 250–259.
214. Miller, G. J., Stapleton, G. E., Hedlund, T. E., and Moffat, K. A. (1995) Vitamin D receptor expression, 24-hydroxylase activity, and inhibition of growth by 1alpha,25-dihydroxyvitamin D3 in seven human prostatic carcinoma cell lines. *Clin. Cancer Res.* **1,** 997–1003.
215. Ly, L. H., Zhao, X. Y., Holloway, L., and Feldman, D. (1999) Liarozole acts synergistically with 1alpha,25-dihydroxyvitamin D3 to inhibit growth of DU 145 human prostate cancer cells by blocking 24-hydroxylase activity. *Endocrinology* **140,** 2071–2076.
216. Walters, M. R., Rosen, D. M., Norman, A. W., and Luben, R. A. (1982) 1,25-Dihydroxyvitamin D receptors in an established bone cell line. Correlation with biochemical responses. *J. Biol. Chem.* **257,** 7481–7484.
217. Boyan, B. D., Sylvia, V. L., Dean, D. D., and Schwartz, Z. (2001) 24,25-(OH)(2)D(3) regulates cartilage and bone via autocrine and endocrine mechanisms. *Steroids* **66,** 363–374.
218. Dean, D. D., Boyan, B. D., Schwart, Z., Muniz, O. E., Carreno, M. R., Maeda, S., and Howell, D. S. (2001) Effect of 1alpha,25-dihydroxyvitamin D3 and 24R,25-dihydroxyvitamin D3 on metalloproteinase activity and cell maturation in growth plate cartilage in vivo. *Endocrine* **14,** 311–323.
219. Schwartz, Z., Pedrozo, H. A., Sylvia, V. L., Gomez, R., Dean, D. D., and Boyan, B. D. (2001) 1alpha,25-(OH)2D3 regulates 25-hydroxyvitamin D3 24R-hydroxylase activity in growth zone costochondral growth plate chondrocytes via protein kinase C. *Calcif. Tissue Int.* **69,** 365–372.
220. Harant, H., Spinner, D., Reddy, G. S., and Lindley, I. J. (2000) Natural metabolites of 1alpha,25-dihydroxyvitamin D(3) retain biologic activity mediated through the vitamin D receptor. *J. Cell Biochem.* **78,** 112–120.
221. Siu-Caldera, M. L., Rao, D. S., Astecker, N., Weiskopf, A., Vouros, P., Konno, K., et al. (2001) Tissue specific metabolism of 1alpha,25-dihydroxy-20-epi-vitamin D3 into new metabolites with significant biological activity: studies in rat osteosarcoma cells (UMR 106 and ROS 17/2.8). *J. Cell Biochem.* **82,** 599–609.
222. Kamao, M., Tatematsu, S., Reddy, G. S., Hatakeyama, S., Sugiura, M., Ohashi, N., et al. (2001) Isolation, identification and biological activity of 24R,25-dihydroxy-3-epi-vitamin D3: a novel metabolite of 24R,25-dihydroxyvitamin D3 produced in rat osteosarcoma cells (UMR 106). *J. Nutr. Sci. Vitaminol. (Tokyo)* **47,** 108–115.
223. Pols, H. A., Van Leeuwen, J. P., Schilte, J. P., Visser, T. J., and Birkenhager, J. C. (1988) Heterologous up-regulation of the 1,25-dihydroxyvitamin D3 receptor by parathyroid hormone (PTH) and PTH-like peptide in osteoblast-like cells. *Biochem. Biophys. Res. Commun.* **156,** 588–594.
224. Van Leeuwen, J. P., Birkenhager, J. C., Vink-van Wijngaarden, T., Van Den Bemd, G. J., and Pols, H. A. (1992) Regulation of 1,25-dihydroxyvitamin D3 receptor gene expression by parathyroid hormone and cAMP-agonists. *Biochem. Biophys. Res. Commun.* **185,** 881–886.
225. Klaus, G., von Eichel, B., May, T., Hugel, U., Mayer, H., Ritz, E., and Mehls, O. (1994) Synergistic effects of parathyroid hormone and 1,25-dihydroxyvitamin D3 on proliferation and vitamin D receptor expression of rat growth cartilage cells. *Endocrinology* **135,** 1307–1315.
226. Krishnan, A. V., Cramer, S. D., Bringhurst, F. R., and Feldman, D. (1995) Regulation of 1,25-dihydroxyvitamin D3 receptors by parathyroid hormone in osteoblastic cells: role of second messenger pathways. *Endocrinology* **136,** 705–712.

227. Armbrecht, H. J., Hodam, T. L., Boltz, M. A., Partridge, N. C., Brown, A. J., and Kumar, V. B. (1998) Induction of the vitamin D 24-hydroxylase (CYP24) by 1,25-dihydroxyvitamin D3 is regulated by parathyroid hormone in UMR106 osteoblastic cells. *Endocrinology* **139,** 3375–3381.
228. Van Leeuwen, J. P., Birkenhager, J. C., Schilte, J. P., Buurman, C. J., and Pols, H. A. (1990) Role of calcium and cAMP in heterologous up-regulation of the 1,25-dihydroxyvitamin D3 receptor in an osteoblast cell line. *Cell Calcium* **11,** 281–289.
229. Huening, M., Yehia, G., Molina, C. A., and Christakos, S. (2002) Evidence for a regulatory role of inducible cAMP early repressor in protein kinase a-mediated enhancement of vitamin D receptor expression and modulation of hormone action. *Mol. Endocrinol.* **16,** 2052–2064.
230. Chen, C., Noland, K. A., and Kalu, D. N. (1997) Modulation of intestinal vitamin D receptor by ovariectomy, estrogen and growth hormone. *Mech. Ageing Dev.* **99,** 109–122.
231. Davoodi, F., Brenner, R. V., Evans, S. R., Schumaker, L. M., Shabahang, M., Nauta, R. J., et al. (1995) Modulation of vitamin D receptor and estrogen receptor by 1,25(OH)2-vitamin D3 in T-47D human breast cancer cells. *J. Steroid Biochem. Mol. Biol.* **54,** 147–153.
232. Van Leeuwen, J. P., Pols, H. A., Schilte, J. P., Visser, T. J., and Birkenhager, J. C. (1991) Modulation by epidermal growth factor of the basal 1,25(OH)2D3 receptor level and the heterologous up-regulation of the 1,25(OH)2D3 receptor in clonal osteoblast-like cells. *Calcif. Tissue Int.* **49,** 35–42.
233. Staal, A., Birkenhager, J. C., Pols, H. A., Buurman, C. J., Vink-van Wijngaarden, T., Kleinekoort, W. M., et al. (1994) Transforming growth factor beta-induced dissociation between vitamin D receptor level and 1,25-dihydroxyvitamin D3 action in osteoblast-like cells. *Bone Miner.* **26,** 27–42.
234. Van Leeuwen, J. P., Birkenhager, J. C., Buurman, C. J., Van Den Bemd, G. J., Bos, M. P., and Pols, H. A. (1992) Bidirectional regulation of the 1,25-dihydroxyvitamin D3 receptor by phorbol ester-activated protein kinase-C in osteoblast-like cells: interaction with adenosine 3',5'-monophosphate-induced up-regulation of the 1,25-dihydroxyvitamin D3 receptor. *Endocrinology* **130,** 2259–2266.
235. Reinhardt, T. A. and Horst, R. L. (1994) Phorbol 12-myristate 13-acetate and 1,25-dihydroxyvitamin D3 regulate 1,25-dihydroxyvitamin D3 receptors synergistically in rat osteosarcoma cells. *Mol. Cell Endocrinol.* **101,** 159–165.
236. Petkovich, P. M., Heersche, J. N., Tinker, D. O., and Jones, G. (1984) Retinoic acid stimulates 1,25-dihydroxyvitamin D3 binding in rat osteosarcoma cells. *J. Biol. Chem.* **259,** 8274–8280.
237. Petkovich, P. M., Heersche, J. N., Aubin, J. E., Grigoriadis, A. E., and Jones, G. (1987) Retinoic acid-induced changes in 1 alpha,25-dihydroxyvitamin D3 receptor levels in tumor and nontumor cells derived from rat bone. *J. Natl. Cancer Inst.* **78,** 265–270.
238. Liel, Y., Kraus, S., Levy, J., and Shany, S. (1992) Evidence that estrogens modulate activity and increase the number of 1,25-dihydroxyvitamin D receptors in osteoblast-like cells (ROS 17/2.8). *Endocrinology* **130,** 2597–2601.
239. Escaleira, M. T., Sonohara, S., and Brentani, M. M. (1993) Sex steroids induced up-regulation of 1,25-(OH)2 vitamin D3 receptors in T 47D breast cancer cells. *J. Steroid Biochem. Mol. Biol.* **45,** 257–263.
240. Ishibe, M., Nojima, T., Ishibashi, T., Koda, T., Kaneda, K., Rosier, R. N., et al. (1995) 17 beta-estradiol increases the receptor number and modulates the action of 1,25-dihydroxyvitamin D3 in human osteosarcoma-derived osteoblast-like cells. *Calcif. Tissue Int.* **57,** 430–435.
241. Liel, Y., Shany, S., Smirnoff, P., and Schwartz, B. (1999) Estrogen increases 1,25-dihydroxyvitamin D receptors expression and bioresponse in the rat duodenal mucosa. *Endocrinology* **140,** 280–285.
242. Sriussadaporn, S., Wong, M. S., Pike, J. W., and Favus, M. J. (1995) Tissue specificity and mechanism of vitamin D receptor up-regulation during dietary phosphorus restriction in the rat. *J. Bone Miner. Res.* **10,** 271–280.
243. Walters, M. R. (1981) An estrogen-stimulated 1,25-dihydroxyvitamin D3 receptor in rat uterus. *Biochem. Biophys. Res. Commun.* **103,** 721–726.
244. Krishnan, A. V. and Feldman, D. (1992) Cyclic adenosine 3',5'-monophosphate up-regulates 1,25-dihydroxyvitamin D3 receptor gene expression and enhances hormone action. *Mol. Endocrinol.* **6,** 198–206.
245. Kurahashi, I., Matsunuma, A., Kawane, T., Abe, M., and Horiuchi, N. (2002) Dexamethasone enhances vitamin D-24-hydroxylase expression in osteoblastic (UMR-106) and renal (LLC-PK1) cells treated with 1alpha,25-dihydroxyvitamin D3. *Endocrine* **17,** 109–118.
246. Yanagisawa, J., Yanagi, Y., Masuhiro, Y., Suzawa, M., Watanabe, M., Kashiwagi, K., et al. (1999) Convergence of transforming growth factor-beta and vitamin D signaling pathways on SMAD transcriptional coactivators. *Science* **283,** 1317–1321.
247. Yanagi, Y., Suzawa, M., Kawabata, M., Miyazono, K., Yanagisawa, J., and Kato, S. (1999) Positive and negative modulation of vitamin D receptor function by transforming growth factor-beta signaling through smad proteins. *J. Biol. Chem.* **274,** 12971–12974.
248. Gurlek, A. and Kumar, R. (2001) Regulation of osteoblast growth by interactions between transforming growth factor-beta and 1alpha,25-dihydroxyvitamin D3. *Crit. Rev. Eukaryot. Gene Exp.* **11,** 299–317.
249. Lindenmuth, D., Van Wijnen, A. J., Penman, S., Stein, J. L., Stein, G. S., and Lian, J. B. (1998) TGF-beta1 modifications in nuclear matrix proteins of osteoblasts during differentiation. *J. Cell Biochem.* **69,** 291–303.
250. Chen, T. L. and Feldman, D. (1984) Modulation of PTH-stimulated cyclic AMP in cultured rodent bone cells: the effects of 1,25(OH)2 vitamin D3 and its interaction with glucocorticoids. *Calcif. Tissue Int.* **36,** 580–585.
251. Pols, H. A., Schilte, H. P., Herrmann-Erlee, N. M., Visser, T. J., and Birkenhager, J. C. (1986) The effects of 1,25-dihydroxyvitamin D3 on growth, alkaline phosphatase and adenylate cyclase of rat osteoblast-like cells. *Bone Miner.* **1,** 397–405.

252. Van Leeuwen, J. P., Birkenhager, J. C., Bos, M. P., van der Bemd, G. J., Herrmann-Erlee, M. P., and Pols, H. A. (1992) Parathyroid hormone sensitizes long bones to the stimulation of bone resorption by 1,25-dihydroxyvitamin D3. *J. Bone Miner. Res.* **7,** 303–309.
253. Li, W. and Farach-Carson, M. C. (2001) Parathyroid hormone-stimulated resorption in calvaria cultured in serum-free medium is enhanced by the calcium-mobilizing activity of 1,25-dihydroxyvitamin D(3). *Bone* **29,** 231–235.
254. Tokuda, H., Kotoyori, J., Suzuki, A., Oiso, Y., and Kozawa, O. (1993) Effects of vitamin D3 on signaling by prostaglandin E2 in osteoblast-like cells. *J. Cell Biochem.* **52,** 220–226.
255. Kozawa, O., Tokuda, H., Kotoyori, J., Suzuki, A., Ito, Y., and Oiso, Y. (1993) Modulation of prostaglandin E2-induced Ca2+ influx by steroid hormones in osteoblast-like cells. *Prostaglandins Leukot. Essent. Fatty Acids* **49,** 711–714.
256. Suzuki, A., Tokuda, H., Kotoyori, J., Ito, Y., Oiso, Y., and Kozawa, O. (1994) Effect of vitamin D3 on prostaglandin E2 synthesis in osteoblast-like cells. *Prostaglandins Leukot. Essent. Fatty Acids* **51,** 27–31.
257. Kozawa, O., Tokuda, H., Kaida, T., Matsuno, H., and Uematsu, T. (1998) Effect of vitamin D3 on interleukin-6 synthesis induced by prostaglandins in osteoblasts. *Prostaglandins Leukot. Essent. Fatty Acids* **58,** 119–123.
258. Menaa, C., Vrtovsnik, F., Friedlander, G., Corvol, M., and Garabedian, M. (1995) Insulin-like growth factor I, a unique calcium-dependent stimulator of 1,25-dihydroxyvitamin D3 production. Studies in cultured mouse kidney cells. *J. Biol. Chem.* **270,** 25461–25467.
259. Wei, S., Tanaka, H., and Seino, Y. (1998) Local action of exogenous growth hormone and insulin-like growth factor-I on dihydroxyvitamin D production in LLC-PK1 cells. *Eur. J. Endocrinol.* **139,** 454–460.
260. Wong, M. S., Tembe, V. A., and Favus, M. J. (2000) Insulin-like growth factor-I stimulates renal 1, 25-dihydroxycholecalciferol synthesis in old rats fed a low calcium diet. *J. Nutr.* **130,** 1147–1152.
261. Canalis, E. and Lian, J. B. (1988) Effects of bone associated growth factors on DNA, collagen and osteocalcin synthesis in cultured fetal rat calvariae. *Bone* **9,** 243–246.
262. Kurose, H., Seino, Y., Yamaoka, K., Tanaka, H., Shima, M., and Yabuuchi, H. (1989) Cooperation of synthetic insulin-like growth factor I/somatomedin C and 1,25-dihydroxyvitamin D3 on regulation of function in clonal osteoblastic cells. *Bone Miner.* **5,** 335–345.
263. Liu, P., Oyajobi, B. O., Russell, R. G., and Scutt, A. (1999) Regulation of osteogenic differentiation of human bone marrow stromal cells: interaction between transforming growth factor-beta and 1,25(OH)(2) vitamin D(3) In vitro. *Calcif. Tissue Int.* **65,** 173–180.
264. Somjen, D., Weisman, Y., and Kaye, A. M. (1995) Pretreatment with 1,25(OH)2 vitamin D or 24,25(OH)2 vitamin D increases synergistically responsiveness to sex steroids in skeletal-derived cells. *J. Steroid Biochem. Mol. Biol.* **55,** 211–217.
265. Chen, F. P., Lee, N., Wang, K. C., Soong, Y. K., and Huang, K. E. (2002) Effect of estrogen and 1alpha,25(OH)(2)-vitamin D(3) on the activity and growth of human primary osteoblast-like cells in vitro. *Fertil. Steril.* **77,** 1038–1043.
266. Eichner, A., Brock, J., Heldin, C. H., and Souchelnytskyi, S. (2002) Bone morphogenetic protein-7 (OP1) and transforming growth factor-beta1 modulate 1,25(OH)2-vitamin D3-induced differentiation of human osteoblasts. *Exp. Cell Res.* **275,** 132–142.
267. D'ippolito, G., Schiller, P. C., Perez-stable, C., Balkan, W., Roos, B. A., and Howard, G. A. (2002) Cooperative actions of hepatocyte growth factor and 1,25-dihydroxyvitamin D(3) in osteoblastic differentiation of human vertebral bone marrow stromal cells. *Bone* **31,** 269–275.
268. Anissian, L., Stark, A., Dahistrand, H., Granberg, B., Good, V., and Bucht, E. (2002) Cobalt ions influence proliferation and function of human osteoblast-like cells. *Acta Orthop. Scand.* **73,** 369–374.
269. Narayanan, R., Smith, C., and Weigel, N. (2002) Vector-averaged gravity-induced changes in cell signaling and vitamin d receptor activity in MG-63 cells are reversed by a 1,25-(OH)(2)D(3) analog, EB1089. *Bone* **31,** 381–388.
270. Bouillon, R., Okamura, W. H., and Norman, A. W. (1995) Structure-function relationships in the vitamin D endocrine system. *Endocr. Rev.* **16,** 200–257.
271. Nishii, Y., Sato, K., and Kobayashi, T. (1993) The development of vitamin D3 analogues for the treatment of osteoporosis. *Osteoporos. Int.* **3(Suppl 1),** 190–193.
272. Tsurukami, H., Nakamura, T., Suzuki, K., Sato, K., HiguchI, Y., and Nishii, Y. (1994) A novel synthetic vitamin D analogue, 2 beta-(3-hydroxypropoxy)1 alpha, 25-dihydroxyvitamin D3 (ED-71), increases bone mass by stimulating the bone formation in normal and ovariectomized rats. *Calcif. Tissue Int.* **54,** 142–149.
273. Uchiyama, Y., HiguchI, Y., Takeda, S., Masaki, T., Shira-Ishi, A., Sato, K., et al. (2002) ED-71, a vitamin D analog, is a more potent inhibitor of bone resorption than alfacalcidol in an estrogen-deficient rat model of osteoporosis. *Bone* **30,** 582–588.
274. Peleg, S., Uskokovic, M., Ahene, A., Vickery, B., and Avnur, Z. (2002) Cellular and molecular events associated with the bone-protecting activity of the noncalcemic vitamin D analog Ro-26–9228 in osteopenic rats. *Endocrinology* **143,** 1625–1636.
275. Miyahara, T., Simoura, T., Osahune, N., Uchida, Y., Sakuma, T., Nemoto, N., et al. (2002) A Highly Potent 26,27-Hexafluoro-1a,25-dihydroxyvitamin D3 on calcification in SV40-transformed human fetal osteoblastic cells. *Calcif. Tissue Int.* **70,** 488–495.
276. Shevde, N. K., Yamamoto, H., Clagett-Dame, M., Plum, L., DeLuca, H. F., and Pike, J. W. (2002) A novel vitamin D analogue exhibits selective anabolic actions in osteoblasts that result in enhanced bone formation. *J. Bone Miner. Res.* **17,** S153.
277. Tam, C. S., Wilson, D. R., Hitchman, A. J., and Harrison, J. E. (1981) Protective effect on vitamin D2 on bone apposition from the inhibitory action of hydrocortisone in rats. *Calcif. Tissue Int.* **33,** 167–172.

278. Sato, F., Ouchi, Y., Okamoto, Y., Kaneki, M., Nakamura, T., Ikekawa, N., and Orimo, H. (1991) Effects of vitamin D2 analogs on calcium metabolism in vitamin D-deficient rats and in MC3T3-E1 osteoblastic cells. *Res. Exp. Med. (Berl.)* **191,** 235–242.
279. Finch, J. L., Dusso, A. S., Pavlopoulos, T., and Slatopolsky, E. A. (2001) Relative potencies of 1,25-(OH)(2)D(3) and 19-Nor-1,25-(OH)(2)D(2) on inducing differentiation and markers of bone formation in MG-63 cells. *J. Am. Soc. Nephrol.* **12,** 1468–1474.
280. Clemens, T. L., Tang, H., Maeda, S., Kesterson, R. A., Demayo, F., Pike, J. W., et al. (1997) Analysis of osteocalcin expression in transgenic mice reveals a species difference in vitamin D regulation of mouse and human osteocalcin genes. *J. Bone Miner. Res.* **12,** 1570–1576.
281. Thomas, G. P., Bourne, A., Eisman, J. A., and Gardiner, E. M. (2000) Species-divergent regulation of human and mouse osteocalcin genes by calciotropic hormones. *Exp. Cell Res.* **258,** 395–402.
282. Lian, J. B. and Stein, G. S. (1993) The developmental stages of osteoblast growth and differentiation exhibit selective responses of genes to growth factors (TGF beta 1) and hormones (vitamin D and glucocorticoids). *J. Oral Implantol.* **19,** 95–105.
283. Gerstenfeld, L. C., Zurakowski, D., Schaffer, J. L., Nichols, D. P., Toma, C. D., Broess, M., et al. (1996) Variable hormone responsiveness of osteoblast populations isolated at different stages of embryogenesis and its relationship to the osteogenic lineage. *Endocrinology* **137,** 3957–3968.
284. Thavarajah, M., Evans, D. B., and Kanis, J. A. (1993) Differentiation of heterogeneous phenotypes in human osteoblast cultures in response to 1,25-dihydroxyvitamin D3. *Bone* **14,** 763–767.
285. Kuroki, Y., Shiozawa, S., Kano, J., and Chihara, K. (1995) Competition between c-fos and 1,25(OH)2 vitamin D3 in the transcriptional control of type I collagen synthesis in MC3T3-E1 osteoblastic cells. *J. Cell Physiol.* **164,** 459–464.
286. Martinez, M. E., Medina, S., Sanchez, M., Del Campo, M. T., Esbrit, P., Rodrigo, A., et al. (1999) Influence of skeletal site of origin and donor age on 1,25(OH)2D3-induced response of various osteoblastic markers in human osteoblastic cells. *Bone* **24,** 203–209.
287. Kim, Y. S., Birge, S. J., Avioli, L. V., and Miller, R. (1987) Cell density-dependent vitamin D effects on calcium accumulation in rat osteogenic sarcoma cells (ROS 17/2). *Calcif. Tissue Int.* **41,** 218–222.
288. Rattner, A., Sabido, O., Massoubre, C., Rascle, F., and Frey, J. (1997) Characterization of human osteoblastic cells: influence of the culture conditions. *In Vitro Cell Dev. Biol. Anim.* **33,** 757–762.
289. Franceschi, R. T. and Young, J. (1990) Regulation of alkaline phosphatase by 1,25-dihydroxyvitamin D3 and ascorbic acid in bone-derived cells. *J. Bone Miner. Res.* **5,** 1157–1167.
290. Ishida, H., Bellows, C. G., Aubin, J. E., and Heersche, J. N. (1993) Characterization of the 1,25-(OH)2D3-induced inhibition of bone nodule formation in long-term cultures of fetal rat calvaria cells. *Endocrinology* **132,** 61–66.
291. Van Leeuwen, J. P., Birkenhager, J. C., Buurman, C. J., Schilte, J. P., and Pols, H. A. (1990) Functional involvement of calcium in the homologous up-regulation of the 1,25-dihydroxyvitamin D3 receptor in osteoblast-like cells. *FEBS Lett.* **270,** 165–167.
292. Sugimoto, T., Kanatani, M., Kano, J., Kaji, H., Tsukamoto, T., Yamaguchi, T., et al. (1993) Effects of high calcium concentration on the functions and interactions of osteoblastic cells and monocytes and on the formation of osteoclast-like cells. *J. Bone Miner. Res.* **8,** 1445–1452.
293. Tanaka, S., Haji, M., Takayanagi, R., Tanaka, S., Sugioka, Y., and Nawata, H. (1996) 1,25-Dihydroxyvitamin D3 enhances the enzymatic activity and expression of the messenger ribonucleic acid for aromatase cytochrome P450 synergistically with dexamethasone depending on the vitamin D receptor level in cultured human osteoblasts. *Endocrinology* **137,** 1860–1869.
294. Takayanagi, R., Goto, K., Suzuki, S., Tanaka, S., Shimoda, S., and Nawata, H. (2002) Dehydroepiandrosterone (DHEA) as a possible source for estrogen formation in bone cells: correlation between bone mineral density and serum DHEA-sulfate concentration in postmenopausal women, and the presence of aromatase to be enhanced by 1,25-dihydroxyvitamin D3 in human osteoblasts. *Mech. Ageing Dev.* **123,** 1107–1114.
295. Petkovich, P. M., Wrana, J. L., Grigoriadis, A. E., Heersche, J. N., and Sodek, J. (1987) 1,25-Dihydroxyvitamin D3 increases epidermal growth factor receptors and transforming growth factor beta-like activity in a bone-derived cell line. *J. Biol. Chem.* **262,** 13424–13428.
296. Gonzalez, E. A., Disthabanchong, S., Kowalewski, R., and Martin, K. J. (2002) Mechanisms of the regulation of EGF receptor gene expression by calcitriol and parathyroid hormone in UMR 106–01 cells. *Kidney Int.* **61,** 1627–1634.
297. Kasperk, C. H., Borcsok, I., Schairer, H. U., Schneider, U., Nawroth, P. P., Niethard, F. U., et al. (1997) Endothelin-1 is a potent regulator of human bone cell metabolism in vitro. *Calcif. Tissue Int.* **60,** 368–374.
298. Schutze, N., Lechner, A., Groll, C., Siggelkow, H., Hufner, M., Kohrle, J., et al. (1998) The human analog of murine cystein rich protein 61 [correction of 16] is a 1alpha,25-dihydroxyvitamin D3 responsive immediate early gene in human fetal osteoblasts: regulation by cytokines, growth factors, and serum. *Endocrinology* **139,** 1761–1770.
299. Skjodt, H., Hughes, D. E., Dobson, P. R., and Russell, R. G. (1990) Constitutive and inducible expression of HLA class II determinants by human osteoblast-like cells in vitro. *J. Clin. Invest.* **85,** 1421–1426.
300. Horowitz, M. C., Coleman, D. L., Ryaby, J. T., and Einhorn, T. A. (1989) Osteotropic agents induce the differential secretion of granulocyte-macrophage colony-stimulating factor by the osteoblast cell line MC3T3-E1. *J. Bone Miner. Res.* **4,** 911–921.
301. Wang, X., Schwartz, Z., Yaffe, P., and Ornoy, A. (1999) The expression of transforming growth factor-beta and interleukin-1beta mRNA and the response to 1,25(OH)2D3' 17 beta-estradiol, and testosterone is age dependent in primary cultures of mouse-derived osteoblasts in vitro. *Endocrine* **11,** 13–22.

302. Lacey, D. L., Grosso, L. E., Moser, S. A., Erdmann, J., Tan, H. L., Pacifici, R., et al. (1993) IL-1-induced murine osteoblast IL-6 production is mediated by the type 1 IL-1 receptor and is increased by 1,25 dihydroxyvitamin D3. *J. Clin. Invest.* **91,** 1731–1742.

303. Shen, V., Cheng, S. L., Kohler, N. G., and Peck, W. A. (1990) Characterization and hormonal modulation of IL-1 binding in neonatal mouse osteoblastlike cells. *J. Bone Miner. Res.* **5,** 507–515.

304. Lacey, D. L., Erdmann, J. M., Tan, H. L., and Ohara, J. (1993) Murine osteoblast interleukin 4 receptor expression: upregulation by 1,25 dihydroxyvitamin D3. *J. Cell Biochem.* **53,** 122–134.

305. Tran, J. M., Kleeman, C. R., and Green, J. (1995) Production of interleukin-6 by osteoblastic cells is independent of medium inorganic phosphate. *Biochem. Mol. Med.* **55,** 90–95.

306. Gruber, R., Nothegger, G., Ho, G. M., Willheim, M., and Peterlik, M. (2000) Differential stimulation by PGE(2) and calcemic hormones of IL-6 in stromal/osteoblastic cells. *Biochem. Biophys. Res. Commun.* **270,** 1080–1085.

307. Littlewood, A. J., Russell, J., Harvey, G. R., Hughes, D. E., Russell, R. G., and Gowen, M. (1991) The modulation of the expression of IL-6 and its receptor in human osteoblasts in vitro. *Endocrinology* **129,** 1513–1520.

308. Romas, E., Udagawa, N., Zhou, H., Tamura, T., Saito, M., Taga, T., et al. (1996) The role of gp130-mediated signals in osteoclast development: regulation of interleukin 11 production by osteoblasts and distribution of its receptor in bone marrow cultures. *J. Exp. Med.* **183,** 2581–2591.

309. Kirkwood, K. L., Dziak, R., and Bradford, P. G. (1996) Inositol trisphosphate receptor gene expression and hormonal regulation in osteoblast-like cell lines and primary osteoblastic cell cultures. *J. Bone Miner. Res.* **11,** 1889–1896.

310. Elford, P. R., Felix, R., Cecchini, M., Trechsel, U., and Fleisch, H. (1987) Murine osteoblastlike cells and the osteogenic cell MC3T3-E1 release a macrophage colony-stimulating activity in culture. *Calcif. Tissue Int.* **41,** 151–156.

311. Krieger, N. S. (1997) Parathyroid hormone, prostaglandin E2, and 1,25-dihydroxyvitamin D3 decrease the level of Na+–Ca2+ exchange protein in osteoblastic cells. *Calcif. Tissue Int.* **60,** 473–478.

312. Krieger, N. S. (1997) Parathyroid hormone, prostaglandin E2, and 1,25-dihydroxyvitamin D3 decrease the level of Na+–Ca2+ exchange protein in osteoblastic cells. *Calcif. Tissue Int.* **60,** 473–478.

313. Jehan, F., Naveilhan, P., Neveu, I., Harvie, D., Dicou, E., Brachet, P., and Wion, D. (1996) Regulation of NGF, BDNF and LNGFR gene expression in ROS 17/2.8 cells. *Mol. Cell Endocrinol.* **116,** 149–156.

314. Veenstra, T. D., Fahnestock, M., and Kumar, R. (1998) An AP-1 site in the nerve growth factor promoter is essential for 1, 25-dihydroxyvitamin D3-mediated nerve growth factor expression in osteoblasts. *Biochemistry* **37,** 5988–5994.

315. Yanaka, N., Akatsuka, H., Kawai, E., and Omori, K. (1998) 1,25-Dihydroxyvitamin D3 upregulates natriuretic peptide receptor-C expression in mouse osteoblasts. *Am. J. Physiol.* **275,** E965–E973.

316. Horwood, N. J., Elliott, J., Martin, T. J., and Gillespie, M. T. (1998) Osteotropic agents regulate the expression of osteoclast differentiation factor and osteoprotegerin in osteoblastic stromal cells. *Endocrinology* **139,** 4743–4746.

317. Hofbauer, L. C., Dunstan, C. R., Spelsberg, T. C., Riggs, B. L., and Khosla, S. (1998) Osteoprotegerin production by human osteoblast lineage cells is stimulated by vitamin D, bone morphogenetic protein-2, and cytokines. *Biochem. Biophys. Res. Commun.* **250,** 776 –781.

318. O'Brien, E. A., Williams, J. H., and Marshall, M. J. (2000) Osteoprotegerin ligand regulates osteoclast adherence to the bone surface in mouse calvaria. *Biochem. Biophys. Res. Commun.* **274,** 281–290.

319. Ito, M., Azuma, Y., Ohta, T., and Komoriya, K. (2000) Effects of ultrasound and 1,25-dihydroxyvitamin D3 on growth factor secretion in co-cultures of osteoblasts and endothelial cells. *Ultrasound Med. Biol.* **26,** 161–166.

320. Karmali, R., Nijs-De Wolf, N., Beyer, I., Hendy, G. N., and Bergmann, P. (1999) 1,25-dihydroxyvitamin D3 inhibits parathyroid hormone-related peptide mRNA expression in fetal rat long bones in culture. *In Vitro Cell Dev. Biol. Anim.* **35,** 296–298.

321. Wang, D. S., Yamazaki, K., Nohtomi, K., Shizume, K., Ohsumi, K., Shibuya, M., et al. (1996) Increase of vascular endothelial growth factor mRNA expression by 1,25-dihydroxyvitamin D3 in human osteoblast-like cells. *J. Bone Miner. Res.* **11,** 472–479.

322. Schlaeppi, J. M., Gutzwiller, S., Finkenzeller, G., and Fournier, B. (1997) 1,25-Dihydroxyvitamin D3 induces the expression of vascular endothelial growth factor in osteoblastic cells. *Endocr. Res.* **23,** 213–229.

323. Wang, D. S., Miura, M., Demura, H., and Sato, K. (1997) Anabolic effects of 1,25-dihydroxyvitamin D3 on osteoblasts are enhanced by vascular endothelial growth factor produced by osteoblasts and by growth factors produced by endothelial cells. *Endocrinology* **138,** 2953–2962.

VI
Skeletal Dysmorphology

22

Role of *Pax3* and *PDGF-α Receptor* in Skeletal Morphogenesis and Facial Clefting

Simon J. Conway

INTRODUCTION AND BACKGROUND

The vertebrate head is one of the most intricately patterned structures and yet little is known of the developmental mechanisms by which the tissues are instructed to grow, fuse, and differentiate to give rise to the mature calcified cranial skeleton. In addition to being an anatomically complex structure, the human head is composed of 22 separate bones, numerous cartilages plus 20 deciduous and 32 permanent teeth *(1)*—the evolution of the vertebrate head is uniquely thought to have used many diverse developmental strategies during its construction *(2)*.

Normal facial development starts with the emergence and migration of cranial neural crest cells that combine with mesodermal cells to establish the facial primordia *(3)*. These primordia consist mainly of a neural crest-derived mesenchyme that is covered by an overlying epithelium. The outgrowth/proliferation of facial primordia from undifferentiated mesenchymal cells into the finely detailed structures of the mature head and face is largely determined genetically. These processes are known to be dependent on an ever-increasing spectrum of signaling molecules, transcription factors, and growth factors, produced by either the overlying instructive epithelium or responding mesenchyme *(4)*. Given these complexities, it is not surprising that craniofacial malformations are the most common birth defects that occur in humans, with facial clefting representing the majority of these defects *(5)*. Significantly, advances in the study of the human face have revealed the genetic and gene-environment basis of numerous common and rare craniofacial disorders. Classification of craniofacial malformations based on clinical phenotypes is sometimes quite different from the genetic findings of patients. Different mutations in a single gene can cause distinct syndromes, and mutations in different genes can cause the same syndrome *(6)*. Craniofacial clefts and the resultant skeletal defects can arise at any stage of development as a result of either genetic or environmental perturbations (or both) that alter the extracellular matrix as well as affect the patterning, migration, proliferation, and differentiation of cells. Given that the skeleton is largely a secondary structure built around other anatomical primordia *(7)*, skeletal defects usually originate when developing facial processes fail to fuse, merge, or interact; in addition, the clefts can range from mild to severe midface clefts that are lethal *in utero*. Facial clefts exist within more than 300 known syndromes, but a complete understanding of the genetics of facial clefting and cranial skeletal morphogenesis has yet to be completely uncovered *(8)*. Significantly, molecular genetics and animal models for human malformations have begun to provide many insights into abnormal development *(9)*.

From: *The Skeleton: Biochemical, Genetic, and Molecular Interactions in Development and Homeostasis*
Edited by: E. J. Massaro and J. M. Rogers © Humana Press Inc., Totowa, NJ

Recent advances in the fields of embryology, evolution, and mouse genetics are combining to radically alter our concepts of normal prenatal craniofacial development. These include concepts of germ layer formation, the establishment of the initial head plan in the neural plate, and the manner in which head segmentation is controlled by regulatory transcription factor activity in neuromeres and their derived neural crest cells *(1,3,10)*. There is also a much better appreciation of ways in which new cell associations are established. For example, the associations are achieved by neural crest cells primarily through cell migration and subsequent cell interactions that regulate induction, growth, and programmed cell death *(2,11–13)*. These interactions are mediated primarily by three groups of regulatory signaling molecules: growth factors/receptors, the steroid/thyroid/retinoic acid superfamily, and extracellular matrix proteins *(14)*. Similarly, advances have been made with respect to our understanding of the mechanisms involved in primary and secondary palate formation, such as growth, morphogenetic movements, and the fusion/merging phenomenon. In addition, much progress has been made on the mechanisms involved in the final differentiation of skeletal tissues *(10)*.

Using mice and chicken as animal models for human malformations (treated with known teratogens or genetically altered) has provided many insights into abnormal development. Numerous genes *(1,3, 15)* have been shown to be expressed within the developing head. Significantly several genes that are expressed at a critical time and in a tissue relevant to head development, which have been altered (either in structure or expression), exhibit a cleft of some type. The six best examples to date are the *Msx1*, *Tgfβ*, *sonic hedgehog* (*Shh*), *PDGF-α receptor*, *Alx3/Alx4* double and *Ap-2* knockouts, in which gene expression supports a role in craniofacial development and the knockouts result in mid-face clefts.

Msx1 is expressed in developing craniofacial structures, including the palate *(3)* and two independent knockouts *(16,17)*, resulting in 100% of the cleft palate. MSX1 is deleted in cases of the human 4p- syndrome, which commonly includes clefts. In the case of Tgfβ3, two independent knockouts result in the phenotype of cleft palate *(18–20)*. Expression data and work showing that exogenous Tgfβ3 can induce palate fusion in the chicken, where the palate is normally cleft *(21)*, further support a role for Tgfβ3 in clefting. Shh is downregulated by teratogenic doses of retinoic acid *(22)*, and targeted gene disruption of Shh results in multiple patterning defects of the head, spinal cord, axial skeleton, and the limbs *(23)*. Early defects are observed in the establishment or maintenance of midline structures, such as the notochord and the floorplate, and later defects include absence of distal limb structures, ventral cell types within the neural tube, the spinal column, most of the ribs, and cyclopia. Defects in all tissues extend beyond the normal sites of Shh transcription, confirming the proposed role of Shh proteins as an extracellular signal required for the tissue-organizing properties of several vertebrate patterning centers *(23)*.

Patch mutant mice *(24)* harbor a deletion, including the platelet-derived growth factor *(PDGF)-α receptor* gene, and exhibit defects of neural crest cells, which adversely affect pigmentation in heterozygotes and cranial bones in homozygotes. To verify the role of the *PDGF-α receptor* during development, mice carrying a targeted null mutation were generated *(25)*. No pigmentation phenotype was observed in heterozygotes, but homozygotes die during embryonic development and exhibit midface clefts similar to those observed in *Patch* mutants. In addition, increased apoptosis was observed along the pathways followed by migrating neural crest cells, indicating that *PDGFs* may exert their functions during early embryogenesis by affecting cell survival and patterning.

Compound mutants of *Alx3* and *Alx4* show severe craniofacial abnormalities that are absent in both *Alx3* and *Alx4* single mutants, as *Alx3/Alx4* double-mutant newborn mice have cleft nasal regions. Most facial bones and many other neural crest-derived skull elements were malformed, truncated, or even absent. The craniofacial defects in *Alx3/Alx4* double-mutant embryos become anatomically manifest around 10.5 days post coitum (dpc), when the nasal processes appear to be abnormally positioned. This is thought to lead to a failure of the medial nasal processes to fuse in the facial mid-line and subsequently to the midface cleft phenotype. Increased apoptosis is localized in the outgrowing frontonasal process in 10.0-dpc double-mutant embryos, which is proposed to be the underlying cause of the subsequent malformations *(26)*. Knockouts of the retinoic acid-dependent transcription factor *Ap-2* resulted in extensive craniofacial and more generalized structural disruptions *(27)*. Similarly, chimeric knockouts for *Ap-2 (28)* suggest a more specific role for this gene in clefting. *Ap-2* also lies near the site of two balanced human translocations at 6p that have cleft lip/palate phenotypes *(29)*.

Additional growth and signaling factors thought to play a role in facial development include *JAGGED1, patched, CREB-binding protein, GLI3, FGFR1, CASK, treacle,* and *FGFR2*. Other transcription factors involved include *DLX5/6* and *Pax3/Pax7*. Extracellular matrix proteins, such as *COL2A1, COL1A2, COL11A2, PIGA, αV integrin, glypican 3, fibrillin,* and *aggrecan*, are essential as well. This ever-expanding catalog of molecules highlights the complex genetics underlying the pathogenesis of facial morphogenesis and the formation of facial clefts *(3)*.

Given that most craniofacial defects appear to have a multifactorial etiology, it is not surprising that various teratogens such as retinoic acid, alcohol, jervine, and cyclopamine have all been shown to cause facial clefting *(5)*. Work on animal models for the retinoic acid syndrome shows that there is major involvement of neural crest cells. Administration of the drug 13-cis-retinoic acid in animals, primarily affects the neural crest cells (which undergo excessive apoptosis). Similarly, a mouse model for the fetal alcohol syndrome, which exhibit a mild form of holoprosencephaly, demonstrates a midline anterior neural plate deficiency leads to olfactory placodes being positioned too close to the midline, and other secondary changes. Genetic variations in *TGF-α, RA receptor-α, NADH dehydrogenase* (an enzyme involved in oxidative metabolism), and *cytochrome P-450* (a detoxifying enzyme), have also been implicated as contributing genetic factors. Cigarette smoking (with the attendant hypoxia) is a probable contributing environmental factor *(10)*. Thus, in addition to providing information on the normal developmental processes that generate and pattern the face, genetic and teratogenic techniques also are beginning to provide insight into the basis for abnormal craniofacial growth *(5)*.

This study describes the identification and analysis of a severe midfacial cleft in a subset of homozygous *Splotch* (Sp^{2H} allele) mutant embryos that have a mutation within *Pax3 (30)*. Additionally, the pathogenesis of the formation of the craniofacial defects in Sp^{2H} mutants is compared with that of the well-characterized *Patch* mutants *(25)*, which have a phenotypically similar midface cleft. We have previously shown that *Pax3* expression is important for normal rib development and that increased apoptosis occurs in the Sp^{2H}/Sp^{2H} mutants thoracic muscles and that it is the reduced and/or deficient thoracic muscles that may contribute to the abnormal skeletogenesis. Additionally, our data suggest that *Pax3* may influence the expression of *PDGF-α receptor* during rib morphogenesis *(31)*. Furthermore, analysis of gene expression markers of lateral sclerotome (*tenascin-C* and *scleraxis*) and myotome (*myogenin, MyoD*, and *Myf5*) in the rib truncations and fusions of the Sp^{2H}/Sp^{2H} embryos revealed a role for *Pax3* in specification of the ventrolateral and posterior parts of the somite *(32)*.

Sp^{2H} mice have a mutation within the *Pax3* DNA-binding transcription factor that is thought to function as a transcriptional repressor (located on human chromosome 2q35 and mouse chromosome 1), and *Patch* mice have a mutation within the *PDGF-α receptor* that has been implicated in control of cell proliferation, survival, and migration (located on human chromosome 4q12 and mouse chromosome 5). Although located on different chromosomes, both these mouse mutants have been widely used as models for the human Velocardiofacial/DiGeorge syndromes *(33,34)*, in which the majority of patients are hemizygous for a deletion of chromosome 22q11 *(35)*. DiGeorge syndrome is a complex human developmental disorder (occurs in 1 of 4000 live births) associated with cardiac outflow tract defects, mild facial dysmorphology, velopharyngeal insufficiency, submucous cleft palate, and thymic/parathyroid hypoplasia/aplasia. DiGeorge is thought to be multifactorial because no one gene is responsible for all clinical defects (because homologous mouse chromosome 22q11 deletions do not completely recapitulate syndrome), and other genes not on chromosome 22 are thought to be downstream effectors *(35)*. Thus, our goal was to determine whether these similar facial clefting phenotypes (but different genetic mutations) are caused by similar mechanisms, in order to begin to understand how patients with very different genetic mutations exhibit similar malformations.

MATERIALS AND METHODS

Animal Breeding, Genotyping, and Determination of Sex

Splotch (Sp^{2H}) homozygous embryos were generated from heterozygous mating of Sp^{2H}/+ mice, and the genotypes were confirmed by polymerase chain reaction (PCR) analysis, as previously described *(36)*. Sp^{2H}/+ mice were bred to the *RARE-lacZ* reporter mice *(37)* that contain a retinoic acid-sensitive promoter/*lacZ* reporter construct as indicator transgenic mice to assess endogenous retinoic acid levels. Embryos were prepared and processed for *lacZ* staining as previously described *(38)*.

Patch heterozygotes on a *C57Bl/6* background (Jackson Laboratories) were backcrossed with *Balb/c* mice for seven generations to generate *Patch*/+ heterozygotes enriched with the *Balb/c* genetic background *(39)*. Two different protocols were used to genotype homozygous *Patch* mutants. First, for embryos on a pure *C57Bl/6* background, Mouse Map Pairs 290 and 201 (D5MIT290 and D5MIT201 Map Pairs; Research Genetics) were used to distinguish between homozygous mutant and wild-type or heterozygote embryos; this method cannot distinguish between heterozygotes and homozygous wild-type embryos. The 201 primer pair (3'-ACCAGTCAAGGACGAATCCTT-5'; 3'-CCCTTTAGCTT CCTCAGGAG-5') amplifies a segment of *PDGF-α receptor* inside the deletion and the 290 primer pair (5'-ACCCAGGCCACAAAAGAAC-3'; 5'-ACCCCTATTCAGTGCCAGG-3') amplifies a region of DNA outside the deletion, thereby serving as a positive control for the presence of genomic DNA. The following program was used for 30 cycles to amplify genomic DNA: denaturation at 94°C for 30 s, annealing at 58°C for 45 s, and extension at 72°C for 30 s. PCR products were run on a 4% agarose gel alongside known controls and homozygous mutants were identified by the presence of the 290 amplified band and the subsequent absence of the 201 band. Wild-type and heterozygous embryos contained both the 201 and 290 bands. Once the *C57Bl/6* heterozygotes were backcrossed onto a *Balb/c* background, all three genotypes of embryos (wild-type, heterozygote, homozygous mutant) could be distinguished from heterozygote matings with PCR primers, which localize to the D5MIT135 region of the mouse locus (3'-CGGAGATTAGGTTTTAGAGGGA-5'; 3'-GGGACAGGAAAGGGACACAT-5'; D5Mit135 Map Pairs, Research Genetics; ref. *40*). PCR conditions were the same as listed above and products were run on a 2% agarose gel alongside known controls.

DNA from all embryos were subjected to PCR sex determination using male and female specific primers designed against X- (*DXNds3*) and Y- (*Sry*, *Zfy*) mouse gene sequences as described *(41)*.

Noon on the day of the finding, a copulation plug was designated 0.5 d of gestation. Pregnant females were killed by cervical dislocation, and the embryos were explanted into Dulbecco's Modified Eagle's Medium (GIBCO) containing 10% fetal calf serum prior to genotyping, fixation, and processing. This investigation conforms to the publication "Guide for the Care and Use of Laboratory Animals" published by the National Institutes of Health (NIH Publication No. 85–23, revised 1985).

Histological Examination

Embryos were fixed by immersion in Bouin's fluid overnight, dehydrated through a graded series of alcohols, and stored in absolute ethanol. Embryos were then cleared in Histoclear and embedded in paraffin wax. Serial sections of 10 μm in thickness were cut on a Leica microtome, stained with hematoxylin and eosin, mounted in DPX, and photographed on a Zeiss Axiophot microscope.

Scanning Electron Microscopy (SEM)

Embryos were isolated in cold phosphate-buffered saline and immersed overnight in a fixative comprising 2% glutaraldehyde and 1% formaldehyde in 0.1 *M* cacodylate buffer (300 mosmol/L). After fixation, hearts were washed overnight in 0.1 *M* cacodylate buffer, postfixed for 1 h in 0.1 *M* cacodylate buffer containing 1% osmium tetroxide, rinsed twice in isotonic 0.1 *M* cacodylate buffer, and then stored in the same buffer. Embryos were then dehydrated through a graded series of ethanols and critical point dried using liquid CO_2 at a temperature of 50°C and pressure of 1400 lb/m^2.

Whole-Mount in Situ *Hybridization and Terminal Deoxynucleotidyl Transferase-Mediated Deoxyuridine Triphosphate-Digoxigenin Nick End Labeling (TUNEL) Analysis of Apoptosis*

Whole-mount *in situ* hybridization was performed using antisense and sense (as negative controls; not shown) probes as described previously *(36)*. Plasmids were linearized with the appropriate restriction enzymes (*AP-2*, ref. *2*; *CRABP1*, ref. *43*; and *Prx2*, ref. *44*) and used as templates to generate digoxygenin both labeled sense and anti-sense RNA probes according to manufacturer's directions (Genius3 kit, Boehringer Mannheim). Embryos were dehydrated through a glycerol/phosphate-buffered saline series and photographed in 40% glycerol.

Embryos were prehybridized according to the whole-mount *in situ* hybridization protocol *(36)*, and subsequently whole-mount TUNEL analysis was performed as described *(45)*.

RESULTS AND DISCUSSION

Derivation of Mice and Characterization of Facial Malformations

The *Splotch* (Sp^{2H}) mice have been backcrossed for eight generations onto a *CBA* genetic background via brother–sister matings. Histological analysis of the resultant embryos from $Sp^{2H}/+$ matings revealed that 99.7% ($n = 47$ litters) of the Sp^{2H}/Sp^{2H} mutants have either spina bifida or exencephaly (or both) neural tube defects and die *in utero* by 14 dpc as a result of associated cardiovascular defects *(30,36,46)*. Interestingly, 11% of the $Sp^{2H}/+$ embryos also exhibit neural tube defects and die at birth (approx 20 dpc). Additionally, it was noted that 9% ($n = 29$ mice at 13.5 dpc) of the Sp^{2H}/Sp^{2H} mutants have severe midface clefts (Fig. 1). Careful re-examination of the Sp^{2H}/Sp^{2H} mutants also revealed that a further 29% of the mutants had small facial blebs (Fig. 2), either on the snout or on the forehead.

The *Patch* (*Ph*) mice were backcrossed for seven generations onto a *Balb/C* genetic background via brother–sister mating. Histological analysis of the resultant embryos from *Ph*/+ mating revealed that 100% ($n = 28$ litters) of the *Ph/Ph* mutants have mid-face clefts (Fig. 1) as previously reported and that 60% of the mutants die at birth (rest of mutants die between 9 and 11.0 dpc as a result of severe hemorrhaging). Detailed histology (not shown) and SEM (Fig. 1) analysis revealed that although both mutants had severe midface clefts, there were anatomical differences. The *Ph* clefts were always accompanied by vascular blood-filled blebbing and were usually more superficial than the Sp^{2H} mutant clefts, which were deep and not accompanied by blood-filled blebs. Additionally, histology revealed that the *Ph* mutant facial cleft was caused by a generalized paucity of mesenchyme within the frontonasal prominence, probably secondary to the reported elevated levels of neural crest-associated apoptosis associated with lack of *PDGF-α receptor* gene *(25)*.

Sp^{2H} *Mutant Facial Clefts Are Gender-Biased But* Ph *Clefts Are Random*

Because it has been reported that cranial defects (exencephaly) can sometimes have a gender prevalence in both humans and mice models, with more females affected than males *(47,48)*, we addressed the question as to whether there was a gender bias. After PCR sex determination of the DNA, the severe midface clefts were found to only be present within the male Sp^{2H}/Sp^{2H} mutants ($n = 29/29$ embryos with midface clefts were male). Additionally, the small facial blebs were only macroscopically observed in male Sp^{2H}/Sp^{2H} mutants (Fig. 2). However, the severe mid-face clefts present within *Ph/Ph* mutants were not statically gender biased ($n = 37$ embryos with mid-face clefts: 16 female, 21 male). This gender bias is significant because it has been previously reported that *Splotch-delayed* (which contain a different mutation of *Pax3*) mice interspecifically bred have significant alterations in skull morphology and are thought to have several genetic modifiers, one being the sex of the mouse *(49)*.

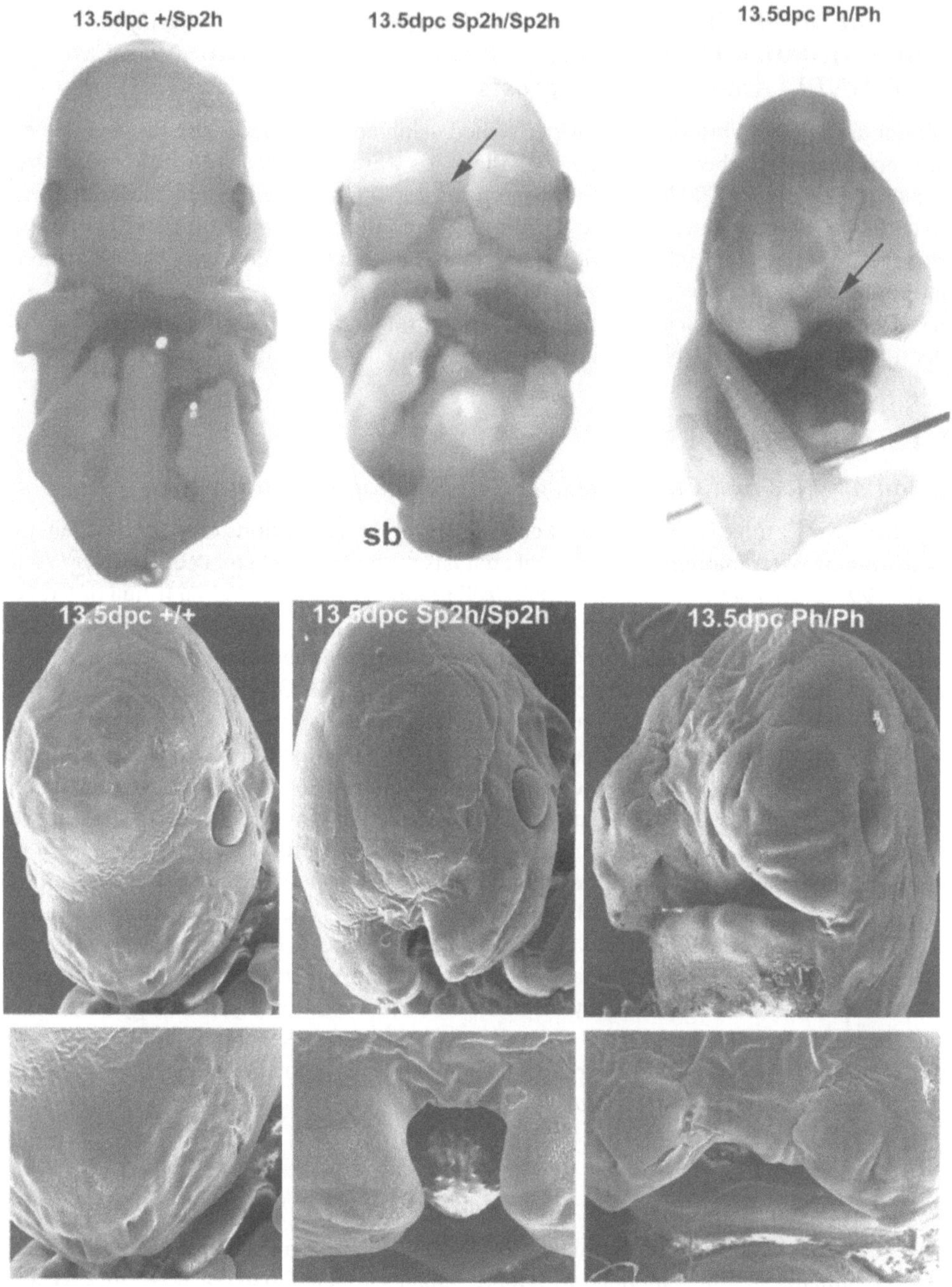

Fig. 1. Major phenotypic abnormalities in mutant embryos. Upper Panel, 13.5-dpc whole embryos viewed frontally. Left embryo is a heterozygous $Sp^{2H}/+$ mutant embryo (tail partially removed to enable clear viewing of face) and homozygous Sp^{2H}/Sp^{2H} mutant (middle embryo) littermates. Note that the homozygote mutant has spina bifida (sb) and a large midface cleft (indicated by arrow) Homozygous *Patch* (*Ph/Ph*) mutant embryo (right embryo) with midface cleft and facial bleeding/edema (indicated by arrow) Lower Panel, SEM images of 13.5-dpc heads viewed frontally, which are enlarged images viewed from above. Wild-type (+/+) and homozygous Sp^{2H}/Sp^{2H} mutant embryos (middle embryo) with mid-face cleft. Note that the tongue is normal, as is the lower jaw. Homozygous *Patch* mutant embryo with mid-face cleft. Note the crumpled appearance of the skin overlying the nasal bridge/forehead region, and that the mid-face cleft is more superficial than the Sp^{2H}/Sp^{2H} mutant cleft.

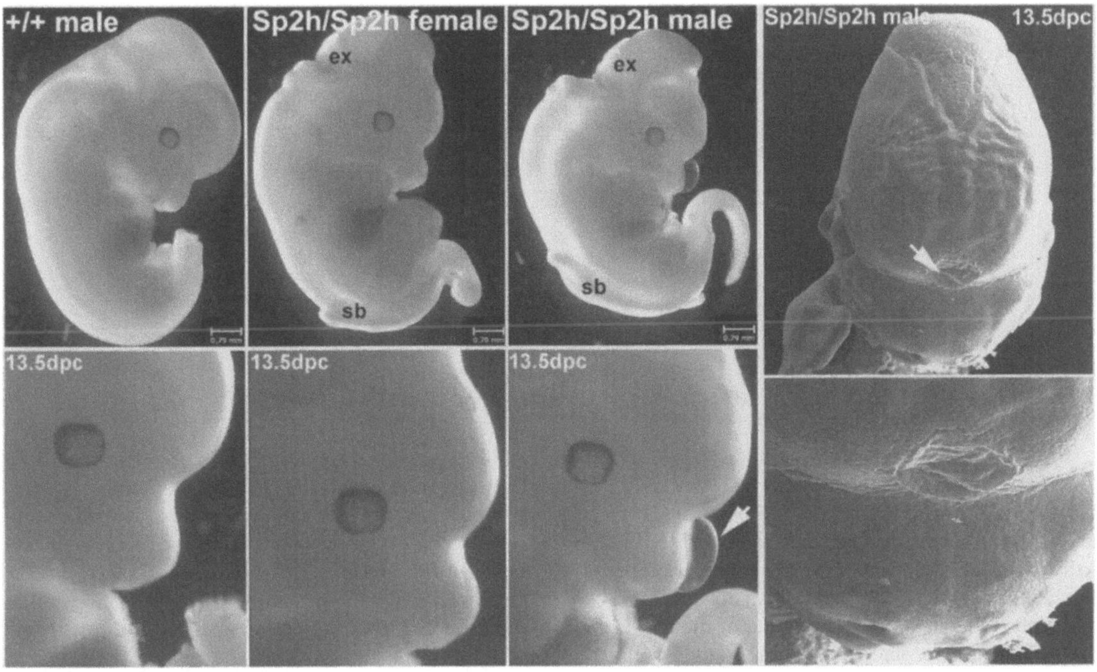

Fig. 2. Subtle phenotypic abnormalities in mutant embryos. Left six panels, 13.5-dpc whole embryos viewed from the left. Note that only the male homozygous Sp^{2H}/Sp^{2H} mutant embryos with spina bifida (sb) and exencephaly (ex) have a small edematous facial bleb (indicated by white arrow), while the homozygous mutant female embryos only exhibit spina bifida and exencephaly. (Bar = 0.79 mm) Right panels, SEM image of 13.5-dpc Sp^{2H}/Sp^{2H} mutant embryo with spina bifida (not visible) and midface bled (indicated by small white arrow), but no exencephaly.

Comparative Pathogenesis of Sp

To define the onset and nature of the facial cleft defect, embryos were analyzed at various stages during development. Histology revealed that facial clefts were present within Sp^{2H}/Sp^{2H} mutant embryos from 9.0 dpc onwards (not shown) and were grossly manifest at 10.0 and 10.5 dpc (Fig. 3). However, facial clefts were not present within *Ph/Ph* mutant embryos until after 11.0 dpc (Fig. 3). This indicates that the underlying mechanisms are clearly different and that the facial cleft in Sp^{2H}/Sp^{2H} mutant embryos occurs prior to cranial neural crest migration and differentiation. Rather, these results indicate that lack of frontonasal neural tube closure of the anterior neuropore is responsible for the formation of the midface cleft. Closure of the neural tube is thought to occur in at least four major sites *(50)* at different times of development. In normal embryos, neural tube closure and craniofacial development is accomplished by concurrent closure of the prosencephalon/mesencephalon boundary (closure point 2) and fusion from the rostral tip of the neural tube (closure point 3) that extends caudally to close the anterior neuropore at around 8.5–9.0 dpc. Thus, in a subgroup of Sp^{2H}/Sp^{2H} mutant embryos, the anterior neuropore remains open, secondarily resulting in formation of the midface cleft defects.

Mechanism Underlying Sp^{2H} *Mutant Facial Clefts*

Facial clefts in *Patch* has been associated with defects in the migration of cranial neural crest cells, either during migration or within the crest cells themselves *(51)*. Additionally, increased apoptosis has been observed within cephalic/branchial arch region of *PDGF-α receptor* knockout embryos *(25)*. Similarly, abnormalities in retinoic acid levels and/or signaling have been shown to be involved in the generation of facial malformations, either by teratogenic studies *(52)* or in transgenically altered

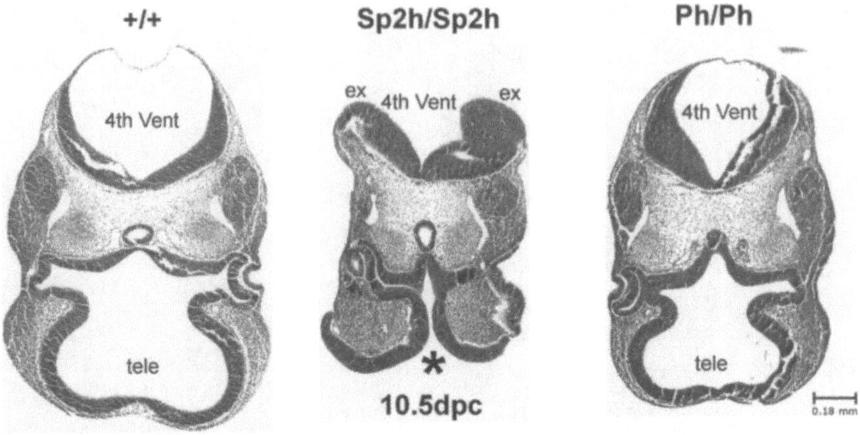

Fig. 3. Histological analysis of the pathogenesis of the midface cleft. Transverse sections through the heads of 10.5-dpc wild-type (+/+), male homozygous (Sp^{2H}/Sp^{2H}), and homozygous *Patch* (*Ph/Ph*) mutant embryos. At 10.5 dpc, the wild-type telencephalic (tele) vesicle is intact within the forehead region and there is a large open chamber. The communication between the optic stalk and intra-retinal space is intact and there is space between the walls of the third ventricle, plus the chamber of the fourth ventricle (4th Vent) is intact. Note that while the *Ph/Ph* mutant head is grossly normal at 10.5 dpc, the Sp^{2H}/Sp^{2H} mutant head is already malformed. There is a large mid-face cleft (indicated by *), the space of the telencephalon and third chamber is missing and the neuroepithelial walls of the telencephalon and third chamber abut each other. Also, this embryo has exencephaly (ex) and the chamber of the fourth ventricle is lost. (Bar = 0.18 mm.)

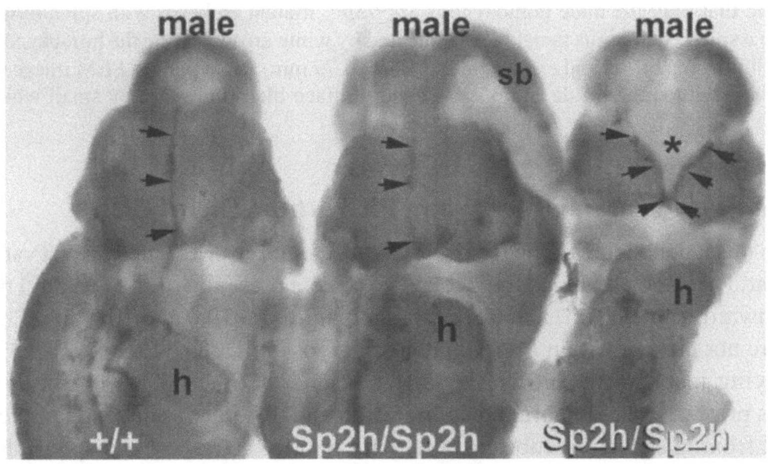

Fig. 4. Apoptotic cell death. TUNEL analysis in wild-type and homozygous (Sp^{2H}/Sp^{2H}) mutant male 10.5-dpc embryos, as detected by the whole death method. The wild-type (+/+) embryo (viewed frontally) has a seam of apoptotic cells along the frontonasal region of the anterior neuropore (indicated by arrowheads), following fusion of the neural folds. Also note that there are normal levels of apoptosis within the heart (h) and in the remodeling somites. There are equivalent levels of apoptotic cells within both the Sp^{2H}/Sp^{2H}) mutant frontonasal regions, even though one mutant (middle embryo) has a closed anterior neuropore and exencephaly (ex) whereas the other mutant (right) has an open anterior neuropore and a mid-face cleft (indicated by *). It is interesting to note that there are still apoptotic cells along the neural folds in the cleft-face mutant, even in the absence of fusion.

mouse mutant models *(28,53)*. In the absence of pronounced cell death, it appears that retinoic acid can possibly produce deleterious effects on the precursors of craniofacial primordia, such as the neural crest, by misexpression of developmentally important genes. Given these results, we addressed the questions as to whether apoptosis was affected in Sp^{2H}/Sp^{2H} mutant embryos, whether endogenous

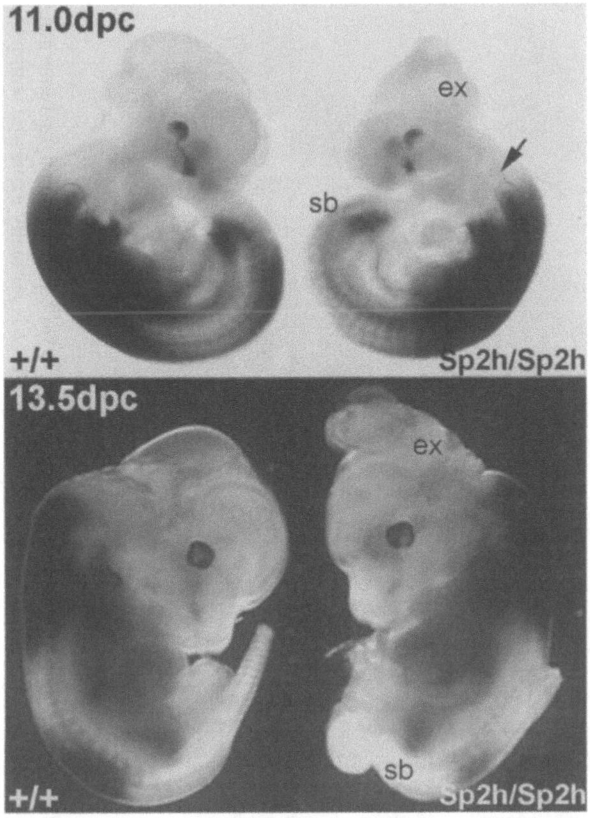

Fig. 5. Analysis of the endogenous levels of retinoic acid within homozygous (Sp^{2H}/Sp^{2H}) mutant embryos. At 11.0 dpc, retinoic acid-mediated *β-gal* staining is prominent along the anterior-posterior axis of the spinal cord, and within the eyes and regions of the frontonasal primordia. Note that in the Sp^{2H}/Sp^{2H} mutant embryos. *LacZ* expression is reduced in the tail (around the region of spina bifida), and there is ectopic staining of one of the vagal branches in the cardiothoracic region (indicated by arrow), but the endogenous levels (as shown by *lacZ* expression) are unchanged in the craniofacial region. A similar pattern of *lacZ* expression is observed in the 13.5-dpc mutants.

levels of retinoic acid were altered in Sp^{2H}/Sp^{2H} mutant embryos, and what role the cranial neural crest play in the pathogenesis of the Sp^{2H}/Sp^{2H}mutant facial clefting.

Apoptotic cell death was examined at 9.5, 10.5, and 13.5 dpc by the "whole death" procedure. No significant difference between wild-type and Sp^{2H}/Sp^{2H} mutant embryos was observed, even when facial clefts were evident (Fig. 4). Both wild-type and Sp^{2H}/Sp^{2H} mutant embryos have a seam of apoptotic cells along the frontonasal region of the anterior neuropore and histological sections through the cephalic region did not reveal any differences in the localization or extent of apoptosis (not shown). This result suggests that mid-face clefts are not caused by elevated apoptotic levels, but are more likely due to a different cause.

Endogenous retinoic acid levels were assessed by breeding the $Sp^{2H}/Sp^{2H}/+$ mice to a retinoic acid responsive reporter mouse, that expresses *β-galactasidase* in the presence of retinoic acid *(37)*. *β-galactasidase* expression was examined at 9.5–13.5 dpc by whole embryo staining, and the levels of expression were unchanged in the Sp^{2H}/Sp^{2H} craniofacial region (Fig. 5). Similarly, retinoic acid signaling and the role of the neural crest were assessed at 9.5–13.5 dpc by using molecular markers. A retinoic acid-responsive transcription factor, Ap-2, *(42)* and *cellular retinoic acid-binding protein-1*

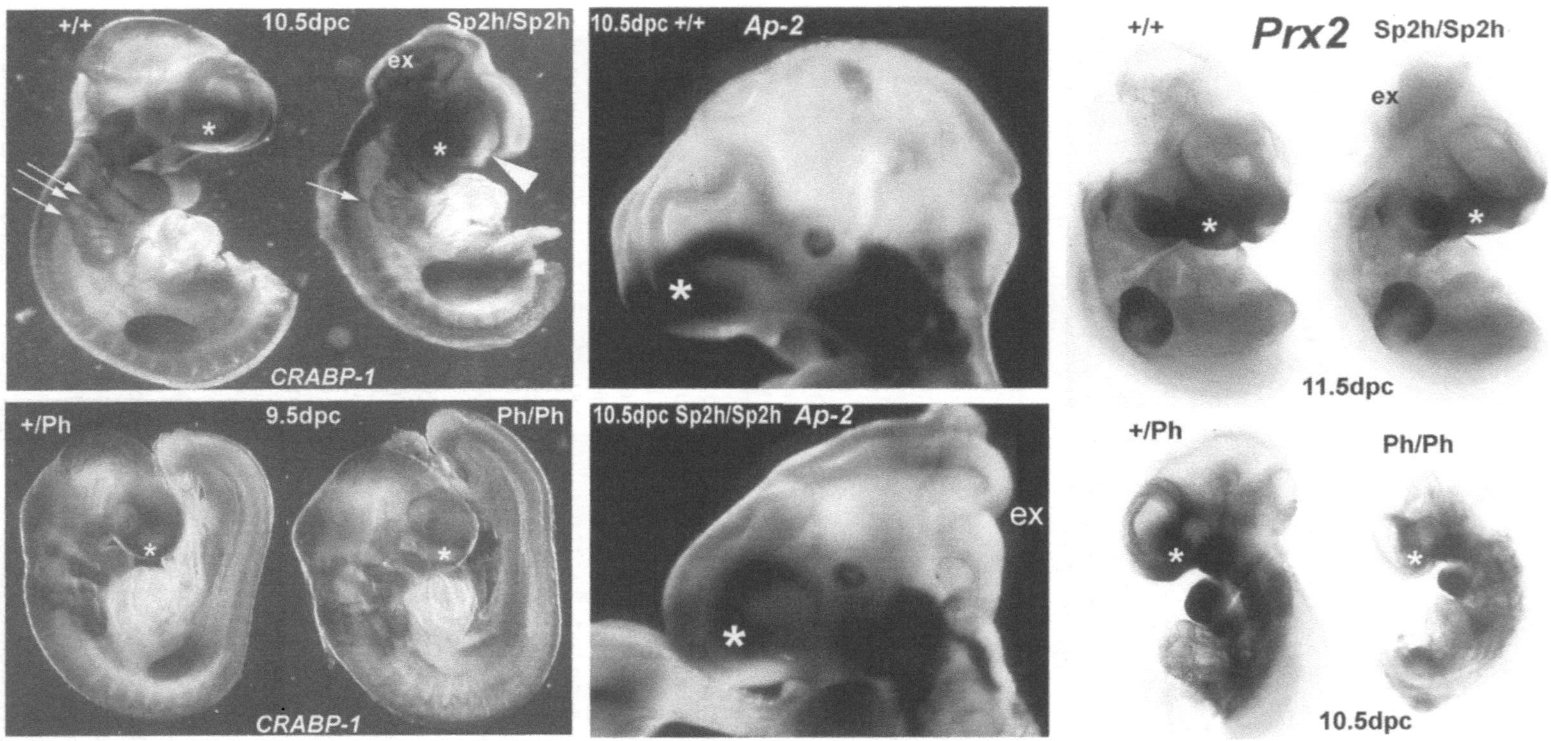

Fig. 6. Expression of neural crest cell marker genes in both Sp^{2H}/Sp^{2H} and *Ph/Ph* mutant embryos. Left panels, Sp^{2H}/Sp^{2H}, *Ph/Ph* mutant, and littermate control embryos were analyzed for *CRABP-1* mRNA expression by whole-mount *in situ* hybridization. Note that *CRABP-1* is normally expressed within the craniofacial region of 10.5-dpc Sp^{2H}/Sp^{2H} mutant embryos (indicated by *) with a midface cleft (indicated by large white arrow head) and exencephaly but that *CRABP-1* is significantly downregulated in 9.5-dpc *Ph/Ph* mutant craniofacial region (indicated by *). Also note that *CRABP-1* is misexpressed within the cardiac neural crest cell region in Sp^{2H}/Sp^{2H} mutant embryo, as instead of the normal three streams of migrating neural crest cells (indicated by three small white arrows in +/+), there is only a single stream of migrating neural crest cells in the mutant embryo (indicated by single small white arrow in mutant) Middle panels, Enlarged Sp^{2H}/Sp^{2H} and wild-type (+/+) littermate control embryo were analyzed for *AP-2* mRNA expression by whole-mount *in situ* hybridization. Note that *Ap-2* is normally expressed within the craniofacial region of 10.5-dpc Sp^{2H}/Sp^{2H} mutant embryo (indicated by *) with exencephaly. Right panels, Sp^{2H}/Sp^{2H}, *Ph/Ph*, mutant and littermate control embryos were analyzed for *Prx2* mRNA expression by whole-mount *in situ* hybridization. Note that *Prx2* is normally expressed within the craniofacial region of 11.5-dpc Sp^{2H}/Sp^{2H} mutant embryos (indicated by *), but that *Prx2* is significantly downregulated in 10.5-dpc *Ph/Ph* mutant craniofacial region (indicated by *).

(*CRABP-1*; ref. *47*) are two genes that respond to retinoic acid that are also expressed within migrating neural crest cells *(30,46)*. Both *Ap-2* and *CRABP-1* expression are unaffected in Sp^{2H}/Sp^{2H} mutant craniofacial region but is downregulated in *Ph/Ph* mutants (Fig. 6).

The aristaless-related homeobox gene *Prx2* is known to be required for normal skeletogenesis and *Prxl/Prx2* double mutants have a reduction or absence of skeletal elements in the skull and face *(54)*. Given this association and that *Prx2* is expressed in neural crest cells as they are undergoing terminal differentiation, we used the *Prx2* molecular marker to determine whether there was a lack of cranial neural crest cells present within the frontonasal primordia. *Prx2* expression was unchanged in the Sp^{2H}/Sp^{2H} mutant embryos but is downregulated in *Ph/Ph* mutants (Fig. 6), suggesting that the Sp^{2H}/Sp^{2H}facial clefts are not caused by a lack of neural crest-derived mesenchyme.

These data suggest that Sp^{2H}/Sp^{2H} mutant midface clefts are not caused by the same neural crest-associated mechanism as in *Ph/Ph* embryos and that neither retinoic acid levels and/or retinoic acid signaling is perturbed within the Sp^{2H}/Sp^{2H} mutant embryo heads. Furthermore, these data indicate that a lack of complete neural fold closure is the underlying cause of the Sp^{2H}/Sp^{2H} craniofacial malformations. Thus, the Sp^{2H}/Sp^{2H} mutant mice provides us with a new model for the study of facial clefting and importantly demonstrates that craniofacial malformations are not solely caused by neural crest-associated defects. It also has been demonstrated that similar abnormal phenotypes can be caused by completely different mechanisms. This will be important when trying to understand the embryological pathogenesis of many clinically complex and diverse human syndromes. Especially as the human genome project continues, the understanding of facial clefting and its syndromes may continue to improve. Such knowledge could advance diagnosis and treatment of the patient and counseling of the affected family *(8)*.

ACKNOWLEDGMENTS

I would like to thank Jian Wang, Rhonda Rogers, Eileen Dickman, and Kristi Singletary for their excellent technical assistance and mouse husbandry. Additionally, we are grateful to Melissa Colbert (Cincinnati Children's Hospital Medical Center) for providing the *RARE-lacZ* reporter mice and Penny Roon for help with the electron microscope. This work was supported by NIH grants HL60714 and HL60104 to S. J. C.

REFERENCES

1. Wilkie, A. O. and Morriss-Kay, G. M. (2001) Genetics of craniofacial development and malformation. *Nat. Rev. Genet.* **2,** 458–468.
2. Thorogood, P. (1993) The problems of building a head. *Curr. Biol.* **3,** 705–708.
3. Schutte, B. C. and Murray, J. C. (1999) The many faces and factors of orofacial clefts. *Hum. Mol. Gene* **8,** 1853–1859.
4. Richman, J. M. and Tickle, C. (1992) Epithelial-mesenchymal interactions in the outgrowth of limb buds and facial primordia in chick embryos. *Dev. Biol.* **154,** 299–308.
5. Young, D. L., Schneider, R. A., Hu, D., and Helms, J. A. (2000) Genetic and teratogenic approaches to craniofacial development. *Crit. Rev. Oral. Biol. Med.* **11,** 304–307.
6. Nuckolls, G. H., Shum, L., and Slavkin, H. C. (1999) Progress toward understanding craniofacial malformations. *Cleft Palate Craniofac. J.* **36,** 12–26.
7. Gruneberg, H. (1975) How do genes affect the skeleton? in *New approaches to the evaluation of abnormal embryonic development* (Neuberg, D. and Merker, H. J., eds.), Georg Thieme, Stuttgart, pp. 354–359.
8. Coleman, J. R. Jr. and Sykes, J. M. (2001) The embryology, classification, epidemiology, and genetics of facial clefting. *Facial Plast. Surg. Clin. North. Am.* **9,** 1–13.
9. Johnston, M. C. and Bronsky, P. T. (1991) Animal models for human craniofacial malformations. *J. Craniofac. Genet. Dev. Biol.* **11,** 277–291.
10. Johnston, M. C. and Bronsky, P. T. (1995) Prenatal craniofacial development: new insights on normal and abnormal mechanisms. *Crit. Rev. Oral. Biol. Med.* **6,** 368–422.
11. Noden, D. M. (1975) An analysis of migratory behavior of avian cephalic neural crest cells. *Dev. Biol.* **42,** 106–130.
12. Le Douarin, N. M., Ziller, C., and Couly, G. F. (1993) Patterning of neural crest derivatives in the avian embryo: in vivo and in vitro studies. *Dev. Biol.* **159,** 24–49.
13. Kontges, G. and Lumsden, A. (1996) Rhombencephalic neural crest segmentation is preserved throughout craniofacial ontogeny. *Development* **122,** 3229–3242.

14. Francis-West, P., Ladher, R., Barlow, A., and Graveson, A. (1998) Signaling interactions during facial development. *Mech. Dev.* **75,** 3–28.
15. Sulik, K. K., Cook, C. S., and Webster, W. S. (1988) Teratogens and craniofacial malformations: relationships to cell death. *Development* **103,** 213–231.
16. Satokata, I. and Maas, R. (1994) *Msx1* deficient mice exhibit cleft palate and abnormalities of craniofacial and tooth development. *Nat. Genet.* **6,** 348–356.
17. Houzelstein, D., Cohen, A., Buckingham, M. E., and Robert, B. (1997) Insertional mutation of the mouse Msx1 homeobox gene by an n*lacZ* reporter gene. *Mech. Dev.* **65,** 123–133.
18. Proetzel, G., Pawlowski, S. A., Wiles, M. V., Yin, M., Boivin, G. P., Howles, P. N., et al. (1995) Transforming growth factor-beta 3 is required for secondary palate fusion. *Nat. Genet.* **11,** 409–414.
19. Kaartinen, V., Voncken, J. W., Shuler, C., Warburton, D., Bu, D., Heisterkamp, N., et al. (1995) Abnormal lung development and cleft palate in mice lacking TGF-beta 3 indicates defects of epithelial-mesenchymal interaction. *Nat. Genet.* **11,** 415–421.
20. Kaartinen, V., Cui, X. M., Heisterkamp, N., Groffen, J., and Shuler, C. F. (1997) Transforming growth factor-beta3 regulates transdifferentiation of medial edge epithelium during palatal fusion and associated degradation of the basement membrane. *Dev. Dyn.* **209,** 255–260.
21. Sun, D., Vanderburg, C. R., Odierna, G. S., and Hay, E. D. (1998) TGFbeta3 promotes transformation of chicken palate medial edge epithelium to mesenchyme in vitro. *Development* **125,** 95–105.
22. Helms, J. A., Kim, C. H., Hu, D., Minkoff, R., Thaller, C., and Eichele, G. (1997) Sonic hedgehog participates in craniofacial morphogenesis and is down-regulated by teratogenic doses of retinoic acid. *Dev. Biol.* **187,** 25–35.
23. Chiang, C., Litingtung, Y., Lee, E., Young, K. E., Corden, J. L., Westphal, H., et al. (1996) Cyclopia and defective axial patterning in mice lacking Sonic hedgehog gene function. *Nature* **383,** 407–413.
24. Gruneberg, H. and Truslove, G. M. (1960) Two closely linked genes in the mouse. *Gen. Res.* **1,** 69–90.
25. Soriano, P. (1997) The PDGF alpha receptor is required for neural crest cell development and for normal patterning of the somites. *Development* **124,** 2691–2700.
26. Beverdam, A., Brouwer, A., Reijnen, M., Korving, J., and Meijlink, F. (2001) Severe nasal clefting and abnormal embryonic apoptosis in *Alx3/Alx4* double mutant mice. *Development* **128,** 3975–3986.
27. Schorle, H., Meier, P., Buchert, M., Jaenisch, R., and Mitchell, P. J. (1996) Transcription factor AP-2 essential for cranial closure and craniofacial development. *Nature* **381,** 235–238.
28. Nottoli, T., Hagopian-Donaldson, S., Zhang, J., Perkins, A., and Williams, T. (1998) AP-2-null cells disrupt morphogenesis of the eye, face, and limbs in chimeric mice. *Proc. Natl. Acad. Sci. USA* **95,** 13714–13719.
29. Davies, A. F., Imaizumi, K., Mirza, G., Stephens, R. S., Kuroki, Y., Matsuno, M., et al. (1998) Further evidence for the involvement of human chromosome 6p24 in the aetiology of orofacial clefting. *J. Med. Genet.* **35,** 857–861.
30. Conway, S. J., Henderson, D. J., Kirby, M. L., Anderson, R. H., and Copp, A. J. (1997) Development of a lethal congenital heart defect in the splotch (Pax3) mutant mouse. *Cardiovascular Res.* **36,** 163–173.
31. Dickman, E. D., Rogers, R., and Conway, S. J. (1999) Abnormal skeletogenesis occurs coincident with increased apoptosis in the Splotch (Sp2H) mutant—putative roles for Pax3 and PDGFRα in rib patterning. *Anat. Rec.* **255,** 353–361.
32. Henderson, D. J., Conway, S. J., and Copp, A. J. (1999) Rib truncations and fusions in the Sp^{2H} mouse reveal a role for *Pax3* in specification of the ventro-lateral and posterior part of the somite. *Dev. Bio.* **209,** 143–158.
33. Magnaghi, P., Roberts, C., Lorain, S., Lipinski, M., and Scambler, P. J. (1998) HIRA, a mammalian homologue of Saccharomyces cerevisiae transcriptional co-repressors, interacts with *Pax3. Nat. Genet.* **20,** 74–77.
34. Maschhoff, K. L. and Baldwin, H. S. (2000) Molecular determinants of neural crest migration. *Am. J. Med. Genet.* **97,** 280–288.
35. Lindsay, E. A. (2001) Chromosomal microdeletions: dissecting del22q11 syndrome. *Nat. Rev. Genet.* **2,** 858–868.
36. Conway, S. J., Henderson, D. J., and Copp, A. J. (1997) *Pax3* is required for cardiac neural crest migration in the mouse: evidence from the (Sp^{2H}) mutant. *Development* **124,** 505–514.
37. Colbert, M. C., Linney, E., and LaMantia, A. S. (1993) Local sources of retinoic acid coincide with retinoid-mediated transgene activity during embryonic development. *Proc. Natl. Acad. Sci. USA* **90,** 6572–6576.
38. Koushik, S. V., Wang, J., Rogers, R., Moskofidis, D., Lambert, L., Creazzo, T., et al. (2001) Targeted inactivation of the sodium-calcium exchanger (Ncx1) results in the lack of a heartbeat and abnormal myofibrillar organization. *FASEB J.* **15,** 1209–1211.
39. Payne, J., Shibasaki, F., and Mercola, M. (1997) Spina bifida occulta in homozygous *Patch* mouse embryos. *Dev. Dyn.* **209,** 105–116.
40. Wehrle-Haller, B., Morrison-Graham, K., and Weston, J. A. (1996) Ectopic *c-kit* expression affects the fate of melanocyte precursors in *Patch* mutant embryos. *Dev. Biol.* **177,** 463–474.
41. Greenlee, A. R., Krisher, R. L., and Plotka, E. D. (1998) Rapid sexing of murine preimplantation embryos using a nested, multiplex polymerase chain reaction (PCR) *Mol. Reprod. Dev.* **49,** 261–267.
42. Mitchell, P. J., Timmons, P. M., Hebert, J. M., Rigby, P. W., and Tjian, R. (1991) Transcription factor AP-2 is expressed in neural crest cell lineages during mouse embryogenesis. *Genes Dev.* **5,** 105–119.
43. Stoner, C. M. and Gudas, L. J. (1989) Mouse cellular retinoic acid binding protein: cloning, complementary DNA sequence, and messenger RNA expression during the retinoic acid-induced differentiation of F9 wild type and RA-3-10 mutant teratocarcinoma cells. *Cancer Res.* **49,** 1497–1504.
44. Kern, M. J., Argao, E. A., Birkenmeier, E. H., Rowe, L. B., and Potter, S. S. (1994) Genomic organization and chromosome localization of the murine homeobox gene *Pmx. Genomics* **19,** 334–340.

45. Conlon, R. A., Reaume, A. G., and Rossant, J. (1995) Notch1 is required for the coordinate segmentation of somites. *Development* **121,** 1533–1545.
46. Conway, S. J., Bundy, J., Chen, J., Dickman, E., Rogers, R., and Will, B. M. (2000) Abnormal neural crest stem cell expansion is responsible for the conotruncal heart defects within the *Splotch* (Sp^{2H}) mouse mutant. *Cardiovasc. Res.* **47,** 314–328.
47. Copp, A. J., Brook, F. A., Estibeiro, J. P., Shum, A. S., and Cockroft, D. L. (1990) The embryonic development of mammalian neural tube defects. *Prog. Neurobiol.* **35,** 363–403.
48. Sah, V. P., Attardi, L. D., Mulligan, G. J., Williams, B. O., Bronson, R. T., and Jacks, T. (1995) A subset of p53-deficient embryos exhibit exencephaly. *Nat. Genet.* **10,** 175–180.
49. Asher, J. H. Jr, Harrison, R. W., Morell, R., Carey, M. L., and Friedman, T. B. (1996) Effects of *Pax3* modifier genes on craniofacial morphology, pigmentation, and viability: a murine model of Waardenburg syndrome variation. *Genomics* **34,** 285–298.
50. Gunn, T. M., Juriloff, D. M., and Harris, M. J. (1995) Genetically determined absence of an initiation site of cranial neural tube closure is causally related to exencephaly in SELH/Bc mouse embryos. *Teratology* **52,** 101–108.
51. Morrison-Graham, K., Schatteman, G. C., Bork, T., Bowen-Pope, D. F., and Weston, J. A. (1992) A PDGF receptor mutation in the mouse (*Patch*) perturbs the development of a non-neuronal subset of neural crest-derived cells. *Development* **115,** 133–142.
52. Morriss-Kay, G. M. and Sokolova, N. (1996) Embryonic development and pattern formation. *FASEB J.* **10,** 961–968.
53. Lohnes, D., Mark, M., Mendelsohn, C., Dolle, P., Decimo, D., LeMeur, M., et al. (1995) Developmental roles of the retinoic acid receptors. *J. Steroid Biochem. Mol. Biol.* **53,** 475–486.
54. ten Berge, D., Brouwer, A., Korving, J., Martin, J. F., and Meijlink, F. (1998) *Prx1* and *Prx2* in skeletogenesis: roles in the craniofacial region, inner ear and limbs. *Development* **125,** 3831–3842.

23
Genetics of Achondroplasia and Hypochondroplasia

Giedre Grigelioniene

PHENOTYPE AND GENETIC DEFECTS

Clinical Features

Achondroplasia and hypochondroplasia are relatively common skeletal dysplasias characterized by disproportionate short stature, rhizomelic shortening of the limbs, and increased head circumference. Short stature and body disproportion are usually severe and uniform in achondroplasia, whereas phenotype in hypochondroplasia varies from severe achondroplasia-like forms to mild shortness and body disproportion. Mild forms of hypochondroplasia are on clinical grounds difficult to differentiate from idiopathic short stature or normal height at the shorter end of the height spectrum.

Achondroplasia

Achondroplasia has a rather constant phenotype and is easily diagnosed at birth because of the infant's short arms and legs, macrocephaly with a relatively small face, depressed nasal bridge, and frontal bossing. The length at birth is slightly decreased (mean at about –1.7 SDS*), and weight is normal. The growth failure usually becomes obvious in a few months and the loss of body height is severe during the first 3 yr of life (Fig. 1; Hertel, N. T., Kaitila, I., and Hagenäs L., manuscript in preparation). The proximal parts of the limbs are especially affected and the short stature is thus called rhizomelic. In contrast with extremities, the length of the trunk is affected to a minor extent. Hands and feet are short and broad because of short metacarpals and phalanges, with the hand having a characteristic appearance that is often called "trident hand." Extension and rotation defects of elbows are common. Muscular hypotonia and ligament laxity are often noticed at birth and later on are associated with delayed gross motor development. The head is larger than normal usually as the result of true megalencephaly, but in some cases it might be combined with hydrocephalus. Intelligence and cognitive development are normal *(1)*. Thoracolumbar kyphosis is common during the first year of life and is replaced by lumbar lordosis when the child begins to walk. Bowed tibia (varus deformity) usually develops during childhood and may require correcting surgery. Narrowing of the foramen magnum is common and may cause neurological symptoms, for example, sleep apnea during infancy. Spinal stenosis may cause neurological symptoms during adulthood. Radiological features include (1) large neurocranium, (2) small slit-shaped foramen magnum, (3) shortened skull base, (4) caudally narrowing interpedicular distance, (5) short broad pelvis, and (6) short thick long bones and are in detail described elsewhere *(2,3)*. Final adult height for males is 118–145 cm and for females, 112–136 cm *(4)*.

*Standard deviation score shows the relationship of the analyzed data to the standard population mean. SDS is the ratio of the difference between body height or segment size of the subject and the 50th percentile value of the population standard for same age and sex to the corresponding standard deviation.

From: *The Skeleton: Biochemical, Genetic, and Molecular Interactions in Development and Homeostasis*
Edited by: E. J. Massaro and J. M. Rogers © Humana Press Inc., Totowa, NJ

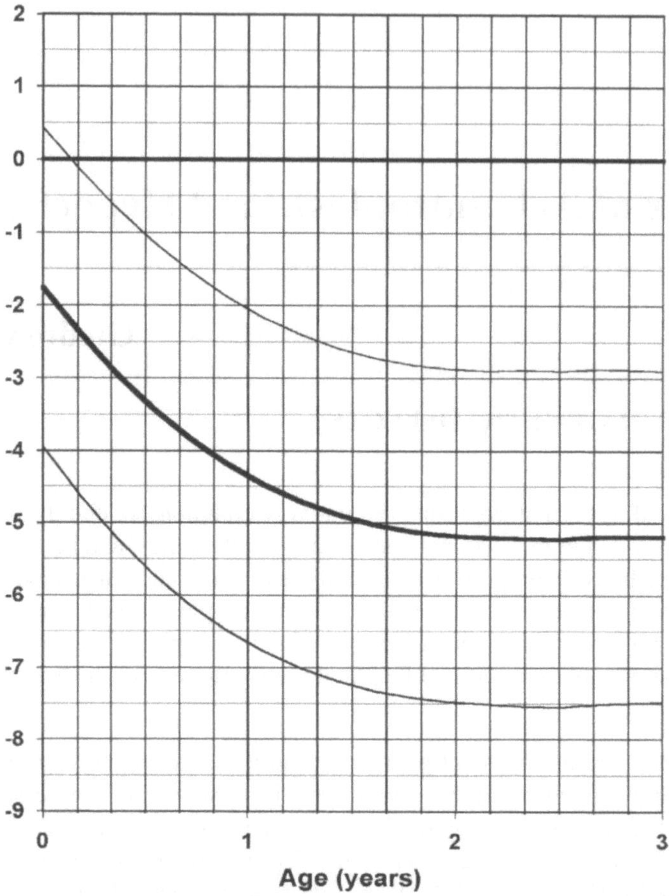

Fig. 1. The loss of the body height expressed in standard deviation score (SDS) in achondroplasia during the first 3 yr of life. The figure is based on 910 measurements from 72 children with achondroplasia and was kindly provided by Hertel et al. (manuscript in preparation).

Hypochondroplasia

Hypochondroplasia is a skeletal dysplasia phenotypically similar to but usually milder than achondroplasia. Because the phenotypic deviations are mild at birth, this dysplasia is usually diagnosed later in childhood. Patients with hypochondroplasia are sometimes characterized as having stocky build, lumbar lordosis, relative macrocephaly with normal facies, *genu varum* (i.e., bowleg), and short broad arms and feet. The diagnosis may be confirmed by radiological examination. The features commonly used for radiological diagnosis of hypochondroplasia are (1) narrowing or unchanged interpedicular distance in the lumbar spine going caudally from L1 to L5, (2) squared shortened ilia, (3) short broad femoral neck, (4) shortening of long tubular bones with mild metaphyseal flare, and (5) mild brachydactyly *(5)*. Some of the above described features may be subtle or absent in milder cases of hypochondroplasia, especially in young children, rendering diagnostic difficulties. Hypochondroplasia-specific metacarpophalangeal profile is available and might be important in confirming the diagnosis *(5,6)*. Body disproportion and short stature is mild in infants and toddlers with hypochondroplasia and usually becomes more obvious with age *(7)*. Absence or decrease of pubertal growth spurt is thought to be common in hypochondroplasia *(8,9)*, but data on this issue are sparse. Final adult height for males is 145–165 cm and for females, 133–151 cm *(8)*. It has to be emphasized that no consensus opinion exists regarding which and how many of the above-described clinical and radiological features must be present to confirm the diagnosis of hypochondroplasia. Consequently, establishing the diagnosis of hypochondroplasia by radiological and clinical-auxological means might be difficult in milder cases. In these cases differentiation among hypochondroplasia, idiopathic short stature, and other skeletal dysplasias with mild short stature and body disproportion (e.g., dyschondrosteosis) should be regarded. In some of these cases, early diagnosis might be possible only on the basis of molecular-genetic examination.

Inheritance

The prevalence of achondroplasia is reported to be 1:10,000–30,000 *(10,11)*, whereas the prevalence of hypochondroplasia is unknown, although probably higher than that of achondroplasia. This could be explained by the phenotypic variability in hypochondroplasia and its overlap with that of normal short stature. Both achondroplasia and hypochondroplasia are inherited in an autosomal-dominant manner. Most cases of achondroplasia and hypochondroplasia are the result of *de novo* mutation. The germ-line frequency of achondroplasia mutation has been estimated to be $5.5–28 \times 10^{-6}$, and the base where this mutation occurs is considered to be among the most mutable nucleotides in the human genome *(12)*. This high mutation rate could be partially explained by the fact that it occurs in a context of CpG dinucleotide. The rate of achondroplasia mutation is slightly increasing with paternal age and has been molecularly confirmed to occur exclusively in the paternal allele *(13,14)*. Gonadal mosaicism has also been reported in a few cases with achondroplasia *(15,16)*. Evidence that hypochondroplasia and achondroplasia were allelic disorders was first suggested by the observation of a child who was born to a hypochondroplastic mother and achondroplastic father *(17)*. This child had clinical and radiological features that were more severe than in heterozygous achondroplasia or hypochondroplasia but milder than in homozygous achondroplasia.

Molecular Genetics

Achondroplasia and hypochondroplasia were mapped to the short arm of chromosome 4 (4p16.3) in 1994, and mutations in the *FGFR3* gene were then rapidly found in both dysplasias *(12,18,19)*. Almost all achondroplasia cases were found to be caused by C1177A or C1177G transversions (according to GenBank accession no. M58051), occurring in the first base of the codon 380, which results in a glycine to arginine substitution (Gly380Arg). This mutation is located in the region coding for the transmembrane domain of the FGFR3. For hypochondroplasia, C1659A and C1659G transversions in the third base of the codon 540, converting it from asparagine to lysine codon (Asn540Lys), have been described in 40–70% of the cases selected for genetical examination *(19–25)*. Other *FGFR3* mutations were later described in a few families with hypochondroplasia. Most of hypochondroplasia mutations are located in the gene region coding for the tyrosine kinase domain of the receptor. The known mutations in the *FGFR3* associated with achondroplasia and hypochondroplasia are summarized in Table 1 and Fig. 2.

It has to be emphasized that in a significant proportion of cases that on clinical and radiological grounds are classified as hypochondroplasia mutations have not yet been identified. Genotyping a few informative pedigrees have excluded the involvement of *FGFR3* in hypochondroplasia phenotype of these families *(6,22,26)*. Thus, hypochondroplasia is a genetically heterogeneous disorder, that is, more than one gene is responsible for this skeletal dysplasia. The actual proportion of locus heterogeneity in hypochondroplasia is difficult to establish because most of the cases are sporadic, which makes genotyping analysis impossible. Sequencing of the whole *FGFR3* gene has been performed only in a few hypochondroplasia cases; thus, some of the yet unidentified mutations still might be localized in this gene.

Genotype–Phenotype Correlation

Given the uniformity of the achondroplasia phenotype, in both physical appearance and radiographic features, it is not surprising that almost 100% of the cases are caused by a single mutation, the Gly380Arg

Table 1
FGFR3 Mutations in Achondroplasia and Hypochondroplasia

Nucleotide triplets	*Codon*	*Reference*	*Comments*
Achondroplasia			
GGC → TGC	Gly375Cys	*(61,62)*	A couple of cases reported so far.
GGG → CGG	Gly380Arg	*(18)*	Less common achondroplasia mutation.
GGG → AGG	Gly380Arg	*(18)*	The most common achondroplasia mutation.
Hypochondroplasia			
AAC → ATC	Asn328Ile	*(63)*	A single family reported.
TC → GTC	Ile538Val	*(64)*	A single family reported.
AAC → AAA	Asn540Lys	*(19–25)*	40–70% of the patients reported in several studies.
AAC → AAG	Asn540Lys	*(20)*	
AAC → AGC	Asn540Ser	*(65)*	A single family reported.
AAC → ACC	Asn540Thr	*(66)*	A single family reported.
AAG → AAT	Lys650Asn	*(43)*	A single individual reported.
AAG → AAC	Lys650Asn	*(43)*	Three unrelated probands reported.
AAG → CAG	Lys650Gln	*(43)*	A single individual reported.

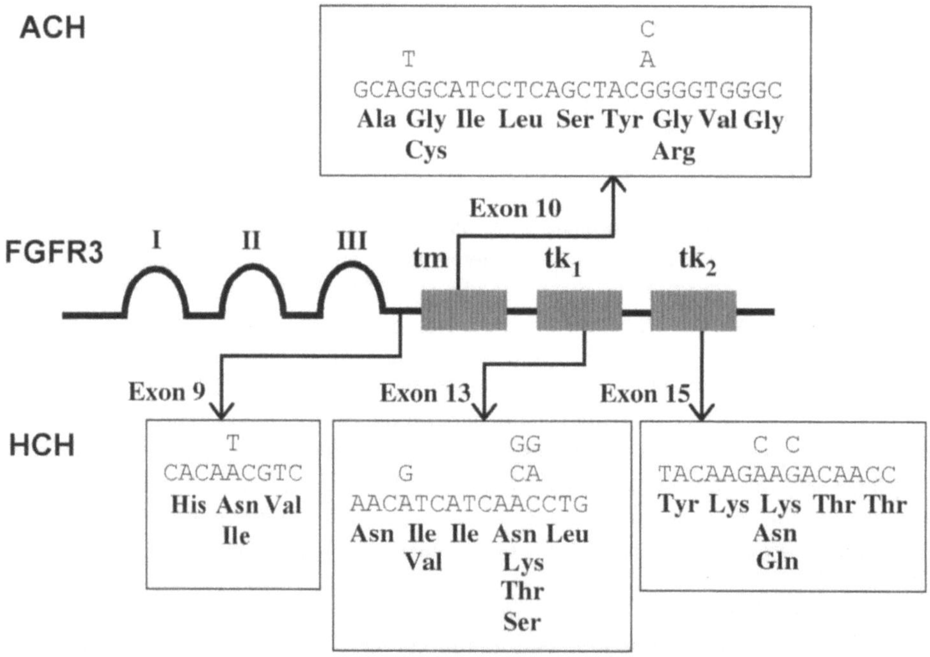

Fig. 2. Mutations responsible for achondroplasia (ACH) and hypochondroplasia (HCH) in the *FGFR3* gene and their corresponding locations in the protein (modified from Bellus et al. *[43]*). FGFR3 protein is drawn schematically and the areas of currently known achondroplasia and hypochondroplasia mutations are shown in detail. tm, transmembrane domain; tk, tyrosine kinase domains; I, II, and III, immunoglobulin-like domains.

substitution. In contrast to the uniformity of achondroplasia, hypochondroplasia is characterized by varying phenotype and genetic heterogeneity. The studies on genotype and phenotype correlation in hypochondroplasia suggest that patients with the Asn540Lys mutation are more disproportionate, have a bigger head circumference, and tend to have more of the characteristic radiological features than those without this mutation *(6,22–24)*. Consequently, the children with the Asn540Lys mutation

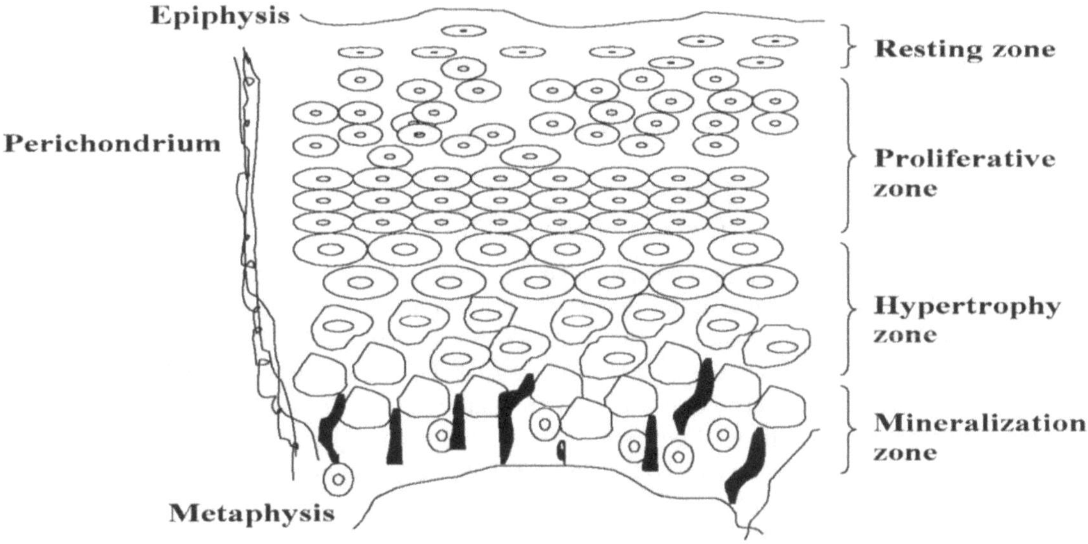

Fig. 3. Schematic representation of the epiphyseal growth plate and its cellular organization.

come to medical attention earlier compared with hypochondroplastic children without this mutation *(24)*. However, considerable phenotype variability has been observed even among the individuals with Asn540Lys mutation *(23,27)*. An individual with hypochondroplasia, cloverleaf skull deformity, and Asn540Lys mutation has been reported, further illustrating the phenotypic heterogeneity in hypochondroplasia *(28)*.

MOLECULAR INTERACTIONS AND DEVELOPMENT OF THE GROWTH PLATE IN ACHONDROPLASIA FAMILY OF SKELETAL DYSPLASIAS

Longitudinal Bone Growth and FGFR3

The template for the longitudinal bone growth is the cartilaginous anlagen of the embryonic bones and epiphyseal growth plates after the endochondral ossification is established. *FGFR3* gene expression has been found in these structures, indicating its importance for skeletal development *(29–31)*. It is has been demonstrated that FGF8 and FGF17 act as FGFR3 ligands during embryonic bone development, whereas FGF2 and FGF9 are involved in the regulation of the growth plate *(32,33)*.

The structure of the growth plate is briefly described below. The growth plate consists of chondrocytes and the extracellular matrix and exhibits spacial polarity. It is divided into four zones: resting, proliferative, hypertrophic and mineralization (Fig. 3). The chondrocytes occupying different zones of the growth plate are in different phases of their life cycle. The stem cells of the resting zone divide and form strictly organized chondrocytic columns in the proliferative zone. The proliferative chondrocytes then increase their volume and form the hypertrophic zone. The hypertrophic chondrocytes mature, stop dividing, and finally undergo a programmed cell death. The extracellular matrix in the end of the hypertrophy zone is mineralized and invaded by blood vessels and bone forming osteoblasts (the mineralization zone). The overall rate of longitudinal bone growth is determined by the progression of the chondrocytes through the aforementioned developmental stages. Thus chondrocyte growth, proliferation, and differentiation (chondrogenesis) in the growth plate are tightly coupled to vascular invasion of the matrix and mineralization (osteogenesis). Many hormones and growth factors control chondrogenesis and osteogenesis. A delicate balance between proliferation and differentiation of chondrocytes and ossification of the epiphyseal growth cartilage is necessary for normal longitudinal bone growth. FGFR3 is one of the key regulators of the longitudinal bone growth and is involved in proliferation, differentiation and apoptosis of chondrocytes as well as ossification of the growth plate. As described below, mutations of the FGFR3 disturb the highly controlled regulation of the growth plate, which results in growth failure and skeletal dysplasia.

Achondroplasia Family of Skeletal Dysplasias Result from Activation of the FGFR3

Mutations in the *FGFR3* gene have been found in rhizomelic skeletal dysplasia syndromes, including achondroplasia, hypochondroplasia, thanatophoric dysplasia, and severe achondroplasia with developmental delay and acanthosis nigricans (SADDAN) *(19,20,34–37)*. These syndromes are now grouped into the achondroplasia family of skeletal dysplasias. The transgenic mouse models with inactivated *Fgfr3* indicated that the receptor is a negative regulator of bone growth because *Fgfr3* knockout mice have longer bones than the wild-type mice *(38,39)*. The phenotypic differences between skeletal overgrowth in *Fgfr3* knockout mice and short stature in *FGFR3*-related human skeletal dysplasias strongly suggested that the mutations responsible for short stature activate the receptor. Indeed, further experiments have demonstrated that FGFR3 activation is responsible for the spectrum of the phenotypes in achondroplasia family of skeletal dysplasias *(40–43)*. Mutations responsible for different clinical entities were found to cluster to certain domains of the receptor. For example, mutations in the extracelullar domain of the receptor are involved in thanatophoric dysplasia type I, whereas mutations in the transmembrane domain of the receptor are responsible for achondroplasia. Interestingly, different amino acid substitutions occurring at the same position can activate the receptor to different levels and the degree of FGFR3 activation correlates to the severity of the clinical phenotype. The Lys650Asn and Lys650Gln mutations causing hypochondroplasia occur in the same codon as mutations reported in thanatophoric dysplasia type II (Lys650Glu) and SADDAN syndrome (Lys650Met). The hypochondroplasia mutations Lys650Asn/Gln cause less severe FGFR3 activation than the mutations described in thanatophoric dysplasia type II and SADDAN *(43)*. Thus, all these studies suggest a correlation between the degree of receptor activation and severity of skeletal dysplasia.

FGFR3 Activation Is Achieved in Several Ways

The mechanisms by which mutations cause the increased level of signaling through FGFR3 are partly different. The thanatophoric dysplasia type I mutation, Arg248Cys, and achondroplasia mutation, Gly375Cys, activate FGFR3 by forming a disulfide linked receptor homodimer, which constitutively stimulate the cells in the absence of ligand *(41,44)*. The achondroplasia mutation (Gly380Arg) has been shown to cause ligand-independent activation of the receptor *(40)*, as well as to increase its responsiveness to the ligand *(42)*. Mutations in the tyrosine kinase domain (Asn540Lys, Lys650Glu, and Lys650Met) are thought to affect the intracellular kinetics of the FGFR3. In cells expressing the mutations of the tyrosine kinase domain the amount of the mature (membrane bound, glycosylated, p170) FGFR3 receptor form is decreased, whereas the immature (intracellular, unglycosylated, p130) exhibits abnormally strong ligand-independent tyrosine phosphorylation *(42)*. Furthermore, the mutant FGFR3 containing the achondroplasia mutations is more resistant to ligand-induced internalization and downregulation compared with that of the wild type, which results in increased receptor levels at the plasma membrane *(44,45)*. This mechanism seems to be involved in thanatophoric dysplasia as well, because increased FGFR3 expression has been observed in the growth plates of thanatophoric dysplasia fetuses *(46)*.

In summary, the increased signaling through FGFR3 in the achondroplasia family of skeletal dysplasias is accomplished in at least three different ways, all resulting in disturbed regulation of the growth plate: (1) ligand-independent (constitutive) activation; (2) increased receptor responsiveness to the ligand; and (3) change in the intracellular kinetics of the receptor.

Overactivation of the FGFR3 Disturbs Normal Cell Development in the Growth Plate

Transgenic animal models for achondroplasia and thanatophoric dysplasia and morphological studies of the growth plates from human thanatophoric dysplasia fetuses have provided some insight on how the overactivation of FGFR3 affects chondrocyte life cycle in the growth plate. The growth plates of the transgenic mice with achondroplasia and thanatophoric dysplasia type II mutations were diminished with significant decrease and disturbed columnar organization of the proliferative zone and shortening of the hypertrophic zone *(44,47–51)*. Moreover, similarly to human thanatophoric dysplasia *(46,52)*, mice with achondroplasia mutation have foci of abnormal vascularization and transverse tunneling of the growth plate cartilage *(51)*. These findings indicate that activating *FGFR3* mutations decrease chondrogenesis and stimulate osteogenesis. This is further supported by data on increased expression of genes related to osteoblast differentiation (osteocalcin, osteopontin and osteonectin) in mice with achondroplasia mutation Gly375Cys *(44)*. Moreover, thanatophoric dysplasia type I mutations have been shown to promote chondrocyte apoptosis *(53)*. Thus, different types of mutations seem to affect different stages of chondrocyte life cycle when causing disturbed longitudinal bone growth.

Interestingly, developmental differences have been observed in the regulation of chondrocyte proliferation by normal and mutant FGFR3. In contrast with both prenatal and postnatal inhibition of differentiation, proliferation of chondrocytes might even be increased prenatally. It was demonstrated that thanatophoric dysplasia type II mutation in mice (Lys644Glu) enhanced chondrocyte proliferation at embryonic day 15 but not at embryonic day 18 *(50)*. In vitro studies of chondrocytes from thanatophoric dysplasia type I fetuses suggest that at least during fetal development, cell differentiation is more affected than cell proliferation *(53)*. The presence of two FGFR3 isoforms with different affinities for FGF1 and FGF2 during chondrogenic differentiation *(54)* further supports the hypothesis that FGFR3 might have different functions during different developmental stages.

Molecular Pathways Used by Normal and Mutant FGFR3

As presented below, activating FGFR3 mutations responsible for the achondroplasia group of skeletal dysplasias involve different signaling pathways. These molecular mechanisms vary not only with regard to mutation type (and thus specific clinical entity) but also depend on developmental period.

Activation of Cell-Cycle Inhibitors and Disturbance of PTHrP/Ihh Signaling Loop

The transgenic animal models as well as expression of both normal and mutated *FGFR3* in cell lines have been used to highlight intracellular signaling pathways, involved in pathogenesis of the achondroplasia family of skeletal dysplasias. The Fgfr3 containing achondroplasia and thanatophoric dysplasia mutations activates STAT1, 5a and 5b (signal transducers and activators of transcription responsible for antiproliferative effects), and ink4 family cell cycle inhibitors and in this way decreases cell proliferation *(44,48,55)*.

Several studies suggest that parathyroid hormone-related protein and Indian hedgehog (PTHrP/Ihh) signaling loop, a major coordinator of the growth plate, is also affected by mutations causing the achondroplasia family of skeletal dysplasias. Sox9 is a target of PTHrP signaling *(56,57)*, and both normal and mutant FGFR3 stimulate expression of the transcription factor Sox9 *(58)*. Sox9 is necessary for differentiation of mesenchyme cells to chondrocytes and subsequently for arresting the transition of chondrocytes from the proliferative to the hypertrophic stage *(56,57)*. Thus, an increased expression of Sox9 in the achondroplasia family of skeletal dysplasias may contribute to decreased hypertrophy of growth plate chondrocytes. Moreover, the signaling pathways for induction of Sox9 and activation of the cell cycle inhibitor STAT1 seem to be independent of each other *(58)*, indicating that several intracellular pathways are involved in the pathogenesis of the achondroplasia family of skeletal dysplasias. In addition, Fgfr3 signaling downregulates the expression of Ihh and bone morphogenetic

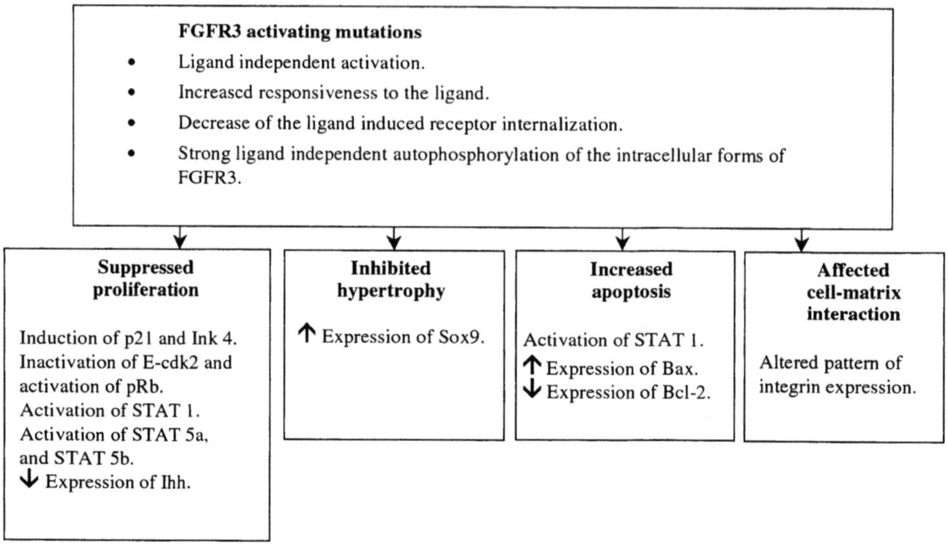

Fig. 4. A schematic summary of cellular and molecular mechanisms involved in the disturbance of bone growth in the achondroplasia family of skeletal dysplasias. Cell cycle progression is regulated by assembly of cyclins, cyclin-dependent kinases (cdk), and cdk inhibitors with subsequent regulation of retinoblastoma protein, pRb. Cells, in this case chondrocytes, are kept in growth arrest by active pRb. pRb can be phosphorylated and by cyclin complex E-cdk2/D-cdk4, which leads to inactivation. Cdks are blocked by so called cell cycle inhibitors, among which p21 has a broad spectrum, whereas ink4 has a narrow spectrum (inhibits only D-cdk4 and D-cdk6). The increased expression of p21 blocks the E-cdk2, which in turn cannot phosphorylate (inactivate) pRb. The active pRb does not allow the cell to enter S-phase. Ihh stimulates chondrocyte proliferation and regulates their longitudinal stacking in the proliferative zone, thus a decreased amount of this factor may cause disorganization of the cellular structure in the growth plate. The regulation of apoptosis involves Bax and Bcl-2 proteins. Bax is a proapoptotic protein, whereas Bcl-2 is an antiapoptotic protein. STATs are also involved in the inhibition of proliferation and in the activation of apoptosis. Integrins provide a link between the extracellular matrix and the cytoskeleton, functioning as important transducers of mechanical stimuli. Integrin binding stimulates intracellular signaling, which can affect gene expression and regulate chondrocyte function. Thus, changes in integrin expression pattern might affect cell-matrix interactions and integrin-related signaling pathways.

protein 4 in transgenic mice with achondroplasia mutation *(47)*. Ihh is known to be impor-tant for the chondrocyte proliferation and their longitudinal stacking in the proliferative zone *(59)*, whereas bone morphogenetic protein 4 might serve as a link coordinating chondrogenesis and osteogenesis in the growth plate.

The above-described activation of the cell cycle inhibitors and downregulation of Ihh contribute to decreased proliferation and affected columnar organization of the chondrocytes, whereas increased expression of Sox9 probably confer decreased hypertrophy of the cells. All these molecular processes explain the morphological changes of the growth plates in human thanatophoric dysplasia as well as in the transgenic models of achondroplasia and thanatophoric dysplasia. Interestingly, neither altered expression of Ihh nor STAT protein activation has been found in prenatal mice with thanatophoric dysplasia II mutation, suggesting that different molecular pathways are important for bone growth during different developmental stages *(50)*.

Activation of MAPK Pathway, Altered Integrin Expression, and Triggering of Apoptosis

One of the important signaling molecules in the tyrosine kinase pathway is mitogen-activated protein kinase. This molecule is activated in a ligand-dependent manner in achondroplasia, hypochondroplasia, and thanatophoric dysplasia *(42,53)*. In contrast to mitogen-activated protein kinase signaling, STAT1 signaling pathway is activated in a ligand-independent manner in thanatophoric dysplasia type I *(53)*. The latter is likely involved in triggering premature apoptosis of the growth plate chon-drocytes by decreasing Bcl-2 levels *(53)*.

Another mechanism involved in the pathogenesis of the achondroplasia is disturbed cell–matrix interaction because chondrocytes containing *FGFR3* with achondroplasia mutation change the pattern of integrin expression *(60)*. Integrins function as a link between the extracellular matrix and the cytoskeleton and can transduce signals into the cells. Consequently, changes in integrin expression affect not only chondrocyte interaction with the surrounding extracellular matrix but also integrin signaling into the cell. Celullar and molecular mechanisms involved in the pathogenesis of the achondroplasia family of skeletal dysplasias are summarized in Fig. 4.

ACKNOWLEDGMENTS

This work has been supported by Foundation of Society for Children Care. Associated Prof. Lars Hagenäs and Dr. Thomas Hertel are gratefully acknowledged for revision of this manuscript.

REFERENCES

1. Hecht, J. T., Thompson, N. M., Weir, T., Patchell, L., and Horton, W. A. (1991) Cognitive and motor skills in achondroplastic infants: neurologic and respiratory correlates. *Am. J. Med. Genet.* **41,** 208–211.
2. Langer, L. O., Jr., Baumann, P. A., and Gorlin, R. J. (1967) Achondroplasia. *Am. J. Roentgenol. Radium Ther. Nucl. Med.* **100,** 12–26.
3. Scott, C. I. Jr. (1976) Achondroplastic and hypochondroplastic dwarfism. *Clin. Orthop.* **Jan./Feb.,** 18–30.
4. Horton, W. A., Rotter, J. I., Kaitila, I., et al. (1977) Growth curves in achondroplasia. *Birth Defects Orig. Artic. Ser.* **13,** 101–107.
5. Hall, B. D. and Spranger, J. (1979) Hypochondroplasia: clinical and radiological aspects in 39 cases. *Radiology* **133,** 95–100.
6. Grigelioniene, G., Eklof, O., Laurencikas, E., Ollars, B., Hertel, N. T., Dumanski, J. P., and Hagenas, L. (2000) Asn540Lys mutation in fibroblast growth factor receptor 3 and phenotype in hypochondroplasia. *Acta Paediatr.* **89,** 1072–1076.
7. Brook, C. G. and de Vries, B. B. (1998) Skeletal dysplasias. *Arch. Dis. Child.* **79,** 285–289.
8. Appan, S., Laurent, S., Chapman, M., Hindmarsh, P. C., and Brook, C. G. (1990) Growth and growth hormone therapy in hypochondroplasia. *Acta Paediatr. Scand.* **79,** 796–803.
9. Bridges, N. A., Hindmarsh, P. C., and Brook, C. G. (1991) Growth of children with hypochondroplasia treated with growth hormone for up to three years. *Horm. Res.* **36,** 56–60.
10. Orioli, I. M., Castilla, E. E., and Barbosa-Neto, J. G. (1986) The birth prevalence rates for the skeletal dysplasias. *J. Med. Genet.* **23,** 328–332.
11. Martinez-Frias, M. L., Cereijo, A., Bermejo, E., Lopez, M., Sanchez, M., and Gonzalo, C. (1991) Epidemiological aspects of Mendelian syndromes in a Spanish population sample: I. Autosomal dominant malformation syndromes. *Am. J. Med. Genet.* **38,** 622–625.
12. Bellus, G. A., Hefferon, T. W., Ortiz de Luna, R. I., Hecht, J. T., Horton, W. A., Machado, M., et al. (1995) Achondroplasia is defined by recurrent G380R mutations of FGFR3. *Am. J. Hum. Genet.* **56,** 368–373.
13. Stoll, C., Roth, M. P., and Bigel, P. (1982) A reexamination on parental age effect on the occurrence of new mutations for achondroplasia. *Prog. Clin. Biol. Res.* **104,** 419–426.
14. Wilkin, D. J., Szabo, J. K., Cameron, R., Henderson, S., Bellus, G. A., Mack, M. L., et al. (1998) Mutations in fibroblast growth-factor receptor 3 in sporadic cases of achondroplasia occur exclusively on the paternally derived chromosome. *Am. J. Hum. Genet.* **63,** 711–716.
15. Bowen, P. (1974) Achondroplasia in two sisters with normal parents. *Birth Defects Orig. Artic. Ser.* **10,** 31–36.
16. Henderson, S., Sillence, D., Loughlin, J., Bennetts, B., and Sykes, B. (2000) Germline and somatic mosaicism in achondroplasia. *J. Med. Genet.* **37,** 956–958.
17. McKusick, V. A., Kelly, T. E., and Dorst, J. P. (1973) Observations suggesting allelism of the achondroplasia and hypochondroplasia genes. *J. Med. Genet.* **10,** 11–16.
18. Shiang, R., Thompson, L. M., Zhu, Y. Z., Church, D. M., Fielder, T. J., Bocian, M., et al. (1994) Mutations in the transmembrane domain of FGFR3 cause the most common genetic form of dwarfism, achondroplasia. *Cell* **78,** 335–342.
19. Bellus, G. A., McIntosh, I., Smith, E. A., Aylsworth, A. S., Kaitila, I., Horton, W. A., et al. (1995) A recurrent mutation in the tyrosine kinase domain of fibroblast growth factor receptor 3 causes hypochondroplasia. *Nat. Genet.* **10,** 357–359.
20. Prinos, P., Costa, T., Sommer, A., Kilpatrick, M. W., and Tsipouras, P. (1995) A common FGFR3 gene mutation in hypochondroplasia. *Hum. Mol. Genet.* **4,** 2097–2101.

21. Bonaventure, J., Rousseau, F., Legeai-Mallet, L., Le Merrer, M., Munnich, A., and Maroteaux, P. (1996) Common mutations in the fibroblast growth factor receptor 3 (FGFR 3) gene account for achondroplasia, hypochondroplasia, and thanatophoric dwarfism. *Am. J. Med. Genet.* **63,** 148–154.
22. Rousseau, F., Bonaventure, J., Legeai-Mallet, L., Schmidt, H., Weissenbach, J., Maroteaux, P., et al. (1996) Clinical and genetic heterogeneity of hypochondroplasia. *J. Med. Genet.* **33,** 749–752.
23. Prinster, C., Carrera, P., Del Maschio, M., Weber, G., Maghnie, M., Vigone, M. C., et al. (1998) Comparison of clinical-radiological and molecular findings in hypochondroplasia. *Am. J. Med. Genet.* **75,** 109–112.
24. Ramaswami, U., Rumsby, G., Hindmarsh, P. C., and Brook, C. G. (1998) Genotype and phenotype in hypochondroplasia. *J. Pediatr.* **133,** 99–102.
25. Tsai, F. J., Wu, J. Y., Tsai, C. H., and Chang, J. G. (1999) Identification of a common N540K mutation in 8/18 Taiwanese hypochondroplasia patients: further evidence for genetic heterogeneity. *Clin. Genet.* **55,** 279–280.
26. Stoilov, I., Kilpatrick, M. W., Tsipouras, P., and Costa, T. (1995) Possible genetic heterogeneity in hypochondroplasia. *J. Med. Genet.* **32,** 492–493.
27. Prinster, C., Del Maschio, M., Beluffi, G., Maghnie, M., Weber, G., Del Maschio, A., et al. (2001) Diagnosis of hypochondroplasia: the role of radiological interpretation. Italian Study Group for Hypochondroplasia. *Pediatr. Radiol.* **31,** 203–208.
28. Angle, B., Hersh, J. H., and Christensen, K. M. (1998) Molecularly proven hypochondroplasia with cloverleaf skull deformity: a novel association. *Clin. Genet.* **54,** 417–420.
29. Wuechner, C., Nordqvist, A. C., Winterpacht, A., Zabel, B., and Schalling, M. (1996) Developmental expression of splicing variants of fibroblast growth factor receptor 3 (FGFR3) in mouse. *Int. J. Dev. Biol.* **40,** 1185–1188.
30. Peters, K., Ornitz, D., Werner, S., and Williams, L. (1993) Unique expression pattern of the FGF receptor 3 gene during mouse organogenesis. *Dev. Biol.* **155,** 423–430.
31. Delezoide, A. L., Benoist-Lasselin, C., Legeai-Mallet, L., Le Merrer, M., Munnich, A., Vekemans, M., et al. (1998) Spatio-temporal expression of FGFR 1, 2 and 3 genes during human embryo- fetal ossification. *Mech. Dev.* **77,** 19–30.
32. Ornitz, D. (2000) Fibroblast Growth Factors, Chondrogenesis, and Related Clinical Disorders, in *Skeletal Growth Factors* (Canalis, E., ed.). Lippincott Williams and Wilkins, Philadelphia, pp. 197–209.
33. Weksler, N. B., Lunstrum, G. P., Reid, E. S., and Horton, W. A. (1999) Differential effects of fibroblast growth factor (FGF) 9 and FGF2 on proliferation, differentiation and terminal differentiation of chondrocytic cells in vitro. *Biochem. J.* **342,** 677–682.
34. Tavormina, P. L., Shiang, R., Thompson, L. M., Zhu, Y. Z., Wilkin, D. J., Lachman, R. S., et al. (1995) Thanatophoric dysplasia (types I and II) caused by distinct mutations in fibroblast growth factor receptor 3. *Nat. Genet.* **9,** 321–328.
35. Burke, D., Wilkes, D., Blundell, T. L., and Malcolm, S. (1998) Fibroblast growth factor receptors: lessons from the genes. *Trends Biochem. Sci.* **23,** 59–62.
36. Bellus, G. A., Bamshad, M. J., Przylepa, K. A., Dorst, J., Lee, R. R., Hurko, O., et al. (1999) Severe achondroplasia with developmental delay and acanthosis nigricans (SADDAN): phenotypic analysis of a new skeletal dysplasia caused by a Lys650Met mutation in fibroblast growth factor receptor 3. *Am. J. Med. Genet.* **85,** 53–65.
37. Vajo, Z., Francomano, C. A., and Wilkin, D. J. (2000) The molecular and genetic basis of fibroblast growth factor receptor 3 disorders: the achondroplasia family of skeletal dysplasias, Muenke craniosynostosis, and Crouzon syndrome with acanthosis nigricans. *Endocr. Rev.* **21,** 23–39.
38. Colvin, J. S., Bohne, B. A., Harding, G. W., McEwen, D. G., and Ornitz, D. M. (1996) Skeletal overgrowth and deafness in mice lacking fibroblast growth factor receptor 3. *Nat. Genet.* **12,** 390–397.
39. Deng, C., Wynshaw-Boris, A., Zhou, F., Kuo, A., and Leder, P. (1996) Fibroblast growth factor receptor 3 is a negative regulator of bone growth. *Cell* **84,** 911–921.
40. Webster, M. K. and Donoghue, D. J. (1996) Constitutive activation of fibroblast growth factor receptor 3 by the transmembrane domain point mutation found in achondroplasia. *EMBO J.* **15,** 520–527.
41. Naski, M. C., Wang, Q., Xu, J., and Ornitz, D. M. (1996) Graded activation of fibroblast growth factor receptor 3 by mutations causing achondroplasia and thanatophoric dysplasia. *Nat. Genet.* **13,** 233–237.
42. Raffioni, S., Zhu, Y. Z., Bradshaw, R. A., and Thompson, L. M. (1998) Effect of transmembrane and kinase domain mutations on fibroblast growth factor receptor 3 chimera signaling in PC12 cells. A model for the control of receptor tyrosine kinase activation. *J. Biol. Chem.* **273,** 35250–35259.
43. Bellus, G. A., Spector, E. B., Speiser, P. W., Weaver, C. A., Garber, A. T., Bryke, C. R., et al. (2000) Distinct missense mutations of the FGFR3 lys650 codon modulate receptor kinase activation and the severity of the skeletal dysplasia phenotype. *Am. J. Hum. Genet.* **67,** 1411–1421.
44. Chen, L., Adar, R., Yang, X., Monsonego, E. O., Li, C., Hauschka, P. V., et al. (1999) Gly369Cys mutation in mouse FGFR3 causes achondroplasia by affecting both chondrogenesis and osteogenesis. *J. Clin. Invest.* **104,** 1517–1525.
45. Monsonego-Ornan, E., Adar, R., Feferman, T., Segev, O., and Yayon, A. (2000) The transmembrane mutation G380R in fibroblast growth factor receptor 3 uncouples ligand-mediated receptor activation from down-regulation. *Mol. Cell. Biol.* **20,** 516–522.
46. Delezoide, A. L., Lasselin-Benoist, C., Legeai-Mallet, L., Brice, P., Senee, V., Yayon, A., et al. (1997) Abnormal FGFR 3 expression in cartilage of thanatophoric dysplasia fetuses. *Hum. Mol. Genet.* **6,** 1899–1906.
47. Naski, M. C., Colvin, J. S., Coffin, J. D., and Ornitz, D. M. (1998) Repression of hedgehog signaling and BMP4 expression in growth plate cartilage by fibroblast growth factor receptor 3. *Development* **125,** 4977–4988.
48. Li, C., Chen, L., Iwata, T., Kitagawa, M., Fu, X. Y., and Deng, C. X. (1999) A Lys644Glu substitution in fibroblast growth factor receptor 3 (FGFR3) causes dwarfism in mice by activation of STATs and ink4 cell cycle inhibitors. *Hum. Mol. Genet.* **8,** 35–44.

49. Wang, Y., Spatz, M. K., Kannan, K., Hayk, H., Avivi, A., Gorivodsky, M., et al. (1999) A mouse model for achondroplasia produced by targeting fibroblast growth factor receptor 3. *Proc. Natl. Acad. Sci. USA* **96,** 4455–4460.
50. Iwata, T., Chen, L., Li, C., Ovchinnikov, D. A., Behringer, R. R., Francomano, C. A., et al. (2000) A neonatal lethal mutation in FGFR3 uncouples proliferation and differentiation of growth plate chondrocytes in embryos. *Hum. Mol. Genet.* **9,** 1603–1613.
51. Segev, O., Chumakov, I., Nevo, Z., Givol, D., Madar-Shapiro, L., Sheinin, Y., et al. (2000) Restrained chondrocyte proliferation and maturation with abnormal growth plate vascularization and ossification in human FGFR-3(G380R) transgenic mice. *Hum. Mol. Genet.* **9,** 249–258.
52. Rimoin, D. L. (1975) The chondrodystrophies. *Adv. Hum. Genet.* **5,** 1–118.
53. Legeai-Mallet, L., Benoist-Lasselin, C., Delezoide, A. L., Munnich, A., and Bonaventure, J. (1998) Fibroblast growth factor receptor 3 mutations promote apoptosis but do not alter chondrocyte proliferation in thanatophoric dysplasia. *J. Biol. Chem.* **273,** 13007–13014.
54. Shimizu, A., Tada, K., Shukunami, C., Hiraki, Y., Kurokawa, T., Magane, N., and Kurokawa-Seo, M. (2001) A novel alternatively spliced fibroblast growth factor receptor 3 isoform lacking the acid box domain is expressed during chondrogenic differentiation of ATDC5 cells. *J. Biol. Chem.* **276,** 11031–11040.
55. Su, W. C., Kitagawa, M., Xue, N., Xie, B., Garofalo, S., Cho, J., et al. (1997) Activation of Stat1 by mutant fibroblast growth-factor receptor in thanatophoric dysplasia type II dwarfism. *Nature* **386,** 288–292.
56. Bi, W., Deng, J. M., Zhang, Z., Behringer, R. R., and de Crombrugghe, B. (1999) Sox9 is required for cartilage formation. *Nat. Genet.* **22,** 85–89.
57. Huang, W., Chung, U. I., Kronenberg, H. M., and de Crombrugghe, B. (2001) The chondrogenic transcription factor Sox9 is a target of signaling by the parathyroid hormone-related peptide in the growth plate of endochondral bones. *Proc. Natl. Acad. Sci. USA* **98,** 160–165.
58. Murakami, S., Kan, M., McKeehan, W. L., and de Crombrugghe, B. (2000) Up-regulation of the chondrogenic Sox9 gene by fibroblast growth factors is mediated by the mitogen-activated protein kinase pathway. *Proc. Natl. Acad. Sci. USA* **97,** 1113–1118.
59. Karp, S. J., Schipani, E., St-Jacques, B., Hunzelman, J., Kronenberg, H., and McMahon, A. P. (2000) Indian hedgehog coordinates endochondral bone growth and morphogenesis via parathyroid hormone related-protein-dependent and -independent pathways. *Development* **127,** 543–548.
60. Henderson, J. E., Naski, M. C., Aarts, M. M., Wang, D., Cheng, L., Goltzman, D., and Ornitz, D. M. (2000) Expression of FGFR3 with the G380R achondroplasia mutation inhibits proliferation and maturation of CFK2 chondrocytic cells. *J. Bone Miner. Res.* **15,** 155–165.
61. Ikegawa, S., Fukushima, Y., Isomura, M., Takada, F., and Nakamura, Y. (1995) Mutations of the fibroblast growth factor receptor-3 gene in one familial and six sporadic cases of achondroplasia in Japanese patients. *Hum. Genet.* **96,** 309–311.
62. Superti-Furga, A., Eich, G., Bucher, H. U., Wisser, J., Giedion, A., Gitzelmann, R., et al. (1995) A glycine 375-to-cysteine substitution in the transmembrane domain of the fibroblast growth factor receptor-3 in a newborn with achondroplasia. *Eur. J. Pediatr.* **154,** 215–219.
63. Winterpacht, A., Hilbert, K., Stelzer, C., Schweikardt, T., Decker, H., Segerer, H., et al. (2000) A novel mutation in FGFR-3 disrupts a putative N-glycosylation site and results in hypochondroplasia. *Physiol. Genomics* **2,** 9–12.
64. Grigelioniene, G., Hagenas, L., Eklof, O., Neumeyer, L., Haereid, P. E., and Anvret, M. (1998) A novel missense mutation Ile538Val in the fibroblast growth factor receptor 3 in hypochondroplasia. Mutations in brief no. 122. Online. *Hum. Mutat.* **11,** 333.
65. Mortier, G., Nuytinck, L., Craen, M., Renard, J. P., Leroy, J. G., and de Paepe, A. (2000) Clinical and radiographic features of a family with hypochondroplasia owing to a novel Asn540Ser mutation in the fibroblast growth factor receptor 3 gene. *J. Med. Genet.* **37,** 220–224.
66. Deutz-Terlouw, P. P., Losekoot, M., Aalfs, C. M., Hennekam, R. C., and Bakker, E. (1998) Asn540Thr substitution in the fibroblast growth factor receptor 3 tyrosine kinase domain causing hypochondroplasia. *Hum. Mutat.* **Suppl 1,** S62–S65.

24

Effects of Boric Acid on *Hox* Gene Expression and the Axial Skeleton in the Developing Rat*

Michael G. Narotsky, Nathalie Wéry, Bonnie T. Hamby, Deborah S. Best, Nathalie Pacico, Jacques J. Picard, Françoise Gofflot, and Robert J. Kavlock

INTRODUCTION

The adult axial skeleton consists of the skull, ribs, and vertebrae. Based on their morphology, the vertebrae can be divided into five distinct regions, that is, the cervical (C), thoracic (T), lumbar (L), sacral (S), and caudal vertebrae. The number of vertebrae in each region varies across species within the vertebrate phylum. In humans, the vertebral column normally consists of 7C, 12T, 5L, 5S, and four or five caudal vertebrae, whereas rodents have 7C, 13T, 6L, 4S and varying numbers of caudal vertebrae.

During embryonic development, positional information determining the craniocaudal identity of the somites, the precursors to the vertebrae, is thought to be conferred by the *hox* genes. They encode transcriptional regulators containing a homeodomain that mediates sequence-specific DNA binding. These genes are clustered in four genomic loci, the HoxA, -B, -C, and -D complexes. Hox expression in the paraxial mesoderm begins early, during gastrulation, before the formation of the somites. Hox genes have overlapping domains of expression in the somites and prevertebrae (PV) that extend from the caudal end of the embryo to a precise cranial limit that is correlated to the linear order of the genes within a given cluster. This expression pattern along the craniocaudal axis of the embryo suggests a combinatorial code according to which the expression of a given combination of hox genes will specify the identity of a vertebral segment *(1–3)*.

Several agents have been reported to induce anomalies of the axial skeleton that resemble homeotic transformations, that is, they induce the transformation of the anatomical structure of a vertebra to that of an adjacent vertebra, thus leading to altered numbers of vertebrae or ribs. Boric acid (BA), an essential plant micronutrient, is widely used industrially (cosmetics, pharmaceuticals, pesticides, glazing, ceramics) and widely distributed. Prenatal exposure to BA has been shown to cause reductions in the number of ribs in rodents *(4–8)* as well as induce a missing cervical vertebra *(7)* with associated

*This document has been reviewed in accordance with the U.S. Environmental Protection Agency policy and approved for publication. Mention of trade names or commercial products does not constitute endorsement or recommendation for use.

From: *The Skeleton: Biochemical, Genetic, and Molecular Interactions in Development and Homeostasis*
Edited by: E. J. Massaro and J. M. Rogers © Humana Press Inc., Totowa, NJ

changes in hox gene expression *(9)*. Although many agents, for example, valproic acid *(10)*, retinoic acid *(11)*, salicylate *(12)*, and acetazolamide *(13)*, have been shown to cause supernumerary ribs in rodents, very few agents cause a reduction in the number of ribs or vertebrae. In addition to BA, agents or conditions in the latter category include arsenate *(14)*, methanol *(15)*, and hyperthermia *(16)*. This unusual effect on axial development has also been associated with changes in homeotic gene expression *(17–19)* as well as deletion of the *bmi-1* proto-oncogene *(20)*. In this study, we describe BA-induced homeotic shifts by characterizing the morphological changes in the axial skeleton of rats after prenatal exposure to BA and also report the changes in hox gene expression associated with BA exposure shown to alter cervical vertebral development.

MATERIALS AND METHODS

Chemicals

BA (H_3BO_3; Lot no. 83H0843) was purchased from Sigma Chemical Co.; purity was reported to be approx 99%. Dosing solutions were prepared in double-distilled deionized water at appropriate concentrations to provide the desired dose (0 or 500 mg/kg) when given at 10 mL/kg.

Animals and Husbandry

For assessment of effects on full-term morphology, timed-pregnant Sprague–Dawley rats were obtained from Charles River, Inc. and individually housed. For assessment of gene expression, male and female Sprague–Dawley rats (Charles River, Inc.) were cohabited overnight and mated females were housed two per cage. All animals were maintained in polycarbonate cages with heat-treated wood shavings supplied as bedding. The day that evidence of mating (i.e., copulatory plug or vaginal sperm) was detected was designated gestation day (GD) 0. The animals were provided feed (Purina Lab Chow no. 5001) and tap water *ad libitum*, and a 12:12 light:dark cycle (lights on at 0600). Room temperature and relative humidity were maintained at 22.2 ± 1.1°C and 50 ± 10%, respectively.

Experimental Design

Animals were assigned to treatment groups using a nonbiased procedure that assured a homogeneous distribution of body weights among groups *(21)*.

Full-Term Morphology

BA was administered at 0 or 500 mg/kg twice daily (b.i.d.; approx 0700 and 1600 h). This experiment was conducted in two blocks. In the first block, rats were dosed with BA on GD 6, 7, 8, or 9; controls received vehicle on GD 6–9. In the second block, rats were dosed on GD 9, 10, or 11; controls received vehicle on GD 9–11. Individual doses were based on GD 6 body weights. Animals were weighed on GD 6–10, 13, 16, and 21. All rats were examined throughout the experimental period for clinical signs of toxicity.

On GD 21, dams were killed by cervical dislocation, and the liver, kidneys, and gravid uterus were weighed. Uterine implantation sites were counted and their relative positions were recorded. Each implantation site was classified as a live fetus, dead fetus, or resorption. Each resorption site was further classified as a macerated fetus, placenta (with no recognizable fetus), metrial gland (with no placenta), or scar. Ovaries from live-bearing dams were examined and corpora lutea were counted. Live fetuses were weighed individually, fixed in 95% ethanol, and subsequently double stained with Alizarin red S and Alcian blue *(22)* for skeletal examination. Nongravid uteri were stained with 10% ammonium sulfide to detect cases of full-litter resorption *(21)*.

Skeletal examinations included evaluation of vertebral, costal, and skull morphology. Each side of the specimen was evaluated independently. The pattern of costal cartilage attachment to the sternum and the number of presacral vertebrae were recorded. The first thoracic vertebra (T1) was defined as the most cephalad vertebra bearing a rib with a prominent costal cartilage. At the thoracolumbar junc-

Table 1
Key Morphological Criteria Used in Assessing Vertebral Regions on GD 21

Vertebral region	*Normal no. of vertebrae*	*Key features*
Cervical	7	
C1 (atlas)	1	Large arch, wide transverse process
C2 (axis)	1	Large arch, spinous process
C3-C5	3	Lateral cartilage
C6	1	Tuberculum anterium, lateral cartilage
C7	1	Lateral cartilage
Thoracic	13	
T1	1	Cranial-most with rib and costal cartilage, rostrad diapophysis
T2	1	Prominent spinous process, rostrad diapophysis
T3-T10	8	High ossified arch, lateral cartilage
T11	1	Blunted ossified arch, reduced lateral cartilage
T12-T13	2	Virtually no lateral cartilage
Lumbar	6	
L1-L3	3	Reduced/absent pleurapophysis
L4-L6	3	Pleurapophysis projecting cephalad

tion, all rib-bearing vertebrae were designated as thoracic, regardless of the length of the rib. The number of C, T, and L vertebrae were recorded for each side. Vertebrae in each region were further classified into subregions (normally represented by C1, C2, C3–5, C6, C7, T1, T2, T3–10, T11, T12–13, L1–3, and L4–6; ref. *22*). The morphological criteria for each subregion are presented in Table 1; the cervical region of normal and abnormal specimens are pictured in Fig. 1. Because variations in the size of the cartilaginous area on the lateral aspects of C3, C7, and T1 were observed in the first block, the extent of the lateral cartilaginous aspect was scored from zero (normal for T1) to four (cartilage spanning the width of the arch, normal for C3 and C7) for the specimens of the second block.

Statistics

Females who died or had only one uterine implantation site were excluded from statistical analyses. The litter was used as the statistical unit for the analysis of data regarding corpora lutea, implantation sites, prenatal loss, fetal weights, and fetal examination findings. Maternal body weights and litter data were analyzed using the General Linear Models procedure in SAS software versions 6.04 and 6.12. Because data from GD-9 exposure and controls were collected in two blocks, data were compared across blocks using General Linear Models. Except for the incidence of fetuses with <6 sternebrae (observed only in the second block), all developmental end points were comparable between blocks. Thus, data from the two blocks were combined. Fetal weights were analyzed with the number of live fetuses as a covariate. Similarly, the number of implantation sites was used as a covariate in the analysis of litter size. When a significant treatment effect was detected by analysis of variance, Student's *t*-test on least-squares means was used for pairwise comparisons between groups. No adjustments were made for multiple comparisons. For vertebral-count distributions, inferential statistical analyses were not conducted; instead, descriptive statistics were calculated for each side based on the numbers of fetuses, not litters, in each group.

Hox *Gene Expression*

Pregnant rats were treated by gavage with BA at 0 or 500 mg/kg, b.i.d. (approx 0900 and 1800 h) on GD 9. Females were killed by cervical dislocation on GD 13.5 and embryos were recovered in

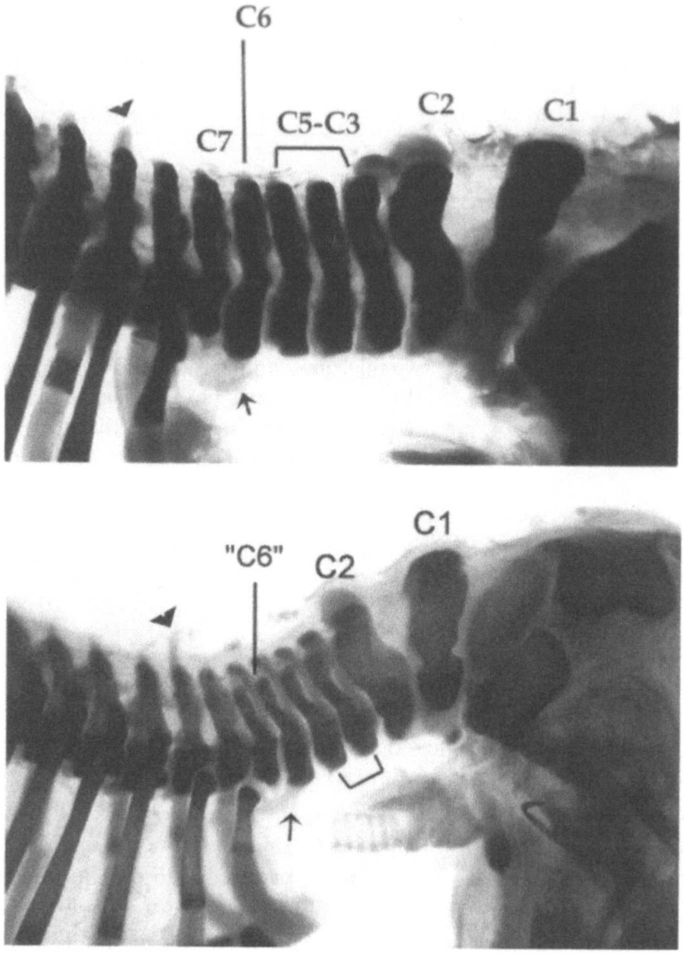

Fig. 1. Top, Control fetal skeleton with forelegs disarticulated to show cervical vertebral subregions: C1 (atlas), C2 (axis), C3–C5, C6 (with tuberculum anterium; arrow), and C7. The spinous process of T2 is also indicated (arrowhead). Bottom, Fetus exposed to boric acid (500 mg/kg b.i.d.) on GD 9. The C3–C5 subregion (bracket) has only two vertebrae rather than the normal complement of three. The C1, C2, "C6" (the fifth vertebra, with tuberculum anterium, arrow), and "C7" (the sixth vertebra) subregions are intact. The spinous process of T2 is also indicated (arrowhead).

phosphate-buffered saline (PBS) from one control and two BA-treated dams. The embryos were dissected from the decidua and membranes and fixed in 4% paraformaldehyde in PBS (pH 7.4) overnight at 4°C. Embryos were washed in PBS and stored in 70% ethanol at room temperature.

In Situ Hybridization (ISH)

Embryos were dehydrated in a graded series of ethanol, cleared in benzene, and embedded in paraffin by standard methods. Approximately 350 serial sagittal 6-µm sections were distributed into seven groups. The first group was stained with toluidine blue, and the remaining slides were each hybridized with a different probe (approx 50 sections/probe/embryo), thus allowing direct comparisons of expression domains of the different genes on neighboring sections of the same embryo *(23)*. Although all embryos were hybridized with the five or six probes, the number of embryos analyzed for each probe

Table 2
Summary of Uterine Findings (Mean ± SE) at GD 21 Cesarean Section

	No. of dams	*Implantation sites*	*Live fetuses*	*Postimplantation loss (%)*	*Fetal weight (g)*
Control	15	12.8 ± 0.4	12.3 ± 0.5	4.6 ± 1.9	5.5 ± 0.1
GD 6	11	13.1 ± 0.5	12.4 ± 0.5	4.6 ± 2.1	5.5 ± 0.1
GD 7	11	13.7 ± 0.4	12.7 ± 0.5	7.5 ± 2.1	5.1 ± 0.1[a]
GD 8	13	13.2 ± 0.6	12.2 ± 0.7	7.5 ± 2.6	5.3 ± 0.1
GD 9	15	13.4 ± 0.3	12.5 ± 0.5	8.2 ± 2.5	5.0 ± 0.1[b]
GD 10	10	13.1 ± 0.4	12.1 ± 0.6	7.8 ± 3.3	4.8 ± 0.0[c]
GD 11	10	12.4 ± 0.7	11.1 ± 1.0	12.3 ± 5.6	4.8 ± 0.2[a]

[a]Significantly different from control value ($p < 0.05$).
[b]Significantly different from control value ($p < 0.01$).
[c]Significantly different from control value ($p < 0.001$).

varied because of processing artifacts on some slides; a minimum of nine embryos were observed for each probe. Analysis was restricted to the expression domain in the PV (the sclerotomal derivatives of the somite).

ISH was performed as described by Duboule and Dolle *(24)* and reviewed by Picard et al. *(23)*. The single-strand antisense RNA probes were synthesized in a standard T7, T3, or SP6 polymerase reaction using 35S-CTP, followed by partial alkaline hydrolysis to reduce the average probe length to the optimal size of approx 150 nucleotides. Sections were pretreated with Proteinase K at 1 µg/mL for 30 min at 37°C. After ISH, the deposit of silver grain was visualized on a microscope using dark field.

Probes

A fragment of the murine homeobox gene *hoxa4* extending from an *Eco*RI site in the second exon until the extremity of the 3' untranslated region was cloned in a pGEM11zf vector (Promega). The probe for *hoxa4* was then synthesized from the extremity of the 3' untranslated region of the gene until a *Bgl*II site located in the second exon. The RNA probe for *hoxd4* was prepared after subcloning a cDNA fragment into a pBluescript KS (+/–) transcription vector (Stratagene). This sequence extended up to 700 bp downstream of the homeobox *Bgl*II site (*Bgl*II–*Hin*dIII fragment; ref. *25*). The probes for *hoxa5*, *hoxc5*, and *hoxc6* were described by Fibi et al. *(26)*, Gaunt et al. *(27)*, and Sharpe et al. *(28)*, respectively. The probe for *hoxa6* was synthesized from a vector provided by P. Gruss and which contained a 1.7 kb *Eco*RI insert in pSP65.

False-Color Display of ISH

To analyze the ISH signal, dark-field sections were visualized using a Laborlux S microscope (Leitz) with an attached CCD camera (TK-890 E, JVC) and were processed using PC-based image analysis software (vidas Res 2.1, Kontron Elektronik). For the expression-level analysis, the image analysis system substituted a false-color look-up table for the 256 gray level look-up table initially used to display the ISH image. Gradients of increasing intensity of expression were thus converted to colors spanning from blue (corresponding to background), to green (a weak signal), to yellow (a clearly visible signal), to red (a very intense, saturated signal). Analyzers of expression levels were blind to treatment.

RESULTS

BA treatment had no effect on prenatal mortality; however, a slight, nonsignificant, increase in postimplantation loss was noted after GD 11 treatment (Table 2). Fetal weights were reduced for groups treated on GD 7, 9, 10, or 11. A variety of malformations (Table 3) involving the axial skeleton (small

Table 3
Summary of Fetal Examination Findings

Treatment	*Control*	*GD 6*	*GD 7*	*GD 8*	*GD 9*	*GD 10*	*GD 11*
No. litters (fetuses)	*17 (211)*	*12 (150)*	*11 (140)*	*13 (162)*	*16 (201)*	*10 (121)*	*10 (111)*
Mean fetal incidence per litter (%)							
<26 presacral vertebrae	0	0.6 ± 1.4	0	8.5 ± 3.0	51.9 ± 6.5[c]	57.2 ± 9.1[c]	0
<7 cervical vertebrae	0	0	0	1.8 ± 1.4	88.3 ± 6.1[c]	0	0
<13 ribs	0	0	0	1.3 ± 1.3	0	55.9 ± 8.4[c]	0
>13 ribs	2.0 ± 1.1	2.4 ± 1.8	6.2 ± 2.4	7.4 ± 1.9	48.2 ± 5.6[c]	0	0
<6 sternebrae	0	0.8 ± 0.8	0	2.7 ± 1.8	15.0 ± 3.2	27.4 ± 8.8[c]	1.5 ± 1.0
Cervical rib	0.4 ± 0.4	0	1.3 ± 0.9	3.8 ± 0.3[a]	4.8 ± 1.5[b]	1.6 ± 1.1	0
Sternoschisis (partial)	0	0	0	0	0	0	0.8 ± 0.8
Sternal agenesis	0	0	0	0	0.5 ± 0.5	0	0
Fused ribs	0.5 ± 0.5	0	0	4.1 ± 1.5[b]	0	3.2 ± 2.4[a]	0
Bifurcated ribs	0	0	0	1.8 ± 0.9[b]	0	0	0
Fused vertebrae	0.5 ± 0.5	0.6 ± 0.6	0	8.9 ± 3.3[b]	1.1 ± 0.7	5.9 ± 2.7[a]	3.3 ± 3.3
Fused mandibles	0	0	0	0	0.5 ± 0.5	0	0
Small orbit	0	0	3.7 ± 2.5	0	0.5 ± 0.5	0	0
Fused costal cartilage	0	0	0	2.0 ± 1.5	18.4 ± 3.3[c]	0	0
Asymmetric L-S junction	0	0.6 ± 0.6	0	3.1 ± 1.7	11.7 ± 3.8[c]	4.6 ± 2.6[c]	0
Vestigial tail	0	0	0	0	0	0.9 ± 0.9[a]	0
Umbilical hernia	0	0	0	0.5 ± 0.5	0	0	0
Agnathia and exophthalmia	0.5 ± 0.5	0	0	0	0	0	0
Extra rib cage, etc.	0	0.6 ± 0.6	0	0	0	0	0
Lateral cartilage score:							
C3	3.9 ± 0.0	–	–	–	3.9 ± 0.1	3.9 ± 0.0	3.8 ± 0.1
C7	3.7 ± 0.1	–	–	–	3.9 ± 0.1	3.9 ± 0.1	3.8 ± 0.1
T1	0.0 ± 0.0	–	–	–	1.0 ± 0.5	0.1 ± 0.1	0.0 ± 0.0

[a]Significantly different from control value ($p < 0.05$).
[b]Significantly different from control value ($p < 0.01$).
[c]Significantly different from control value ($p < 0.001$).

orbit, partial sternoschisis, sternal agenesis, fused or bifurcated ribs, fused vertebrae, and fused mandibles) were similar to findings in earlier experiments *(7)* and were attributed to BA treatment. Both the GD 8 and GD 9 groups had low, but significant, incidences of (rudimentary) cervical ribs. Isolated cases of malformations observed included agnathia with exophthalmia (one control fetus), umbilical hernia (one GD 8-exposed fetus), and vestigial tail (one GD 10-exposed fetus). Also, one GD 6-exposed fetus had exencephaly, ablepharia, agnathia, an extra rib cage, two extra scapulae, and one extra forelimb.

The most noteworthy effects of BA were alterations in the numbers of vertebrae, ribs, and sternebrae. Although treatment on GD 6, 7, 8, or 11 generally had no such effect, exposure on GD 9 or 10 resulted in dramatic, but strikingly different, alterations in the axial skeleton. In the GD 9 group, about 90% of the fetuses (15 of 16 litters) had only six cervical vertebrae (Fig. 2). Based on the placement of the tuberculum anterium (normally on C6), the deficient region was usually C3–C5 (Fig. 1), with C7 or C6 being affected less frequently. Morphology on the right side of the vertebrae indicated that 61, 27, and 1% of the fetuses were deficient at C3–C5, C7, and C6, respectively. Although vertebral asymmetry was sometimes observed, similar incidences (70, 20, and 0%, respectively) were seen on the left side. Alterations in the attachment pattern of the costal cartilage to the sternum were also evident and fused costal cartilage were observed in approx 10% of the progeny. Examination of the lateral aspects of the arches of C3, C7, and T1 showed significant changes in the last of these vertebrae. Although T1 (by our working definition) bore a rib with a prominent costal cartilage, this vertebra sometimes had a lateral cartilaginous aspect characteristic of a cervical vertebra. It is important to note, however, that the vertebra with a prominent spinous process (a defining feature for T2) was always situated immediately caudal to the vertebra defined as T1 regardless of the amount of cartilage present on the lateral aspect. The GD 9 group also exhibited, though less frequently, supernumerary thoracic ("lumbar") ribs, (rudimentary) cervical ribs, <6 sternebrae, and asymmetric lumbosacral (L–S) junction (Table 2). Despite the increased incidence of supernumerary ribs, approximately one half of the fetuses had reduced numbers of presacral vertebrae.

Progeny exposed on GD 10 also had increased incidences of <6 sternebrae, <26 presacral vertebrae, and asymmetric L–S junction; unlike the other groups, however, the GD 10 group had nearly 60% incidence of progeny with less than 13 ribs (Fig. 2). The most frequently deficient thoracic subregion was T11 (44% of the fetuses), followed by the T3–10 (12% of the fetuses), and T12–13 subregions (5% of the fetuses); T1 and T2 were present in all fetuses.

In our examination of GD-13.5 hox gene expression, control and treated embryos showed similar expression profiles for *hoxd4*, *hoxa4*, *hoxa5*, and *hoxc5* (Fig. 3). For *hoxd4*, the cranial limit of expression was observed in PV1 for all embryos; however, the signal in PV1 was weak or just above the limit of detection. For *hoxa4*, the cranial border of expression was weakly labeled in PV2 in 4 of 11 control embryos and 6 of 13 treated embryos. The *hoxa4* transcript was strongly expressed in PV3 and caudad for all embryos. For *hoxa5*, a control embryo was unique in that a signal was detected just above the detection limit in PV2. For the remaining control and treated embryos, the cranial boundary of expression was PV3; however, for 6 of 10 controls and 4 of 13 treated embryos, the signal in PV3 was weak. For *hoxc5*, all embryos showed a gradient of expression from PV2 (1 of 11 controls, 6 of 13 treated), PV3 (9 of 11 controls, 7 of 13 treated), or PV4 (1 of 11 control) increasing to full intensity in PV8.

For *hoxc6* and *hoxa6*, BA shifted the cranial border of expression cranially on GD 13.5 (Fig. 3). Among treated embryos, the maximum intensity of expression of *hoxc6* was detected in PV9 in 10 of 11 embryos, whereas none of the control embryos presented a maximum intensity of expression in that PV. Increasing gradients of expression with a cranial boundary at PV7 or PV8 were evident in the treated embryos and at PV8 or PV9 in controls. For *hoxa6*, all 11 treated embryos showed a signal with a maximum intensity in PV10, whereas all control embryos presented such an expression in PV11. Increasing gradients of expression with a cranial boundary at PV9 or PV10 were observed in controls, and at PV7, PV8, or PV9 in treated embryos.

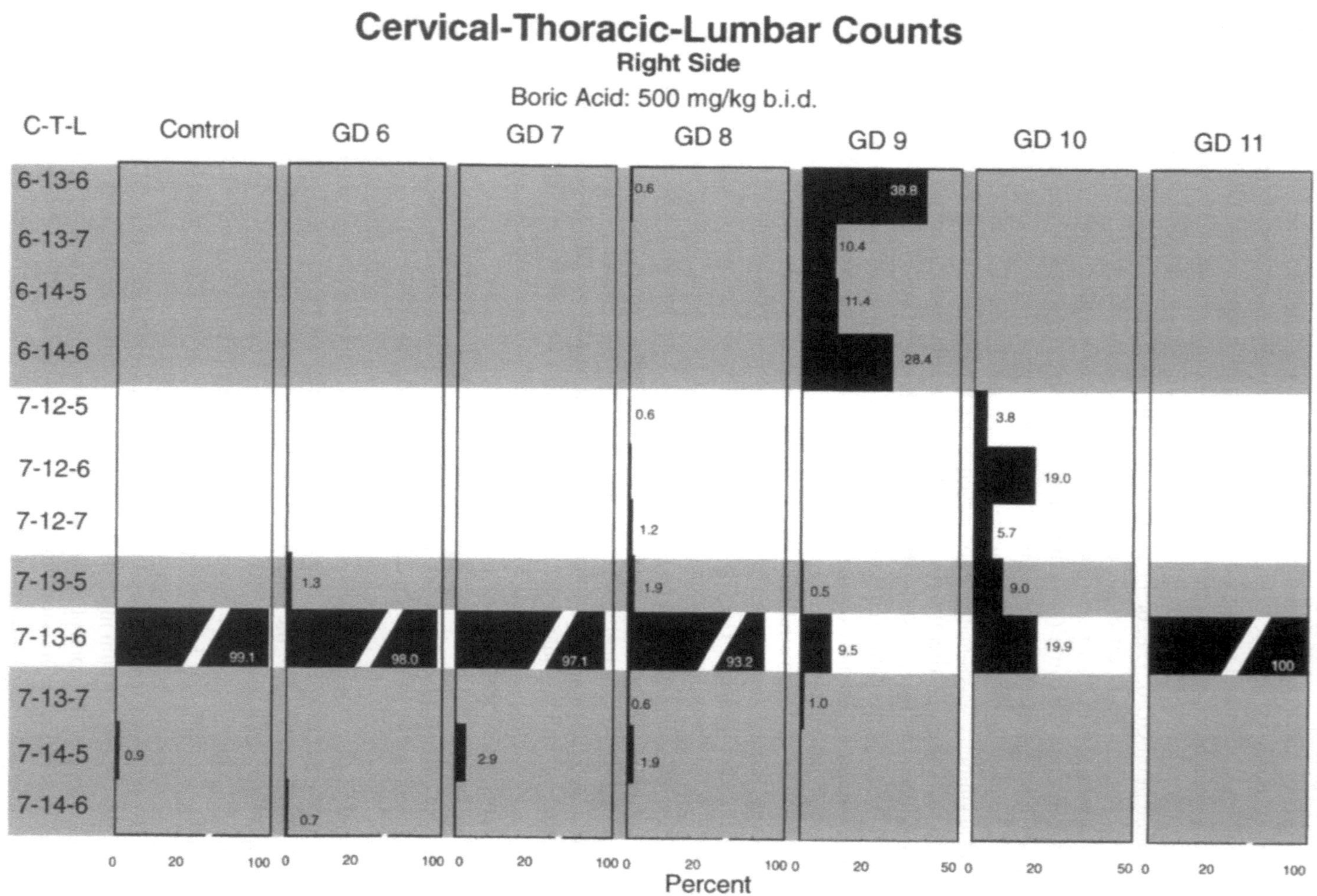

Fig. 2. Incidences of fetuses with different cervical–thoracic–lumbar (C–T–L) vertebral patterns (counts) after BA exposure on different days of gestation. For example, 100% of fetuses exposed on GD 11 had the normal C–T–L vertebral pattern of 7-13-6, that is, 7 C, 13 T, and 6 L vertebrae. These graphs present data for the right side of the fetus only. Although the right and left sides of any given fetus were not necessarily symmetrical, the left-side profiles were very similar to the right-side profiles shown here.

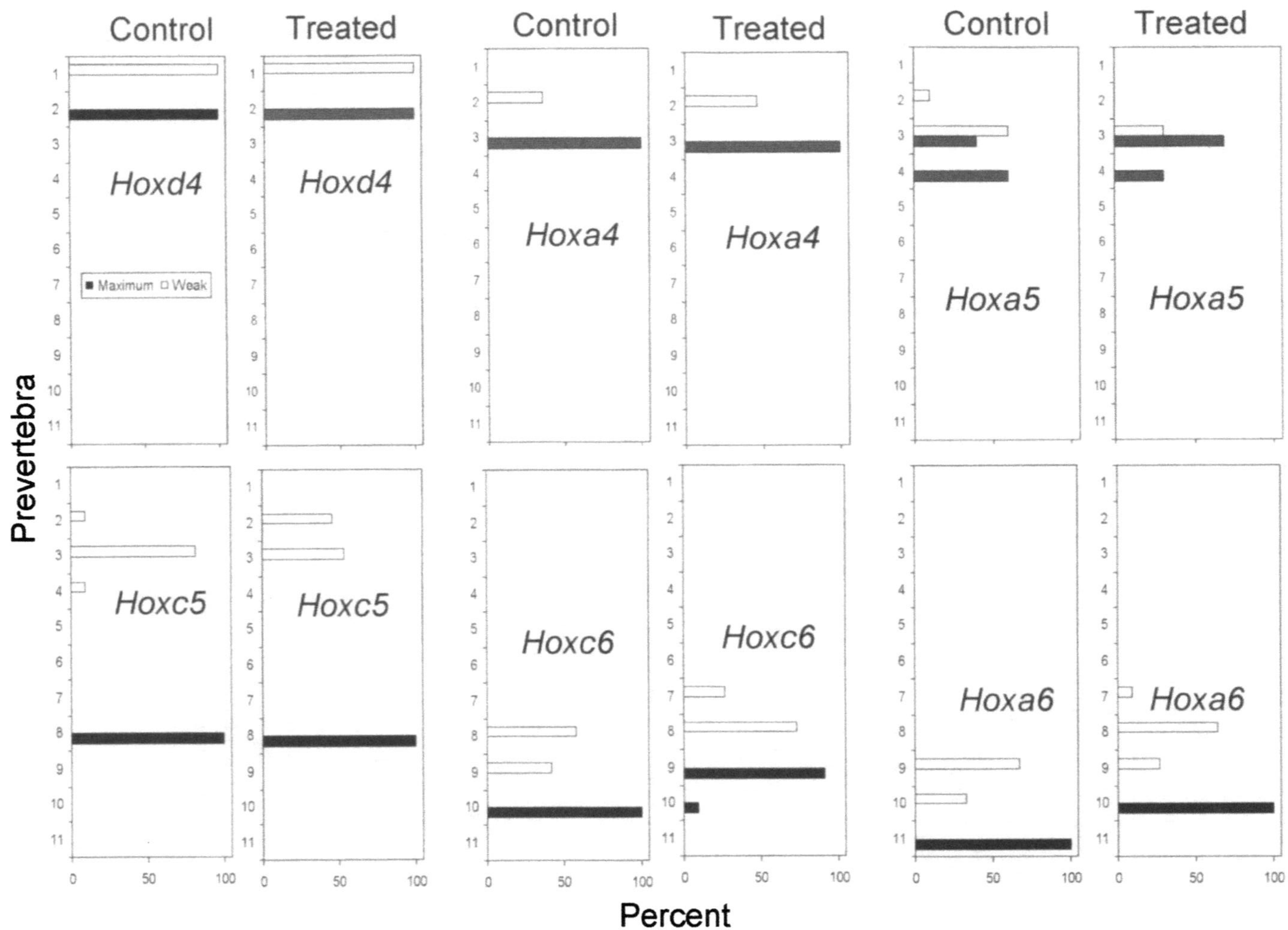

Fig. 3. Percent incidence of embryos showing a cranial border of gene expression of *hoxd4*, *hoxa4*, *hoxa5*, *hoxc5*, *hoxc6*, and *hoxa6* genes in prevertebrae of control and BA-treated GD 13.5 embryos. Bars represent the incidence of embryos with a cranial border of expression at the indicated prevertebra; solid bars reflect the cranial border of a signal of maximum intensity whereas open bars reflect the cranial border of a weaker signal. Note that the cranial border of expression of *hoxc6* and *hoxa6* genes is shifted in the BA-treated embryos when compared with control embryos.

DISCUSSION

As reported by others *(4,5,8)*, BA administration caused distinct effects on the developing rodent axial skeleton. The single-day dosing regimen also demonstrated discrete periods of axial development. Although GD 6 exposure had no developmental effects, and treatment on GD 7 and 11 caused only relatively mild developmental toxicity (reduced fetal weights), treatments on GD 8, 9, and 10 disrupted axial development. GD 8 exposure induced cervical ribs and rib or vertebral malformations, but only treatment on GD 9 or 10 dramatically altered numbers of vertebrae, ribs, or sternebrae. GD 9 exposure yielded a high penetrance (approx 90%) of a missing cervical vertebra whereas GD 10 exposure resulted in a missing thoracic or lumbar vertebra. Close examination of vertebral morphology indicated a missing vertebra usually in the C3–C5 region for the GD 9-exposed fetuses; missing C7 or, less frequently, C6 was also seen in this group. Although the majority of GD 10 fetuses had a missing vertebra, the penetrance was not as high as in the GD 9 group. The most frequently affected vertebral regions in the GD 10 group were, in decreasing order, T11, T3–10, and T12–13; T1 and T2 were unaffected. These findings suggest an impact of BA on the fundamental control mechanisms that define the positional identity of the somites and, consequently, the vertebrae.

Homeotic genes that are known to confer positional information in the cervical and the cranial-most thoracic regions include *hoxd4*, *a4*, *a5*, *c5*, *c6*, and *a6*; we hypothesized that their expression may be affected by GD-9 exposure to BA. Because GD-9 exposure yielded a highly localized effect on the cervical region, with high penetrance (approx 90%), and with little else effected, we used this exposure regimen as an experimental model for investigating BA's possible effects on homeotic gene expression. Comparison of expression patterns between BA-exposed embryos and controls revealed a shift in the expression domain of two genes, *hoxc6* and *hoxa6* on GD 13.5. According to the hox code, these shifts are likely to result in posterior transformation of cervical vertebrae later in development, without altering the total number of vertebrae. This is consistent with the observed morphological defects at GD 21 after similar BA exposure, suggesting that these hox gene alterations are indeed part of the dysmorphogenic cascade resulting from BA exposure.

In control GD-13.5 embryos, five genes are expressed in PV8 (T1): *hoxd4*, *a4*, *a5*, *c5*, and *c6*. In embryos exposed to BA, a one-PVor a one- to two-PV cranial shift of the cranial boundary of expression of *hoxc6* and *hoxa6*, respectively, was observed. Therefore, in exposed embryos, the same combination of five genes is expressed in PV7 (C7). In the same way, in control embryos, the six genes studied are expressed in PV9 (T2). In exposed embryos, we observed the expression of these genes in PV8 (T1). Thus, the cranial shift of the cranial boundary of *hoxc6* and *hoxa6* leads to a modification of the hox code that may explain the posterior transformation of C7 to T1, and of T1 to T2 observed in full-term fetuses exposed to BA. However, our data do not directly explain the two other vertebral patterns observed on GD 21, namely the absence of C6 or a deficiency in the C3–C5 region. This suggests that BA may induce shifts in the expression of genes acting spatially and temporally upstream of *hoxa6* and *hoxc6* and that the modifications observed here reflect the cascade of misexpression of these genes. Among candidate genes are the upstream hox genes, such as paralogs 4 and/or 5, as well as pattern-regulating genes other than those studied here. The similar incidences of embryos with a cranial shift of *hoxa6* and *hoxc6* expression, and of fetuses with six cervical vertebrae support an association between the altered gene expression and the full-term phenotype.

Comparative analyses that map hox gene expression boundaries to morphological regions in the chick and mouse embryo showed that gene expression patterns are consistently correlated with morphology *(29)*. In other words, specific hox genes are always expressed at specific morphological boundaries along the craniocaudal axis regardless of changes in the number of segments that contribute to each morphological region in different species of vertebrates. Notably, the cranial border of expression of *hoxc6* is in the first thoracic PV of mice (somite 12), chicks (somite 19), and geese (somite 21). Moreover, in all amniotes, the T1 segment is the caudal-most segment to contribute a spinal nerve to the branchial plexus; *hoxc6* expression is always aligned with this segment, indicating that the axial level of *hoxc6* expression is morphologically conserved between all these species *(29)*. Therefore, the cranial shift of one PV in the expression domain of *hoxc6* may explain the cranial shift of the cervicothoracic transition observed in BA-exposed fetuses. The maximum intensity of expression of *hoxc6* was detected in PV9 in 91% of the embryos exposed to BA whereas none of the control embryos presented a maximum intensity of expression in that PV. It is interesting to note that the percentage of GD 21 fetuses with six cervical vertebrae is similar to the percentage of BA-treated embryos that presented a shift in the maximum level of expression of *hoxc6*.

Changes observed in the cervical vertebrae after treatment suggested an action of BA on expression of specific hox genes. The present work further supports the hypothesis that BA-induced axial skeletal alterations involve early modifications of hox gene expression. Several mechanisms may underlie the BA-induced changes in such gene expression. BA may act directly on hox gene expression via a cofactor or indirectly via upstream regulators of hox genes. Possible candidates include the mouse homologues of the Polycomb group genes or Cdx proteins, repressor, and activators of hox genes, respectively. Indeed, knockout mutants for the M33 gene (mouse Pc gene) showed homeotic transformations of the axial skeleton similar to those described after BA exposure *(30)*. Alternatively, BA could interfere with critical physiological process during development. A transient arrest of cell proliferation in somites or presomitic mesoderm has already been associated with skeletal defects induced by hyperthermia. These homeotic-type defects were also associated with a shift in the cranial limit of expression for some hox genes *(31)*.

To pursue these different hypotheses, further investigations should include work on the effects of BA on additional hox genes, upstream regulator genes, and cell proliferation. The study of hox expression patterns in other research models, for example, embryonic carcinoma cells treated with BA or retinoic acid, may also provide complementary information regarding the ability of BA to alter hox expression as well as induce homeotic transformations.

ACKNOWLEDGMENTS

We are indebted to P. Gruss and P. Sharpe for kindly providing plasmids. We thank Mary C. Cardon, Harriette P. Nichols, and Marian Ebron-McCoy for excellent technical assistance in embryo dissection and specimen processing. We also thank Drs. P. Hartig and J.E. Andrews for their contributions to this project. This work was supported in part by the Grant 3.4551.99 of the Fonds de la Recherche Scientifique Médicale (Belgium) to the Belgian team. The research described in this article has been supported by the United States Environmental Protection Agency through contract 8D1401NAFX to the Université Catholique de Louvain.

REFERENCES

1. Duboule, D. and Morata, G. (1994) Colinearity and functional hierarchy among genes of the homeotic complexes. *Trends Genet.* **10,** 358–364.
2. Kessel, M. and Gruss, P. (1991) Homeotic transformations of murine vertebrae and concomitant alteration of Hox codes induced by retinoic acid. *Cell* **67,** 89–104.
3. Krumlauf, R. (1993) Mouse Hox genetic functions. *Curr. Opin. Genet. Dev.* **3,** 621–625.
4. Heindel, J. J., Price, C. J., Field, E. A., Marr, M. C., Myers, C. B., Morrissey, R. E., et al. (1992) Developmental toxicity of boric acid in mice and rats. *Fundam. Appl. Toxicol.* **18,** 266–277.
5. Heindel, J. J., Price, C. J., and Schwetz, B. A. (1994) The developmental toxicity of boric acid in mice, rats, and rabbits. *Environ. Health Perspect.* **102(Suppl. 7),** 107–112.
6. Allen, B. C., Strong, P. L., Price, C. J., Hubbard, S. A., and Daston, G. P. (1996) Benchmark dose analysis of developmental toxicity in rats exposed to boric acid. *Fundam. Appl. Toxicol.* **32,** 194–204.
7. Narotsky, M. G., Schmid, J. E., Andrews, J. E., and Kavlock, R. J. (1998) Effects of boric acid on axial skeletal development in rats. *Biol. Trace Elem. Res.* **66,** 373–394.
8. Cherrington, J. W. and Chernoff, N. (2002) Periods of vertebral column sensitivity to boric acid treatment in CD-1 mice in utero. *Reprod. Toxicol.* **16,** 237–243.
9. Wéry, N., Narotsky, M. G., Pacico, N., Kavlock, R. J., Picard, J. J., and Gofflot, F. (2003) Defects in cervical vertebrae in boric acid-exposed rat embryos are associated with anterior shifts of *hox* gene expression domains. *Birth Defects Res. (Part A) Clin. Mol. Teratol.* **67,** 59–62.

10. Narotsky, M. G., Francis, E. Z., and Kavlock, R. J. (1994) Developmental toxicity and structure–activity relationships of aliphatic acids, including dose–response assessment of valproic acid in mice and rats. *Fundam. Appl. Toxicol.* **22,** 251–265.
11. Kessel, M. (1992) Respecification of vertebral identities by retinoic acid. *Development* **115,** 487–501.
12. Wickramaratne, G. A. (1988) The post-natal fate of supernumerary ribs in rat teratogenicity studies. *J. Appl. Toxicol.* **8,** 91–94.
13. Beck, S. L. (1983) Assessment of adult skeletons to detect prenatal exposure to acetazolamide in mice. *Teratology* **28,** 45–66.
14. Beaudoin, A. R. (1974) Teratogenicity of sodium arsenate in rats. *Teratology* **10,** 153–157.
15. Connelly, L. E. and Rogers, J. M. (1997) Methanol causes posteriorization of cervical vertebrae in mice. *Teratology* **55,** 138–144.
16. Kimmel, C. A., Cuff, J. M., Kimmel, G. L., Heredia, D. J., Tudor, N., Silverman, P. M., et al. (1993) Skeletal development following heat exposure in the rat. *Teratology* **47,** 229–242.
17. Kessel, M., Balling, R., and Gruss, P. (1990) Variations of cervical vertebrae after expression of a Hox-1.1 transgene in mice. *Cell* **61,** 301–308.
18. Small, K. M. and Potter, S. S. (1993) Homeotic transformations and limb defects in Hox A11 mutant mice. *Genes Dev.* **7,** 2318–2328.
19. Charité, J., de Graaff, W., Shen, S., and Deschamps, J. (1994) Ectopic expression of Hoxb-8 causes duplication of the ZPA in the forelimb and homeotic transformation of axial structures. *Cell* **78,** 589–601.
20. van der Lugt, N. M., Domen, J., Linders, K., et al. (1994) Posterior transformation, neurological abnormalities, and severe hematopoietic defects in mice with a targeted deletion of the bmi-1 proto-oncogene. *Genes Dev.* **8,** 757–769.
21. Narotsky, M. G., Brownie, C. F., and Kavlock, R. J. (1997) Critical period of carbon tetrachloride-induced pregnancy loss in Fischer-344 rats, with insights into the detection of resorption sites by ammonium sulfide staining. *Teratology* **56,** 252–261.
22. Narotsky, M. G. and Rogers, J. M. (2000) Examination of the axial skeleton of fetal rodents. *Methods Mol. Biol.* **135,** 139–150.
23. Picard, J. J., Clotman, F., Van Maele-Fabry, G., Menegola, E., Bastin, A., and Giavini, E. (1997) Alterations in expression domains of developmental genes induced in mouse embryos exposed to valproate, in *Methods in Developmental Toxicology/Biology* (Klug, S., Thiel, R., eds.), Blackwell Wissenschafts-Verlag, Berlin, pp. 161–176.
24. Duboule, D. and Dolle, P. (1989) The structural and functional organization of the murine HOX gene family resembles that of Drosophila homeotic genes. *EMBO J.* **8,** 1497–1505.
25. Gaunt, S. J., Krumlauf, R., and Duboule, D. (1989) Mouse homeo-genes within a subfamily, Hox-1.4, -2.6 and -5.1, display similar anteroposterior domains of expression in the embryo, but show stage- and tissue-dependent differences in their regulation. *Development* **107,** 131–141.
26. Fibi, M., Zink, B., Kessel, M., et al. (1988) Coding sequence and expression of the homeobox gene Hox 1.3. *Development* **102,** 349–359.
27. Gaunt, S. J., Coletta, P. L., Pravtcheva, D., and Sharpe, P. T. (1990) Mouse Hox-3.4: homeobox sequence and embryonic expression patterns compared with other members of the Hox gene network. *Development* **109,** 329–339.
28. Sharpe, P. T., Miller, J. R., Evans, E. P., Burtenshaw, M. D., and Gaunt, S. J. (1988) Isolation and expression of a new mouse homeobox gene. *Development* **102,** 397–407.
29. Burke, A. C., Nelson, C. E., Morgan, B. A., and Tabin, C. (1995) Hox genes and the evolution of vertebrate axial morphology. *Development* **121,** 333–346.
30. Core, N., Bel, S., Gaunt, S. J., Aurrand-Lions, M., Pearce, J., Fisher, A., et al. (1997) Altered cellular proliferation and mesoderm patterning in Polycomb-M33-deficient mice. *Development* **124,** 721–729.
31. Li, Z. L. and Shiota, K. (1999) Stage-specific homeotic vertebral transformations in mouse fetuses induced by maternal hyperthermia during somitogenesis. *Dev. Dyn.* **216,** 336–348.

25

Toxicant-Induced Lumbar and Cervical Ribs in Rodents

John M. Rogers, R. Woodrow Setzer, and Neil Chernoff

INTRODUCTION

The design of "Segment II" developmental toxicity studies involves exposure of pregnant rodents or rabbits to dosages of test chemical up to and including at least one that is maternally toxic. Adverse developmental effects noted in these studies may be induced by direct *in utero* exposure of the embryo to the test agent or its metabolite(s) and/or indirect effects because of compound-induced maternal toxicity. Standard developmental toxicity bioassays in rodents include a detailed examination of the near-term fetal skeleton in single-stained (alizarin red for ossified bone) or double-stained (alizarin red plus Alcian blue for cartilage) specimens. Lumbar supernumerary ribs (LSNRs) lateral to the 21 vertebra (first lumbar, L1), are common finding in such studies, and have been categorized as "rudimentary" (shorter) or "extra" (longer) by some investigators using various criteria (refs. *1–3*; Fig. 1). Cervical supernumerary ribs (CSNRs), ribs lateral to the seventh vertebra (seventh cervical, C7), are less common than LSNRs, but still often observed in rodent developmental toxicity bioassays.

A broad spectrum of chemical agents, including valproic acid *(4)*, retinoic acid *(5)*, salicylate *(6)*, acetazolamide *(7)*, and bromoxynil *(8,9)* have been shown to cause LSNRs in rodents. However, LSNRs also exhibit a high background incidence in commonly used strains of rats and mice, and background rates vary over time *(10)*. In mice, LSNRs have been associated with maternal toxicity induced by diverse chemicals *(11–13)*, and Chernoff and coworkers have demonstrated that maternal-restraint stress in mice causes elevations in the incidence of LSNRs *(14,15)*. These findings, along with the question of whether LSNRs have any adverse effects on health, have made the interpretation of the significance of LSNRs for human risk assessment controversial.

Wickramaratne *(6)* concluded that salicylate-induced LSNRs in rats were transient, subsequently becoming part of the transverse process of the first lumbar vertebra. However, Foulon et al. *(16)* followed the fate of salicylate-induced LSNRs in rats by radiography from birth to adulthood and reported that although rudimentary LSNRs were transient, the incidence of offspring with extra LSNRs was the same at birth and adulthood. We have reported that fetal LSNR induced in rats by the herbicide bromoxynil appeared to be transient, whereas in contrast, some bromoxynil-induced LSNRs in mice appeared to persist postnatally (refs. *8* and *9*). In agreement with the results of Foulon et al. *(16)*, bromoxynil-induced LSNRs in rats were mostly rudimentary, whereas those that persisted in mice were extra LSNRs. Beck *(7)* reported that LSNRs induced prenatally by acetazolamide also persist to adulthood in mice.

From: *The Skeleton: Biochemical, Genetic, and Molecular Interactions in Development and Homeostasis*
Edited by: E. J. Massaro and J. M. Rogers © Humana Press Inc., Totowa, NJ

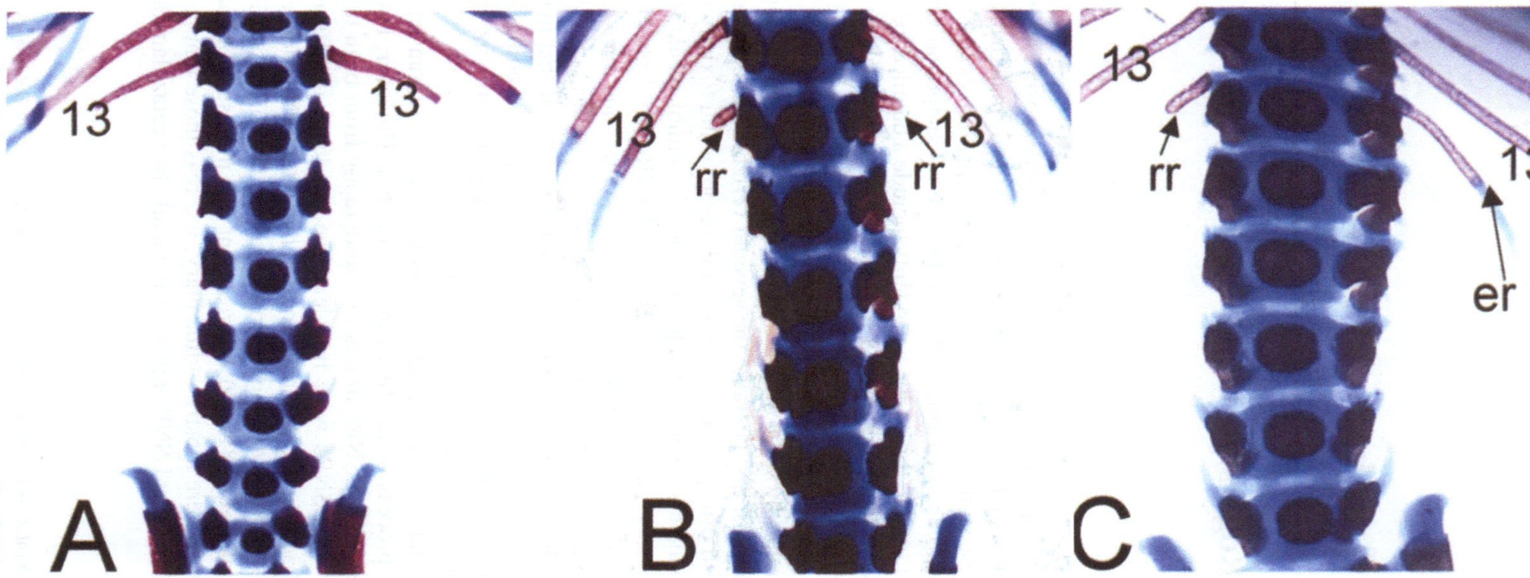

Fig. 1. LSNRs in term rodent fetuses. Skeletons were stained with Alizarin red S for bone and Alcian blue for cartilage. **A**, An untreated CD-1 mouse fetus with the normal number of 13 thoracic ribs, with the13th pair labeled. **B**, An untreated CD-1 mouse fetus with bilateral rudimentary LSNR (rr) on lumbar vertebra one. Thirteenth thoracic ribs are also labeled. **C**, Fetus from a Sprague–Dawley rat dam treated with valproic acid showing a rudimentary LSNR (rr) on one side and an extra LSNR (er) on the other side. Thirteenth thoracic ribs are also labeled.

Lumbar ribs are relatively rare in humans, but studies have indicated adverse health effects associated with their occurrence. Symptomology associated with lumbar ribs primarily consists of pain in the lumbar region *(17)* and a tendency for L4–5 degeneration *(18)*.

CSNRs have been induced in mice or rats by various maternal chemical treatments, including tri-*n*-butyltin *(19)*, nitrous oxide *(20)*, mitomycin-C *(21)*, methanol *(22,23)*, and boric acid *(24)*. CSNRs, similar to LSNRs, occur in various lengths in rodents, ranging from ossification sites to full ribs connected to the sternum distally. Background rates for CSNRs in laboratory species are variable, but most spontaneous CSNRs in rodents consist of ossification sites or very short ribs. No categorization of CSNRs by length has been proposed to date.

Cervical ribs have been associated with adverse health effects in humans. The most common effect of cervical ribs is thoracic outlet disease *(25–28)*, a condition characterized by compression of and diminished blood flow in the subclavian artery and vein and carotid arteries, and displacement of the stellate ganglia, sympathetic ganglia, and C7–T1 nerve roots. Symptomology of these anomalies is both vascular and neurological. The vascular effects include cerebral and distal embolism *(29–32)*, whereas neurological symptoms include extreme pain *(33)*, migraine *(34)*, and Parkinson's disease symptoms *(27)*. A family exhibiting cervical ribs across two generations was described by Schapera *(35)*, indicating that a genetic component may be involved in some instances.

Human CSNRs have been shown to be associated with an increased risk of cancer *(36)*. Schumacher et al. *(37)* studied a series of 1000 children with malignancies and investigated the occurrence of skeletal anomalies in this population. They found a highly significant correlation of CSNRs and other rib anomalies with a series of cancers. The specific cancers and the percentage of cancer patients with anomalous ribs included leukemia (27%), brain tumor (27%), neuroblastoma (33%), soft tissue sarcoma (25%), and Wilm's tumor (24%). These relationships may be caused by effects on a gene or genes that play a role in the development of the axial skeleton and is/are also a component/s of the cellular pathways that lead to cancer. Anbazhagan and Raman *(38)* hypothesized that alterations in homeobox genes that are known to be important in the development of the axial skeleton may also be critical in the etiology of cancer in children.

Effects on axial skeletal development have been associated with changes in homeobox (*Hox*) gene expression *(39–42)* as well as deletion of the *bmi-1* proto-oncogene *(43)*. Shifting of the anterior boundary of *Hoxa-10* expression in a posterior direction has been associated with lumbar ribs in mice after prenatal exposure to retinoic acid *(44)*. Retinoic acid treatment of pregnant mice on gestation day 7 results in posteriorization of cervical vertebrae, including CSNRs. Homeotic transformations reported to occur concurrently with CSNRs in fetuses of retinoic acid-treated dams include splits and/or fusions of the atlas (C1) or axis (C2) and displacement of the tubercula anterior (ventral vertebral processes) to C5 from their normal position on C6 *(5,44)*.

CHEMICALLY INDUCED LUMBAR RIBS: SIZE DISTRIBUTION AND DOSE RESPONSE

Kimmel and Wilson *(1)* observed a bimodal distribution of lengths of LSNRs induced in rat fetuses by maternal treatment with acetazolamide or actinomycin D. These authors defined two size classes: rudimentary, less than half the length of the ipsilateral 13th thoracic rib; and extra, at least half the length of the ipsilateral 13th thoracic rib. These authors concluded that the two classes of LSNRs were different phenomena. In further support of this conclusion, they found that extra LSNRs were induced in a dose–response fashion, whereas rudimentary LSNRs were not. Despite these early findings concerning the interpretation of fetal LSNRs in developmental toxicity studies, current studies generally do not report lengths or size categories for LSNRs. More recently, Foulon et al. *(2)* examined the induction and size distribution of LSNRs induced by salicylate in rats. These investigators also reported a bimodal distribution of LSNR lengths and also referred to the short and long LSNRs as rudimentary and extra, respectively. They found that a ratio of the length of the thirteenth to the

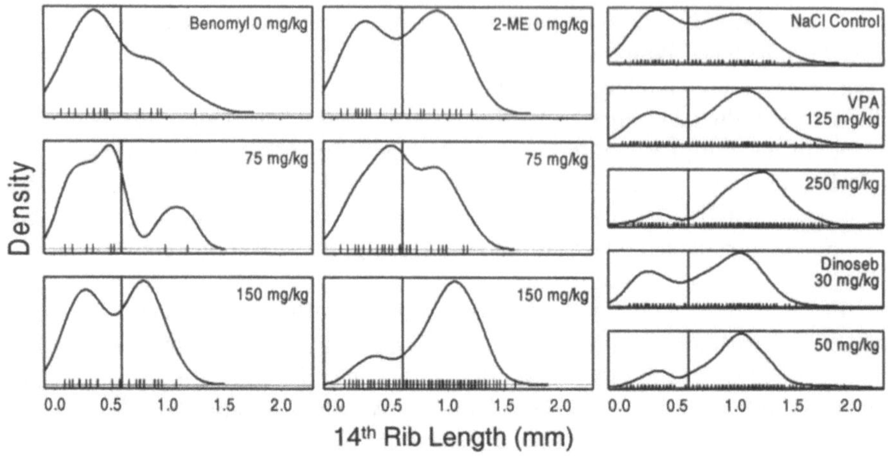

Fig. 2. Size distribution of LSNRs in litters of dams treated with benomyl (0, 75, 150 mg/kg/d), 2-methoxyethanol (2-ME; 0, 75, 150 mg/kg/d), valproic acid (VPA; 0 [saline], 125, 250 mg/kg/d), or dinoseb (0 [saline], 30, 50 mg/kg/d) on GD 7 and 8. Hashmarks on the inside of the *x*-axis represent individual cases of LSNR and density represents a smoothed function of the regional frequency of LSNR lengths. The vertical line at 0.6 mm indicates the point taken to separate the two populations of LSNR in our study.

fourteenth rib of 0.35 separated the two populations better than did the ratio of 0.5 used by Kimmel and Wilson *(1)*.

We designed a study to examine spontaneous and chemically induced LSNRs in fetal CD-1 mice using diverse developmental toxicants. The chemicals chosen were benomyl, dinoseb, 2-methoxyethanol and valproic acid. Benomyl is a benzimidazole carbamate fungicide that is teratogenic in rats and mice when administered by oral gavage *(45)*; dinoseb is a dinitrophenol herbicide shown to induce LSNRs in CD-1 mice *(13,46)*; 2-methoxyethanol is an industrial solvent that produces multiple skeletal anomalies in mice *(47)*; and valproic acid is an anticonvulsant drug and human teratogen that is also teratogenic in multiple laboratory species *(48)*. We determined the size distribution of LSNRs and the dose responses for different size classes of chemically induced LSNRs. We found that, similar to the phenomenon reported for rats by Kimmel and Wilson *(1)* and Foulon et al. *(2)*, LSNR lengths in mice were bimodally distributed both in controls and in all chemically treated groups (Fig. 2). The two size classes of LSNR had different dose responses. The incidence of the rudimentary LSNRs was independent of dose, whereas the incidence of extra LSNR showed a clear dose response (Fig. 3). Thus, size classification of LSNRs in developmental toxicity studies may provide a clearer indication of their toxicological significance. The extant literature indicates that extra LSNRs are a significant toxicological finding, while the significance of rudimentary LSNRs appears questionable.

BROMOXYNIL-INDUCED LUMBAR RIBS IN MICE AND RATS: EVALUATION OF POSTNATAL PERSISTENCE

Bromoxynil, a broad-spectrum herbicide, causes LSNRs in offspring of treated rats or mice *(8,9)* in the absence of other anomalies or overt maternal toxicity. The postnatal persistence of LSNRs in controls and of those induced by maternal bromoxynil treatment was studied by Chernoff et al. (Fig. 4; ref. *9*). Control fetuses in both rats and mice exhibited rudimentary LSNRs (11% in mice and 13% in rats), but the incidence at postnatal day (PD) 40 was zero in both species. In litters of pregnant mice treated with 96.4 mg/kg/d bromoxynil on gestation day (GD) 6–15, the incidence of LSNR was similar across the different age groups examined (approx 45% in term fetuses and 42% in offspring at PD 40). A significant reduction in the incidence of rudimentary LSNR was observed in both species between PD 20 and PD 40. The incidence of LSNR in offspring of pregnant rats treated with bromoxynil was

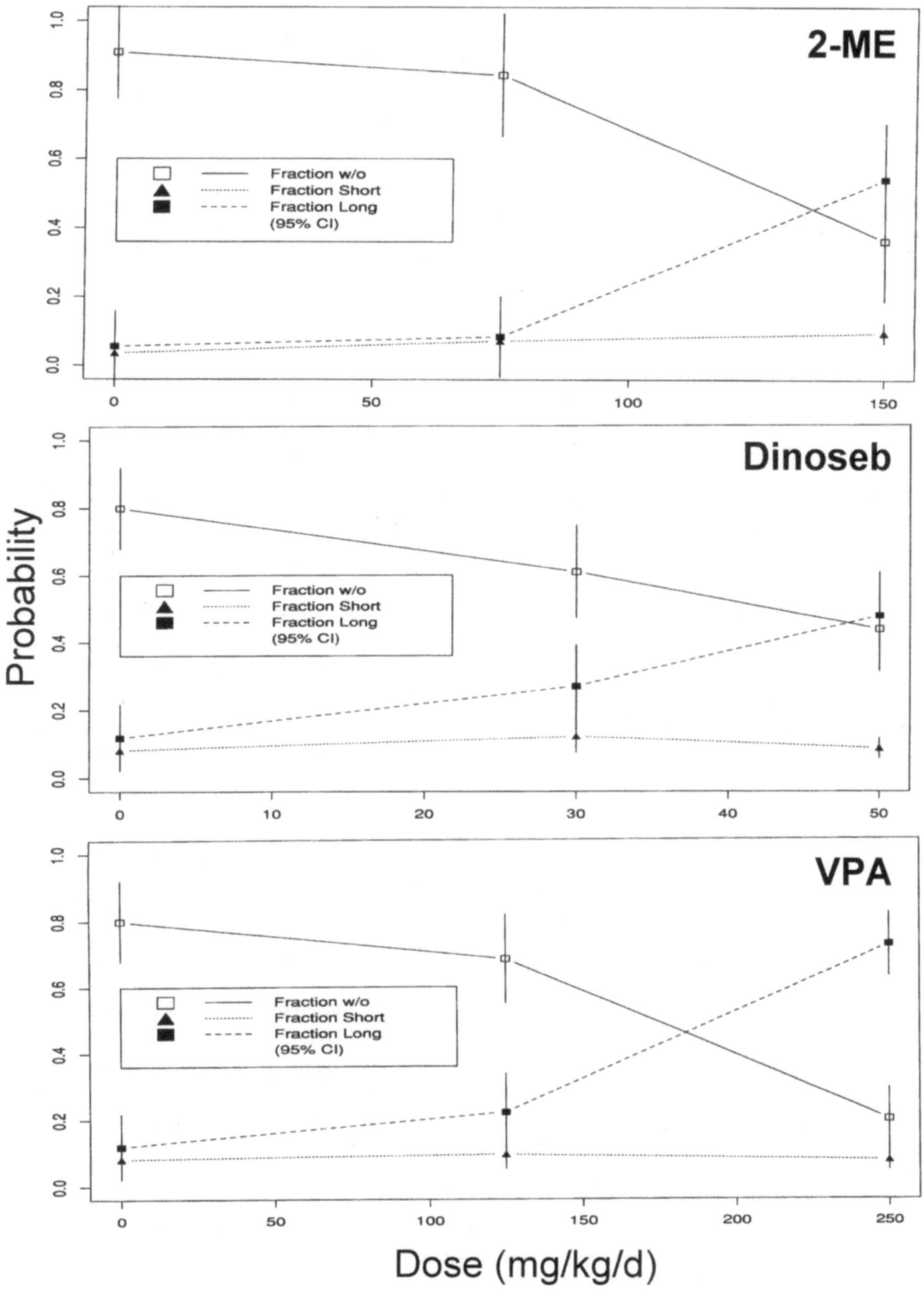

Fig. 3. Dose–response for the incidence of fetuses with no, short (rudimentary), or long (extra) LSNRs in litters of dams treated with 2-methoxyethanol (2-ME; 0, 75, 150 mg/kg/d), dinoseb (0 [saline], 30, 50 mg/kg/d), or valproic acid (VPA; 0 [saline], 125, 250 mg/kg/d) GD 7 and 8. Error bars are 95% confidence intervals.

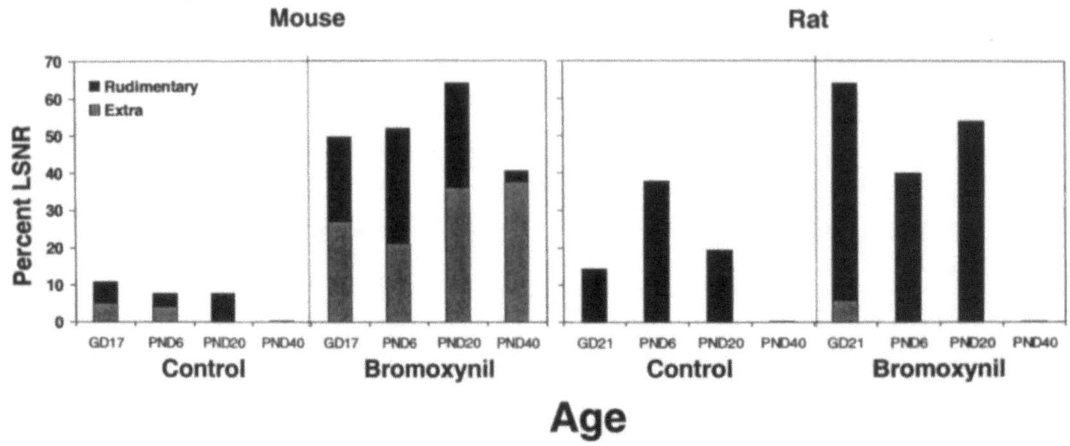

Fig. 4. The incidence of bromoxynil-induced LSNRs in fetuses and offspring of CD-1 mice and Sprague–Dawley rats treated on GD6–15. In both species there was a significant ($p < 0.01$) increase in LSNR in fetuses at term (GD17 and 20 in mouse and rat, respectively). In the mouse, extra LSNRs persisted through postnatal day (PND) 40, whereas the incidence of rudimentary ribs decreased sharply between PND20 and PND40. The incidence of rudimentary LSNRs decreased similarly in the rat between PND20 and PND40. There was only a low incidence of extra LSNRs in bromoxynil-treated rat fetuses at term.

similar in term fetuses (62%) and PD 20 pups (55%), but the incidence dropped to zero by PD 40. It is important to note that approx 50% of the lumbar ribs in mouse fetuses were extra ribs by the criterion of being at least half the length of the 13th rib, whereas in rat fetuses more than 90% of the lumbar ribs were rudimentary. The authors also noted that 95% of the lumbar ribs observed in mice on PD 40 were categorized as extra. These results again support the idea that rudimentary and extra LSNRs are two different phenomena, the former being transient and the latter being persistent. These findings reinforce the contention that it is important to differentiate the two classes of LSNRs and that they have different implications for risk assessment. It is interesting to note that a similar lack of persistence for short ribs appears to exist for CSNRs in humans. The fetal incidence of CSNR ranges between 19 and 63% *(49,50)*, whereas the adult incidence is greatly reduced, with incidences of 0.04–4.5% having been reported *(37,51)*. It has been hypothesized that fetal CSNRs may be ossification sites that become part of the transverse processes of the cervical ribs *(52)*.

METHANOL-INDUCED CERVICAL RIBS AND VERTEBRAL ANOMALIES

The effects of inhaled methanol during pregnancy were first studied by Nelson and coworkers *(22)*. Sprague–Dawley rats were exposed to 5,000, 10,000, or 20,000 ppm methanol for 7 h/day. Maternal exposure to 20,000 ppm methanol resulted in decreased fetal weight and significant increases in external, visceral and skeletal malformations. Skeletal malformations were the most prevalent and included abnormalities of the basicranium and the vertebra, including an increase in the incidence of fetuses with CSNRs.

Rogers et al. *(23)* studied the effects of methanol exposure (filtered air or 1000, 2000, 5000, 7500, 10,000, or 15,000 ppm methanol) during pregnancy in CD-1 mice under conditions similar to those used for rats by Nelson et al. *(22)*. No maternal toxicity was attributed to methanol although the exposure procedure per se reduced maternal weight gain in all groups, including the filtered air-exposed mice, compared to unhandled controls. This study demonstrated that CD-1 mice were more sensitive to the developmental toxicity of methanol than were Sprague–Dawley rats. The incidence of fetuses with CSNRs was increased in a dose-related fashion at 2000 ppm methanol and above. Cleft palate, exencephaly, and skeletal defects were observed at 5000 ppm and above. The skeletal anomalies observed,

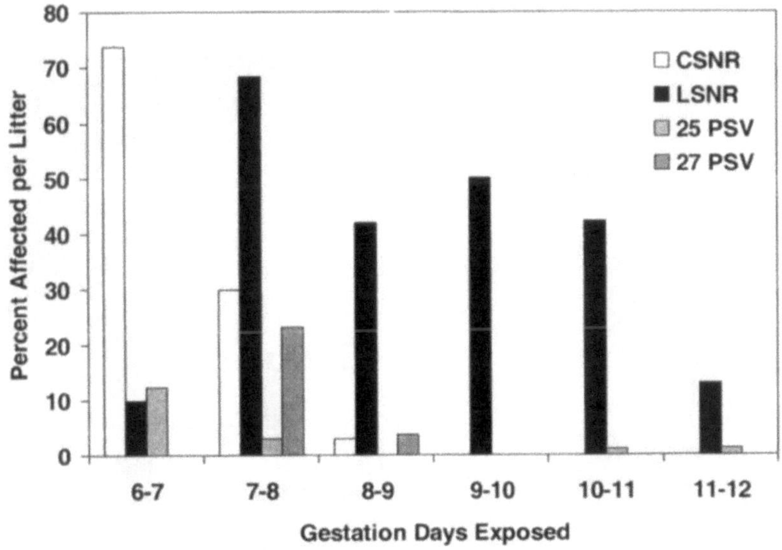

Fig. 5. Critical periods for CSNRs and LSNRs in CD-1 mouse fetuses examined at term. Pregnant CD-1 mice were exposed to 10,000 ppm methanol by inhalation for 7 h/d on two consecutive days as indicated. Peak induction of CSNR occurred with exposure on GD 6–7, with incidence of CSNR falling rapidly with later exposures. The peak induction of LSNRs occurred with exposure on GD 7–8, continued at 40–50% with exposures on GD 8–9, 9–10, and 10–11, and fell to about 12% with GD 11–12 exposure. Background rate of LSNR in CD-1 mice in our hands ranges from approx 5–15%. Also shown is the incidence of fetuses per litter with 25 or 27 presacral vertebrae (PSV; 26 is normal). Effects on the number of PSV suggest that methanol is interfering with the process of segmentation in the embryo.

including CSNRs, were similar to those observed in rats by Nelson et al. *(22)*. The effects of methanol administered by oral gavage during pregnancy in CD-1 mice were also studied by Rogers et al. *(23)*. Mice were given twice daily dosages of 2 g/kg methanol, 7 h apart, on GD 6–15. Effects observed were similar to those observed after inhalation exposure (cleft palate, exencephaly, skeletal defects including CSNR and resorptions).

The developmental phase specificity for the adverse effects of exposure to inhaled methanol in pregnant CD-1 mice has been examined. Single or 2-d exposures to 10,000 ppm methanol during the period of GD 5–13 were performed by Rogers and Mole *(53)*. Two-day exposures were performed beginning on each of GD 6–12 (e.g., the latest exposure was on GD 12–13) and single-day exposures were on each of GD 5–9. Peak blood methanol concentration after a single exposure was approx 4 mg/mL, and blood levels returned to baseline within about 24 h. Peak sensitivity to cleft palate occurred with 2-d exposure on GD 7–8 or 1-d exposure on GD 7. Exencephaly occurred with 2-d exposure on GD 6–7 through GD 8–9 (peak GD 6-7) and 1-d exposure on GD 5 through GD 8 (peak GD 7). The critical periods for skeletal defects were progressively later going from more anterior to more posterior structures affected. The critical single-day exposure period for exoccipital defects was GD 5, for atlas defects GD 5 or 6, and for axis defects, lower cervical defects, and supernumerary lumbar ribs, GD 7. The peak 2-d exposure period for CSNRs was GD 6–7 and for LSNRs was GD 7-8 (Fig. 5). Approximately 12% of fetuses had only 25 presacral vertebrae (one less than normal) with methanol exposure on GD 6–7, and about 22% of fetuses had 27 presacral vertebrae (one more than normal) with methanol exposure on GD 7–8.

The skeletal abnormalities observed by Rogers and Mole *(53)*, including splits and duplications of the atlas and axis (Fig. 6B), CSNRs (Fig. 6B,D,F), and abnormal number of presacral vertebrae, were suggestive of disruption of embryo segmentation and/or segment identity. These skeletal malformations

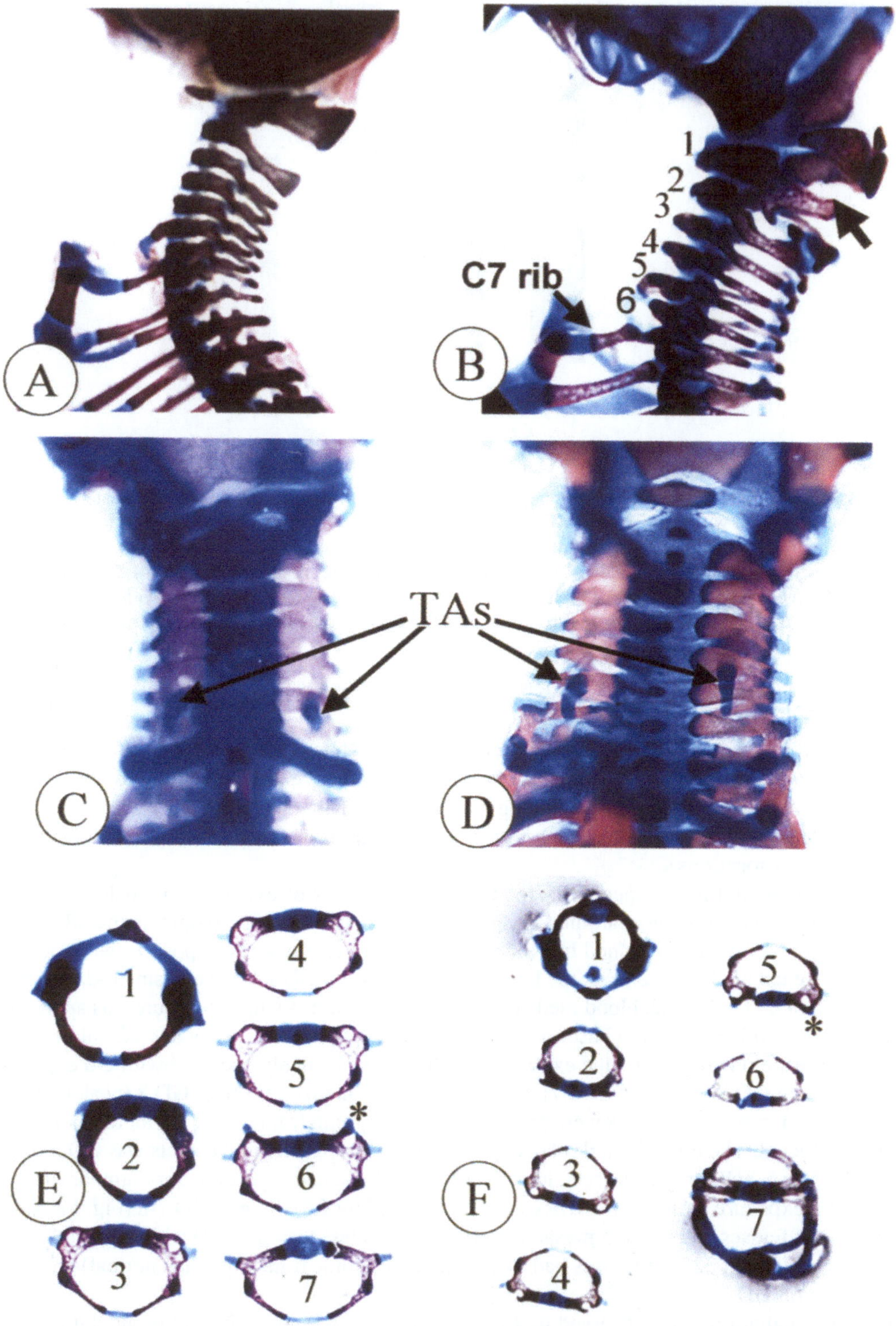
A
B
C7 rib
1
2
3
4
5
6
C
D
TAs
E
1
2
3
4
5
6
7
*
F
1
2
3
4
5
6
7
*

were examined in greater detail by Connelly and Rogers *(54)*. Methanol (5 g/kg) was administered orally to CD-1 mice on GD 7, fetuses were collected on GD 18, and fetal skeletons were double-stained for bone and cartilage. Anatomical landmarks identifying specific cervical vertebrae were examined, including the tubercula anterior normally found on C6 and various foramina and other features evident in disarticulated cervical vertebrae. The number of free (e.g., ventrally unattached) ribs and ribs attached to the sternum were counted, and CSNRs were categorized as partial or full (i.e., attached to the sternum). Methanol caused homeotic shifts of segment identity. Specifically, a posteriorization of vertebral elements, especially in the cervical region, was observed. That is, some vertebrae had structural features normally found on the next vertebra posteriad. Methanol-treated fetuses often had cartilaginous tubercula anterior on C5 rather than their normal position on C6, and full ribs attached to the sternum were observed on C7 (Fig. 6B,D,F). Further, morphological abnormalities of the atlas and axis (fusions, splits, duplications; Fig. 6B) gave the appearance of disrupted segmentation. The process(es) underlying these striking skeletal alterations is unknown, but similar phenotypes have been observed in mice in which homeobox gene function has been ablated (e.g., ref. *42*).

SUMMARY

A wide variety of chemical and physical agents are capable of disrupting the normal development of the axial skeleton in rodents when administered to the pregnant female during sensitive periods of gestation. One of the most common anomalies reported in standard developmental toxicity bioassays is the presence of supernumerary ribs. These can occur at the cervicothoracic border (C7) or the thoracolumbar border (L1). Mice are known to have a high background incidence of lumbar ribs (LSNRs) whereas cervical ribs (CSNRs) occur less frequently in controls. Low incidences of both of these anomalies have been reported in human populations and are associated with adverse health effects. In humans, CSNRs are the cause of thoracic outlet disease, a condition characterized by vascular and neurological symptoms due to diminished blood flow and compression of critical nerves. An intriguing association between CSNRs and a number of pediatric cancers has been reported. The incidence of LSNRs in humans is less than CSNRs. Here too, the anomalous ribs are associated with adverse health effects, specifically lower back pain and/or degeneration of lumbar vertebrae 4 or 5. The size distribution of LSNRs in rats and mice indicates that this anomaly is comprised of two populations differing in size and fate during pre- and postnatal growth. Using a ratio 0.35 for the length of the 14th to the 13th rib allows for good separation of these two populations in both species. The smaller (rudimentary) LSNRs most often are not affected by maternal treatment, whereas the larger (extra) LSNRs are induced in a dose-dependent manner. Rudimentary LSNRs do not persist postnatally and are no longer seen by PD 40 in mice and rats; it has been hypothesized that they are absorbed into the lateral process of the vertebrae. In contrast to rudimentary ribs, observations to date indicate that extra ribs are permanent structures. The basic mechanism(s) involved in the formation of supernumerary ribs are unknown. There is evidence that alterations in developmental genes can affect the number of ribs formed, but the relevance of these findings to xenobiotic- and stress-induced supernumerary ribs is currently unknown.

Fig. 6. *(opposite page)* Cervical vertebrae in the mouse fetus at GD 18. **A**, Side view, control (normal) fetus. There are seven cervical vertebrae (C1–C7), and the tubercula anterior are on C6. **B**, Side view, fetus from a dam treated with methanol on gestation day 7. C1 and C2 are fused and abnormally shaped, the tubercula anterior are abnormally positioned on C-5, and there is a full rib (attached to the sternum ventrally) on C7. **C**, Ventral view, control (normal) fetus. Tubercula anterior are on C6 bilaterally, C7 has no rib, and the first rib is on T1. **D**, Front view, fetus from a dam treated with methanol on GD 7. The tubercula anterior on the left side of the fetus is misplaced on C5, whereas the tubercula anterior on the right side is in the correct position on C6. There is a full bilateral rib on C7. **E**, Disarticulated cervical vertebrae from a control (normal) fetus. The tubercula anterior are on C6 (asterisk), and there is no rib on C7. **F**, Disarticulated cervical vertebrae of a fetus from a dam treated with methanol on GD 7. The tubercula anterior are abnormally located on C5 (asterisk) and C7 has a full rib attached to it.

REFERENCES

1. Kimmel, C. A. and Wilson, J. G. (1973) Skeletal deviations in rats: malformations or variations? *Teratology* **8,** 309–315.
2. Foulon, O., Girard, H., Pallen, C., Urtizberea, M., Repetto-Larsay, M., and Blacker, A. M. (1999) Induction of supernumerary ribs with sodium salicylate. *Reprod. Toxicol.* **13,** 369–374.
3. Rogers, J. M., Setzer, R. W., Branch, S., and Chernoff, N. (2003) Chemically-induced supernumerary lumbar ribs in CD-1 mice: size distribution and dose response. *Birth Defects Res., Part B,* in press.
4. Narotsky, M. G., Francis, E. Z., and Kavlock, R. J. (1994) Developmental toxicity and structure-activity relationships of aliphatic acids, including dose-response assessment of valproic acid in mice and rats. *Fundam. Appl. Toxicol.* **22,** 251–265.
5. Kessel, M. (1992) Respecification of vertebral identities by retinoic acid. *Development* **115,** 487–501.
6. Wickramaratne, G. A. (1988) The post-natal fate of supernumerary ribs in rat teratogenicity studies. *J. Appl. Toxicol.* **8,** 91–94.
7. Beck, S. L. (1983) Assessment of adult skeletons to detect prenatal exposure to acetazolamide in mice. *Teratology* **28,** 45–66.
8. Rogers, J. M., Francis, B. M., Barbee, B. D., and Chernoff, N. (1991) Developmental toxicity of bromoxynil in rats and mice. *Fundam. Appl. Toxicol.* **17,** 442–447.
9. Chernoff, N., Rogers, J. M., Turner, C. I., and Francis, B. M. (1991) Significance of supernumerary ribs in rodent developmental toxicity studies: postnatal persistence in rats and mice. *Fundam. Appl. Toxicol.* **17,** 448–453.
10. Chernoff, N., Rogers, E., Carver, B., Kavlock, R., and Gray, L. E. (1979) The fetotoxic potential of municipal drinking water in the mouse. *Teratology* **19,** 165–70.
11. Khera, K. S. (1984) Maternal toxicity-a possible factor in fetal malformations in mice. *Teratology* **29,** 411–416.
12. Khera, K. S. (1985) Maternal toxicity: a possible etiological factor in embryo-fetal deaths and fetal malformations of rodent-rabbit species. *Teratology* **31,** 129–153.
13. Kavlock, R. J., Chernoff, N., and Rogers, E. H. (1985) The effect of acute maternal toxicity on fetal development in the mouse. *Teratog. Carcinog. Mutagen.* **5,** 3–13.
14. Beyer, P. E. and Chernoff, N. (1986) The induction of supernumerary ribs in rodents: role of the maternal stress. *Teratog. Carcinog. Mutagen.* **6,** 419–429.
15. Chernoff, N., Miller, D. B., Rosen, M. B., and Mattscheck, C. L. (1988) Developmental effects of maternal stress in the CD-1 mouse induced by restraint on single days during the period of major organogenesis. *Toxicology* **51,** 57–65.
16. Foulon, O., Jaussely, C., Repetto, M., Urtizberea, M., and Blacker, A. M. (2000) Postnatal evolution of supernumerary ribs in rats after a single administration of sodium salicylate. *J. Appl. Toxicol.* **20,** 205–209.
17. Steiner, H. A. (1943) Roentgenologic manifestations and clinical symptoms of rib abnormalities. *Radiology* **40,** 175–178.
18. MacGibbon, B. and Farfan, H. F. (1979) A radiologic survey of various configurations of the lumbar spine. *Spine* **4,** 258–266.
19. Noda, T., Morita, S., Yamano, T., Shimizu, M., Nakamura, T., Saitoh, M., and Yamada, A. (1991) Teratogenicity study of tri-n-butyltin acetate in rats by oral administration. *Toxicol. Lett.* **55,** 109–115.
20. Fujinaga, M., Baden, J. M., and Mazze, R. I. (1989) Susceptible period of nitrous oxide teratogenicity in Sprague-Dawley rats. *Teratology* **40,** 439–444.
21. Inouye, M. and Kajiwara, Y. (1988) Teratogenic interactions between methylmercury and mitomycin C in mice. *Arch. Toxicol.* **61,** 192–195.
22. Nelson, B. K., Brightwell, W. S., MacKenzie, O. R., Khan, A., Burg, J. R., Weigel, W. W., and Goad, P. T. (1985) Teratological assessment of methanol and ethanol at high inhalation levels in rats. *Fundam. Appl. Toxicol.* **5,** 727–736.
23. Rogers, J. M., Mole, M. L., Chernoff, N., Barbee, B. D., Turner, C. I., Logsdon, T. R., et al. (1993) The developmental toxicity of inhaled methanol in the CD-1 mouse, with quantitative dose-response modeling for estimation of benchmark doses. *Teratology* **47,** 175–188.
24. Cherrington, J. W. and Chernoff, N. (2002) Periods of vertebral column sensitivity to boric acid treatment in CD-1 mice in utero. *Reprod. Toxicol.* **16,** 237–243.
25. Henderson, M. S. (1914) Cervical rib. Repot of thirty-one cases. *Am. J. Orthop. Surg.* **11,** 408–430.
26. Nguyen, T., Baumgartner, F., and Nelems, B. (1997) Bilateral rudimentary first ribs as a cause of thoracic outlet syndrome. *J. Natl. Med. Assoc.* **89,** 69–73.
27. Fernandez-Noda, E. I., Nunez-Arguelles, J., Perez Fernandez, J., Castillo, J., Perez Izquierdo, M., and Rivera Luna, H. (1996) Neck and brain transitory vascular compression causing neurological complications, results of surgical treatment on 1,300 patients. *J. Cardiovasc. Surg. (Torino)* **37,** 155–166.
28. Sanders, R. J. and Hammond, S. L. (2002) Management of cervical ribs and anomalous first ribs causing neurogenic thoracic outlet syndrome. *J. Vasc. Surg.* **36,** 51–56.
29. Bearn, P., Patel, J., and O'Flynn, W. R. (1993) Cervical ribs: a cause of distal and cerebral embolism. *Postgrad. Med. J.* **69,** 65–68.
30. Short, D. W. (1975) The subclavian artery in 16 patients with complete cervical ribs. *J. Cardiovasc. Surg.* **16,** 135–141.
31. Connell, J. L., Doyle, J. C., and Gurry, J. F., (1980) The vascular complications of cervical rib. *Aust. N. Z. J. Surg.* **50,** 125–130.
32. Hood, D. B., Keuhne, J., Yellin, A. E., and Weaver, F. A. (1997) Vascular complications of thoracic outlet syndrome. *Am. Surg.* **63,** 913–917.

33. Evans, A. L. (1999) Pseudoseizures as a complication of painful cervical ribs. *Dev. Med. Child. Neurol.* **41,** 840–842.
34. Saxton, E. H., Miller, T. Q., and Collins, J. D. (1999) Migraine complicated by brachial plexopathy as displayed by MRI and MRA: aberrant subclavian artery and cervical ribs. *J. Natl. Med. Assoc.* **91,** 333–341.
35. Schapera, J. (1987) Autosomal dominant inheritance of cervical ribs. *Clin. Genet.* **31,** 386–388.
36. Galis, F. (1999) Why do almost all mammals have seven cervical vertebrae? Developmental constraints, Hox genes and cancer. *J. Exp. Zool.* **285,** 19–26.
37. Schumacher, R., Mai, A., and Gutjahr, P. (1992) Association of rib anomalies and malignancy in childhood. *Eur. J. Pediatr.* **151,** 432–434.
38. Anbazhagan, R. and Raman, V. (1997) Homeobox genes: molecular link between congenital anomalies and cancer. *Eur. J. Cancer* **33,** 635–637.
39. Kessel, M., Balling, R., and Gruss, P. (1990) Variations of cervical vertebrae after expression of Hoxa-1.1 transgene in mice. *Cell* **61,** 301–308.
40. Small, K. and Potter, S. (1993) Homeotic transformations and limb defects in Hox A11 mutant mice. *Genes Dev.* **7,** 231–238.
41. Charité, J. W., de Graaff, W., Shen, S., and Deschamps, J. (1994) Ectopic expression of Hoxb-8 causes duplication of the ZPA in the forelimb and homeotic transformation of axial structures. *Cell* **78,** 589–601.
42. Kmita, M., Duboule, D., anad Zakany, J. (2004) Molecular genetic analysis of the role of the HoxD complex in skeletal development, in *The Skeleton: Biochemical, Genetic and Molecular Interactions in Development and Homeostasis* (Massaro, E. J. and Rogers, J. M., eds.), Humana Press, Totowa, NJ, pp. 101–112.
43. van der Lugt, N. M., Domen, J., Linders, K., van Roon, M., Robanus-Maandag, E., te Riele, H., et al. (1994) Posterior transformation, neurological abnormalities, and severe hematopoietic defects in mice with a targeted deletion of the bmi-1 proto-oncogene. *Genes Dev.* **8,** 757–769.
44. Kessel, M. and Gruss, P. (1991) Homeotic transformations of murine vertebrae and concomitant alteration of Hox codes induced by retinoic acid. *Cell* **67,** 89–104.
45. Kavlock, R. J., Chernoff, N., Gray, L. E. Jr., Gray, J. A., and Whitehouse, D. (1982) Teratogenic effects of benomyl in Wistar rat and CD-1 mouse, with emphasis on route of administration. *Toxicol. Appl. Pharmacol.* **62,** 44–54.
46. Branch, S., Rogers, J. M., Brownie, C. F., and Chernoff, N. (1996) Supernumerary lumbar rib: manifestation of basic alteration in embryonic development of ribs. *J. Appl. Toxicol.* **16,** 115–119.
47. Horton, V. L., Sleet, R. B., John-Greene, J. A., and Welsch, F. (1985) Developmental phase-specific and dose-related teratogenic effects of ethylene glycol monomethyl ether in CD-1 mice. *Toxicol. Appl. Pharmacol.* **80,** 108–118.
48. Schardein, J. L. (2000) *Chemically Induced Birth Defects*, Third Ed. Marcel Dekker, Inc., New York.
49. Bagnall, K. M., Harris, P. F., and Jones, P. R. (1984) A radiographic study of variations of the human fetal spine. *Anat. Rec.* **208,** 265–270.
50. McNally, E., Sandin, B., and Wilkins, R. A. (1990) The ossification of the costal element of the seventh cervical vertebra with particular reference to cervical ribs. *J. Anat.* **170,** 125–129.
51. Etter, L. E. (1944) Osseous abnormalities in the thoracic cage seen in forty thousand consecutive chest photoroentgenograms. *Am. J. Roentgenol.* **51,** 359–363.
52. O'Rahilly, R., Muller, F., and Meyer, D. B. (1990) The human vertebral column at the end of the embryonic period proper. 3. The thoracicolumbar region. *J. Anat.* **168,** 81–93.
53. Rogers, J. M. and Mole, M. L. (1997) Critical periods for the developmental toxicity of inhaled methanol in the CD-1 mouse. *Teratology* **55,** 364–372.
54. Connelly, L. E. and Rogers, J. M. (1997) Methanol causes posteriorization of cervical vertebrae in mice. *Teratology* **55,** 138–144.

26
Experimental Skeletal Dysmorphology
Risk Assessment Issues

Rochelle W. Tyl, Melissa C. Marr, and Christina B. Myers

INTRODUCTION

The two components of formal risk assessment are hazard identification and risk assessment. Hazard can be defined as the intrinsic capacity of an agent to do harm. Risk can be defined as the assessment of whether an agent will produce adverse outcomes to the species of interest under relevant exposure conditions. The critical aspect of risk is relevant exposure, by a relevant route, at relevant doses or concentrations, during sensitive life stages (i.e., timing of exposure), and for appropriate durations. Laboratory animal studies are critical for the risk component. The doses for the animal studies at which effects are observed or not observed are then compared with the exposures from all sources (e.g., feed, water, air) as measured, calculated, or modeled of the species of interest, to calculate a margin of exposure (MOE). The larger the MOE, the less concern. The species of interest is usually, but not always, humans (e.g., increasing attention to environmental risk assessments).

An early attempt to graphically visualize the risk process is presented in Fig. 1 *(1)*. It presents the process as one-way and essentially linear. A more recent version is presented in Fig. 2 *(2)*, wherein the risk assessment process is represented as iterative and interactive between hazard identification (science-based basic research) and risk assessment (science-based applied research). Formal risk assessment requires animal data from relevant studies compliant with regulatory test guidelines and (ideally) performed under Good Laboratory Practice principles and regulations. Submission of animal studies, as part of an extensive submission package, is required to obtain US Food and Drug Administration (FDA) approval for marketing a drug and to obtain labeling approval from the US Environmental Protection Agency (EPA) Federal Insecticide, Fungicide, and Rodenticide Act (FIFRA) to market a pesticide. Requirements for EPA Toxic Substances Control Act premanufacturing notices are minimal (*see* Table 1).

TESTING GUIDELINE STUDIES

The prenatal development of the skeletal system is currently assessed only in a developmental toxicity study (FDA nomenclature: Phase or Segment II study, old terminology: teratology study, EPA and Organization for Economic Cooperation and Development [OECD] designation: prenatal developmental toxicity study). All so-designated studies share a similar study design: exposure to maternal animals of two species (rodent: rat or mouse, and nonrodent: usually rabbit) during the pregnancy,

From: *The Skeleton: Biochemical, Genetic, and Molecular Interactions in Development and Homeostasis*
Edited by: E. J. Massaro and J. M. Rogers © Humana Press Inc., Totowa, NJ

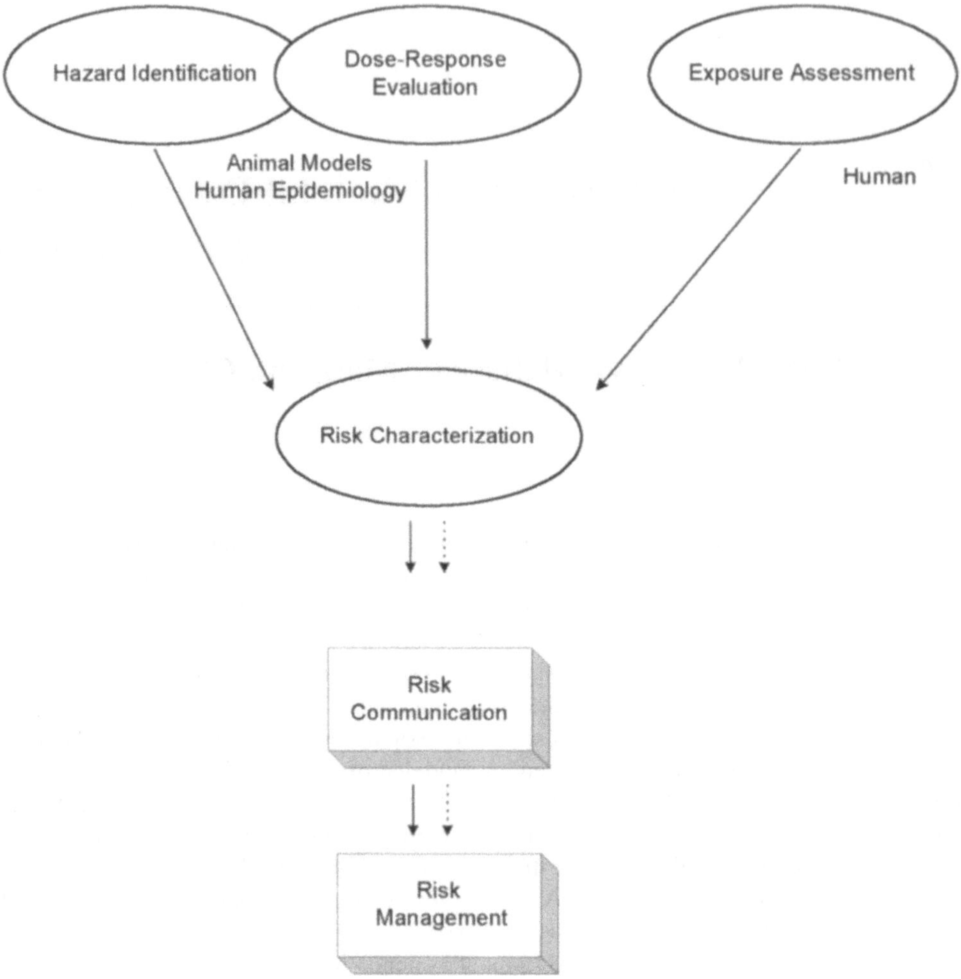

Fig. 1. Risk assessment paradigm *(1)*.

termination of the dams/does just before expected parturition (birth), and necropsy of maternal and fetal organisms. The number of ovarian corpora lutea (postovulation follicles) is counted as a measure of the number of eggs ovulated. The number and uterine location of total uterine implantations (as a measure of the number of conceptuses which have implanted in the uterine wall), and the number of resorptions (early *in utero* deaths) and dead and live fetuses are also recorded. Fetuses are counted, weighed, sexed, examined externally (100% per litter), examined viscerally by various methods on fresh or fixed specimens (50% per litter for rodents, 100% for rabbits), and examined skeletally (50% intact [not decapitated] fetuses per litter for rodents, 100% [50% intact, 50% decapitated] for rabbits). Earlier testing guidelines *(3–5)* and current FDA testing guidelines *(6)* specified examination of ossified skeletal components only, after staining the fetal carcasses with alizarin red S *(7–10)*. Current EPA *(11)* and OECD *(12)* testing guidelines specify examination of both ossified and cartilaginous skeletal components, with methods of visualization left to the performing laboratory. Almost all laboratories use a double staining technique before examination, with alizarin red S for bony components and Alcian blue for cartilaginous components *(13–15)*. There are currently no testing guidelines that evaluate the postnatal development of the skeletal system, although there are a number of focused studies that have done so *(16–19)*.

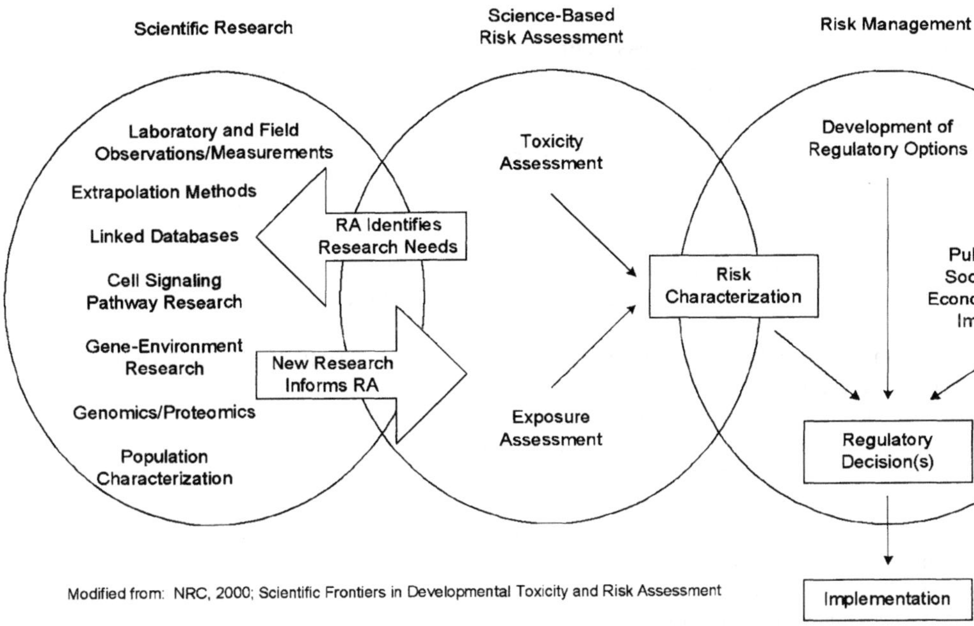

Fig. 2. New risk assessment/risk management paradigm *(2)*.

Prior to 1998, regulatory testing guidelines for developmental toxicity assessments specified exposure from gestational day (GD) 6 (time of implantation of conceptuses into the uterine lining) to the end of major organogenesis (closure of the secondary palate), GD 15 for rodents, and GD 18 *(4)* or 19 *(3)* for rabbits. Current International Conference on Harmonization guidelines *(20)* have retained this duration of exposure. Recent EPA *(11,21)*, FDA *(6)*, and OECD *(12)* testing guidelines specify exposure beginning after implantation is complete (or on the day of insemination; see below) and continuing until the day before scheduled sacrifice at term. This corresponds to GD 6 (or 0) through 19 (or 20) for rats, GD 6 (or 0) through 17 (or 18) for mice, and GD 6 (or 0) through 28 (or 29) for rabbits. The day vaginal sperm or a copulation plug is found (rodent) or mating is observed (rabbit) is designated GD 0.

The rationale for starting exposures after implantation is complete is based on two possible confounding scenarios:

- If the initial (parent) test material is teratogenic and the metabolite(s) is not, and if metabolism is induced by exposure to the parent compound, then exposure beginning earlier than implantation (with concomitant induction of enzymes and enhanced metabolism) will result in the conceptuses being exposed to less of the teratogenic moiety, and the study may be falsely negative.
- If the test chemical and/or metabolite(s) interfere with implantation, then exposure prior to implantation will result in few or no conceptuses available for examination at term.

However, there are situations when initiation of exposure should begin before uterine implantation. These include the following:

- For exposure regimens that are anticipated to result in slow systemic absorption (e.g., topical application, subcutaneous injection or insertion of an osmotic mini-pump for continuous infusion, or dosing via feed or water), steady-state or maximal blood levels may not be attained until the very end (or beyond) of major organogenesis if exposures begin on GD 6 or 7.
- For materials that are known to have cumulative toxicity (due to build-up of chemical and/or insult) after repeated exposures, exposure should begin on GD 0 (or earlier) so the conceptuses are developing in a fully affected dam.

Table 1
Regulated Materials Requiring Risk Assessment

1. U.S. FDA (Food and Drug Administration)
   a. Food additives (preservatives, flavorings, dyes, etc.)
   b. Vitamins, not "natural products" (biologically active)
   c. Food substitutes (e.g., fat substitutes, artificial sweeteners)
   d. Pharmaceuticals (biologically active)
   e. Veterinary pharmaceuticals (biologically active)
   f. Food use pesticides (biologically active)
   g. Food use chemicals (e.g., chemical wrapping, artificial sausage skins, etc.)
   h. Medical devices

NOTE: Attention to mechanism, human focus: disease state, clinical trials (IND [investigational new drug], NDA [new drug application], FDA approval)

2. U.S. EPA (Environmental Protection Agency)
   a. U.S. FIFRA (Federal Insecticide, Fungicide and Rodenticide Act)
      i. Pesticides (biologically active)
      ii. Food use pesticides (biologically active)
      iii. Biological pesticides (e.g., BT—*Bacillus thuringiensis*)
      iv. Biochemical pesticides (biologically active)
      v. Engineered plants (e.g., transgenic plants make pesticidal chemicals or are otherwise resistant to pests; GMOs [genetically modified organisms])

NOTE: Attention to nontarget species, environmental migration, contamination, transformation, bioaccumulation, etc. (registration and labeling, reregistration, data "call-ins")

   b. U.S. TSCA (Toxic Substances Control Act)
      i. Commodity chemicals (use based on physio-chemical properties)
         —Paints, paint thinners, inks, plasticizers, plastics, medical supplies, PVC piping, solvents, carpets, car parts, chemical intermediates, etc.
      ii. Options the Agency uses to obtain/require animal testing
         —Test rules
         —Negotiated test agreements
         —Voluntary submissions/programs (e.g., HPV [High Production Volume] initiative)

NOTE: Minimal information required for PMN (premanufacturing notice), SNUR (significant new use registration); EPA has 90 d to respond to submission

- For materials that are known to deplete essential components, such as vitamins, minerals, cofactors, etc., exposures should begin early enough so that the dam is in a depleted state by the start of organogenesis (or by GD 0).
- For materials that are innocuous as the parent chemical but that are metabolized to teratogenic forms, exposures should begin early enough so that postimplantation conceptuses are exposed to maximal levels of the teratogenic metabolites.
- For test materials that are known not to interfere with implantation, so exposure can encompass the entire gestational period and offspring will be available for examination.

The previous specification for cessation of exposure prior to term allowed for a postexposure recovery period for both the dam and the fetuses, and an assessment could be made regarding whether the observed maternal effects (body weights, clinical observations) are transient or permanent. However, the fetal evaluations take place only at term, and there is no commonly employed way to detect early adverse effects on the conceptus that resolve (are repaired, or compensated for, or result in *in utero* demise) earlier in gestation. What was observed at term was the net result of the original insult and any repair or compensation that occurred subsequently in the dam and conceptus after a post-exposure period. Thus, no detailed necropsy information on the dam was obtained during the exposure period (unless satellite females were used), and there was no way to distinguish effects during exposure from those occurring afterward. Most germane to this chapter, the fetal skeleton primarily develops during the fetal period, so the previous maternal exposure period ended prior to fetogenesis, and the fetal skeleton developed after maternal exposure had ended. The new developmental toxicity testing guidelines require exposure until term, which includes the postembryonic fetogenesis period.

The rationale for continuing exposure until term includes the following:

- Maternal exposure until term is a better model for human exposure than exposure only during a portion of gestation with abrupt cessation at the end of embryogenesis.
- Maternal responses at term with continued exposure (e.g., changes in organ weights, hematology, clinical chemistry, histopathology) can be better interpreted in terms of causality; there is no confounding maternal postexposure period for compensatory changes to occur.
- Many systems continue to develop in the fetal period, both in terms of increases in cell size and number, and of differentiation of specialized cells, tissues, organs, and systems (e.g., skeletal, central nervous, pulmonary, renal, gastrointestinal, etc.). The effects on these processes occurring in the presence of continued maternal exposure will be manifested at term (for most of the systems) and will not be confounded by compensatory processes that may occur in a postexposure period.
- The male fetal reproductive system is established and differentiates internally and externally *in utero*, beginning on GD 13–14 in rodents, so effects may occur from continued exposure to possible endocrine-active or reproductively toxic compounds by other mechanisms and may be detected. However, at term, only the testes and epididymides can be reasonably assessed, and most effects are not discernible until weaning, puberty, or adulthood (such as morphological and/or functional effects on accessory sex organs, adult testicular spermatogenesis, and epididymal sperm transit, etc.).

Recently in the authors' laboratory, a comparison was made of parameters of maternal and developmental effects in control CD® (Sprague–Dawley) rat dams dosed by oral gavage from GD 6 through 15 vs CD® rat dams dosed from GD 6 through 19 (22). Although the GD 6 through 15 dosing was employed for earlier studies (1992–1997) and the GD 6 through 19 dosing was predominantly used for more recent studies (1996–1998), there was an overlap in time between studies using the different dosing durations.

The authors concluded that the longer dosing regimen with no recovery period resulted in significant depression of maternal body weight and weight gain end points, as well as a reduction in fetal body weights. Presumably, the stress of continued handling and dosing was responsible for these differences. The three vehicles used (methylcellulose, corn oil, and water) were equally represented in both data sets. The concern was whether dosing with a potentially toxic test material would result in even further reductions because of a synergistic effect of the longer dosing period and the toxicity of the test material. The unexpected decrease in the number of implants and live fetuses may be the result of the differences in times of performance of the two groups of studies. In the early 1990s, Charles River Laboratories selected all offspring from larger litters (i.e., rather than a set number per litter, regardless of litter size) as breeders, so that the average litter size rose. In the latter 1990s, a more balanced selection program was instituted [the CD®(SD) "international gold standard"] to halt and reverse the increasing litter sizes and to minimize spontaneous differences in CD® rats in the different Charles River breeding facilities. The decreased incidence of hydronephrosis (a common malformation), as well as enlarged lateral ventricles of the brain and of rudimentary ribs on Lumbar I (both variations), may represent genetic drift in this strain over the years evaluated. The relative developmental delay of the fetal skeleton, evidenced by the increased incidences of dumbbell cartilage and bipartite ossification centers in the thoracic centra, was likely because of decreased fetal body weights at term in the litters under the longer dosing regimen (i.e., the fetuses are delayed in late gestational development but are appropriate in the development of their systems, especially the skeletal system, for their size; ref. *23*).

Any embryofetal adverse outcome must be interpreted in the context of maternal toxicity. This is especially true of the development of the skeletal system because fetal well being (e.g., body weight) is absolutely dependent on maternal well-being. Therefore, the maternal animals should be evaluated in-life for at least clinical signs of toxicity, body weights, body weight gains, and feed and/or water consumption (as g/d and g/kg body weight/d). At maternal necropsy, body and organ weights are essential, including gravid uterine weight, so gestational/treatment period weight gain, minus the contribution of the gravid uterus, can be calculated as a measure of maternal toxicity separate from any embryofetal toxicity (e.g., reduced numbers of fetuses/litter and/or reduced fetal body weights/litter will result in reduced gravid uterine weight which, in turn, will cause reduced maternal body weight in the intact female) as well as at least a gross evaluation of organs.

ADVERSE *IN UTERO* EMBRYOFETAL OUTCOMES

There are four general categories of adverse *in utero* embryofetal outcomes:

1. **Prenatal death**, including preimplantation loss (the difference between the number of eggs ovulated and the number of conceptuses implanted) and postimplantation loss (the difference before the number of conceptuses implanted and the number of live fetuses at term; nonlive implantations include resorptions, indicative of early postimplantation demise, and dead fetuses, indicative of late postimplantation demise).
2. **Fetal malformations and variations**, including individual alterations; alterations by system; pooled external, visceral, and skeletal alterations; and all alterations. Usually, the alterations are separated into malformations and variations for summarization and analysis. See below for a discussion of the definitions and characteristics of malformations and variations.
3. **Developmental delays or growth retardation**, including reduced body weights and reduced ossification, especially in those areas which ossified late, which are frequently associated with immaturity or delayed development (reduced fetal body weight) caused by toxicity. For example, typical skeletal delays include reduced ossification in fore- and hindpaw bony structures, such as metacarpals, metatarsals (hand, foot), and phalanges (fingers, toes); carpals and tarsals (wrist and ankle), are usually not ossified in terms of rodents or rabbits; caudal vertebrae, pubis (but usually not ilium or ischium), skull plates, sternebrae (especially 5 [last to ossify], 6, 2, or 4 in that order), and cervical centra (especially 1; last to ossify; *see* the section titled Term Rodent Skeletal Components and Historical Control Incidences of Fetal Skeletal Malformations and Variations in this chapter). In addition, other evidence of delays includes enlarged renal pelvis in rats *(24)*, reduced size of organs (e.g., liver or lung lobes, etc.) or other structures (e.g., long bones of the limbs), and dilated lateral ventricles (without tissue compression) of the cerebrum. Developmental delays or growth retardation also includes delayed organ development (reduced size and/or level of differentiation).
4. **Functional deficits**, which are not assessed in a developmental toxicity study design. They can be assessed in postnatal offspring exposed prenatally, which is done in other study designs.

CLASSIFICATION OF FETAL MALFORMATIONS AND VARIATIONS

In the test animal and human literature on malformations, there is no case to date where a teratogenic agent causes a new, never-before-seen malformation. What is detected is an increase in the incidence of the malformation(s) above that seen in the general population in humans and that seen in historical and concurrent control groups for animal studies. The current view is that teratogenic agents act on susceptible genetic loci and/or on susceptible developmental events. Therefore, the response seen is influenced by the genetic background and will vary by species, strain, stock/colony, or race (in the case of humans) and individual (the last is more variant in, and therefore more relevant to, genetically heterogeneous populations than in and to inbred strains). The outcome is also influenced by timing and duration of exposure.

There is genetic predisposition to certain malformations that characterizes specific species, strains, races, and individuals. Historical control data are indispensable (along with concurrent controls) to determine the designation and occurrence of the present finding(s) in the context of the background "noise" of the population on test or at risk.

The general considerations for designation of a finding as a malformation, a variation, or a delay are imprecise, may vary from study to study and teratologist to teratologist, are relatively arbitrary, and are not necessarily generally accepted. However, the following are the general classification criteria for skeletal findings currently used in the authors' laboratory (refs. *25* and *26*; *see also* Figs. 7–15 in this chapter).

Malformations

- Incompatible with or severely detrimental to postnatal survival (e.g., exencephaly, anencephaly, spina bifida, cleft palate, ectopia cordis, gastroschisis, missing limbs [amelia])
- Involves replication, reduction (if extreme), or absence of essential structure(s) or organs (e.g., missing, extra, or small limbs, digits, ribs, other skeletal components)
- Abnormal fusion of skeletal components (long bones of appendages, digits, ribs, etc.), dichiria (double hand), sympodia (fusion of legs), craniostenosis (abnormal/accelerated closure of anterior/posterior fontanelles and suture margins of skull plates), syndactyly (fused digits), vertebral scoliosis, cleft or "lobster claw" hand
- Skeletal components unossified in an abnormal pattern (e.g., cleft sternum)
- Result from partial or complete failure to migrate, close, or fuse (e.g., cleft palate, cleft lip, facial clefts, forked ribs, open neural tube, exencephaly, anencephaly, spina bifida, cranioraschisis)
- May include syndromes of otherwise minor anomalies
- Exhibit a concentration- or dose-dependent increased incidence (and/or severity) across dose groups, with a quantitative and/or qualitative change across dose groups (e.g., meningocele → meningomyelocele → meningoencephalocele → exencephaly; foreshortened face → facial cleft → facial atresia; short tail → no tail → anal atresia; short rib → missing rib; brachydactyly (short digits) → oligodactyly (absence of some digits) → adactyly (absence of all digits); missing distal limb bones (hemimelia) → missing distal and some proximal limb bones → amelia (missing limbs)
- Rare in concurrent and historical control fetuses
- Cervical ribs

Transitional Findings

These may be upgraded to "malformation" or downgraded to "variation" status, depending on severity and/or frequency of occurrence.

- Nonlethal and generally not detrimental to postnatal survival
- Generally irreversible
- Frequently may involve reduction or absence of nonessential structures (e.g., innominate or brachiocephalic artery, as long as the subclavian artery to the arm and common carotid artery to the head are still present)
- Frequently may involve reduction in number or size (if extreme) of nonessential structures or may involve their absence
- Exhibit a dose-dependent increased incidence

Variations

- Nonlethal and not detrimental to postnatal survival
- Generally reversible or transitory, such as wavy rib, extra rib (especially rudimentary)
- May occur with a high frequency and/or may not exhibit a dose-related increased incidence (e.g., extra ribs on Lumbar I in mouse, rat, and rabbit fetuses)
- Detectable change (if not extreme) in size of specific structures (subjective); e.g., shortened long bones of forelimb (humerus, radius, ulna, and/or hind limb femur, tibia, fibula), reduced renal papilla, small/large/accessory spleen, short rib (XIII in rodents, XII in rabbits), etc.

Please note that there is less variability in the development of the fetal skeleton the closer to term it is evaluated (i.e., if the term sacrifice is on GD 21 for rats, GD 18 for mice, and GD 31–32 for rabbits, rather than on GD 20 for rats, GD 17 for mice, and GD 28–30 for rabbits), but the risk of delivery before scheduled sacrifice is much greater. In addition, the sacrifice order must be random or selection of one from each dose group in rotation. If the dams and their fetuses are necropsied by group, there will be uncorrectable confounding. If done in the order of high, mid, low, and control groups, then there will be a "dose"-related reduction in fetal body weight and skeletal ossification due to the timing of sacrifice (independent of any treatment-related effects), since late gestation, even a few hours close to term, is the time of rapid growth and development, especially of the fetal ossified skeleton *(27)*.

Skeletal defects may be primary (intrinsic to the cells and tissues that will form the skeletal components) or they may be secondary to a defect in another system that impacts on the development of associated skeletal components. Examples of the first situation are cleft sternum, cleft or "lobster claw" hand, duplication or loss of limb components (if not caused by amniotic band syndrome), etc. Examples of the second situation are exencephaly (when the overgrowth of the brain is considered primary, causing subsequent failure of the skull plates to form), spina bifida (where the initial failure of the neural folds to fuse into a closed neural tube subsequently prevents normal formation of the associated vertebrae), etc.

The skeletal system is formed of two types of bones: (1) the flat, plate-like bones of the face, cranial vault, and scapulae are dermal elements that develop directly in a connective tissue membrane (i.e., "membranous bone"); and (2) the deeper, three-dimensional bones go through a membranous phase, then form as cartilaginous anlagen, and then finally the cartilaginous structures are replaced by bone-forming cells (osteoblasts and osteocytes) and extracellular bony matrix (i.e., cartilage replacement bone). The genesis of the rat skeleton has been previously described *(28–30)*.

With the new regulatory requirement for identifying and evaluating both cartilaginous and bony components of the fetal skeleton, knowledge of the status and nomenclature of both types of components at term is essential (excellent sources are ref. *31* for the rat, mouse, and rabbit; refs. *32* and *33* for the rabbit; ref. *34* for the mouse, etc.). The designation of skeletal malformations and variations, especially in the vertebral column, are now primarily based on the status of the cartilaginous components. If the cartilage is abnormal or variant, then the ossified bone that develops will follow the cartilaginous form and be abnormal variant. Examples of fetal malformations at term under this classification include fused cartilage:lumbar centrum; unilateral cartilage, unilateral ossification center:lumbar centrum; bipartite cartilage, dumbbell ossification center:lumbar centrum; split sternal cartilage; fused rib cartilage; rib cartilage attached to sternum; discontinuous rib cartilage; bipartite cartilage, normal ossification center/dumbbell ossification center/unossified ossification center:thoracic centrum, and so on.

In contrast, if the cartilage is normal, then unossified ossification centers in thoracic centra are designated as variations. If the cartilage is dumbbell, then unossified dumbbell or bipartite ossification sites in the thoracic and lumbar centra are also designated as variations. If cartilage is present for other bones (such as the pubis), even though there is incomplete ossification, the findings are designated as variations.

TERM RODENT SKELETAL COMPONENTS AND HISTORICAL CONTROL INCIDENCES OF FETAL SKELETAL MALFORMATIONS AND VARIATIONS

The fetal skeletal components, which ossify last during late gestation, are the most sensitive to insult and are, therefore, usually the most affected by (and associated with) maternal and other embryofetal toxicity *(33,35)*. These skeletal regions include the fetal skull (the GD 20 rat skull is illustrated in Fig. 3), the ribs and sternum (the GD 20 rat clavicle, ribs, and sternum are illustrated in Fig. 4), and the distal appendages (the rat GD 20 fore- and hind-paws are illustrated in Fig. 5). The complete fetal rat skeleton on GD 20 is presented in Fig. 6. Note the large anterior and posterior fontanelles in the GD 20 skull (Fig. 3), the predominantly cartilaginous rib cage in the GD 20 thorax (Fig. 4), and the pattern of ossification of units of the fore- and hind paws (Fig. 5). The bones of the wrist (carpals) and ankle (tarsals) are not yet ossified in the GD 20 rat. The bones of the hand (metacarpals) and foot (metatarsals) are ossified to a variable extent, with the forepaw usually ahead of the hindpaw in ossification. In Fig. 5, four of the five metacarpals and three of the five metatarsals are ossified. The phalangeal bones are also ossified to a variable extent in the GD 20 rat. There are ossification sites in the proximal phalanges of digits II and III of the forepaw, and no ossification sites yet in any phalanges of the digits in the hindpaw. The alizarin red S stained tips of the digits are the nails (not bones). A beautiful and detailed colored atlas of the double-stained fetal skeletons of Jcl:ICR mice on GD 18, Wistar rats on GD 21, and Kbl:JW rabbits on GD 28 is strongly recommended for the reader's review *(31)*.

Historical control fetal incidences of malformations and variations have been published periodically to aid in the interpretation of findings in a particular study and to illustrate the background incidence of effects of interest in rats *(36–41)*, in mice *(37,38,42)*, and in rabbits *(38,40,42–45)*. Historical

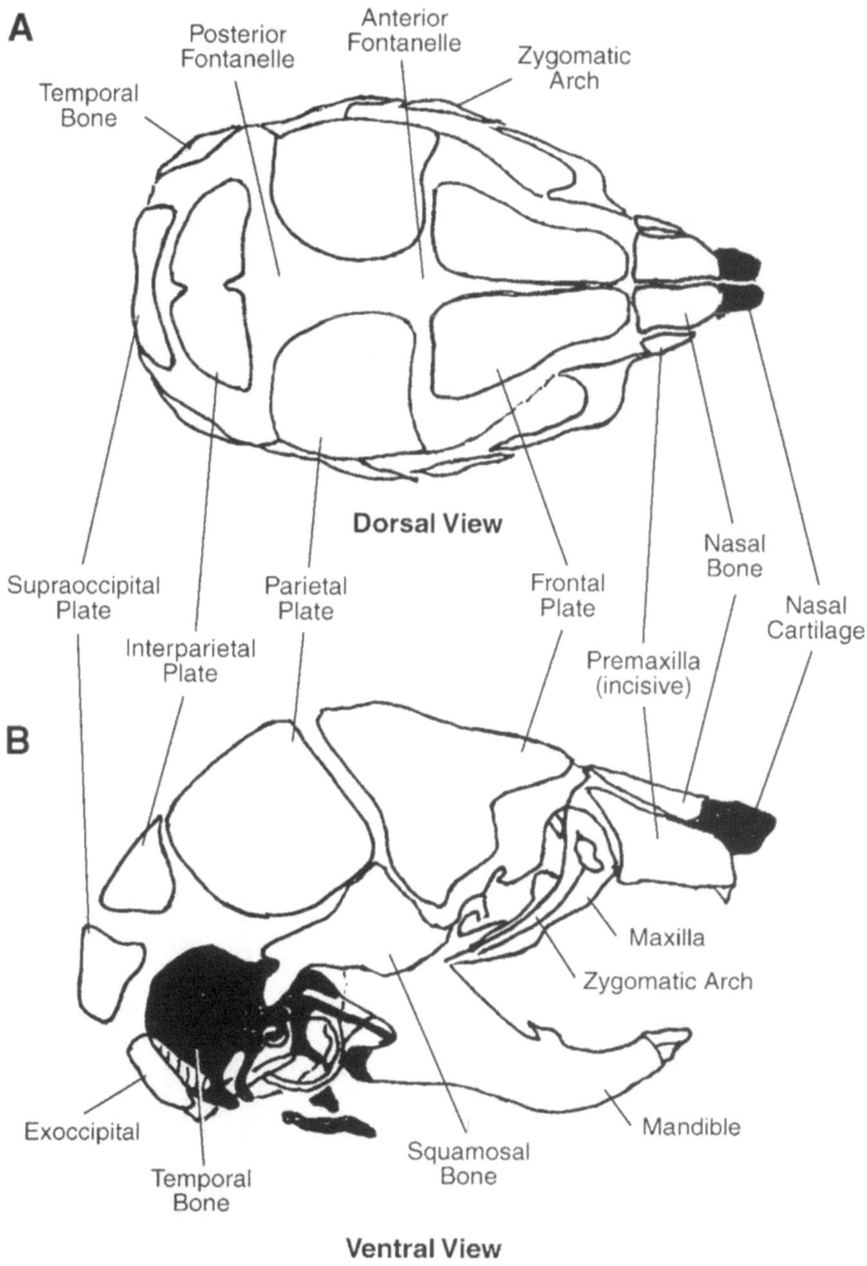

Fig. 3. Rat gestational day 20 cranium. **A**, Dorsal view; **B**, ventral view. Ossified bone is clear, cartilaginous bone is black (modified from ref. *31* with permission).

control fetal skeletal malformations and variations from the authors' laboratory are presented to illustrate the changing incidences over time within specific stocks and strains of rats, mice, and rabbits. These changing incidences are caused by founder effects, genetic drift, and spontaneous fluctuations (causes unknown) and are presented to make the point that concurrent and historical control data are absolutely essential to place the fetal skeletal findings in treatment groups in a given study in the proper context and to provide the background for deciding whether the effects are biologically and toxicologically significant (whether or not they are statistically significant). This information will

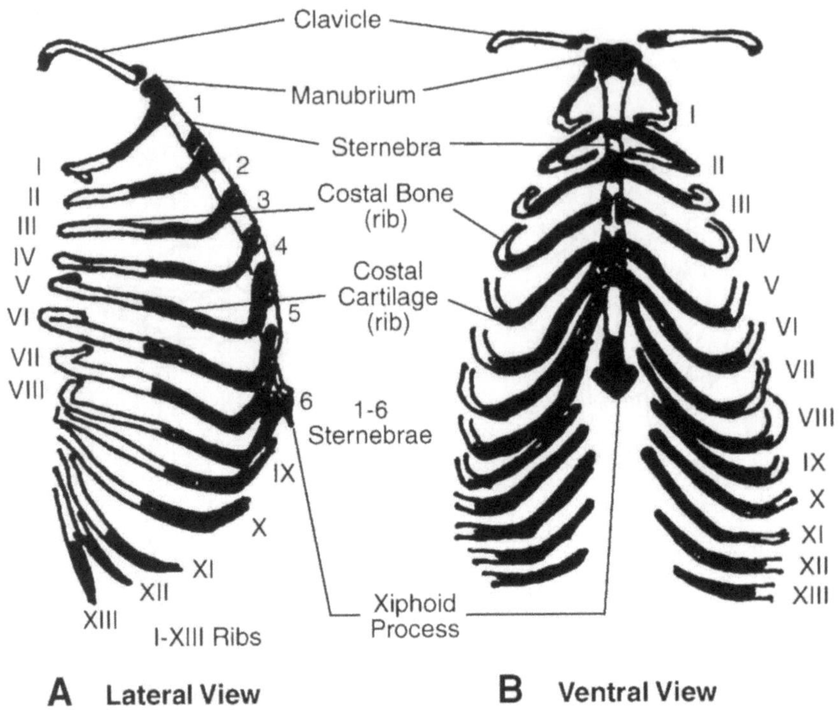

Fig. 4. Rat gestational day 20 rib cage. **A**, Lateral view; **B**, ventral view. Ossified bone is clear, cartilaginous bone is black (modified from ref. *31* with permission).

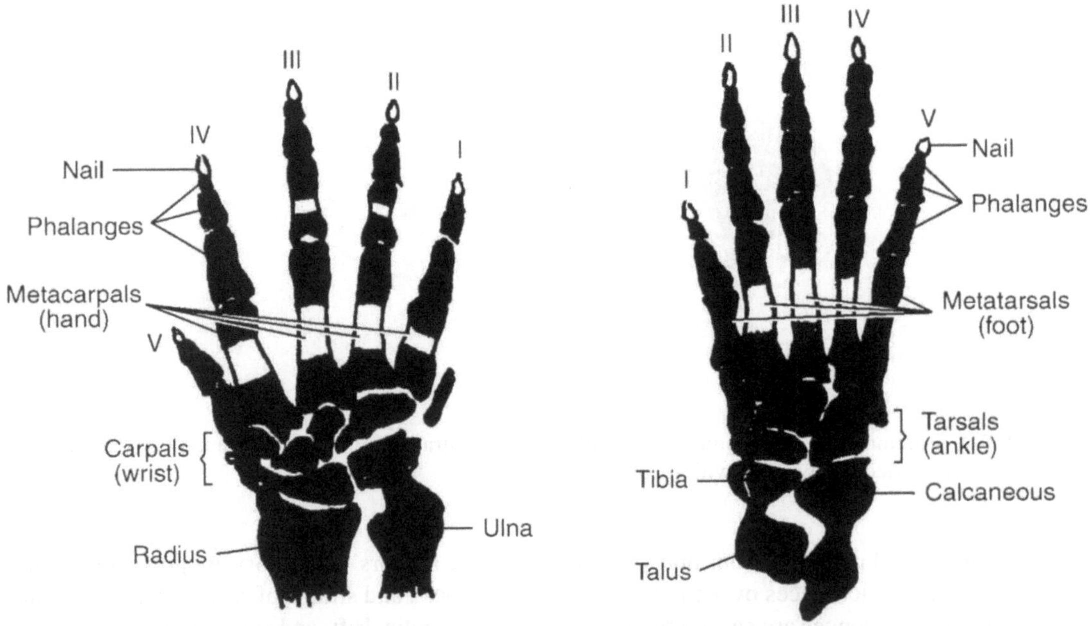

Fig. 5. Rat gestational day 20 appendages. **A**, Forepaw, dorsal view; **B**, hindpaw, dorsal view. Ossified bone is clear, cartilaginous bone is black (modified from ref. *31* with permission).

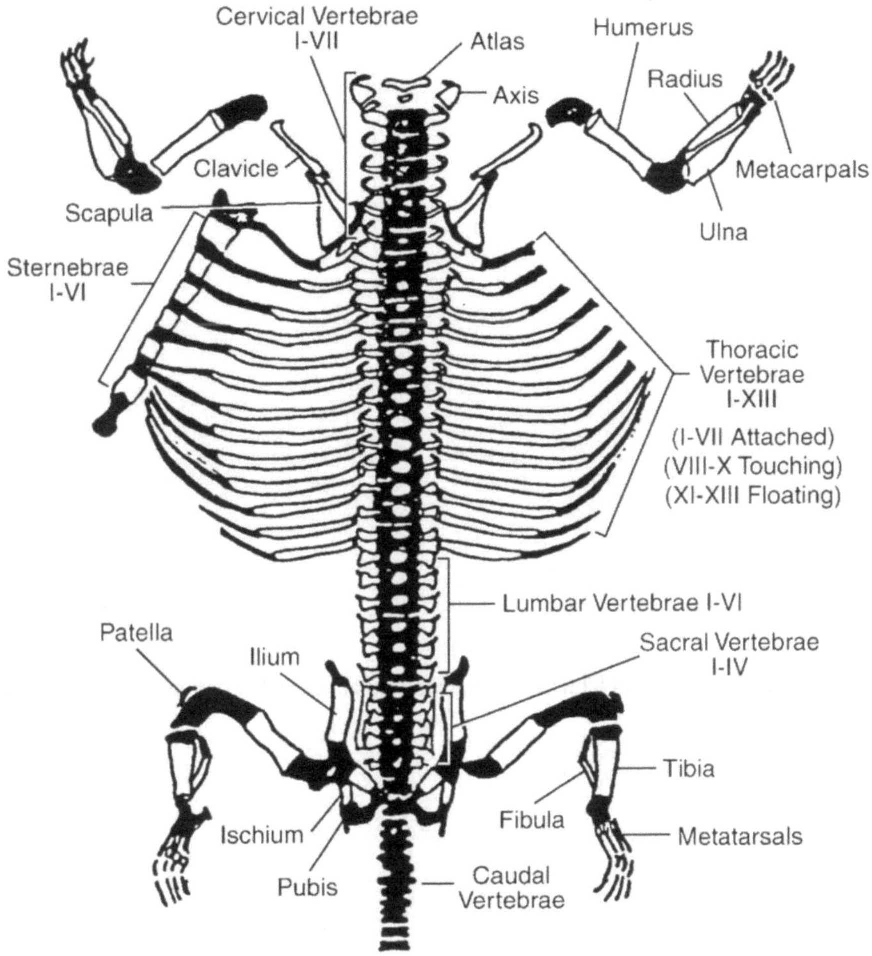

Fig. 6. Rat gestational day 20 axial and appendicular skeleton. Ossified bone is clear, cartilaginous bone is black (from refs. *25* and *26* with permission).

also inform subsequent risk assessment procedures and decisions (*see* below) based on the most sensitive, biologically relevant end points in the animal model.

The historical control data from the authors' laboratory are based on three CD-1® (Swiss) mouse studies with 70 dams and 841 fetuses evaluated on GD 17 (date of copulation plug = GD 0), 28 CD® (Sprague–Dawley) rat studies with 652 dams and 10,033 fetuses evaluated on GD 20 (date of vaginal sperm = GD 0), and 11 New Zealand White rabbit studies with 224 does and 1800 fetuses evaluated on GD 30 (date of maternal breeding = GD 0). The rats and mice were all obtained from Charles River Laboratories (Raleigh, NC; Portage, MI; and New York facilities). The rabbits were all obtained from Covance Laboratories (Denver, PA; previously known as Hazleton Research Products [HRP], Inc.). Figures 7 through 9 provide data on the fetal incidence of all skeletal malformations and variations over time in rats (Fig. 7), mice (Fig. 8), and rabbits (Fig. 9). In general, the incidence of skeletal malformations is always lower than the incidence of skeletal variations, and the peaks and troughs of malformations do not mirror the peaks and troughs of variations (and vice versa). The incidences of both parameters vary greatly over time, with no apparent trends. Pooling the control incidences across

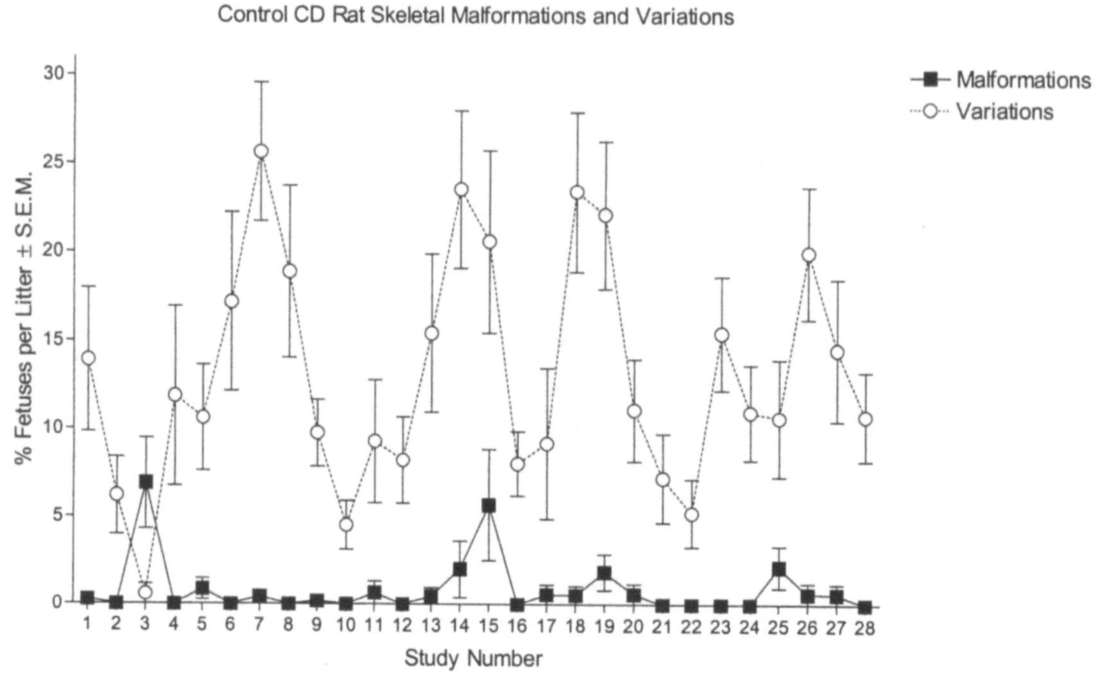

Fig. 7. Historical incidence of total fetal rat skeletal malformations and variations on gestational day 20 (over 28 studies).

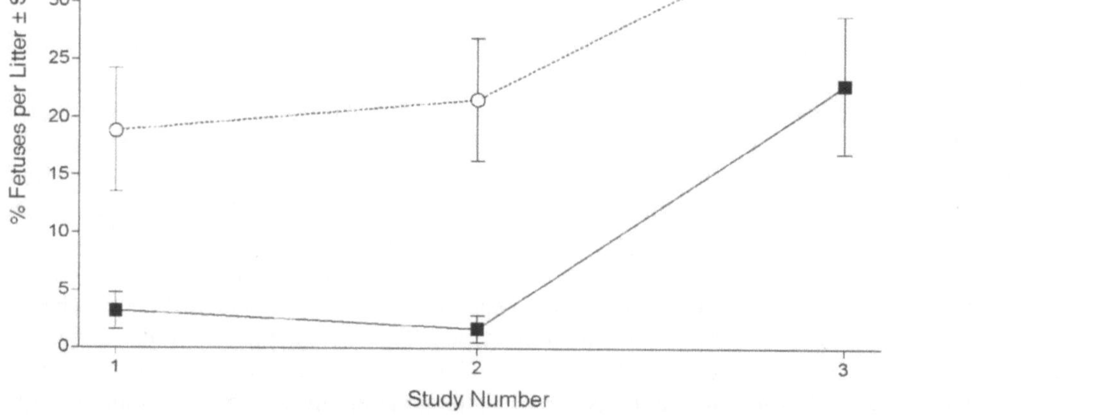

Fig. 8. Historical incidence of total fetal mouse skeletal malformations and variations on gestational day 17 (over three studies).

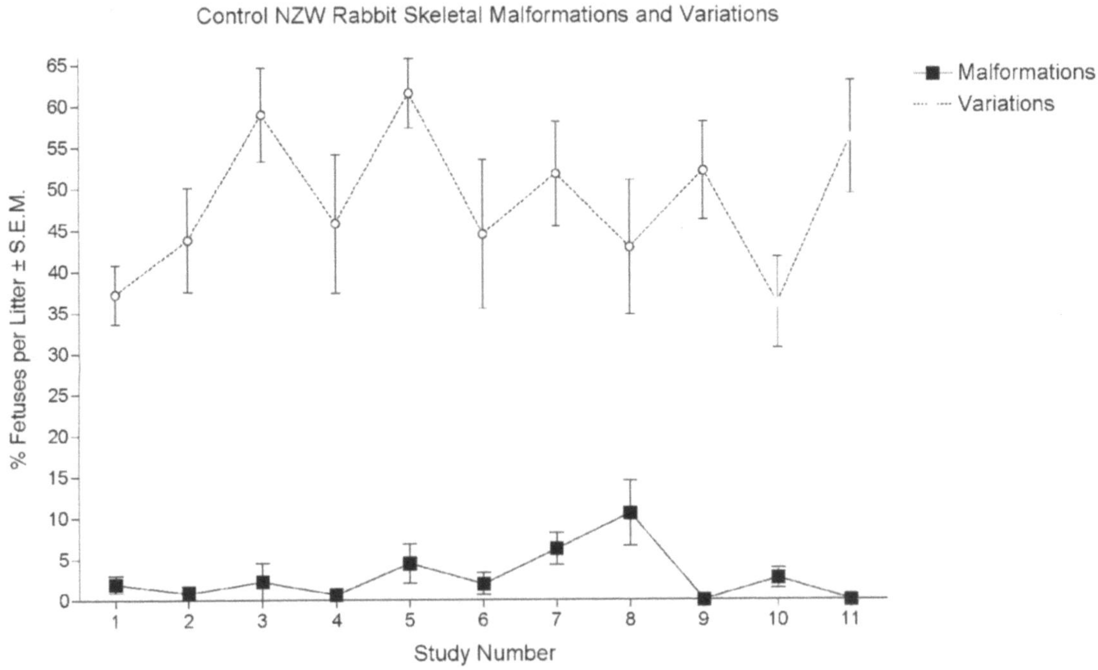

Fig. 9. Historical incidence of total fetal rabbit skeletal malformations and variations on gestational day 30 (over 11 studies).

many studies is not recommended since it obscures the fluctuations over time and precludes the use of historical control values around the time of the study of interest (the most appropriate range to consider).

The incidences of the most common skeletal malformations (A) and variations (B) in control fetuses in studies over time are presented in Figs. 10 through 12 (for rats, Fig. 10; for mice, Fig. 11; for rabbits, Fig. 12). Interestingly, the predominant areas affected for malformations and variations in all three species are the ribs and sternebrae. All three species exhibit relatively comparable ranges of incidences of skeletal malformations and variations, although rabbits and mice exhibit higher incidences of skeletal malformations than do rats (except for study 3 in rats performed in 1990).

The incidences of extra rib(s) on lumbar centrum I (the most common fetal skeletal variations in all three species) are presented for rudimentary (bilateral, left, or right; A series) or full or supernumerary (bilateral, left, or right, B series) in Figs. 13 through 15 (for rats, Fig. 13; for mice, Fig. 14; for rabbits, Fig. 15). The extra rib(s) on lumbar I are considered variations in the authors' laboratory, with lumbar I with a rib equivalent to thoracic vertebra XIV in rats and mice and thoracic vertebra XIII in rabbits. The incidence of each entry in each species varies from 0.0% to relatively robust values (expressed as percent fetuses with rib on lumbar I). The incidence of rudimentary extra ribs is higher than full extra ribs for rats (Fig. 13) but the reverse for mice (Fig. 14) and rabbits (Fig. 15). The incidence of bilateral extra ribs (full and rudimentary) is higher than the incidence for unilateral extra ribs (full and rudimentary) for rats (Fig. 13) and mice (Fig. 14), and for full ribs (Fig. 15B) but not rudimentary ribs (Fig. 15A) for rabbits. Note that for the rat, the incidences of full and rudimentary rib(s) on lumbar I are higher in studies 1–19 (1989–1996) and are much lower in studies 20–28 (1997–present). This shift is approximately concurrent with the establishment by Charles River of the International Gold Standard (IGS) CD rat.

Marr et al. *(18)* exposed CD rats on GD 6 through 15 during gestation to ethylene glycol (EG) by gavage and followed the incidences and types of EG-induced fetal skeletal malformations and variations

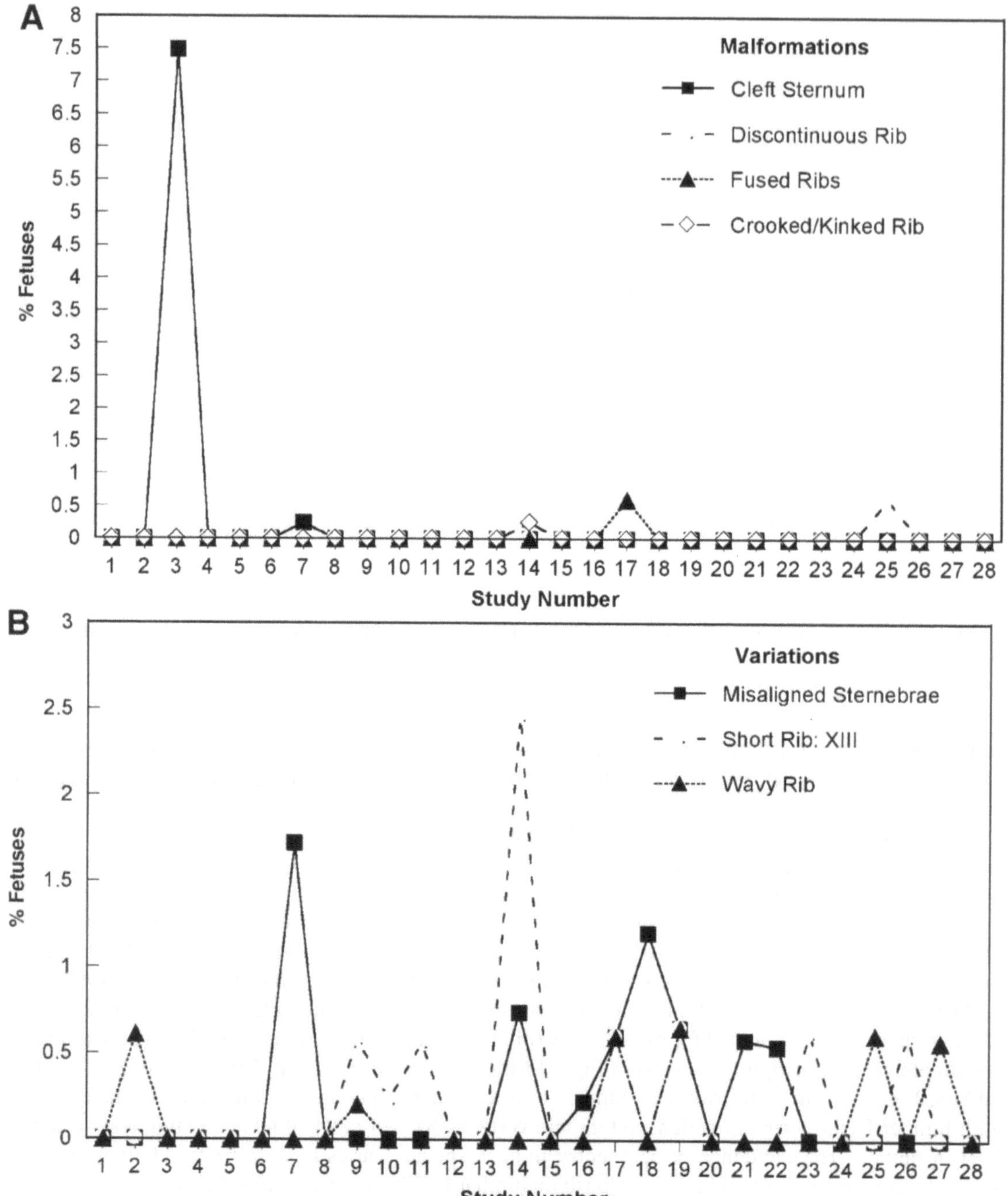

Fig. 10. A, Historical incidence of selected fetal rat rib cage skeletal malformations on gestational day 20 (over 28 studies); **B**, historical incidence of selected fetal rat rib cage skeletal variations on gestational day 20 (over 28 studies).

(including lumbar ribs) from GD 18 to adulthood on postnatal day (PND) 63. Chernoff et al. *(46)* exposed rats and mice on GD 6 through 15 during gestation to bromoxynil by gavage and followed the incidence of lumbar ribs (rudimentary and supernumerary) to PND 40. In rats in both studies, the skeletal alterations, including lumbar ribs (predominantly rudimentary), resolved essentially entirely

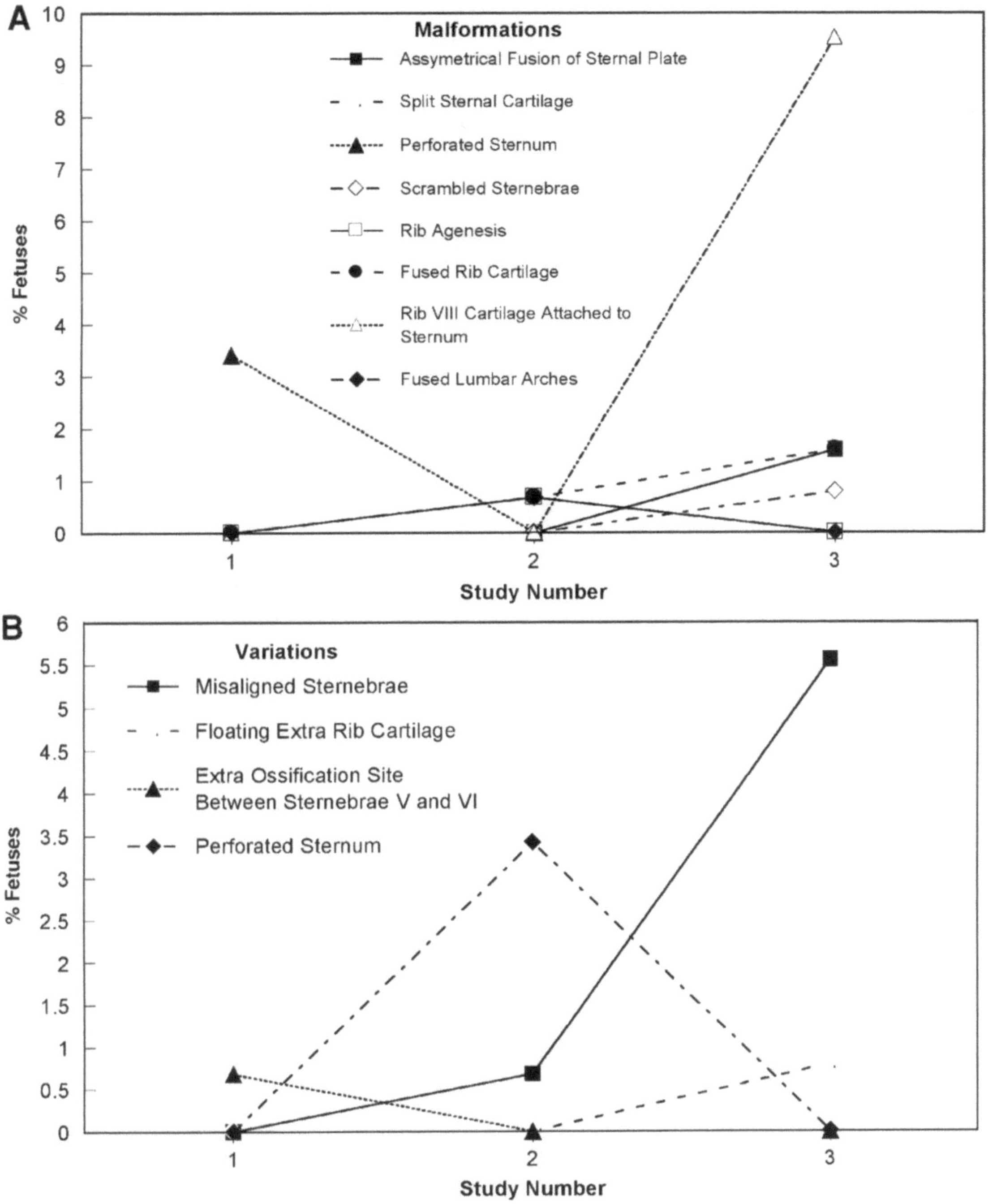

Fig. 11. A, Historical incidence of selected fetal mouse rib cage and vertebral arch skeletal malformations on gestational day 17 (over three studies); **B**, historical incidence of selected fetal mouse rib cage skeletal variations on gestational day 17 (over three studies).

by the last evaluation day. In the mice, with approx 50% of the extra lumbar ribs classified as "extra" (i.e., full, not rudimentary), the lumbar ribs persisted at approximately the same incidence through PND 40 *(46)*. These results suggest that the rudimentary and extra (full) lumbar ribs may be two different phenomena, with lumbar rudimentary ribs transient, becoming incorporated into the arches of

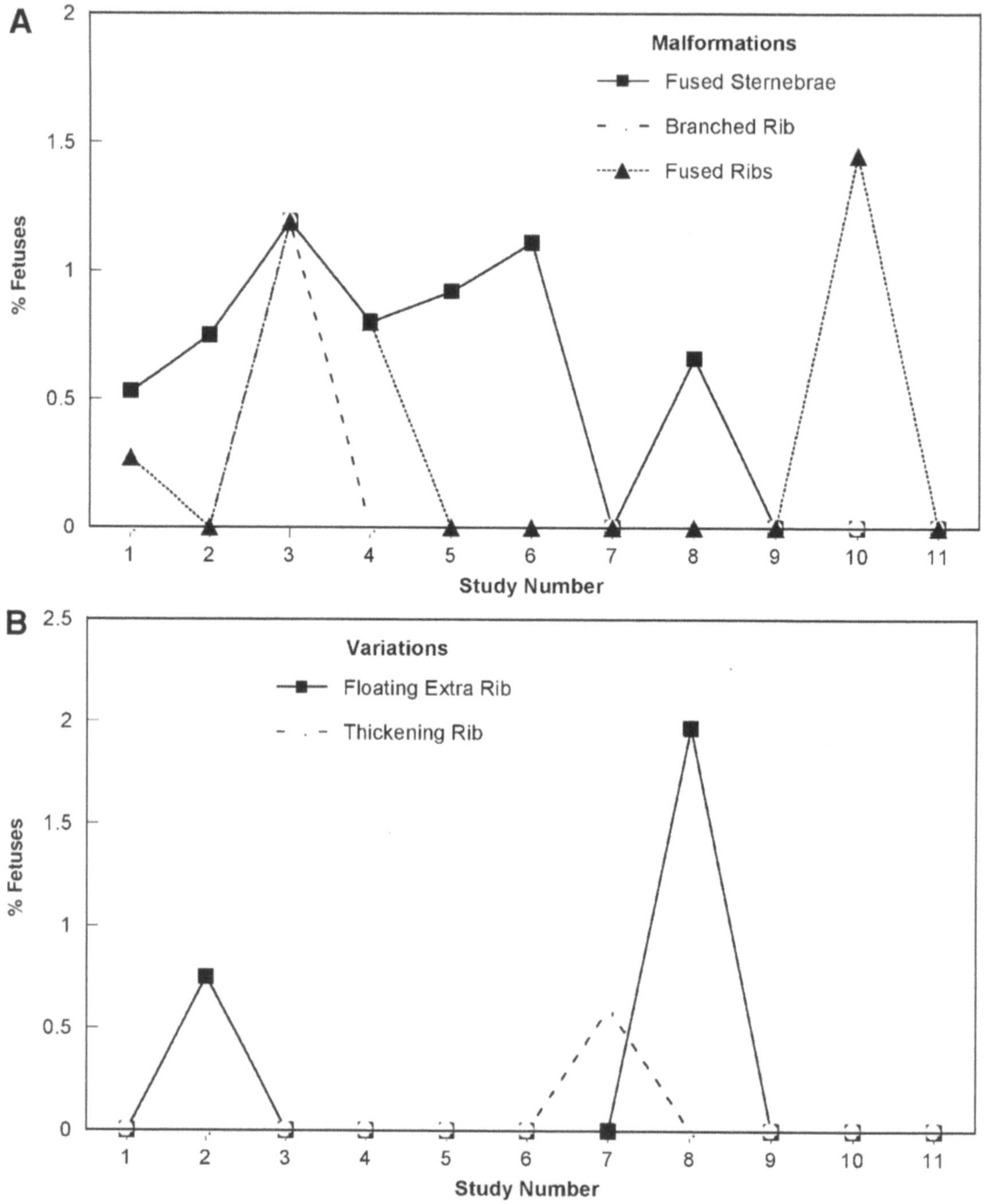

Fig. 12. A, Historical incidence of selected fetal rabbit rib cage skeletal malformations on gestational day 30 (over 11 studies); **B**, Historical incidence of selected fetal rabbit rib cage skeletal variations on gestational day 30 (over 11 studies).

Lumbar Centrum I and with the full lumbar ribs permanent, at least in mice *(47)*. There may be species differences *(48)*, such that the rat differs from the mouse in postnatal skeletal plasticity and differences in fate, and/or whether the rudimentary and/or full rib is spontaneous in origin or due to induction by a chemical or physical agent.

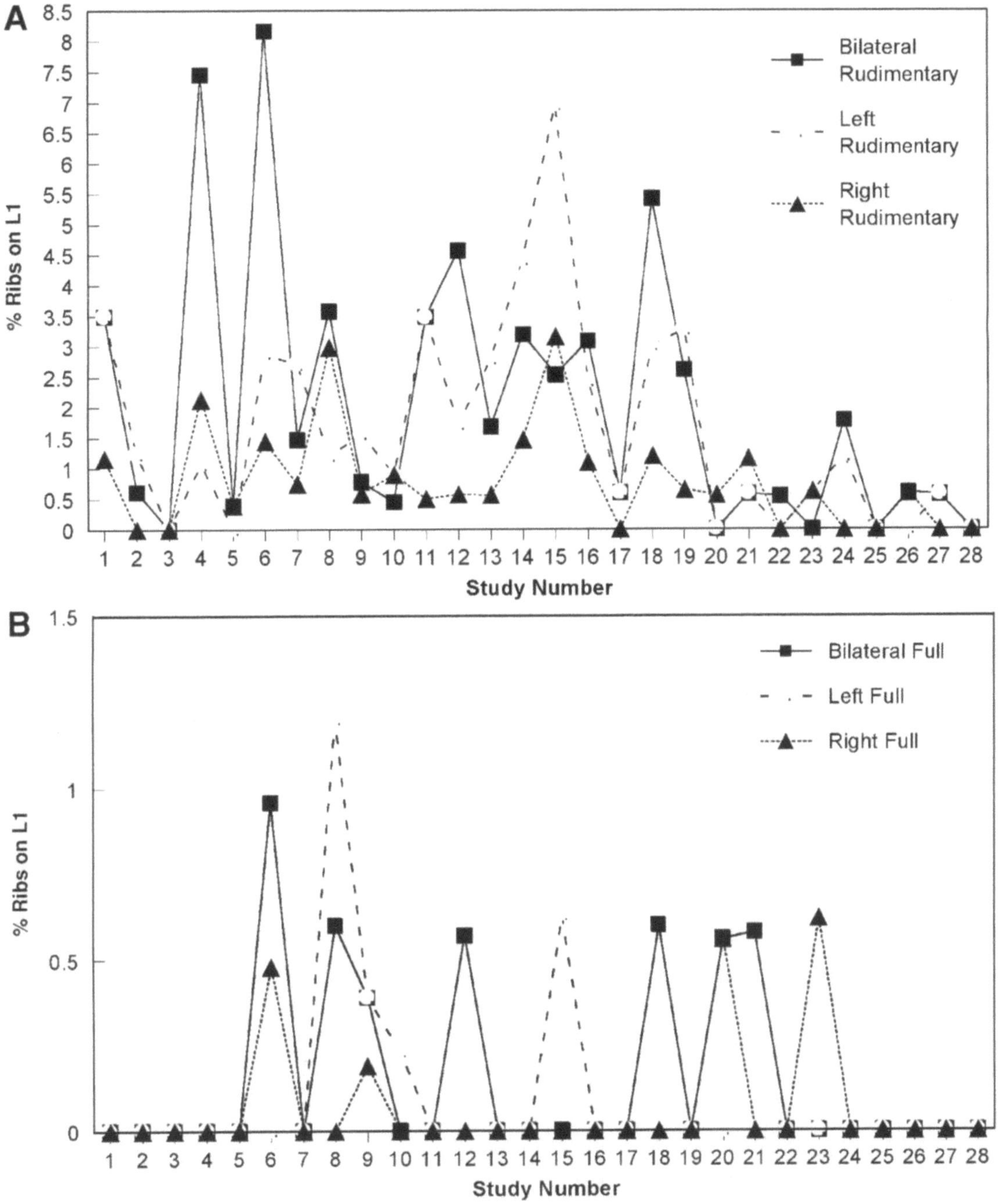

Fig. 13. Historical incidence of extra ribs in the fetal rat on gestational day 20 (over 28 studies). **A**, Rudimentary ribs; **B**, full ribs.

The anticipation, usually justified, is that the test material (if fetotoxic in general) will result in increased incidences of skeletal malformations and/or variations in a dose–response pattern, even if there is a dose-related decrease in fetal body weights, and may predict the likelihood of more profound skeletal effects at higher doses *(49)*. Many test materials and physical states have been shown

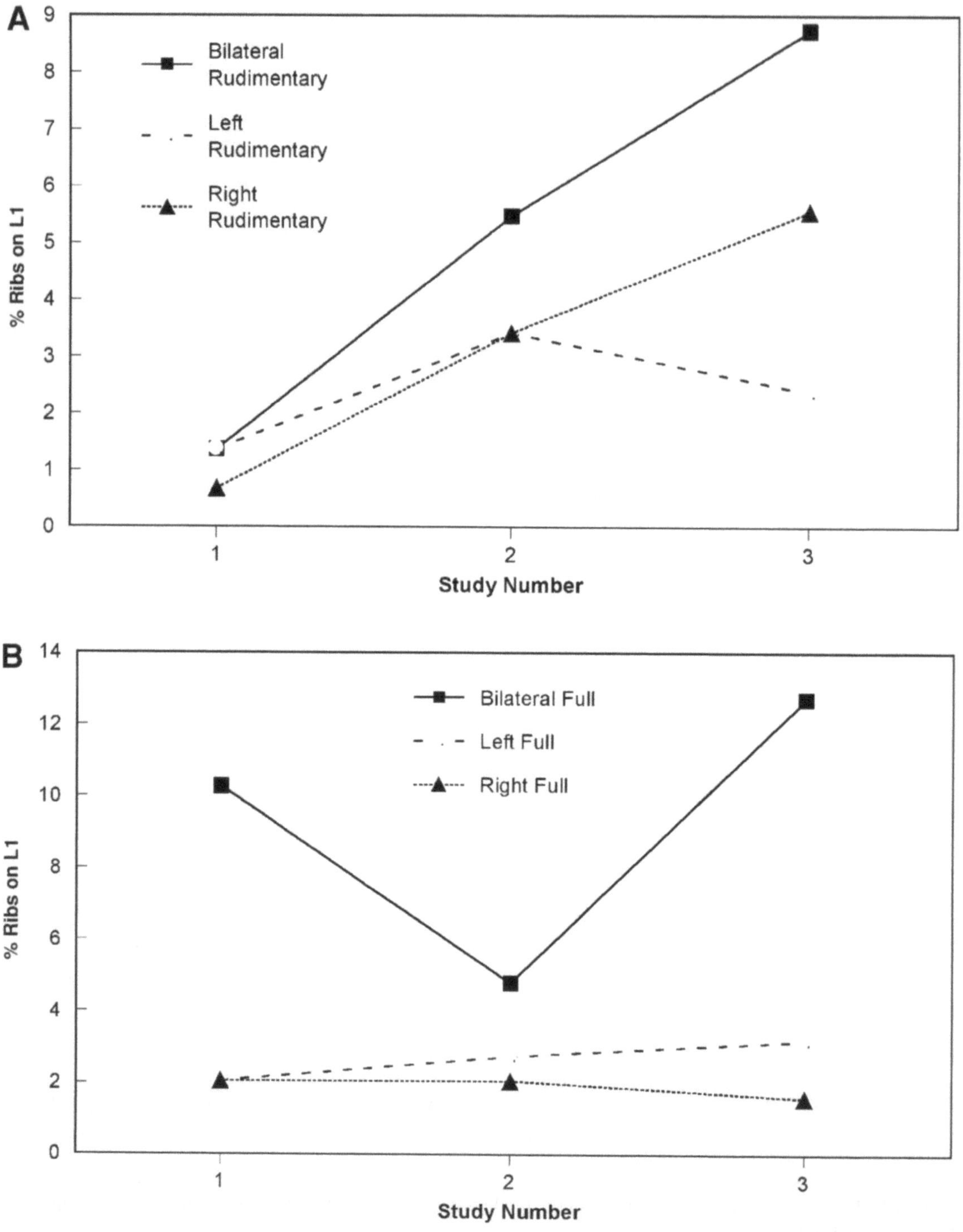

Fig. 14. Historical incidence of extra ribs in the fetal mouse on gestational day 17 (over three studies). **A**, Rudimentary ribs; **B**, full ribs.

to increase fetal skeletal variations and malformations, including lumbar ribs, in a dose-response pattern, for example, ethylene glycol *(18,50–54)*, valproic acid *(55,56)*, heat *(57)*, vitamin A *(58)*, methanol *(59,60)*, and bromoxynil (only lumbar ribs; refs. *46,61*).

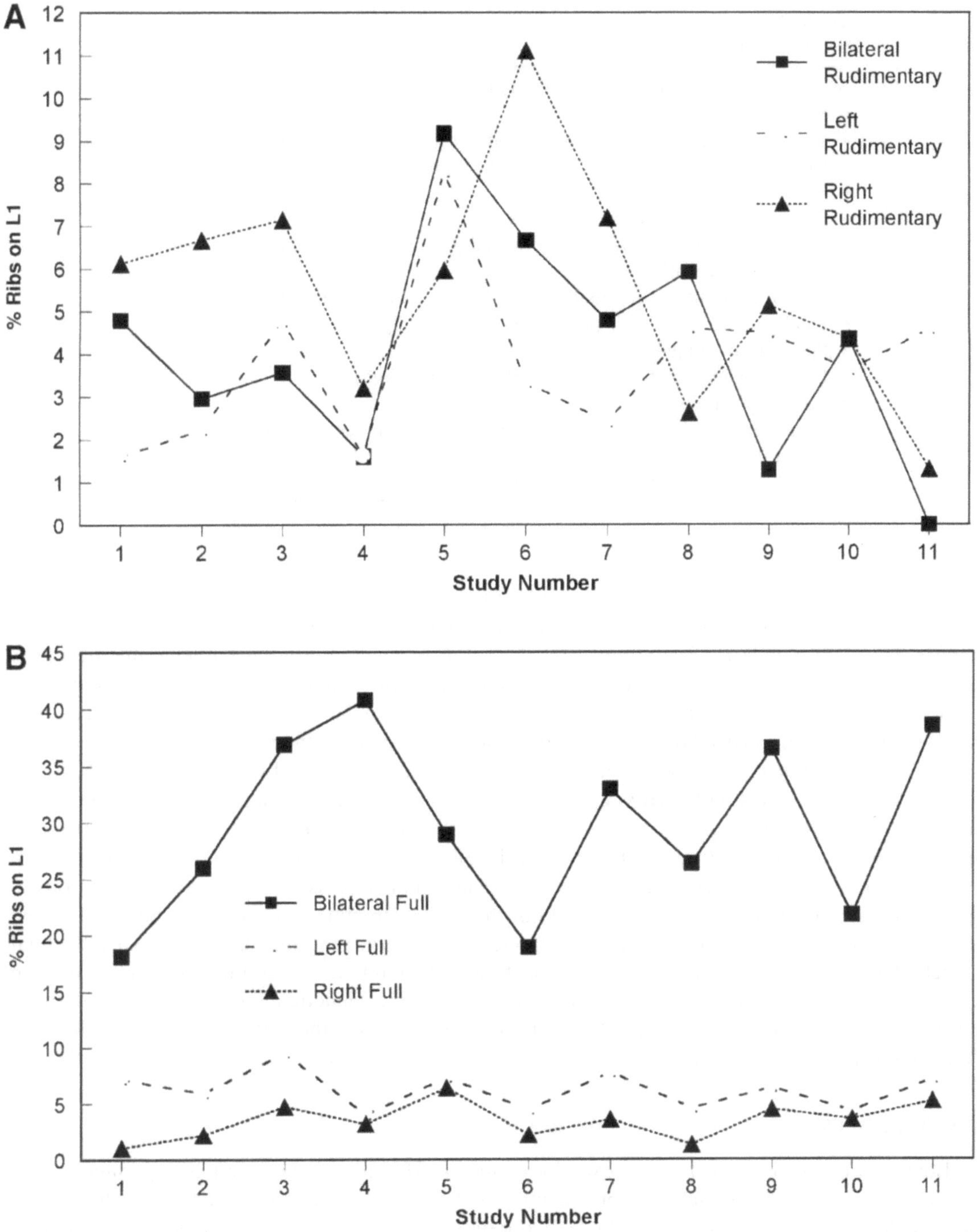

Fig. 15. Historical incidence of extra ribs in the fetal rabbit on gestational day 30 (over 11 studies). **A**, Rudimentary ribs; **B**, full ribs.

One striking exception is the skeletal response in fetal CD-1® mice and rats (but not NZW rabbits; ref. *62*) to gestational exposure to dietary boric acid *(63–70)*. With increasing dietary concentrations in ppm (and therefore increasing dose in mg/kg/d) in the presence of dose-related decreases in fetal

Table 2
Studies to Identify Hazard

In vitro/ex vivo scenarios with limited end points
• Mechanism(s) of action
• Molecular assessment of receptor binding/transcriptional activation
• Up/downregulation of gene activity (gene products)
In vivo scenarios
• Focused, limited exposure regimens
• Varied routes of administration, oral and parenteral (iv, sc, ip, etc.)
• Worse-case scenarios
• ADME (absorption, distribution, metabolism, elimination), bioaccumulation
• Small number of animals per group (and per study)
• Specialized, unique protocols
• One or limited number of dose levels (typically high)
• Specific endpoints
• Objectives: to identify mechanism(s) of action and identify endpoints
—Not designed to evaluate risk
—Not designed to determine NOAELs and LOAELs

body weight, the incidence of extra ribs (full and/or rudimentary) on lumbar I was significantly decreased. The explanation for this finding with boric acid, with exposure to methanol *(71)* and with exposure to bromoxynil *(61)*, is still under investigation. It may represent just another manifestation of systemic fetal toxicity or it may represent a very specific effect on the highly conserved homeobox (so-called Hox) patterning genes that determine the cephalocaudal boundaries of the cervical, thoracic, lumbar, sacral, and caudal portions of the vertebral column and their associated characteristics, such as ribs on thoracic vertebrae and the shapes of the vertebrae in the different regions *(46,48,72–75)*. This proposed effect on the Hox regulatory genes is most likely epigenetic (i.e., not mutational in origin), affecting transcriptional (or posttranscriptional) or translational (or post-translational) events in the production and, therefore, the function of the Hox regulatory protein(s) *(76,77)*. Mutations in Hox genes *(78)* or proto-oncogenes *(79)* can also cause homeotic-axial skeletal transformations in mice. The identification of the mechanism(s) of this effect (treatment-related reduced or increased incidences of extra ribs on lumbar I) would determine whether the test article is a specific fetal skeletal teratogen or a general maternal and/or developmental toxicant. In fact, maternal stress can cause supernumerary (extra) ribs in rats and mice *(74,80,81)*. Genetic alterations (e.g., mutations, clastogenesis, trisomies) can also result in patterning alterations in the vertebral skeleton in humans (e.g., trisomy 13, refs, *82–84*; trisomy 21, ref. *85*; trisomy 18, ref. *86*; and triploid fetuses, ref. *87*).

ENDPOINTS

Both hazard- and risk-based studies examine endpoints. Hazard-based research is important to identify new hazardous test materials; explore, identify, and define new endpoints; evaluate mechanism(s); and to enhance risk-based evaluations (Table 2). For rigorous risk-based studies, endpoints used (Table 3) must exhibit the following:

- Reproducibility: within the initial laboratory (intralaboratory) and among laboratories (interlaboratory); reliability.
- Robustness: present after comparable routes of exposure (e.g., various oral routes; responses may differ by parenteral routes) and at the same routes and doses over time; is not dependent on unique conditions (e.g., intrauterine position, etc.).
- Sensitivity: not insensitive (spontaneous variability too great); not too sensitive (greatly affected by confounders).

Table 3
Studies to Assess Risk

In vivo intact animal studies
- In vivo exposures
- In laboratory animal models (to predict human risk)
- In organisms in ecosystems as "canaries in the mine" (to predict human risk) or to determine ecotoxicity risk, per se
- Formalized apical study designs
- Mimic routes, doses, and durations of real, predicted, or modeled exposures in species of interest
- Large number of animals per group (and per study)
- Protocols compliant with regulatory guidelines
- Performed under appropriate Good Laboratory Practice standards and regulations (ideally)
- Specific and apical endpoints
- Objectives: to identify animal NOAELS and LOAELs
  —Not designed to identify mechanism
  —Not designed to identify initial target site

- Relevance: biologically plausible; related to adverse effects of interest.
- Consistency: occurs in the presence of effects in other related, relevant endpoints (if possible) at the same dose, routes, etc.

RISK ASSESSMENT PROCESS

Table 2 presents the characteristics of hazard-based studies. They are important to inform the risk-based studies in terms of providing information on new endpoints and possible mechanisms prior to risk-based studies and also to answer specific questions, investigate specific findings, etc., identified in robust, risk-based studies in an interactive process. Because these studies are specific and focused, they can evaluate and interpret specific effects.

Table 3 presents the characteristics of risk-based studies. These are important to provide the data on which formal risk assessment is based. Because they are apical studies (with many end points, exposure during sensitive life stages, robust group sizes, etc.), they can identify adverse outcomes but usually not specific mechanisms. These studies are designed to identify and provide the regulators the NOAELs (no observable adverse effect levels) for maternal and embryofetal toxicity. This is the highest dose in the study at which there are no statistically or biologically significant effects. In the absence of a NOAEL, a LOAEL (lowest observable adverse effect level) can be used, with additional safety factors to define a "safe" dose or concentration for the species of interest. The LOAEL is the lowest dose in the study at which there are statistically or biologically significant treatment-related effects.

The NOAEL is usually divided by 10 (to extrapolate from the animal model to humans; inter-species variability) × 10 (to encompass and protect sensitive subpopulations of humans; intraspecies variability) to calculate a reference dose for developmental toxicity (RfD_{DT}). If a LOAEL is used, an additional safety factor (or uncertainty factor $\leq$10) is placed in the denominator to extrapolate from the LOAEL to the presumed NOAEL. The RfD_{DT} is assumed to be below the threshold for an increase in adverse developmental effects in humans and is used, along with human exposure assessments, for risk characterization. The ratio of the most sensitive endpoint NOAEL from the most-sensitive species to the estimated human exposure level from all potential sources is defined as the MOE. The MOE is also used for risk characterization; the higher it is (the greater the disparity between the animal NOAEL and human exposures), the less concern and the lower the considered risk.

The characteristics/limitations of NOAELs (and LOAELs) are as follows:

- It is obviously experimentally derived and therefore dependent on the statistical power of the study which is, in turn, dependent on the number of animals employed, the number of dose groups, and the route of administration.
- It is also dependent on the number, relevance, and sensitivity of the parameters (endpoints) examined.
- It uses only the one dose (the NOAEL or LOAEL) and there is no way to factor in the shape of the dose-response curve (shallow or steep), etc.
- Its presence implies a "threshold," that is, a dose at and below which no statistically significant and/or biologically relevant adverse effects are observed in "any adequate developmental toxicity study," with the same study design limitations listed above. This is an experimental threshold, with the implication that there is a population threshold.

The limitations of the NOAEL/LOAEL approach (above) have prompted development of an alternative approach. The benchmark dose (BMD) approach (now used by the EPA) uses a software program to factor in the shape of the dose–response curve and intercalates or extrapolates a dose with lower and upper bound values which will result in an increase over the control value (of typically 1%, 5%, or 10%) for the effect(s) of interest. This is then used in place of the LOAEL or NOAEL for the subsequent step in formal risk assessment (i.e., determination of the reference dose and MOE).

Fetal body weight by sex per litter is typically considered the most sensitive endpoint in a developmental toxicity study, because the variability is small and is a continuous variable. However, skeletal findings, in the context of concurrent and historical control data, are powerful and sensitive indicators of treatment-related, statistically and biologically significant adverse outcomes.

The official position of the EPA and other federal and international regulatory agencies is that any of the adverse outcomes are equally bad, and that the most sensitive outcomes will determine the study NOAEL (or BMD). The rationale is that there is no guarantee that the effects observed in the animal model will be the same as those observed in humans (or another species of concern). In addition, in the absence of information on the relevance of the animal model and/or the end points evaluated, the safest default is to use the most sensitive animal model and the most sensitive indicator.

RISK ASSESSMENT ISSUES

Issues about the risk assessment process and outcome can be separated into scientific and regulatory areas with some overlap. They are relevant to any parameter or endpoint, but for this chapter, the discussion focuses on their relevance to fetal skeletal parameters.

Scientific Issues

The scientific issues include the following:

- Is the finding biologically plausible? By this we mean, is there a temporal association between exposure and outcome? Is there a biologically meaningful relationship between the timing of exposure and the location and type of effect observed? Does the initiation of the adverse finding occur before, during, or after (if there is a postexposure period) the exposure period? Is there a mechanistic basis for the adverse finding?
- Do other chemicals with similar physicochemical properties or biological activities cause similar adverse findings? Is there a structure–activity relationship such as with the ethylene glycol-based ethers or with the phthalates?
- Is there consistency and reproducibility of the exposure(s) and adverse outcome(s)? Do the endpoints predict or reflect adverse outcome? Are they appropriate to assess risk?
- Is there a dose–response pattern? Does the incidence and/or severity of adverse finding increase with dose? Is there a shift in the response with dose? If so, is the shift biologically plausible? For example, incidence of fetal malformations may increase in the mid dose but decrease in the top dose, accompanied with an increase in the incidence of *in utero* deaths at the top dose. Does a reduction in live fetuses per litter affect the incidence statistically and/or biologically? What if the incidence of skeletal variations goes down with increasing dose? For example, exposure to dietary boric acid during gestation in rats and mice (but not rabbits) results in a dose-related decrease in the incidence of extra ribs on Lumbar I (associated with dose-related decreases in fetal body weights; refs. *62* and *65*). If the incidence of skeletal variations goes down with increasing dose, but the incidence of skeletal malformations goes up with increasing dose,

do the skeletal variations at the lower doses predict the skeletal malformations at the higher doses? Are the skeletal malformations at the far end of the continuum of skeletal effects for the same bones or areas as the skeletal variations *(88)*?

- What is known about the animal model? Is this species/strain the most appropriate surrogate for humans? Is there similarity between the animal model and humans in terms of ADME (absorption, distribution, metabolism, elimination), systemic exposure (and toxicity), blood levels (and associated toxicity) of the test material, target organs, calculated dose at the target, etc.? Are the ADME characteristics of the test material in the animal model known? Are the ADME characteristics of the test material in humans known? Without pharmacokinetic/toxicokinetic data in the animal model and the human, it is difficult (if not impossible) to extrapolate results (routes, doses, effects) from animal models to humans with any scientific rigor, and one is forced to use default assumptions and uncertainty factors.
- Extrapolation from route to route, from high doses to low human-relevant doses, from short- to long- or long- to short-term exposure durations, is critical to risk assessment and should be based on scientific data, if at all possible, rather than on default assumptions.
- Does the adverse finding occur only in the presence of maternal toxicity? Is that important? The initial definition of a teratogen by Staples *(89)* specified that the fetal effects had to occur in the absence of maternal effects to define the test material as teratogenic. The current EPA view is that the interpretation of the fetal effects as secondary to the maternal effects (or not) is dependent on the type and severity of the maternal vs fetal effects. It is reasonable and scientifically defensible to interpret altered fetal skeletal ossification (only reduced? reduced and/or abnormal ossification?), associated with reduced fetal body weights in the presence of reduced maternal body weight gain, as likely secondary to the maternal toxicity causing the fetal toxicity, especially if the reductions in maternal and fetal body weights are reasonably comparable. It may not be reasonable or scientifically defensible to interpret major skeletal (or other) fetal malformations, whether or not associated with reduced fetal body weights, in the presence of reduced maternal weight gain on the order of 10% (statistically significant but not profound), as likely secondary to maternal toxicity. It is more likely that these latter major fetal malformations were not caused by the maternal toxicity, but that these endpoints represent separate and independent pleiotropic responses from the test material at the same dose(s). The interpretation of cause and effect must be made on a case-by-case basis.
- Should temporary/transient effects be viewed differently than permanent effects? The Segment II protocol currently does not include a postnatal component. However, we know that:
  - In the postnatal period, extra ribs (especially rudimentary ones) on lumbar I become incorporated into the arches of the vertebral centra *(17)*.
  - In the postnatal period, wavy ribs resolve *(90–92)*.
  - In the postnatal period, there is tremendous plasticity in the perinatal skeleton (EG-induced skeletal malformations and variations are present in term fetuses and pnd 4 and 21 postnatal offspring, but are essentially gone by pnd 63; ref. *18*).
  - In the postnatal period, dilated renal pelves can resolve *(24)*.
  - In the postnatal period, dilated lateral ventricles of the cerebrum resolve if there is no tissue compression (which may indicate hydrocephaly).
  - In the postnatal period, ventricular septal defects can spontaneously heal if they are small.
- Should cervical and lumbar ribs be viewed in the same way? The present authors are convinced that cervical ribs are a malformation, based on rarity in animal models and possible consequences (e.g., interference with blood flow or nerve tracts to the brain). Conversely, lumbar ribs are common in animal models and appear to resolve postnatally and/or have no adverse consequences and should be considered variations in animal models. In contrast to animal models, cervical ribs are more common than lumbar ribs in humans, but they also may have adverse consequences in the postnatal human.

Both cervical and lumbar ribs are reported in the human literature *(93,94)*, with evidence of lumbar ribs in a Neanderthal specimen *(95)*, a prehistoric skeleton *(96)*, and of cervical and lumbar ribs in a young woman of the 12th century AD *(97)*. A number of studies evaluating human fetal accessory ribs have reported a high prenatal incidence of cervical ribs (19%, ref. *98*; to 63%, ref. *99*), relative to the incidence of lumbar ribs (1.1%, ref. *98*; to 2.2% ref. *100*). These incidences are in contrast with the postnatal incidences of cervical (but not lumbar) ribs in children and adults. The percentage of patients with cervical ribs ranged from 0.04% *(101)* to 4.5% (based on only nine patients; ref. *102*), much lower than the prenatal incidence. The incidence of lumbar ribs in postnatal humans was similar to that in prenatal humans (0.04%, ref. *103* to 15.8%, ref. *104*).

With the large differences between prenatal and postnatal incidences in cervical ribs, it is likely that the prenatal rib on cervical vertebra 7 becomes incorporated into the lateral arches of this vertebral body *(47)*. In fact, cervical ribs can be considered as relatively common in pre- and perinatal humans *(105–108)*. They can occur spontaneously or be inherited as an autosomal-dominant mutation *(109)*. Cervical ribs are associated with adverse health effects in humans. The most common effect is thoracic outlet disease *(101,110,111)*, characterized by compression of the subclavian artery and vein and of the carotid arteries, and therefore diminished blood flow to and from the arms and to the head, and by displacement of the stellate ganglia, sympathetic ganglia, and C7-T1 nerve roots. The vascular consequences include cerebral and distal embolism *(112–115)*. The neurological consequences include extreme pain *(116)*, migraine *(117)*, and Parkinson's disease-like symptoms *(111)*.

The possible consequences of lumbar ribs primarily consist of pain in the lumbar region *(103)* and a tendency for L4–5 degeneration *(104)*.

  — Do cervical and/or lumbar ribs represent changes in Hox gene designated borders of the vertebral column? That is, do they represent indications of misfunction of fundamental (and evolutionally conserved) patterning genes?
  — If so, are they more than just variations? Do they indicate toxicologically and teratogenically relevant changes in gene expression with possibly far-reaching consequences?

- A strong association has been reported between the presence of axial skeletal anomalies (especially cervical ribs) and cancer in two studies. In one, evaluation of basal cell carcinoma syndrome often included multiple skeletal and rib anomalies *(118)*. Schumacher et al. *(102)* also reported a highly significant correlation of rib anomalies (especially cervical ribs) with a series of cancers in 1000 children. The percentage of cancer patients with a specific type of anomalies (cervical ribs) was leukemia (27%), brain tumor (27%), neuroblastoma (33%), soft tissue sarcoma (25%), and Wilm's tumor (24%). These associations may be due to effects on genes that play a role in development of the axial skeleton and are also components of the cellular pathways that, when deranged, result in childhood cancers. Again, the homeobox genes may be involved *(47,76)*.
- Are increased incidences of specific skeletal variations predictors of increased incidences of specific skeletal malformations at higher doses? In the authors' laboratory, the incidence of total skeletal variations is usually not a predictor of increased incidence of total skeletal malformations at the same or higher doses (although it is dependent on the test material evaluated). Is the presence of ribs on cervical-7 and/or lumbar-1 predictive of a risk for childhood cancer (both from altered homeobox gene structure and/or function)?

Regulatory Issues

The regulatory issues include the following:

- Adequate data to perform risk assessment are defined by the EPA as from in vivo standardized developmental toxicity studies (preferably in two species), unless there are compelling human data.
- The official EPA position is that any of the adverse outcomes are equally "bad," and the most sensitive outcome will determine the NOAEL or BMD.
- Is there a threshold?
  - — Experimental threshold is a dose at and below which no statistically significant and/or biologically relevant adverse effects are observed in "any adequate developmental toxicity study" (experimentally derived).
  - — Population threshold is a dose at and below which no adverse effects would be observed in any and all groups of rats, mice, rabbits, etc. This is based on the study data and is dependent on the number of animals used, the number of dose groups, route of administration, the number and sensitivity of the endpoints examined in addition to the statistical power of the study.
  - — There may be no threshold for changes at the level of the gene or cell, but there may be a threshold for an "adverse" effect; how the term "adverse" is and will be defined is very important (and very contentious). Are the changes at the cellular or molecular level within the homeostatic range?
- Role of mechanistic data
  - — In vitro/ex vivo mechanistic data cannot drive risk assessment; it can (and should) inform risk assessment.
  - — Mechanistic data will aid in understanding structure–activity relationships (SARs) and in predicting risk for new compounds, based on SARs (especially three-dimensional quantitative [3D-Q] SARs) in the same chemical class.

CONCLUSIONS

Evaluation of the fetal skeleton (both cartilaginous and bony components) at term is a major component of developmental toxicity studies in animal models, which are required for registration of drugs under the FDA and pesticides under EPA FIFRA (as well as for marketing in other countries under OECD and International Conference on Harmonization testing guidelines). Adverse fetal skeletal findings include frank malformations, variations, and developmental delays. The location, incidence, and severity of the adverse fetal skeletal findings are important considerations during the risk assessment process. Risk assessment is performed to establish whether exposure to the test chemical, by relevant routes of exposures at relevant doses, during sensitive life stages (timing of exposure), and for short- or long-term exposure (duration of exposure), will result in adverse effects in the species of interest, including humans, based almost always on data from animal studies. The determination of a reference dose (a dose at and below which no apparent risk is anticipated) and the margin of exposure (both based on animal data) are used to characterize the risk, communicate the risk, and to manage the risk. Risk management includes the decision on whether the test material can be marketed as a drug (with the animal studies and clinical trials in humans performed during drug development and submitted to the FDA for registration of the drug), whether it can be registered as a pesticide (again, based on pre-use submission packages for EPA FIFRA), or whether it should be removed from the marketplace (if the studies are performed during postmarketing surveillance for drugs or pesticides, or under voluntary action or test rules for chemicals regulated under EPA Toxic Substances Control Act). If the test material is or can be marketed, then risk management will also involve determination of the efficacious versus the toxic dose (for pesticides) or therapeutic margin (for drugs), safe levels of human and/or environmental exposure (from food, water, and soil contamination, etc.), development of personal or manufacturing plant-wide protective measures, and minimization of exposures to humans and other nontarget species to an acceptable level (e.g., calculation of an "acceptable daily intake" [ADI] for pesticides). Risk assessment issues are both scientific and regulatory and include the interpretation of the adverse outcomes as primary or secondary to maternal or other fetal toxicity, the appropriateness (or sensitivity) of the animal model for extrapolation to humans, and the reproducibility, robustness, sensitivity, consistency, and relevance of the endpoints in the animal models to determination of the risk to humans.

ACKNOWLEDGMENTS

The authors wish to thank the technical staff at RTI whose performance of Segment II studies in rats, mice, and rabbits over the years made this chapter possible. In addition, we would like to thank Ms. Sharon Davis of RTI for assistance with Figs. 3–6 and 10–15 and Ms. Cathee Winkie for her patient and accurate typing (and retyping...) of this manuscript.

REFERENCES

1. National Research Council (NRC) (1983) Committee on the Institutional Means for the Assessment of Risks to Public Health. *Risk Assessment in the Federal Government: Managing the Process.* Commission on Life Sciences, NRC, National Academy Press, Washington, DC, pp. 17–83.
2. National Research Council (NRC) (2000) *Scientific Frontiers in Developmental Toxicity and Risk Assessment.* Committee on Developmental Toxicology, Board on Environmental Studies and Toxicology, NRC, National Academy Press, Washington, DC, p. 27.
3. U.S. Environmental Protection Agency (1982) OPP Guideline 83-3, Teratogenicity Study, Pesticide Assessment Guidelines, Subdivision F, Hazard Evaluation, Human and Domestic Animals, Office of Pesticides and Toxic Substances, Washington, DC.
4. U.S. Food and Drug Administration (1982) *Toxicological Principles for the Safety Assessment of Direct Food Additives and Color Additives Used in Food* ("Redbook"), Appendix II, Guidelines for teratogenicity testing in rat, hamster, mouse, and rabbit, US FDA, Washington, DC, p. 108.
5. Organisation for Economic Cooperation and Development (OECD) (1983) Guidelines for Testing of Chemicals, No. 414. Teratogenicity [C(83)44 (final)].

6. U.S. Food and Drug Administration (FDA) (2000) "Redbook 2000." *Toxicological Principles for the Safety of Food Ingredients*. Center for Food Safety and Applied Nutrition, Office of Premarket Approval (CFSAN, OPA), July 20, 2000.
7. Dawson, A. B. (1926) A note on the staining of the skeleton of cleared specimens with alizarin red S. *Stain Tech.* **1,** 123–124.
8. Crary, D. D. (1962) Modified benzyl alcohol clearing of alizarin-stained specimens without loss of flexibility. *Stain Tech.* **37,** 124–125.
9. Peltzer, M. A. and Schardein, J. L. (1966) A convenient method for processing fetuses for skeletal staining. *Stain Tech.* **41,** 300–302.
10. Barrow, M. V. and Taylor, W. J. (1969) A rapid method for detecting malformations in rat fetuses. *J. Morphol.* **127,** 291–306.
11. US Environmental Protection Agency (EPA) (1998) Office of Prevention, Pesticides and Toxic Substances (OPPTS), Health Effects Testing Guidelines, OPPTS 870.3700, Prenatal Developmental Toxicity Study (Final Guideline, August, 1998).
12. Organisation for Economic Cooperation and Development (OECD) (2001) OECD Guideline for the Testing of Chemicals Proposal for Updating Guideline 414: Prenatal Developmental Toxicity Study. Adopted January 22, 2001.
13. Monie, I. W. (1965) *Dissection Procedures for Rat Fetuses Permitting Alizarin Red Staining of Skeleton and Histological Study of Viscera*. Supplement to Teratology Workshop Manual, pp. 163–173.
14. Inouye, M. (1976) Differential staining of cartilage and bone in fetal mouse skeleton by Alcian blue and alizarin red S. *Congenit. Anomal.* **16,** 171–173.
15. Kimmel, C. A. and Trammel, C. A. (1981) A rapid procedure for routine double staining of cartilage and bone in fetal and adult animals. *Stain Technol.* **56,** 271–273.
16. Fritz, H. and Ness, R. (1970). Ossification of rat and mouse skeletons in the perinatal period. *Teratology* **3,** 331–337.
17. Wickramarante, G. A. de S. (1988) The postnatal fate of supernumerary ribs in rat teratogenicity studies. *J. Appl. Toxicol.* **8,** 91–94.
18. Marr, M. C., Price, C. J., Myers, C. B., and Morrissey, R. E. (1992) Developmental stages of the CD (Sprague-Dawley) rat skeleton after maternal exposure to ethylene glycol. *Teratology* **46,** 169–181.
19. Thiel, R., Dillman, I., Schimmel, A., Bochert, G., Chahoud, I., and Neubert, D. (1989) Aspects of designing postnatal studies. III. Persistence of skeletal anomalies induced prenatally (abstract). *Teratology* **40,** 300.
20. U.S. Food and Drug Administration (1994) International Conference on Harmonization (ICH), Guideline for detection of toxicity to reproduction for medicinal products, Section 4.1.3, study for effects on embryo-fetal development. *Fed. Regist.* 59(183), 48749, September 22, 1994.
21. U.S. Environmental Protection Agency (EPA) (1997) 40CFR Part 799, Toxic Substances Control Act Test Guidelines; Final Rule. Section 799.9370, TSCA prenatal developmental toxicity. *Fed. Regist.* **62(158),** 43832–43834 (Friday, August 15, 1997).
22. Marr, M. C., Myers, C. B., Price, C. J., Tyl, R. W., and Jahnke, G. D. (1999) Comparison of maternal and developmental endpoints for control CD® rats dosed from implantation through organogenesis or through the end of gestation. *Teratology* **59,** 413.
23. Kimmel, G. L., Kimmel, C. A., and Francis, E. Z. (1987) Evaluation of maternal and developmental toxicity. *Teratogen. Carcinogen. Mutagen.* **7,** 203–338.
24. Woo, D. C. and Hoar, R. M. (1972) "Apparent hydronephrosis" as a normal aspect of renal development in late gestation of rats: the effect of methyl salicylate. *Teratology* **6,** 191–196.
25. Tyl, R. W. and Marr, M. C. (1996) Developmental toxicity testing methodology, in *Handbook of Developmental Toxicology*, Chapter 7 (Hood, R. D., ed.), CRC Press, Boca Raton, FL, pp. 175–225.
26. Tyl, R. W. and Marr, M. C. (2003). Developmental toxicity testing methodology, in *Handbook of Developmental Toxicology*, Chapter 7, Second Edition (Hood, R. D., ed.), CRC Press, Boca Raton, FL, in press.
27. Rodwell, D. E. (2000) The effect of cesarean section on fetal body weights in rats on developmental toxicity studies (abstract no. 1393). *Toxicologist* **54,** p. 297.
28. Spark, C. and Dawson, A. B. (1928) The order and time of appearance of centers of ossification in the fore- and hindlimbs of the albino rat, with special reference to the possible influence of the sex factor. *Am. J. Anat.* **41,** 411–445.
29. Strong, R. M. (1928) The order, time and rate of ossification of the albino rat (mus norvegicus albinus) skeleton. *Am. J. Anat.* **36,** 313–355.
30. Walker, D. G. and Wirtschafter, Z. T. (1957) *The Genesis of the Rat Skeleton*. Charles C. Thomas, Springfield, IL.
31. Yasuda, M. and Yuki, T. (1996) *Color Atlas of Fetal. Skeleton of the Mouse, Rat, and Rabbit*. Ace Art Co., Osaka, Japan.
32. Hartman, H. A. (1974) The fetus in experimental teratology, in *The Biology of the Laboratory Rabbit* (Weisbroth, S. H., Flatt, R. E., and Kraus, A. L., eds.), Academic Press, New York, pp. 92–153.
33. Fritz, H. (1974) Prenatal ossification in rabbits as indicative of fetal maturity. *Teratology* **11,** 313–320.
34. Beck, S. L. (1983) Assessment of adult skeletons to detect prenatal exposure to acetazolamide in mice. *Teratology* **28,**45–66.
35. Aliverti, V., Bonanomi, L., Giavini, E., Leone, V. G., and Mariani, L. (1979) The extent of fetal ossification as an index of delayed development in teratogenic studies on the rat. *Teratology* **20,** 237–242.
36. Banerjee, B. N. and Durloo, R. S. (1973) Incidence of teratological anomalies in control Charles River CD strain rats. *Toxicology* **1,** 151–154.

37. Perraud, J. (1976) Levels of spontaneous malformations in the CD rat and the CD-1 mouse. *Lab. Anim. Sci.* **26,** 293–300.
38. Fritz, H., Grauwiler, J., and Himmler, H. (1978) Collection of control data from teratological experiments in mice, rats, and rabbits. *Arzneim-Forsch/Drug Res.* **28,** 1410–1413.
39. Charles River Laboratories (1988) Embryo and Fetal Developmental Toxicity (Teratology) Control Data in the Charles River Crl:CD® BR Rat. Charles River Laboratories, Inc., Wilmington, MA.
40. Midwest Teratology Association (1992). *Historical Control Project 1988–1992: Skeletal Findings on Sprague-Dawley CD® Rats and New Zealand White Rabbits.* Parke-Davis Pharmaceutical Research, Ann Arbor, MI.
41. Woo, D. C. and Hoar, R. M. (1979) Reproductive performance and spontaneous malformations in control Charles River CD rats: a joint study by MARTA (abstract). *Teratology* **19,** 54A.
42. Palmer, A. K. (1972) Sporadic malformations in laboratory animals and their influence in drug testing, in *Drugs and Fetal Development. Adv. Biol. Med.* (Klingsberg, M. A., ed.), **27,** 45–60.
43. Cozens, D. D. (1965) Abnormalities of the external form and of the skeleton in the New Zealand white rabbit. *Food Cosmet. Toxicol.* **3,** 695–700.
44. Stadler, J., Kessedjian, M. J., and Perraud, J. (1983) Use of the New Zealand white rabbit in teratology: incidence of spontaneous and drug-induced malformations. *Food. Chem. Toxicol.* **21,** 631–636.
45. Woo, D. C. and Hoar, R. M. (1982) Reproductive performance and spontaneous malformations in control New Zealand white rabbits: a joint study by MARTA (abstract). *Teratology* **25,** 82A.
46. Chernoff, N., Rogers, J. M., Turner, C. I., and Francis, B. M. (1991) Significance of supernumerary ribs in rodent developmental toxicity studies: postnatal persistence in rats and mice. *Fundam. Appl. Toxicol.* **17,** 448–453.
47. Tyl, R. W., Chernoff, N., Myers, C. B., Narotsky, M. G., and Rogers, J. M. (2003) Abnormal patterning, in *Interpretation of Skeletal Variations for Human Health Risk Assessment,* ILSI Press, Washington, DC, in press.
48. Chernoff, N. (1990) Studies on maternal toxicity, formation of supernumerary ribs, and evidence for embryonic repair of xenobiotic-induced cellular injury (Abstract F5). *Teratology* **42,** 18A.
49. Kimmel, C. A. and Wilson, J. G. (1973) Skeletal deviations in rats: malformations or variations. *Teratology* **8,** 309–316.
50. Tyl, R. W., Price, C. J., Marr, M. C., Myers, C. B., Seely, J. C., Heindel, J. J., and Schwetz, B. A. (1993) Developmental toxicity evaluation of ethylene glycol by gavage in New Zealand White rabbits. *Fundam. Appl. Toxicol.* **20,** 402–412.
51. Tyl, R. W., Ballantyne, B., Fisher, L. C., Fait, D. L., Savine, T. A., Dodd, D. E., et al. (1995) Evaluation of the developmental toxicity of ethylene glycol aerosol in the CD rat and CD-1 mouse by whole-body exposure. *Fundam. Appl. Toxicol.* **24,** 57–75.
52. Tyl, R. W., Ballantyne, B., Fisher, L. C., Fait, D. L., Dodd, D.E., Klonne, D. R., et al. (1995) Evaluation of the developmental toxicity of ethylene glycol aerosol in CD-1 mice by nose-only exposure. *Fundam. Appl. Toxicol.* **27,** 49–62.
53. Tyl, R. W., Fisher, L. C., Kubena, M. F., Vrbanic, M. A., and Losco, P. E. (1995). Assessment of the developmental toxicity of ethylene glycol applied cutaneously to CD-1 mice. *Fundam. Appl. Toxicol.* **27,** 155–166.
54. Price, C. J., Kimmel, C. A., Tyl, R. W., and Marr, M. C. (1985). The developmental toxicity of ethylene glycol in rats and mice. *Toxicol. Appl. Pharmacol.* **81,** 113—127.
55. Kessel, M. (1992) Respecification of vertebral identities by retinoic acid. *Development* **115,** 487–501.
56. Narotsky, M. G., Francis, E. Z., and Kavlock, R. J. (1994) Developmental toxicity and structure-activity relationships of aliphatic acids, including dose-response assessment of valproic acid in mice and rats. *Fundam. Appl. Toxicol.* **22,** 251–265.
57. Kimmel, C. A., Cuff, J. M., Kimmel, G. L., Heredia, D. J., Tudor, N., Silverman, P. M., et al. (1993) Skeletal development following heat exposure in the rat. *Teratology* **47,** 229–242.
58. Hayes, W. C., Cobel-Geard, S. R., Hanley, T. R., Murray, J. S., Freshour, N. L., Rao, K. S., et al. (1981) Teratogenic effects of vitamin A palmitate in Fischer 344 rats. *Drug Chem. Toxicol.* **4,** 283–295.
59. Nelson, B. K., Brightwell, W. S., MacKenzie, D. R., Khan, A., Burg, J. R., Weigel, W. W., et al. (1985) Teratologic assessment of methanol and ethanol at high inhalation levels in rats. *Fundam. Appl. Toxicol.* **5,** 727–736.
60. Rogers, J. M., Mole, M. L., Chernoff, N., Barbee, B. D., Turner, C. I., Lugsdon, T. R., et al. (1993) The developmental toxicity of inhaled methanol in the CD-1 mouse, with quantitative dose-response modeling for estimation of benchmark doses. *Teratology* **47,** 175–188.
61. Rogers, J. M., Francis, D. M., Barbee, B. D., and Chernoff, N. (1991) Developmental toxicity of bromoxynil in rats and mice. *Fundam. Appl. Toxicol.* **17,** 442–447.
62. Price, C. J., Marr, M. C., Myers, C. B., Seely, J. C., Heindel, J. J., and Schwetz, B. A. (1996) The developmental toxicity of boric acid in rabbits. *Fundam. Appl. Toxicol.* **34,** 176–187.
63. Heindel, J. J., Price, C. J., Field, E. A., Marr, M. C., Myers, C. B., Morrissey, R. E., et al. (1992) Developmental toxicity of boric acid in mice and rats. *Fundam. Appl. Toxicol.* **18,** 266–277.
64. Heindel, J. J., Price, C. J., and Schwetz, B. A. (1994) The developmental toxicity of boric acid in mice, rats, and rabbits. *Environ. Health Perspect.* **102(Suppl 7),** 107–1121.
65. Price, C. J., Strong, P. L., Marr, M. C., Myers, C. B., and Murray, F. J. (1996) Developmental NOAEL and postnatal recovery in rats fed boric acid during gestation. *Fundam. Appl. Toxicol.* **32,** 179–193.
66. Price, C. J., Strong, P. L., Murray, F. J., and Goldberg, M. M. (1997) Blood boron concentrations in pregnant rats fed boric acid throughout gestation. *Reprod. Toxicol.* **11,** 833–842.
67. Price, C. J., Strong, P. L., Murray, F. J., and Goldberg, M. M. (1998) Developmental effects of boric acid in rats related to maternal blood boron concentrations. *Biol. Trace Element Res.* **66,** 359–372.

68. Narotsky, M. G., Hamby, B. T., Mitchell, D. S., and Kavlock, R. J. (1995) Effects of boric acid on axial skeletal development in rats (Abstract No. P58). *Teratology* **51,** 192.
69. Narotsky, M. G., Hamby, B. J., Best, D. S., and Kavlock, R. J. (1996) Effects of single-day boric acid treatment on axial skeletal development in rats (Abstract No. 70). *Teratology* **53,** 101.
70. Narotsky, M. G., Schmid, J. E., Andrews, J. E., and Kavlock, R. J. (1998) Effects of boric acid on axial skeletal development in rats. *Biol. Trace Element Res.* **66,** 373–394.
71. Connelly, L. E. and Rogers, J. M. (1997) Methanol causes posteriorization of cervical vertebrae in mice. *Teratology* **55,** 138–144.
72. Kessel, M., Balling, R., and Gruss, P. (1990) Variations of cervical vertebrae after expression of a Hox-1.1 transgene in mice. *Cell* **61,** 301–308.
73. Charite, J. W., de Graaff, W., Shen, S., and Deschamps, J. (1994) Ectopic expression of Hoxb-8 causes duplication of the ZPA in the forelimb and homeotic transformation of axial structures. *Cell* **78,** 589–601.
74. Beyer, P. E. and Chernoff, N. (1986) The induction of supernumerary ribs in rodents: role of maternal stress. *Teratog. Carcinog. Mutag.* **6,** 419–429.
75. Daston, G. P. and Overmann, G. J. (1996) Lumbar ribs associated with posteriorization of Hoxa-10 expression in salicylate-treated mouse embryos (abstract). *Teratology* **53,** 85.
76. Anbazhagan, R. and Raman, V. (1997) Homeobox genes: molecular link between congenital anomalies and cancer. *Eur. J. Cancer* **33,** 635–637.
77. Jegalian, B. G. and DeRobertis, E. M. (1992) Homeotic transformations in the mouse induced by overexpression of a human Hox3.3 transgene. *Cell* **71,** 901–910.
78. Small, K. M. and Potter, S. S. (1993) Homeotic transformations and limb defects in Hox A11 mutant mice. *Genes Dev.* **7,** 2318–2328.
79. van der Lugt, N. M., Domen, J., Linders, K., van Roon, M., Robanus-Maandag, E., Riele, H., et al. (1994) Posterior transformation, neurological abnormalities, and severe hematopoietic defects in mice with a targeted deletion of the bmi-1 proto-oncogene. *Genes Dev.* **8,** 757–769.
80. Chernoff, N., Kavlock, R. J., Beyer, P. E., and Miller, D. (1987) The potential relationship of maternal toxicity, general stress, and fetal outcome. *Teratog. Carcinog. Mutagen.* **7,** 241–253.
81. Chernoff, N., Miller, D. B., Rosen, M. B., and Mattscheck, C. L. (1988) Developmental effects of maternal stress in the CD-1 mouse induced by restraint on single days during the period of major organogenesis. *Toxicology* **51,** 57–65.
82. Pettersen, J. C., Koltis, G. G., and White, M. J. (1979) An examination of the spectrum of anatomic defects and variations found in eight cases of trisomy 13. *Am. J. Med. Genet.* **3,** 183–210.
83. Kjaer, I. and Fischer Hansen, B. (1997) Cervical ribs in fetuses with Ullrich-Turner syndrome. *Am. J. Med. Genet.* **71,** 219–221.
84. Kjaer, I., Keeling, J. W., and Fischer Hansen, B. (1997) Pattern of malformations in the axial skeleton in human trisomy 13 fetuses. *Am. J. Med. Genet.* **70,** 421–426.
85. Keeling, J. W., Hansen, B. F., and Kjaer, I. (1997) Pattern of malformations in the axial skeleton in human trisomy 21 fetuses. *Am. J. Med. Genet.* **68,** 466–471.
86. Kjaer, I., Keeling, J. W., and Hansen, B. F. (1996) Pattern of malformations in the axial skeleton in human trisomy 18 fetuses. *Am. J. Med. Genet.* **65,** 332–336.
87. Kjaer, I., Keeling, J. W., Smith, N. M., and Hansen, B. F. (1997) Pattern of malformations in the axial skeleton in human triploid fetuses. *Am. J. Med. Genet.* **72,** 216–221.
88. Kimmel, C. A. and Wilson, J. G. (1973) Skeletal deviations in rats: malformations or variations. *Teratology* **8,** 309–316.
89. Staples, R. E. (with concurrence of J. G. Wilson) (1975) Chapter 4. Definition of teratogenesis and teratogen, in *Methods for Detection of Environmental Agents That Produce Congenital Defects* (Shepard, T. H., Miller, J. R., and Marois, M, eds.), Proceedings of the Guadeloupe Meeting, Elsevier, New York, pp. 25–26.
90. Nishimura, M., Lizuka, M., Iwaki, S., and Kast, A. (1982) Repairability of drug-induced "wavy ribs" in rat offspring. *Arzneim-Forsch./Drug Res.* **32,** 1518–1522.
91. Hayasaka, I., Tamaki, F., Uchiyama, K., Kato, Z., and Murakami, K. (1985) Azosemide-induced fetal wavy ribs and their disappearance after birth in rats. *Cong. Anom.* **25,** 121–127.
92. Kast, A. (1994) "Wavy Ribs." A reversible pathologic finding in rat fetuses. *Exp. Toxicol. Pathol.* **46,** 203–210.
93. Sycamore, L. K. (1944) Common congenital anomalies of the bony thorax. *Am. J. Radiol.* **51,** 593–599.
94. Bohutova, J., Kolar, J., Vitovec, J., and Vyhnanek, L. (1980) Accessory caudal axial and pelvic ribs. *ROFO Fortschr Geb Rontgenstr Nuklearmed* **133,** 641–643.
95. Ogilvie, M. D., Hilton, C. E., and Ogilvie, C. D. (1998) Lumbar anomalies in the Shanidar 3 Neandertal. *J. Hum. Evol.* **35,** 597–610.
96. Wilbur, A. K. (2000) Possible case of Rubinstein-Taybi syndrome in a prehistoric skeleton from west-central Illinois. *Am. J. Med. Genet.* **91,** 56–61.
97. Usher, B. M. and Christensen, M. N. (2000) A sequential developmental field defect of the vertebrae, ribs, and sternum, in a young woman of the 12th century AD. *Am. J. Phys. Anthropol.* **111,** 355–367.
98. Bagnall, K. M., Harris, P. F., and Jones, P. R. (1984) A radiographic study of variations of the human fetal spine. *Anat. Rec.* **208,** 265–270.
99. McNally, E., Sandin, B., and Wilkins, R. A. (1990) The ossification of the costal element of the seventh cervical vertebra with particular reference to cervical ribs. *J. Anat.* **170,** 125–129.

100. Noback, C. R. and Robertson, G. G. (1951) Sequence and appearance of ossification centres in human skeletons during the first five prenatal months. *Am. J. Anat.* **89,** 1–28.
101. Henderson, M. S. (1914) Cervical rib. Report of thirty-one cases. *Am. J. Orthop. Surg.* **11,** 408–430.
102. Schumacher, R., Mai, A., and Gutjahr, P. (1992) Association of rib anomalies and malignancy in childhood. *Eur. J. Pediatr.* **151,** 432–434.
103. Steiner, H. A. (1943) Roentgenologic manifestations and clinical symptoms of rib abnormalities, *Radiology* **40,** 175–178.
104. MacGibbon, B. and Farfan, H. F. (1979) A radiologic survey of various configurations of the lumbar spine. *Spine* **4,** 258–266.
105. Bardeen, C. R. (1909) Vertebral regional determination in young human embryos. *Anat. Rec.* **2,** 99–105.
106. Davis, D. B. and King, J. C. (1938) Cervical rib in early life. *Am. J. Dis. Child.* **56,** 744–755.
107. Meyer, D. B. (1978) The appearance of "cervical ribs" during early human fetal development. *Anat. Rec.* **190,** 481.
108. O'Rahilly, R., Muller, F., and Meyer, D. B. (1990) The human vertebral column at the end of the embryonic period proper. 3. The thoracic columbar region. *J. Anat.* **168,** 81–93.
109. Schapera, J. (1987) Autosomal dominant inheritance of cervical ribs. *Clin. Genet.* **31,** 386–388.
110. Nguyen, T., Baumgartner, F., and Nelems, B. (1997) Bilateral rudimentary first ribs as a cause of thoracic outlet syndrome. *J. Natl. Med. Assoc.* **89,** 69–73.
111. Fernandez Noda, E. I., Nunez-Arguelles, J., Perez Fernandez, J., Castillo, J., Perez Izquierdo, M., and Rivera Luna, H. (1996) Neck and brain transitory vascular compression causing neurological complications, results of surgical treatment on 1,300 patients. *J. Cardiovasc. Surg. (Torino)* **37,** 155–166.
112. Short, D. W. (1975) The subclavian artery in 16 patients with complete cervical ribs. *J. Cardiovasc. Surg.* **16,** 135–141.
113. Connell, J. L., Doyle, J. C., and Gurry, J. F. (1980) The vascular complications of cervical rib. *Aust. NZ J. Surg.* **50,** 125–130.
114. Beam, P., Patel, J., and O'Flynn, W. R. (1993) Cervical ribs: a cause of distal and cerebral embolism. *Postgrad. Med. J.* **69,** 65–68.
115. Hood, D. B., Keuhne, J., Yellin, A. E., and Weaver, F. A. (1997) Vascular complications of thoracic outlet syndrome. *Am. Surg.* **63,** 913–917.
116. Evans, A. L. (1999) Pseudoseizures as a complication of painful cervical ribs. *Dev. Med. Child. Neurol.* **41,** 840–842.
117. Saxton, E. H., Miller, T. Q., and Collins, J. D. (1999) Migraine complicated by brachial plexopathy as displayed by MRI and MRA: aberrant subclavian artery and cervical ribs. *J. Natl. Med. Assoc.* **91,** 333–341.
118. Ferrier, P. F. and Hinrichs, W. L. (1967) Basal-cell carcinoma syndrome. *Am. J. Dis. Child.* **113,** 538–545.

Index

A

B

P

MIX
Papier aus verantwortungsvollen Quellen
Paper from responsible sources
FSC® C105338

If you have any concerns about our products,
you can contact us on
ProductSafety@springernature.com

In case Publisher is established outside the EU,
the EU authorized representative is:
Springer Nature Customer Service Center GmbH
Europaplatz 3, 69115 Heidelberg, Germany

Printed by Libri Plureos GmbH
in Hamburg, Germany